Finding the
Right
Treatment

Finding the Right Treatment

MODERN AND ALTERNATIVE MEDICINE

A Comprehensive Guide to Getting
the Best of Both Worlds

JACQUELINE KROHN, MD, MPH

FRANCES A. TAYLOR, MA

Hartley & Marks
PUBLISHERS

Published by
HARTLEY & MARKS PUBLISHERS INC.

P. O. Box 147   3661 West Broadway
Point Roberts, WA   Vancouver, BC
98281   V6R 2B8

LIBRARY OF CONGRESS CATALOGING-IN-PUBLICATION DATA

Krohn, Jacqueline, 1950-
Finding the right treatment / Jacqueline Krohn, Frances A. Taylor.
p.   cm.
Includes bibliographical references and index.
ISBN 0-88179-166-0
1. Medicine, Popular.   2. Alternative medicine.   I. Taylor,
Frances A., 1938–   . II. Title.
RC81.K875   1998
610—dc21   98-28774
CIP

Design and composition by The Typeworks
Set in SABON

NOTICE TO THE READER

This book is meant to be a source of information for those who are interested in learning about modern and alternative medicine, including their various components and treatments. Every person has different health problems and issues, based on age, sex, lifestyle, health status, genetics, diet, psychological state, and spiritual maturity. Our intent is to share our experience and offer guidelines to help you become more informed about your health care choices and options. In cooperation with your physician and other health care providers, you can then take the necessary steps to maintain optimum health. This book is sold with the understanding that the publisher is not engaged in rendering medical or other professional services. If medical or expert assistance is required, the services of a competent professional should be sought. Neither the authors nor the publisher takes medical or legal responsibility for the reader who uses the contents of this book as a prescription.

DEDICATION

To our families, both immediate and extended:

Particularly our husbands who endured our writing another book and without whose patience, support, and help neither our work nor our writing would be possible.

And our parents and siblings whose enthusiasm and encouragement never fails to cheer us on!

ACKNOWLEDGEMENTS

Our sincere thanks to:

Our office staff for the extra steps they took in enabling the office to run smoothly while we were writing this book, as well as the encouragement they always offer us.

Cheryl Sedlacek for her word processing labors on the computer.

Alice Kernodle and Susan Deininger for their many fact-finding phone calls.

Jeanette Meadows for her painstaking proofreading, and Angie Chipera for the many tasks she performed on our behalf.

Steven Carter, who so capably did the technical read-through.

Elizabeth McLean, our editor, whose enthusiasm, curiosity, insight, and thoroughness assures our readers an easily understood text..

The staff of Hartley & Marks, especially Susan Juby, whose expertise enabled the production of this book.

Our colleagues, in both modern and alternative medicine, whose work, research, and publications allowed us to write this book.

CONTENTS

FOREWORD

Perhaps you or I or a family member has a few symptoms that just won't go away on their own. We've tried the home remedies we know; they haven't worked this time. What to do? Should we go to the medical doctor at the "health plan?" It's likely we'll get an accurate diagnosis, especially if it turns out to be something serious...but unless surgery is required, we'll likely get a prescription for the latest patent medication, and we know that our bodies don't bother us with symptoms because of patent deficiencies.

We've been seeing, hearing, and reading much more about that "alternative medicine" thing...what a grab bag! Diets, vitamins, minerals, herbs, massage, aromatherapy, chiropractors, naturopaths, homeopaths, acupuncturists...the list seems to go on and on. From all the media talk, it appears there's something to it. We sure are hearing a lot more about alternatives to "modern medicine." What part is relevant to those nagging symptoms? Will it be more helpful than that patent medicine, or a waste of time and money?

In *Finding the Right Treatment,* Dr. Jacqueline Krohn and Frances Taylor show us how to take the best (and most likely to help) from the apparent deluge of alternative health care information, while not abandoning the useful and still valuable help to be obtained from conventional medicine. Their comprehensive text covers not only the major alternative therapies, but also gives useful background concerning modern medicine—hospitals, surgery, radiation, chemotherapy, and patent medications. It's the information we need to make intelligent choices about our health care.

On a much larger scale, these same questions are being asked—and answered—throughout our health care system. Although progress is slow and in its very early stages, integration of alternative health care into the mainstream is proceeding. Perhaps the first examples are birthing centers, which are now an established part of the obstetrics programs of most major hospitals. Birthing centers have removed the normal process of birth from the operating room, returning it to a more natural, home-like setting, while not giving up the operating room and emergency procedure backup. A few pioneering hospitals and medical centers have added acupuncture to their regular programs. Many other programs are being considered.

The process of integrating alternative health care with modern medical practice is a very necessary one. Despite resistance from the medical staff of many hospitals, it will happen within the next decade or two. The reasons are varied, but some of the more important ones are the high and still-rising cost of modern health care, as well as its dangers and hazards, ably and accurately described by Dr. Krohn and Frances Taylor. Alternative health care appears to offer many more promising and long-lasting treatments, especially for chronic, non-emergency situations, and they're usually less costly, too. Hospitals as well as doctors' offices in the not-too-distant future will be considerably different places than they are today, including the best of alternative health care along with more conventional approaches.

However, until this process of integration is complete and running smoothly, we need to do the integration of alternative and modern treatments for ourselves. This book will help considerably in that process.

—Jonathan V. Wright, MD
Medical Director, Tahoma Clinic
Kent, Washington

PREFACE

It was the best of times, it was the worst of times,
it was the age of wisdom, it was the age of foolishness...

These lines from *A Tale of Two Cities* by Charles Dickens could be describing medicine in North America today. It is the best of times in some ways, in that technology in medicine is at an all-time high, and intricate treatments and surgical procedures can save lives that could previously not be saved. In other ways, it is the worst of times with the overtreatment by and dependence on pharmaceuticals that do not cure and are mainly palliative. It is the age of wisdom in that knowledge of the human body and its biochemistry are ever increasing, but it is also the age of foolishness in that methods that are both nontoxic and that heal are rejected by modern medicine.

In working with patients we have become ever more cognizant of the conflicts between modern medicine and alternative medicine. Patients are torn between the dogma and inflexibility of both disciplines. Their confusion increases as each side pitches its philosophy, and the decision of which treatment to follow becomes difficult if not almost impossible. One of the main purposes of this book is to teach the readers the weaknesses and strengths of both modern medicine and alternative medicine. Some of the material presented may be surprising to many people, because negative aspects of some medical treatments and procedures are not known by the public and some physicians.

The other purpose of this book is to contribute to the reader's store of knowledge regarding common health problems and possible treatments, both modern and alternative. We are not advocating abandoning either modern medicine or alternative medicine, but selecting the best from both disciplines, including both prevention and treatment. You must select the treatment that will best help your health problem and allow you to heal. Wise decisions require knowledge and informed actions.

Jacqueline Krohn, M.D., M.P.H., C.Hom.
Frances A. Taylor, M.A., C.Hom.
Los Alamos, New Mexico
—1999

Introduction

All of us have health challenges from time to time and must seek the help of a health care professional. Today we have a larger choice of these professionals than at any other time in history. We can consult not only the practitioners of modern medicine, but those who practice many other forms of medical treatments as well—such as Chinese medicine, Ayurvedic medicine, homeopathy, naturopathy, and chiropractic. In addition, we can make use of alternative therapies that employ bodywork, herbs, nutrients, sound, light, color, aroma, and magnets.

However, most people seek the help of a modern medicine practitioner when they have a health problem. While modern medicine (and its technology) can achieve more than ever before, the advice and services it provides are not always healing. Treatment of the chronically and terminally ill is often inadequate, and the incidence of iatrogenic (physician-caused) diseases is high. Diagnostic tests are costly and overused, and sophisticated diagnostic procedures can themselves cause illness and even death. The administration of pharmaceuticals has its own set of problems, including incorrect prescribing, overprescribing, drug interactions, reactions to medications, and adverse side effects. North Americans spend more on health care than do the people of any other country in the world—but we do not have the best health, nor the longest life spans.

People are looking for and need an acceptable degree of relief at an affordable cost. If their present medical care is not providing them the relief they need, they have several options:

- they can give up hope and live with their symptoms;
- they can continue to seek relief within modern medicine; or
- they can seek treatment from practitioners of alternative medicine as well, when it is appropriate.

Many of our current diseases are lifestyle diseases—by-products of modern life. Today we have more exposures to a myriad of toxins and stresses than at any other time in history: our mind, eyes, ears, nose, skin, organs, and immune system are adversely affected. Our bodies are miraculous and resilient, though, and they have the power to heal and self-repair if given the chance.

Modern medicine knows very little about lifestyle diseases, and only minimally acknowledges the innate healing capacity of the body. As people have begun to realize that conventional medicine has limitations, interest in alternative medicine has grown. However, many people have not had the opportunity to learn about alternative therapies, nor have they tried them. The purpose of this book is to give people information about their health care choices, because only informed people can make informed choices. Neither modern medicine nor alternative medicine should be abandoned in favor of the other, but there should be freedom to choose the treatment and practitioner best suited to solve a particular health problem.

Finding the Right Treatment discusses common health problems, listing the treatments provided for them by modern medicine, as well as those offered by alternative therapies. Both major divisions of modern medicine (surgery and medicine) are discussed, and an overview of the work of the modern medical laboratory is provided. Pharmaceuticals—the main treatment tools of modern medicine—are described in some detail, and hospitalization, surgery, and vaccinations are considered.

Alternative medicine is also discussed, and many of the available alternative therapies are described. In general, alternative therapies emphasize prevention and look for causes, rather than just treating symptoms. In many cases, alternative therapies use hands-on treatment techniques, as well as low-toxicity medications such as herbs, homeopathic remedies, and nutrients. In many cases people can learn to carry out alternative healing methods themselves.

Health is not the absence of disease, but rather an interconnected web of emotional, physical, psychological, social, and spiritual conditions. Without good health, the quality of life suffers. With adequate information on health choices, and the broad range of therapies now available, there is no reason not to enjoy the happiest, healthiest life possible. Make good health for you and your family your special mission and passion!

PART I

Modern Medicine

CHAPTER I

Overview

From the beginning of time, people have developed illnesses, broken bones, sustained wounds, and delivered children—and early humans sought help from the physicians of their time in dealing with these events, just as we do today. The first physicians were medicine men and shamans. Medicine and religion were intertwined, and medical treatment emphasized the spiritual aspects of disease. However, even the earliest healers offered treatments that were practical as well. They administered medications (of variable effectiveness), performed crude surgical operations, and applied splints to broken limbs.

The earliest written record of the practice of medicine dates back to the Babylonians in 2250 BC, and the oldest surviving record of Egyptian medical practice is the Ebers Papyrus, which originated around 1550 BC. This document lists diseases together with their recommended remedies, and describes the proper incantations that were to accompany the remedies. Some of the healing methods they used are still in use, but in modern form. For example, the papyrus suggests bandaging moldy bread over a wound to prevent infection—and some of our modern antibiotics are produced from molds.

The early Greeks, who separated medicine from religion, were the first to formulate the principles of scientific medicine. By the sixth century BC, they had developed a rational approach to medicine that combined observation, reasoning, a systematic approach, philosophical assumptions, and logical deductions. They also developed the first theory of pathology—the doctrine of the "humors"—which said that an excess or deficiency of one of the four "humors" (blood, phlegm, yellow bile, or black bile) affected health, as well as mood and disposition. Illness was considered to result from an imbalance among the humors; treatment was designed to re-establish balance and harmony among them.

For centuries, the favorite treatment to restore that balance was bleeding, which was used to treat almost every condition. Galen, a Greek physician who lived from 130 to 201 AD, even bled for complications caused by bleeding. The most common method of bleeding was to open a vein and divert blood from the problem area, but sometimes bleeding was accomplished by using freshwater leeches. At first, physicians performed all the bloodletting until around 1000 AD, when the university schools of medicine were organized. Bloodletting then became the task of surgeons and barber-surgeons, who had no academic training and were therefore considered below physicians in status.

Over time, a hierarchy of medical skills developed. Physicians prescribed diets and medications, and supervised treatment programs. Surgeons removed tumors, repaired rectal fistulas, sutured holes in the intestines, and performed plastic surgery on the lips and nose. Barber-surgeons treated external ulcers, pulled teeth, gave enemas, did bleeding and cupping, and set fractures (in addition to their barbering duties). Apothecaries dispensed medications.

The divisions of modern medicine had their origins in this old distribution of tasks among physicians, surgeons, barber-surgeons, and apothecaries.

Modern medicine, as discussed in this book (also called conventional, traditional, orthodox, or Western medicine), includes both allopathy (standard medical care) and osteopathy. Osteopathy, which was established by Andrew Taylor Still of Missouri in the late 19th century, is considered by some to be "alternative." However, people trained in both disciplines become primary care physicians, and their pharmacology and medical specialties are identical. In the United States, osteopaths (DOs) and allopaths (MDs) take the same state board examinations. Both groups are licensed to practice throughout the United States, and they often practice side by side on the same hospital staffs. Allopaths are licensed to practice throughout Canada, while osteopaths are licensed in parts of Canada.

Both allopathic and osteopathic medicine identify "health" as the maintenance of normal values with respect to blood pressure, body temperature, pulse, respiratory rate, visual acuity, auditory threshold, electrolyte balance, height, weight, and many other factors. Adherence to or variation from normal values is determined through laboratory testing.

Despite their similarities, there is a difference in philosophy between allopathic and osteopathic physicians. Osteopaths accept the interrelationship of all parts of the body in maintaining health, and they believe that the body has the capacity to heal itself. They therefore seek to correct imbalances, in order to permit the body to heal. As well, part of osteopathic philosophy holds that strains or dislocations in the skeletal system affect the structural integrity of the body and result in disease. The curriculum in osteopathic medical colleges includes courses on the correction of such dislocations, in addition to courses that parallel those given at allopathic medical colleges. Some osteopaths use manipulation in their practice, while others rarely use it; a few osteopathic physicians use manipulation techniques extensively.

MAJOR DIVISIONS

There are two major divisions in modern medicine: medicine and surgery. Both medicine and surgery include a number of subdivisions or specialties. In order to work in those specialties, physicians are required to complete additional training beyond the initial four years of medical school (from two to six years, depending on the specialty). Physicians who complete the academic training for a specialty are called "board eligible." When they pass their extensive written and oral board exams, they are called "board certified." A physician who does not have a specialty is called a general practitioner.

Medicine

Physicians who are certified in medicine do no surgery (or only limited small surgery, such as removing cysts and moles). Medicine includes many specialties, each dealing with a particular organ system, family of diseases, or life stage. For example, a cardiologist specializes in conditions affecting the heart and major blood vessels; an oncologist focuses on the diagnosis and treatment of cancers; and a geriatrician deals with the special health needs of older people. Other specialists who work within medicine include allergists (who treat allergies and immune system problems), dermatologists (who treat skin conditions), pediatricians (who care for infants, children, and adolescents), psychiatrists (who deal with emotional and mental problems), and family practitioners, whose specialty replaces the position of general practitioner, treating all members of the family.

Surgery

Surgeons deal with diseases or conditions that require surgical treatment. There are various subdivisions within surgery, including general surgery and subspecialties that deal with particular parts of the body. These include neurosurgery (brain and nerves), thoracic surgery (chest), vascular surgery (blood vessels), and orthopedic surgery (bone structures). Anesthesiology, otolaryngology (ear, nose and throat), ophthalmology (care of the eye), and urology (diseases of the urinary tract) are also considered surgical specialties.

Working within specialties allows physicians to become highly skilled in their own area of expertise. By the same token, however, specialization makes modern medicine rather compartmentalized, and encourages physicians to focus on their particular "specialty area," rather than on the patient as a whole. In reality, the functions of the body are all interrelated, and an extensive series of checks and balances helps to maintain physical integrity and homeostasis.

EVALUATION

Modern medicine excels in the practice of emergency medicine: it manages trauma better than any other system of medicine, and diagnoses and treats medical and surgical emergencies extremely well. Bone fractures, chest pain, and high fevers are handled with efficiency. Acute heart attack victims and people who have been in major accidents are frequently saved by a quick-acting emergency room staff.

Modern medicine achieves good results in correcting body damage and birth defects with cosmetic and reconstructive surgery. It is very successful in replacing damaged hips and knees, which relieves pain and restores function to these joints. It also effectively repairs hernias, late stage cataracts, and, to some degree, herniated discs. Bleeding ulcers can usually be handled well by modern medicine.

In addition, modern medicine is able to successfully treat most acute bacterial infections with antibiotics, and, to a lesser extent, parasitic and fungal infections. People now recover from pneumonias that used to be fatal, and meningitis, encephalitis, and endocarditis can be treated effectively. Modern medicine also has a large measure of success in diagnosing and treating hormonal deficiencies.

Obstetrical complications that used to put both mothers and babies at risk are dealt with safely by modern obstetrical care. Neonatal care allows high-risk babies to live, and in many cases to develop normally.

Great strides have been made in mapping human genes and relating the findings to genetic diseases and birth defects. As a result, the probability of a couple having a child with a genetic disease (Huntington's chorea, Down's syndrome, Tay-Sachs disease, muscular dystrophy, Friedreich's ataxia, and other conditions) can be predicted, allowing prospective parents to have genetic counseling and make reproductive decisions. Counseling also allows adults to know their own likelihood of developing a genetically controlled disease later in life.

For a few cancers (such as early colon cancer, testicular cancer, lymphomas, and childhood leukemia), modern medicine has some effective treatments. For cancers resistant to chemotherapy and not accessible to surgery, it has no answers—and in most cases, manages these cancers poorly. Modern medicine has inadequate success in treating viral infections, and manages many gastrointestinal and skin conditions poorly. Most types of mental illness or psychosomatic illnesses are not well handled by modern medical approaches, and most forms of autoimmune disease or allergy cannot be handled adequately using modern medical techniques.

While modern medicine can diagnose complex medical problems well, it is generally unsuccessful in treating chronic degenerative diseases. Treatment for these conditions is usually limited to control of symptoms. Such an approach can allow symptoms to become chronic. Modern medicine can do little for chronic back pain, chronic pain, arthritis, or the effects of stress. Since the treatment of chronic disease now accounts for 85 percent of the health care bill, it is obvious that the health care problems faced by a great many people are not adequately dealt with by modern medicine.

Because of the discovery that many diseases are caused by germs, modern medicine has come to consider disease as an invasion by an "enemy" that must be defeated in battle. Treatment is often viewed as the use of weapons of war. Because the "enemy" must be defeated at all costs, even dangerous treatments are legitimized. In some cases treatments can be worse than the original illness, and they may backfire and stimulate greater activity and virulence on the part of the "enemy."

There is little attention paid to repairing imbalances that may have allowed the disease to develop in the first place, or to finding means to support the natural defenses of the body. This is unfortunate, because illness is a breakdown in homeostasis adaptive responses—not an enemy that has to be defeated. In many cases modern medicine fails to acknowledge the interrelationships within the body, and it only minimally acknowledges the innate healing power of the human body and mind. For true healing to occur, any medical treatment must consider these factors.

Medicine has traditionally had two functions; preventing disease, and curing it once it has occurred. However, today modern medicine basically manages symptoms and medical emergencies, with little emphasis on promoting a lifetime of optimal wellness. The "preventative" aspects of modern medicine consist of regular physicals, X-rays, and lab work. While these procedures have value, allowing early detection of disease, they are not true preventative medicine. They do not stop problems from developing, but only survey the patient's current state of health. This focus of modern medicine is misplaced, because preventable illness may account for as much as 70 percent of all health care costs in North America.

Because most of the focus of modern medicine is on the cure of disease, most patients have come to expect treatment via a "magic bullet." Patients want to be *given* a cure, and expect to expend very little or no effort themselves to effect improvement in their own health.

True preventative medicine teaches people how to live well and how *not* to get sick. It utilizes the concepts of eating a healthy diet, taking nutritional supplements, exercising, living in a healthy environment, and using detoxification methods when indicated. Spiritual health is emphasized along with physical health. Prevention of disease is seen as the primary goal of alternative medicine, with treatment of disease a secondary approach.

CONSTRAINTS ON MODERN MEDICINE

Modern medicine functions under a number of constraints, many of them a result of the field's development history:

- *The focus of modern medicine is on disease, rather than on health.* The experience of medicine is skewed toward illness and its cure, creating an illusion that the physician has control over life and death. There is little sense of the healing capacity of the body, and the patient's ability to help the body achieve and maintain health. As well, little attention is paid to the roles of family, the work environment, diet, stress, lifestyle factors, and emotional and spiritual issues in maintaining health or causing illness.
- *Modern medical schools are organized into organ-specific departments that fail to consider the body as a whole.* In medical school, students focus on one organ system at a

time—as if that system functioned independently of other parts of the body. If a student goes on to become a specialist, he or she must choose one organ or system for further study. All this has the effect of compartmentalizing medicine, and causing physicians to take a very narrow view of health care. This is not logical or practical, because while the body is made up of many parts, it functions as a whole; a change or problem in one part affects the entire body.

- *Modern medicine exists within a cost-driven health care system.* To control costs, doctors are pressured to run their offices on an assembly line. They see as many patients as possible in as short a time as possible, and this contributes further to the view that patients are merely a collection of body parts. The most economically feasible way to practice medicine is simply to address the dominant problem presented by the patient—usually by prescribing a medication that controls symptoms, but may or may not treat the cause of the problem.

- *Most physicians practice under fear of malpractice accusations, either by patients or their peers.* Many caring and innovative physicians have been ridiculed by their peers and censured by medical societies and hospital boards for providing their patients with "cutting edge of medicine" treatment. Some of them have given up their fresh approaches to medicine. This is unfortunate, for many of these treatments are of value to patients.

- *Most medical schools, like so many other educational institutes, are rigid in their expectations of students.* Independent thinking is discouraged, and material to be learned is presented rather dogmatically. There is a strong bias that if a treatment is not taught in medical school, it is of no value.

Physicians tend to look upon health conditions as either "present" or "not present," and

patients as either "well" or "not well." In fact, a person does not go from health to illness—for example, from normal thyroid function to hypothyroidism—in one day. The breakdown of health is a gradual process, but a day full of stress can "bring out" the symptoms of hypothyroidism, since emotional stress, an illness, or an injury can seriously affect the secretion of an already poorly functioning endocrine gland.

The average physician is not a scientist, but may be quick to label as "unscientific" a treatment or practice without evaluating its effectiveness. Most physicians have very little understanding of statistics, and are unable to read medical literature critically. In addition, the professional journals that physicians read are not iconoclastic: they tend to reflect received opinion. If an article is submitted that questions widely accepted treatment protocols, it is less likely to be published. Consequently, physicians are not always exposed to a complete overview of current scientific studies and treatments.

PARADIGMS

Historically, both science and medicine have experienced paradigm shifts; moments at which the existing rules and theories have failed to explain the outcomes of experiments and research. Whole new world views have had to be adopted in order to create a better "match" with the new evidence.

But such new ideas are often met with much resistance, and in this respect modern medicine is no exception. Those who have worked within the old paradigms all their lives feel threatened by new ideas, because they call into question entire careers and perhaps a lifetime of scientific work. New theories tend to attract mostly the scientists and physicians of the upcoming generation.

Physicians (and scientists generally) do not usually reject an old paradigm, even when they discover that it does not explain new information. They will generally try to modify the old theory to eliminate inconsistencies, and will only adopt a new paradigm under conditions of intellectual crisis.

Conversion to a new paradigm occurs slowly: a few physicians and scientists learn to see medicine and science differently, and they become less committed to the rules of the old paradigm. People in both camps use the same language, but different meanings are attached to terms, and communication between proponents of the two paradigms is imperfect. The superiority of one theory over another cannot be proved in debate. Theory must be tested against research data— and research is carried out only when the new paradigm has gained sufficient strength so that there is competition for the allegiance of the scientific or medical community.

Medicine is now entering a paradigm shift, in which the ideas of alternative medicine are being introduced to the public at large. Predictably, there is resistance. The medical establishment targets doctors who introduce natural (and often less costly) methods, regardless of how safe and effective they are. Alternative medicine threatens modern medicine, because it involves a major shift in scientific thought. Consequently, orthodox medicine has attempted to suppress new treatment ideas.

It takes a great deal of courage and independent thinking for a physician to depart from established treatment practices. When physicians stray from conventional approaches, they often meet with hostility from other physicians—and as we all know, peer pressure is a very powerful force. Furthermore, most physicians are kind, caring individuals. They do not reject new or alternative treatment out of lack of concern for their patients, but because it does not fit their paradigm. They reject these treatments because "there are no adequate studies" of the treatment, or because "studies done in other countries are not as rigorous as those done in North America." They believe the treatment *cannot work,* and if the patient gets better, they assume the

placebo effect was responsible for the cure. And being human, they may feel hurt that the patient did not "believe in them" enough to continue with their suggested treatment, especially if they have spent extra time with the patient and done special research regarding the patient's problem. They also may feel that resorting to alternative treatment prevents the patient from receiving the "proper treatment" offered by modern medicine.

DOUBLE-BLIND STUDIES

For all these reasons, most physicians refuse to accept the validity of new treatments unless they have been proven by double-blind studies. A double-blind (placebo-controlled) study is one in which two groups of patients are treated, an experimental group and a control group. Only the people in the experimental group are given the medicine being tested. Those in the control group are given a placebo, an inert pill that looks identical to the one being tested. No one in contact with either group knows which patients are in the experimental group and which are in the control group; only an off-site researcher has that information. This type of study is considered the "gold standard" of clinical medicine.

Modern medicine is critical of many alternative treatments and theories because there have been no double-blind studies proving their efficacy. Yet most of the orthodox medicines and technologies used today have never undergone double-blind studies. The Office of Technology Assessment (OTA), a research branch for the United States Congress, found that "only 10 to 20 percent of all medical procedures currently used in medical practice have been shown to be efficacious by controlled trial." The OTA notes as well that some of the procedures which have supposedly been proven effective are based on flawed research. (*Assessing The Efficacy And Safety Of Medical Technologies.* #052-003-00593-0, Government Printing Office.)

In theory, the double-blind study seems logical, important, and scientifically correct; however, this has not proved to be the case in practice. Often it is impossible to find a true control group for a study, and many incorrect conclusions have been reached in studies in which the control was flawed.

Far more effective has been the clinical trial method, introduced in the 1600s by Sir Thomas Sydenham. This method calls for the patient to be described accurately, the treatment to be applied, and the outcome evaluated. Modern medicine refuses to accept "anecdotal" evidence derived from the clinical trial method as legitimate. Hopefully this will change in the near future, as outcome evaluation of treatment is now being performed by mainstream medical organizations.

CHOOSING A PHYSICIAN

There are many knowledgeable, competent, kind, and caring physicians who are open to new ideas—as well as some who are more rigid in their views. To enjoy the best possible health, you must make an educated, informed choice of health care professionals. Your goal is to select people whose training and background can best help you deal with your particular health needs. Whether you are basically healthy or have major health issues, you will need a primary care physician as the basis of your health care team. However, you may also want (and need) to consult health care professionals from other fields of expertise, including alternative medicine.

In the United States, many people now have a limited choice of primary care physicians through Health Maintenance Organizations (HMOs) and Preferred Provider Organizations (PPOs). Many HMOs and PPOs have only a small number of physicians under contract. All members of the HMO must see those physicians. Members of PPOs can see another physician but will receive a lower reimbursement from the organization. People who have fee-for-service insurance sometimes are required to choose their physicians from among those who have a contract with the insurance company. Using a physician outside your insurance plan's list can significantly reduce or even void insurance payments. These limitations can make it difficult for you to choose the best possible primary care physician for your needs.

When you are choosing a physician, look for someone you feel is a kind person, and is concerned about you and your health. Such a person will be easy to talk to, and will listen to you and truly hear what you have to say. You should not feel rushed through your appointments, and you should be involved in any decision-making about your care. Your primary care physician should know when to refer you to another professional or a specialist, and should be open to new ideas about health care. He or she should not rely solely on drugs for treatment, but should propose non-pharmaceutical treatments such as diet, physical therapy, bodywork, exercise, and nutrition.

Your physician should be able to explain your health problems and their treatment possibilities without either overwhelming you with technical language or talking down to you. Your calls should be returned within a reasonable time, and you should be confident that your physician is willing to consult with any other health care professionals you see.

If you do not know any of the physicians in your HMO or on your insurance list, talk to your friends, co-workers, and relatives to see if any of them can suggest a good doctor. Your dentist, pharmacist, or another health care professional may also be able to help you. Once you have made a tentative choice of physicians, make a consultation appointment and discuss your health concerns and goals. This can be a great help in deciding whether you have made the right choice or should keep looking.

Even if your physician does not agree with all of your views, open and honest communication can overcome many problems. Each of you can learn from the other, and many times sincere discussion can stimulate a curiosity and an interest that can lead both doctor and patient to broaden their views.

If you feel uneasy about a treatment your physician proposes to you, do not hesitate to get a second or even a third opinion. For any treatment to be successful, the patient's understanding and compliance are essential. Should your physician refer you to a specialist with whom you do not feel comfortable, or whose proposed treatment worries you, again get a second or third opinion. You must feel at ease with any physician you see, and with any treatment proposed for you.

CHAPTER 2

Pharmaceuticals

Modern medicine is heavily dependent on pharmaceuticals, because once a diagnosis is made, treatment is carried out almost exclusively through the administration of pharmaceuticals (medicinal drugs). A drug is any physiologically active substance that is used for the prevention, diagnosis, or treatment of disease.

The science of drugs is called pharmacology, a word derived from an ancient Greek term meaning both "medicine" and "poison." All drugs, no matter how beneficial, can become poisons in high doses. Their potential toxicity is the main drawback of drugs, and many patients experience negative side effects. Such side effects may be as mild as heartburn, nausea, drowsiness, or hives; or they may be severe and cause damage to organs, or even death.

HISTORY

Primitive peoples developed an ancient pharmacology by learning to treat diseases with plant remedies. As medicine progressed, the pharmacopoeia available to practitioners increased. Water was first on the list of all remedies. In addition to cleansing and cooling, it served as a vehicle for introducing other remedies to the body. A long list of other "medicines" was also used, including minerals, resinous materials, wine, honey, waxes and greases, and milk of all kinds. Urines from many animal species were at one time or another employed as treatment substances.

Although much of the knowledge of early medications has been lost over the centuries, some of it has been passed down through folklore, and some exists in ancient books that have survived the ages. The first medical pharmacopoeia was written by the Chinese emperor Shen Nung in 2735 BC. It listed all of the then-known medications. In Europe, the first Materia Medica (text on medicinal substances) was written by the Greek army surgeon Dioscorides in 77–78 AD. It contained a description of 600 plants and plant substances, and was considered an authoritative work up to the 17th century. Galen refined the use of herbal medicine, using infusions (made by soaking herbs) and decoctions (made by boiling herbs). He carefully identified the variety and age of the botanical materials he used—which was the beginning of purity control in drugs.

The early Arabs made several great contributions to medicine. They are credited with inventing the processes of distillation, crystallization, and sublimation, all techniques that are still used in medicine and pharmacology today. They were also the originators of pharmacies (previously, physicians made up and dispensed their own prescriptions), and they were the first to have teaching hospitals, complete with libraries and lecture halls.

As medical knowledge increased, new information about healing plants and other medications was recorded. The *Nuovo Receptaris* was published in Florence in 1498 AD, and pharmacopoeia were published in Nuremberg in 1535, Basel in 1561, Augsburg in 1564, and London in 1618. These books provided standards of purity and preparation methods for various drugs, as well as descriptions of the plant and mineral specimens used. The Danish Pharmacopoeia, first published in 1772, is the world's oldest continuously published materia medica.

Until the 1800s, most drugs were given by mouth, either as crude ground-up preparations of plant material, or in the form of herbal extracts, tinctures, and teas. Neither contents nor doses were standardized, and the use of a particular plant for a given condition was justified only by tradition and ritual, rather than by clinical studies.

In 1803, a German pharmacist extracted morphine from opium—the first extraction of a pharmacologically active chemical substance from plant material. From the middle of the 19th century onward, intense efforts were made to isolate and purify the active substances of healing plants. As time went by, interest in treating with the herbs themselves diminished, and scientists focused on extracting active chemical substances—and patenting and marketing them. With that shift in emphasis, the foundations of modern pharmacology were laid.

DEVELOPMENT OF MODERN DRUGS

Many of the drugs in current use today come from plants, or are synthetic variants of compounds originally found in plants. According to Dr. Norman K. Farnsworth of the University of Illinois, 121 commonly used prescription drugs are derived from plants, while other familiar drugs are metabolic products of molds. Drugs in these two groups make up 60 to 70 percent of all drugs in use today.

New drugs are developed in research institutes and in laboratories—usually labs attached to pharmaceutical companies. Chemists synthesize these drugs, and then correlate their molecular structures with their biological activity. After exhaustive studies in the laboratory, the drugs are sent for clinical trials involving laboratory animals and human volunteers. Such trials are usually held at university teaching hospitals, but some are run from the offices of participating physicians. Drug trials are designed to eliminate the "placebo response," in which symptoms are relieved simply as a response to the idea that "medicine cures." Researchers believe that if a new drug does not perform any better than the placebo, the drug is discredited and useless.

PROBLEMS WITH DRUG TESTING

Although clinical trials can be an excellent way of evaluating new drugs, there are still problems with how such trials are handled. Often, the trials are run for only a very short time—perhaps only a few weeks, rather than the months or years that most people assume are involved. Consequently, side effects are often not evident before the drug is released, and become obvious only after the drug is in public use.

Furthermore, the profile of the patients on whom drugs are tested is often skewed. Most drugs are tested on people who are basically healthy, but who have one health problem—the one being studied. In the real world, many patients must deal with more than one health problem. In addition, drugs may not be tested equally on males and females, or on people from different racial or age groups. For example, children and women of child-bearing age are seldom included in drug studies. Only 42 percent of the drugs used for pediatric patients in the United States have been tested on children.

Because drugs are tested individually, there are virtually no studies on drug interactions. Most drug interaction problems are discovered only when a patient takes more than one drug and side effects occur. Reports then begin to occur in the literature—but unfortunately, this may be too late for some patients.

UNDERSTANDING DRUG NAMES

All drugs are given three different names. One of them is a complicated chemical name that has meaning only to a trained chemist. The second is the generic name, which is usually an easy-to-pronounce contraction of the chemical name. The generic name of a drug is not capitalized.

The manufacturer also gives each drug a proprietary name, which is registered as a trademark; this name is capitalized and followed by the trademark symbol (®). After many years, however, the proprietary name of a frequently used drug may be adopted into common usage—for instance, aspirin is actually a proprietary name.

DRUG PATENTS

In the United States, after extensive testing, new drugs are submitted to the Federal Drug Administration (FDA) for approval. In Canada, new drugs are submitted to the Health Protection Branch (HPB) of Health Canada. After examining the records and performing tests of their own, the FDA and the HPB will license the drug for sale by prescription only. In both the United States and Canada, new drugs are protected by patent for 20 years. During that period the drug companies market the product and recover their developmental expenses, which usually run into millions of dollars.

Once the patent has expired, other companies can market the drug, but they must use the generic name for their product, rather than the patented proprietary name. In producing the generic form of a drug, other companies cannot mimic the dosage, shape, or color of the original product. Generic drugs may or may not be equivalent therapeutically to the original drug. Although the active ingredients may be chemically identical, inert fillers, binders, and excipients can alter the rate at which the body absorbs

the drug. Nevertheless, many generic drugs are just as effective as proprietary drugs. No drug, whether proprietary or generic, is utilized identically by all patients. Biochemical individuality creates variability in the way drugs are processed by the body, so one drug may be better for a given patient, a different one for another.

After a drug with few side effects and a very small chance for error in dosage has been in use for some time, the FDA or HPB may determine that it can safely be sold to the public without a physician's prescription. The manufacturers then apply for permission to market the drug as a non-prescription, proprietary drug. Such a drug will be widely advertised, and sold as an over-the-counter (OTC) preparation. Aspirin and ibuprofen are examples of this type of drug.

Drug companies provide incentives to physicians for prescribing their drugs. Employees of the pharmaceutical manufacturers, called "detail" men and women, call on physicians to dispense free samples, stationery, and pens, as well as information about their latest products.

In the U.S., it is now legal for drug companies to advertise their prescription drugs to the general public. Drug companies spend millions of dollars in ad campaigns to promote their drugs to the public, encouraging patients to ask their doctor to prescribe the advertised drug. The companies claim that this direct-to-consumer advertising builds bridges between the patients, health care providers, and the health care system. However, consumer groups (such as Public Citizen's Health Research Group, based in Washington, D.C.) feel that this kind of advertising has led to misinformed physicians, misinformed patients, and an increase in the writing of unnecessary prescriptions.

TREATMENT WITH PHARMACEUTICALS

Many medications prescribed by physicians are very helpful; some are life saving. Other medications merely cover up an illness, disguising its symptoms, or they may substitute one problem for another. There is no question, however, that in many cases prescribing medications is an effective and desirable method of treating disease.

Unfortunately, physicians sometimes use medications to control disease without having any idea what caused the disease in the first place. For example, when a patient has rheumatoid arthritis, we treat the inflammatory response, often without attempting to discover why the body is having that response. Medication helps to control the inflammation, but such treatment is at best control of symptoms—not a cure. If the oil light on a car flashes, you can take out the bulb; this will control the symptom, but does nothing to solve the problem. While symptom control is important for the comfort of the patient, it is vital that the underlying causes of an illness be investigated.

PROBLEMS WITH MEDICATIONS

Even when a medication is appropriately prescribed, problems can occur. For example, the medication may be ineffective because of an error in manufacturing, processing, storage, or shipping. If drugs interact with one another, with certain foods, or with alcohol, there may be unpleasant or dangerous side effects. As well, a patient may have an idiosyncratic reaction to a drug. Some drugs alter mood and behavior, and there have been cases of attempted suicide following ingestion of prescription drugs. Where there has been inadequate patient education, people sometimes do not understand the effects and hazards of their medications. Finally, drugs for which approval is given hastily, or withdrawal is delayed, can create problems for patients.

Many drugs produce an immediate helpful effect—but because they also destroy or alter an enzyme that is necessary for proper balance in the body, over time an imbalance is created that can make matters worse. For example, diuretics lower blood pressure by forcing the body to retain less water. However, the body then manufactures chemicals that make blood pressure rise again, and higher doses of diuretic (or other medications) are needed to lower it. Similarly, sleeping pills become less and less effective over time, and insomnia thus becomes more and more difficult to treat.

There is no drug without contraindications or side effects. Drug reactions can vary from insignificant to serious; they can be obvious or hidden; and they may occur immediately or be delayed. A drug reaction can be caused by:

- a physician's error (the right drug can accidentally be given to the wrong patient, or in the wrong dosage);
- action on the part of the patient (taking the wrong dose, failing to take the drug, taking the drug incorrectly, or storing the drug incorrectly);
- the nature of the drug itself; or
- interactions with other drugs or substances.

More than two million Americans become seriously ill every year because of toxic reactions to correctly prescribed medications, taken properly. According to a 1977 study carried out jointly by scientists from the United States government and the University of Toronto in Ontario, about 137,000 Americans and 3,500 Canadians die from these reactions every year.

Among the many symptoms that can be caused by reactions to drugs are skin rashes, allergic reactions, anaphylactic shock, blood pressure changes, overgrowth of bacteria or yeast, organ damage, edema, dizziness, headache, joint pain, eye damage, lung disease, kidney stones, seizures, heart problems, vomiting, respiratory problems, paralysis, psychosis, neurological symptoms, coma, and death.

According to Arthur Freese, author of *Managing Your Doctor: How to Get the Best Possible Medical Care*, adverse reactions to prescribed medications result in approximately 1.5 million patient visits to doctors' offices each year. Most physicians continue to depend on treatment with drugs because they believe that the benefit-to-risk ratio for the vast majority of commonly used drugs is reasonable.

PROTECTING YOURSELF

If you need to take a pharmaceutical (either a prescription drug or an over-the-counter drug), you should be certain that you understand:

- the reason you have been given the drug;
- whether the drug is expected to be curative or palliative;
- the correct dosage, and the conditions under which you are to take the drug (with food or on an empty stomach);
- the cost of the drug, and the convenience of taking it;
- the time(s) of day and frequency that you are to take it;
- the length of time for which you are to take it;
- what to do if you miss a dose;
- the contraindications for taking the drug (other drugs you may be taking—either prescription or OTC—alcohol, etc.);
- whether you have any physical condition that precludes your taking the drug;
- possible side effects of the drug, particularly as they may impact on your activity level and sleep—and what to do if they occur;
- the types of binders, fillers, and excipients used in manufacturing the drug; and
- the drug's effectiveness over the long term, and its impact on your overall quality of life.

Ask the pharmacist for the information insert that is packaged with every drug, and read it carefully before you start taking the medication. If you have any questions, ask the pharmacist or your physician (or both) for more information. Never use a medication for purposes not indicated by your physician. Never give your medication to another person.

Protect yourself against medications that may have been tampered with (both prescription and OTC drugs):

- Inspect the package or bottle for tampering signs such as broken seals, open or damaged wrapping, and puncture holes.
- Inspect the medication for discoloration, unusual odor, or other suspicious conditions.
- Check with your pharmacist or physician if you have any doubts regarding a medication.

Observe the following safety precautions:

- Keep all medicine out of the reach of children.
- Check with your doctor or a pharmacist before adding a new medication to those you are already taking (and before giving a child an additional medication).
- Never assume you remember the dose of a medicine. Check the label each time.
- Never take or give a medicine when you are not alert or cannot see clearly.
- Never take someone else's medication.
- Do not store medicine near a dangerous substance that could be taken by mistake.
- Store medication in the original container that identifies it and gives dosage information.
- Carefully read OTC medication labels, checking for dose, ingredients, proper uses, directions, precautions, and expiration dates.
- Discard outdated medications.

AVOIDING THE USE OF DRUGS

All drugs, no matter how useful, have potentially damaging side effects. Modern medicine tends to overuse drugs and invasive procedures while ignoring natural approaches to restoring health. For example, most forms of high blood pressure, and type II diabetes, result from an unhealthy lifestyle—but they are generally treated with pharmaceuticals, rather than by correcting lifestyle choices.

Natural approaches to health restoration enhance the body's inherent ability to heal itself. If these methods are made a part of a person's life, many health problems can be avoided, and most of those that do occur can be treated without drugs. For almost every problem for which drugs are prescribed, there is a non-pharmaceutical solution that might work better. The following approaches can help avoid the use of drugs.

Live a healthy lifestyle:

- Eat a balanced diet of pure foods that are free of pesticides, additives, and preservatives.
- Maintain a regular schedule and get the amount of sleep your body requires.
- Drink at least eight 8-ounce glasses of water each day.
- Avoid alcoholic beverages and use carbonated soft drinks only occasionally, if at all.
- Minimize consumption of all kinds of sugar.
- Exercise regularly.
- Pay attention to the mind-body-spirit interaction, and nurture your spirit by activities appropriate to your belief system.

Take nutritional supplements:

- Take a well-rounded multiple vitamin/mineral preparation.
- Take extra antioxidants as determined by your toxic exposures and health risks.
- Take bowel tolerance vitamin C daily. (See page 372.)
- Take extra supplements as determined by your specific health needs. (For more information on this, see Part 3, Common Health Problems.)

CHAPTER 3

The Laboratory

The modern medical laboratory performs the diagnostic tests ordered by physicians; some laboratories are attached to hospitals, while others are run as independent businesses. There are general laboratories that do the more common diagnostic tests, and specialized laboratories that carry out tests that are not commonly ordered and that require very sophisticated equipment. The specialized labs receive specimens from all over the country, and may perform the tests in batches, as they receive sufficient samples.

Most medical laboratories are under the supervision of a pathologist (a physician who has a completed a specialty in pathology, the branch of medicine that deals with the structural and functional changes caused by disease).

USES OF THE LABORATORY

Laboratories are generally divided into departments or divisions, according to the types of tests performed. These departments and a typical example of the kinds of tests they carry out include:

- clinical chemistry (chemistry profiles, urinalysis);
- clinical hematology (complete blood count and other blood tests);
- immunology (blood grouping and typing);
- microbiology (microorganism culture and identification);

- serology (tests for venereal disease or mononucleosis); and
- cytology or histology (identification of cells and tissues).

Physicians order lab tests for a variety of reasons. Laboratory tests are intended to confirm suspected diagnoses as well as to monitor patient status. The tests are not meant to be a substitute for the observations of the physician and a careful patient history. However, sometimes a patient may have vague, puzzling symptoms that do not fit any specific clinical picture. Under those circumstances, laboratory tests can help to rule out some diseases and point toward the true problem.

Tests are also run for other reasons. For example, when an abnormal finding is reported, the test will be repeated as a check on accuracy. Sometimes medical colleagues, a patient, or family member will press for a test to be done, or there may be a medico-legal need to have certain test results. There may be a need to establish a baseline, or hospital policy may require that certain tests be carried out. Less legitimate reasons for ordering tests include personal or hospital profit, curiosity, insecurity, habit, or frustration at having no medical help to offer a patient.

Many physicians today feel that they must practice "defensive medicine" (including ordering a battery of lab tests, whether or not they are necessary) so that should they be sued, they can testify in court that they considered every possibility in their diagnosis and treatment. According to the American Medical Association, the cost of such defensive medicine is over $20 billion annually in the United States alone.

COMMON LABORATORY TESTS

A great many diagnostic laboratory tests are available in North America and are commonly ordered by physicians. The most frequently ordered tests are urinalysis, SMAC-20, and complete blood count (CBC). These are discussed below, so that you will know why your physician may have ordered a given test, and will be better able to understand the implications of the results. (Other laboratory tests are discussed under Common Health Problems.)

URINALYSIS

A urinalysis may be the most commonly ordered lab test. It is usually performed as part of a general physical examination, and is often a part of any hospital admission procedure. The urinalysis can be helpful in the detection of kidney or metabolic disorders; it is useful in diagnosing diseases of the urinary system and in following the course of their treatment; and it can detect disorders in other parts of the body, such as metabolic or endocrine abnormalities in which there is normal kidney function.

Urine is examined under a microscope to look for red blood cells, white blood cells, epithelial cells (cells from the lining of the bladder and urethra), casts (conglomerations of cells indicating kidney disease), and bacteria. If bacteria are found, a urine culture may be done to diagnose the type of bacteria involved.

Glucose usually appears in the urine when serum glucose exceeds the capacity of the kidney to filter it. This is an indication of diabetes mellitus. Urine glucose tests are used as a screen to detect and confirm diabetes, and to monitor diabetes control.

Protein in the urine is called proteinuria. Combined with microscopic examination of urinary sediment, detection of protein in the urine provides the basis for differential diagnosis of kidney disease.

Hematuria refers to blood in the urine. Fewer than 3 percent of healthy persons have minute numbers of red blood cells in their urine. A higher than normal level of red blood cells suggests the possibility of bacterial infection, kidney disease, cancer, or other disease. White blood cells in the urine suggest inflammation or bladder or kidney infection.

SMAC-20

The most common laboratory panel performed is the SMAC-20 (Sequential Multiple Analyzer for Chem-20) or Chem-20 test. This is a comprehensive automated blood test, which measures electrolytes, proteins, enzymes, nutrients, and waste products—the main constituents of plasma (the fluid in which the blood cells are suspended).

When SMAC-20 results are reported, both normal values and the patient's levels are listed. Levels for some enzymes are lower in women than in men, and levels for some chemistries are different for children than they are for adults—yet only one set of "normal values" is listed. If several tests on the SMAC are abnormal, then more specialized tests can be performed. If you are ill, a normal SMAC does not mean that you are not ill—it just means that the SMAC-20 test was not the right test to identify your problem. Likewise, a normal SMAC-20 does not guarantee that you are healthy.

COMPLETE BLOOD COUNT (CBC)

Blood is composed of plasma (a liquid) and specialized cells, including red blood cells, white blood cells, and platelets. If blood is allowed to stand without clotting, the cells sink to the bottom, and then can be counted. A complete blood count is typically done by a machine called a Coulter counter.

Red Blood Cell Count

Red blood cells contain hemoglobin, a protein that carries oxygen to the cells of the body. Anemia is one of the disorders that is diagnosed through a red blood count (RBC), expressed as hemoglobin or hematocrit. The hematocrit measures packed red blood cells as a percentage of the total volume of blood. Hemoglobin content and the size of red blood cells can be used in differentiating among several types of anemia.

Stained Red Blood Cell Examination

For this test, which identifies variations and abnormalities in erythrocyte size, shape, structure, hemoglobin content, and staining properties, a stained blood smear is studied under a microscope. The test aids in diagnosing anemia, thalassemia (hereditary anemia), and leukemia. It is also an indicator for the effects of radiation and chemotherapy.

Differential White Blood Cell Count

The differential white blood cell count indicates how many of each of the several kinds of white blood cells (leukocytes) exist in a given unit of blood.

White blood cells help to fight off infection. A high white blood count is often a sign of bacterial infection, but can also indicate appendicitis, leukemia, trauma, allergy, and even pregnancy. Specific types of white blood cells are found in different diseases and will change in increased or decreased proportion to the severity of the signs and symptoms of the disease.

Platelets

Platelets are the smallest cells in the blood and their activity is necessary for blood clotting. A deficiency of platelets can lead to impaired clot retention or prolonged bleeding. Abnormally high levels of platelets occur in cancer, heart disease, acute infections, cirrhosis, and chronic pancreatitis, as well as other conditions.

ERROR IN LABORATORY TESTS

Diagnosis and treatment procedures are frequently based on laboratory results. While all labs endeavor to be accurate, there are many sources of error in laboratory tests, and in the reporting of results. For example, errors can occur:

- in the labeling of samples;
- in typing reports and entering codes;
- through improper handling of samples;
- because a sample is of inadequate size for testing;
- because of a delay in delivery of the sample to the laboratory;
- because the test was conducted under improper conditions;
- because the sample was contaminated; or
- because of human error on the part of laboratory technicians.

Other factors can also affect the accuracy of the results of laboratory tests—for instance, some tests require that a patient take nothing by mouth for a prescribed period of time before the test is run, but sometimes patients fail to do this. Test results may also be skewed if a patient:

- takes drugs or supplements prior to the test;
- exercises excessively;
- is subject to stress and anxiety;
- fails to take a medication that is part of the test (or fails to take it at the proper time);
- has an illness that affects test results;
- is pregnant;
- is on a diet, or has a deficiency disease or a malabsorption problem; or
- is on long-term intravenous therapy.

As a result, at least one-fourth of all laboratory test results in the United States are incorrect, giving false positives or false negatives, according to Dr. Stephen Fulder, author of *How to Survive Medical Treatment*. False positives can cause a patient to be given additional tests (often more invasive ones) or even inappropriate treatment. False negatives can mean that a patient receives no treatment—which can be dangerous or fatal.

Also, normal laboratory values are based on average values within the general population. Sometimes, however, values that are slightly off the "normal levels" are in fact normal for a given individual. Lab results that are slightly unusual have led to misdiagnosis of serious problems, and resulted in additional intensive and invasive testing that was not necessary.

RISKS OF LABORATORY AND DIAGNOSTIC TESTS

Most laboratory tests involve little or no risk in themselves, but taking the necessary sample may create some problems.

- A vein or artery can be punctured when blood is drawn, an infection can develop at the puncture site, or a large hematoma (bruise) can form there. It is preferable to do all studies on one blood sample, rather than using many.
- All tests that involve withdrawal of body fluid by needle for analysis in the laboratory pose the danger of an infection developing at the puncture site. As well, the body can be damaged if the procedure is not carried out properly. Such tests include removal of fluid from joints (arthrocentesis), bone, womb (amniocentesis), and spinal column (spinal tap), and removal of bone marrow (bone marrow aspiration).

AVOIDING UNNECESSARY LABORATORY TESTS

It is important to have a primary care physician you see regularly and who knows you, so that he or she can accurately interpret test results based on a knowledge of your general health. If your physician orders laboratory tests for you, use the following guidelines to avoid unnecessary tests and mistaken diagnosis.

- Be skeptical of test results that indicate health problems for which you have no symptoms. Laboratory tests (except for screening and predictive tests) should be used to confirm a diagnosis and explain the reasons for existing symptoms.
- Be skeptical of any diagnosis that is based solely on laboratory tests. Ask for a repeat test of any abnormal results, and if possible have the tests done at another lab. Allow some time to elapse between tests, in case the abnormal results were caused by a passing phenomenon.
- Request a second opinion if your physician advises additional, invasive tests on the basis of lab test results that indicate you have a condition for which you have no symptoms. Take your lab test report with you, but allow the second physician to perform needed reconfirmation tests.
- Ask that the original test results, as well as the proposal for additional invasive tests, be thoroughly discussed with you. You need to know the mechanics of invasive tests, as well as their possible risks.
- You will be asked to sign an informed consent for any laboratory or diagnostic test performed, but be wary of signing an informed consent that allows for "...other measures that may be necessary." Such "other measures" should always be clearly identified in the form before you sign it.

CHAPTER 4

The Hospital and Emergency Room

Most communities regard their hospitals as healing institutions, and there are many instances in which the hospital is, in fact, life-saving. While healing can and does take place in a hospital, being admitted to the hospital can also be hazardous to your health. Unfortunately, the delivery of health care has become big business, and it is often highly technical and very impersonal. This contributes to the increase in hospital-caused mistakes in medications, surgery, and laboratory results; the spread of infections; and other problems. Poor communication between patient and staff, or staff and physicians, accounts for many errors. Carelessness or incompetence on the part of both physicians and hospital staff is another source of error.

In the United States, changes in health care insurance have also caused changes in hospital care. The services that HMOs will cover in hospitals are sometimes minimal, as are the number of "authorized" hospital days permitted for almost any given condition. Prior approval from HMOs is required for all hospital admissions or procedures, and in some instances for emergency room visits.

With a population that is both growing and aging, hospitalizations are increasing yearly, putting stress on hospital staff and facilities. It is imperative that patients (and their families) educate themselves so that they can become active participants on their health care team. Patient knowledge and participation in health care can assist in reducing errors at the hospital, helping to ensure safe and proper treatment and an uneventful recovery.

DIVISIONS OF THE HOSPITAL

A hospital usually has several divisions, each with its own distinct function. Depending on its size, the hospital may have:

- an emergency room or unit equipped to handle medical emergencies;
- inpatient floors, where patients are cared for;
- a surgical unit, where surgeries are performed and post-surgical patients are cared for;
- an ob-gyn (obstetrics-gynecology) unit, where babies are delivered and gynecological patients are treated;
- a medical laboratory in which diagnostic laboratory tests are performed;
- a radiology unit in which radiological tests are performed and treatments are carried out;
- a dietetic division that is responsible for feeding patients and staff;
- an environmental department, which manages both an engineering staff and a housekeeping staff;
- a pharmacy that dispenses medications to inpatients (and in some instances to outpatients); and

- a business office that handles patient billing and insurance and looks after hospital finances.

Some larger hospitals may also have a physical therapy unit, an occupational therapy unit, a respiratory therapy unit, and a social services unit. There may also be separate pediatric and psychiatric units.

HOSPITAL STAFF

Hospitals are staffed by the physicians who practice in the community, and who have applied for and been granted hospital privileges. Depending on the hospital, these physicians will be MDs or DOs; in a few cases (in the United States) NDs are on staff, and (in Canada) the staff may include chiropractors.

In the United States, there may also be physician's assistants (PA or RPA) on the staff; these are college graduates who have completed an accredited PA program of two to two and one-half years. They must pass a nationally administered exam, and their duties are to provide primary care under the supervision of a physician. There are some physician's assistants who enter into specialties and provide care under the supervision of a specialist. Physician's assistants write notes, order tests, and in some states may write prescriptions and dispense controlled substances such as narcotics and pain killers.

Nurse practitioners in the United States have the equivalent of a Master's degree in nursing, with a specialty in some aspect of primary care. They do not normally work in the hospital, but may take call for their supervising physician.

Registered nurses (RNs)—who have either a two-year or a four-year college nursing degree, depending on their state or province—make up the main body of the hospital nursing staff. There will also be licensed practical or vocational nurses (LPNs or LVNs) on staff, who have had one or two years of training (again, depending on the state or province). Nurse's aides (or assistants) and orderlies complete the patient care staff.

Large university hospitals that are associated with a medical school will also have on staff students in varying stages of their training. These include medical students, interns, residents, nursing students, and students of medical technology, respiratory therapy, physical therapy, radiology technology, and occupational therapy, all of whom are completing the clinical requirements of their training. These students work under the direct supervision of physicians, teachers, and department heads.

CHOOSING A HOSPITAL

If you live in a larger community or close to a city, you may be able to choose which hospital you wish to use. If you have time before you must enter the hospital, you should research all available hospitals carefully.

There are two conditions that have to be met if you are to enter a particular hospital: first, your physician or the specialist who is to treat you must be on the staff of the hospital. As well, in the United States a hospital must participate in your insurance plan if you are to be covered for your stay there.

If a given hospital (or hospitals) meets those two conditions, make a trip to the hospital(s) and investigate the following:

- Are the hospital and grounds clean and well maintained?
- Are the visiting hours liberal and reasonable?
- Are the hospital rules and regulations reasonable?
- Are the patient rooms neat and clean?
- Are there windows that can be opened to admit fresh air?
- Is the room air conditioned, and are there individual thermostats?
- Are there call buttons both at the patient bed and in the bathroom?
- Is there enough staff on duty?

- What is the noise level, both in the halls and in patient rooms?
- Are there provisions for a relative or a friend to stay with the patient?

HOSPITAL ADMISSIONS

Patients are admitted to the hospital to receive specialized care that is not possible, or that would be difficult to provide, at home. They are admitted on an emergency or a non-emergency basis, directly from the emergency room or from a physician's office, or they may enter on a planned schedule for surgery or for medical procedures or tests.

Some patients require intensive nursing care, and may be admitted to the intensive care unit, cardiac care unit, or neonatal intensive care unit, depending on the hospital setup and the particular health problem of the patient. People who are not as severely ill are considered "regular admissions" and will be admitted to the general hospital floor—which may provide wards, semi-private rooms, or private rooms.

Unless you enter the hospital on an emergency basis, avoid being admitted on a weekend, as very little will happen—but hospital charges will accrue!

SCHEDULED ADMISSIONS

If you are scheduled for admission to the hospital, there are several things you can do ahead of time to make your hospital visit go more smoothly.

First, call the hospital business office and discuss hospital financial policies. Find out what your insurance will and will not pay for. Ask whether there is any paperwork or information you need to bring with you when you are admitted.

As well, ask about the hospital's ability to meet any special needs you may have. For example, people with allergies will have special dietary and environmental requirements. The business office will refer you to the specific hospital divisions or departments with whom you need to make arrangements. It is very important that any necessary changes and modifications are discussed and agreed on before you are admitted.

Packing for the Hospital

When you pack for the hospital, take your pajamas or gown, robe, and slippers. Though you will probably be wearing a hospital gown at first, later in your stay you may want and need your own bedclothes. Leave your watch, jewelry, other valuables, and money at home; you will not need them, and they could be stolen from your room.

Do not bring electrical appliances that must be plugged into the hospital outlets. These can interfere with hospital equipment, and sparks from inappropriately wired appliances can be dangerous. If you need to take something of this nature (for instance, an air cleaner), have it approved by the hospital engineer before you enter the hospital.

Pack the medications and vitamins that you take daily. Your physician must place an order in your chart allowing you to use your own vitamins and medications; you may have to surrender them to the nurses to administer. If you have not arranged for this, you will have to take the substances provided by the hospital, and they will be more expensive.

Take family pictures if having them with you cheers you up. However, do not keep them in an expensive frame that could be stolen.

PAPERWORK

When you arrive at the hospital, you or a family member will be asked to sign several forms— even for an emergency admission. *Read everything you are asked to sign very carefully before you sign it.* If you have questions, make sure they are answered before you sign.

In the United States, the paperwork you will be asked to sign will include a financial agreement, which will assign your insurance benefits to the hospital. It will also state that you agree to pay any charges your insurance does not cover.

At any hospital, you will be given a Release of Information form; signing this form allows the hospital to give other physicians (and your insurance company) information about your health and the procedures performed at the hospital. An Informed Consent form gives the hospital permission to perform the planned procedures on you, and informs you of any problems that could be involved. Finally, you will be asked to fill out a History form, which consists of general and specific questions about your health history. This gives the hospital information about any medical problems you may have (past and present) and makes them aware of any medication allergies and problems you may have. *Be certain you tell the absolute truth on this document.* Full disclosure is essential for safe and effective treatment.

You will also be asked if you have a "living will" or a "durable power of attorney" on file at the hospital. A living will indicates what you want to be done (or not done) if you are dying and unable to make your wishes known. A durable power of attorney gives the person you designate the authority to make decisions for you, if you should be unable to do so. These documents are called "advance medical directives" and express your wishes regarding management of your health care. In the United States, if you do not have these documents on file, you will be asked to indicate where copies are located, or requested to put copies on file. In Canada, the papers are optional.

When the paperwork has been completed, you will be given an identification wrist band that you will wear during your entire hospital stay; this allows the staff to identify you even if you are unconscious. Check all of the information on the band carefully, to be certain it is all correct. Once you get to your room and hospital procedures have started, it will be too late to change the information. Be certain your name and the name of your physician are spelled correctly, and that any initials that may have been used are correct. In some hospitals patients are assigned a permanent number that is used each time they enter the hospital or use the laboratories. If you know your hospital number, check it also.

You should be given some type of patient handbook that contains a "Patient's Bill of Rights," adopted by the American Hospital Association. This bill of rights states that you have a right to good care, information, courtesy, privacy, dignity, respect, and the opportunity to make your own decisions. If you are not given a copy, you should ask for one. Study its provisions and as your hospital stay progresses, be certain that these rights are being respected.

HOSPITAL CARE

Before you go to the hospital, have your doctor give you a general summary of what will be done for you and to you while you are in the hospital. Ask who is authorized to do the various procedures planned for you. Ask if any of your recent tests and procedures can be used, instead of having them repeated in the hospital. Remind your physician of any special needs you have that should be noted in your chart, or for which special orders are needed. Nurses must strictly adhere to the written and verbal orders of the physician; having all of the correct orders written ahead of time can both save time and prevent mistakes.

When you enter the hospital, your own physician will be the attending physician—but it is possible that your care may be turned over to another physician or to a specialist. In the United States each physician who sees you will charge a separate fee. If you are in a university hospital where there are students, interns, and residents on staff, be sure you know the status of each person who sees you.

When any of the hospital staff comes into your room, find out who they are and what their status is. Introduce yourself by name and ask, "Is that (medication or procedure) really meant for me?" before you allow them to administer anything to you. Some patients have found it a helpful measure to write their name on poster board and tape it to the wall over the head of their bed. (A few hospitals even provide a bulletin board for this purpose.) You may also want to write information about allergies or chronic medical problems on the poster board.

When you get to the hospital floor, ask which nurse is assigned to your care. Have this nurse come in and talk to you about what general schedule and outcomes are expected during your hospitalization. You need to know the goals for your hospitalization, and you need to make your own expectations known. If your room is not satisfactory, speak up at this initial meeting with your nurse. If you wait before making any problems known, it may be too late to do anything about them.

RISKS OF HOSPITALIZATION

Although you will be going into the hospital for treatment of a health problem, being in the hospital can in itself create other health problems. Be certain that your hospitalization is absolutely necessary, and that the procedures you need are not available in any other setting. Once you are in the hospital, take all possible steps to minimize the dangers, and have a designated friend or relative watch out for you if there is to be a period during which you may not be able to do so. Children cannot watch out for themselves, so parents of hospitalized children must take responsibility for seeing that their child's hospital care is carried out properly.

HOSPITAL DIET

Nearly everyone is aware of the importance of diet in maintaining and promoting health. When you are admitted to the hospital, your diet is taken over by the hospital. Many patients are malnourished because of their illness by the time they are admitted to the hospital. Their nutritional needs will be increased by their illness and/or surgery, and malnutrition will interfere with healing and recovery. Malnutrition will also increase their susceptibility to infection, illness, and death.

In spite of the attention paid to hospital diets, they are often deficient. A recent survey (*New England Journal of Medicine* in 1996) of 57 United States teaching hospitals showed that 40 percent of them served massive amounts of fats, extremely salty food, and food low in fiber. In several studies, done in British, American, and Canadian hospitals, an alarmingly large number of patients were found to be malnourished (McWhirter and Pennington, *British Medical Journal,* 1994; Werbach, *Townsend Letter for Doctors & Patients,* June 1997; Butterworth, *Nutrition Today,* 1974).

Discuss diet with your physician before you go to the hospital. While you are in the hospital, if you feel your nutritional needs are not being met, discuss your concerns with your physician and the hospital dietitian. Ask your physician if your family may bring appropriate or additional food to you. You must be certain that any food you consume will not adversely affect your condition, and your physician must determine that.

Even when sincere efforts are made by the hospital kitchen to send you the food ordered by your physician, errors do occur. Check your tray carefully each time it is brought to you. You should be familiar enough with your medical condition and your nutritional needs that if you are brought the wrong tray you can identify it before you eat the food.

If you are scheduled for surgery or a procedure that requires fasting, do not eat during the prescribed time, even if you should be given a tray by mistake.

NOSOCOMIAL INFECTIONS

Infections acquired while in the hospital are called nosocomial infections. Hospital-acquired infections of surgical wounds, the lungs, and the urinary tract affect 5 to 6 percent of all hospital patients. According to the Centers for Disease Control (CDC) in Atlanta, these infections kill 1 percent of the patients who contract them, and contribute to the death of another 3 percent. Many of the organisms that cause nosocomial infections are increasingly resistant to antibiotics, and the illnesses they cause are very difficult to treat.

The organisms that cause these infections are carried from patient to patient by the staff, including doctors, nurses, and other hospital workers, largely because the staff simply fail to wash their hands between patient visits. According to the June 11, 1981 issue of the *New England Journal of Medicine,* intensive care nurses and physicians washed their hands between patient contacts only 40 percent of the time. Physicians were the worst offenders and washed their hands only 28 percent of the time. Hand washing is the single most important procedure in preventing the transfer of infection between patients.

All patients should gently remind staff to wash their hands before touching them. This should always be done, even if the patient is in a private room. It becomes particularly important when another patient in the room has an infection. If you have a hospital roommate who has an infection of any kind, or whose regular visitors have an infection, make every effort to be moved to another room. If this is not possible, you or your family must be very vigilant in seeing that all staff wash their hands—especially if they have done something for the person with the infection before they turn to you.

Infections can strike anyone who enters a hospital, even people who are there for minor procedures or invasive laboratory tests. Needles, tubes, and catheters all provide avenues through which organisms can enter the body, and the debilitated condition and impaired immune defenses of many patients increase their chances of getting an infection. To minimize the possibility, ask that procedures involving the use of needles, tubes, and catheters be performed as

infrequently as possible, and when done, discontinued as soon as possible. Again, make sure that hands are washed before anyone touches you for any reason.

DRUG REACTIONS

Hospitalized patients may receive as many as nine courses of drug therapy while they are in the hospital. In the United States, this results in six million immediate adverse reactions, as reported by Dr. Hershel Jick in the *New England Journal of Medicine* in 1974, and an unknown number of delayed and long-term effects each year. These can be caused by a number of factors:

- the wrong drug can be administered;
- the right drug can be given, but in an incorrect dose;
- a drug can be given by the wrong route, or at the wrong time;
- a drug can be given to the wrong patient;
- a patient can be allergic to a particular drug, or to a certain combination of drugs; or
- an intravenous solution can be incorrectly mixed.

When you are in the hospital, ask your doctor what medications will be prescribed for you. When a member of the staff comes in to give you medication, ask what the medication is and what dose you are to receive. If they name a drug or dosage that your physician has not mentioned to you, ask them to check further and confirm that it is indeed the right medication and the correct dose before you take it. Know what your medication looks like, and if the dose offered you does not look like similar medication doses you have taken previously (and there has been no change in medication ordered), again, ask the staff to check further. Always mention your name to the person bringing you your medication, to be certain you are not receiving medication intended for someone else.

After you take a medication, if you have any unusual sensations, report them to the nursing staff immediately. Symptoms you should report are a flushing sensation, chills, headache, chest pain or pressure, problems breathing, dizziness, itching, nausea, or vomiting. *Do not delay reporting these symptoms* in hopes that they will go away, because these are symptoms that should not happen in response to medication.

You should also know at what time you are to receive medication, and if it is not brought to you at the scheduled time, you should ask the nurse about it. On the other hand, if someone tries to give you the same dose of medication twice, you should be able to tell them who gave you the first dose and when. For this reason, it is very important that you know the names of all the nurses and other staff members who are taking care of you. It is a good idea to keep a written record of all your medication information, as it is easy to forget.

The same precautions should be observed if you are receiving intravenous medications. Be sure you know what is in your IV, even if it is just saline solution. The IV bottle or bag should be labeled with your name, the name of the medication, and the dose. If you cannot trust your memory, write down this information, as well as how often you are to receive it. Report immediately any unexpected symptoms that may develop with your IV, including pain, a burning sensation, dizziness, confusion, numbness, itching, tightness in your chest, difficulty breathing, or shortness of breath.

IATROGENIC DISEASES AND CONDITIONS

An iatrogenic disease is one that is either caused by the actions of a physician, or made worse by such actions. For example, you could contract an illness through an infected blood transfusion, or could be harmed by surgery done at the incorrect site. Other common sources of iatrogenic illness are: use of a procedure which a physician has not mastered; errors in diagnosis—and consequent treatment for the wrong condition; and the prescription of incorrect or harmful medication. Human error—caused by ignorance, care-

lessness, haste, lack of focus, or fatigue—can also result in iatrogenic conditions.

Discussing your condition and treatment plan in detail with your physician will help reduce the possibility of acquiring an iatrogenic disease. Medicine has double checks built into many of its procedures to prevent errors, but human beings inevitably make mistakes; the more safety checks that are available, the better. Your knowledge is an excellent safety check, and your knowledgeable family (or a friend) can be on guard for you when you are unable to monitor things for yourself. Parents must ensure the safety of their hospitalized children.

OTHER PROBLEMS

Other difficulties can arise while you are in the hospital, and you should be prepared to deal with them appropriately. For example, if you have a true emergency (such as unexpected bleeding) and no one responds to your call button, phone the main number of the hospital, report the problem to the hospital operator, and ask him or her to find someone to help you. Having a family member or a friend stay with you while you are critically ill can be a protection for you; they can go for help if no one responds to your call button.

Most hospitals and their staff members make every effort to give safe and effective patient care, but even in the best of hospitals problems can arise. Most problems can be solved with honest effort on the part of everyone involved. If there are problems you and your family cannot solve, call the hospital's patient representative, whose job is to help resolve patients' problems. If there is no patient representative, or if the representative cannot or will not help with the problem, call the hospital administrator.

DISCHARGE FROM THE HOSPITAL

When your physician determines that you have recovered sufficiently to return to your home, you will be discharged from the hospital. Most physicians will tell both you and the staff when you will be going home, at least 24 hours in advance of your departure. Most hospitals will give you written instructions, and a nurse or technician will discuss them with you before you leave. You will be asked to initial a copy of these instructions to signify that they have been explained to you. Be certain that you understand them before you initial them.

In addition to giving you special care instructions, the discharge instructions should tell you when you may resume your normal diet, return to work, resume your exercise regimen, and resume sexual intercourse. You should be told when you are to visit the doctor for a follow-up visit, as well as how to recognize signs and symptoms that could indicate trouble. You should also be given a written medication schedule to follow at home; if you are not, ask for one.

Be sure you understand when a "hospital day" begins—if you will be charged for an extra day starting at noon, you may want to request that you be allowed to leave earlier in the day, before the next day's charges accrue.

Take home everything that is yours, as well as all the things that you have paid for (such as your hospital kit, mattress foam, and respiratory aids). Do not take home hospital-dispensed pharmaceuticals unless you can be certain that they are free. The hospital drugs will cost far more than the same medication purchased at your neighborhood pharmacy, and unless it is an unusual drug that only the hospital pharmacy is likely to have, your physician can write a prescription that you can have filled later.

LEAVING AGAINST MEDICAL ADVICE

There are rare instances in which you may want to leave the hospital before your physician feels that you are ready to do so. However, you would be leaving against medical advice, and this is not a step you should take without careful

consideration. During an illness, people sometimes do not think as clearly as they normally do. They sometimes feel they have recovered when they have not, or feel they must get back to work as soon as possible or they will lose their job. Hospital care may be unacceptable for a variety of reasons: a staff member may be incompetent or unpleasant, approved vitamins and minerals may not be supplied, or food from home may not be delivered.

If you find yourself in such a situation, you should discuss your displeasure and concerns with your family, your physician, the hospital administrator, and the patient representative. Only if the problems remain unresolved should you consider leaving the hospital against medical advice. There *are* instances in which the need to leave the hospital is real, but fortunately, these are rare.

If you do decide to leave, you will be asked to sign a form stating that you are leaving the hospital A.M.A. (Against Medical Advice). *Read this form carefully before you sign it.* Many such forms state that you are losing all rights to bring suit against the hospital should your condition worsen, and in some instances you may run the risk of being dropped by your insurance company. It is best to have your lawyer see the form and discuss the situation, before you take any action. After your lawyer has read the form and approved your signing it, you can make your plans to leave.

Before you sign the document, write on the bottom or sides of the document all of the reasons you are leaving. Do not put these reasons on a separate sheet that could be lost. Also state that you are not giving up your right to sue. Enlist the help of your attorney to assist you in dealing with the hospital bill, and contact your insurance company. Write letters (approved by your lawyer) to the hospital administrator and your insurance company, explaining in detail your complaints and your reasons for leaving.

THE EMERGENCY ROOM

Most hospitals maintain an emergency room where acute emergencies and trauma are cared for. Except in very small hospitals, the emergency room is a separate unit of the hospital, with its own staff. People who go to a hospital emergency room for care are either treated and released (if the necessary follow-up care can be done at home) or (if they have a serious condition) are given critical care immediately and then admitted to the hospital.

Since the 1980s, emergency room standards in the United States have been set by the American College of Surgeons' Committee on Trauma. At a Level I trauma center (the highest-rated type of center), all trauma staff have had special training that allows them to diagnose and treat serious problems rapidly. There is always staff on duty, and specialized equipment is always available and ready. At a Level II trauma center, the staff may not be in the hospital at all times, but will be available within 30 minutes of an emergency alert.

In Canada, standards for both emergency room and hospital care are set by the Canadian Council on Health Services Accreditation.

While any physician—even an intern or a resident—might be of help in the emergency room, you will get the best care if the emergency room physician is a board-certified specialist in emergency medicine. Treating emergencies frequently requires using procedures that the ordinary physician may only rarely (or never) perform. Emergency duty is challenging; the cases treated are frequently difficult, and it is impossible to predict what the next emergency will be. It is important that an emergency room physician have all the skills needed to handle a variety of complex situations.

Many nurses have extra emergency room training as well. Nurses are frequently responsible for triage (determining the order in which patients should be seen). Patients with life-threatening symptoms will always be treated before those presenting with lesser emergencies.

CHOOSING AN EMERGENCY ROOM

A good emergency room and its waiting room will be clean. The waiting room will have seating for the patients and their families, with easy access to restrooms, fountains, snack and drink machines, and telephones. These facilities are important, because people sometimes have to spend hours at the emergency room. There should be security guards, because victims and perpetrators of violence frequently need emergency care, and that means there may be weapons present. There should also be guards who can accompany you to dark parking lots at night (particularly in cities).

Be familiar with the emergency rooms in your area, and know what conditions each does and does not treat. For example, not all emergency rooms are set up to handle pediatric emergencies. Some units are set up for cardiovascular emergencies (such as heart attack and stroke) while others are not.

In the United States, be certain that the hospital whose emergency room you use is on your insurance plan. Most HMOs and PPOs try to keep their subscribers out of the emergency room as much as possible. Should you go to the emergency room of a hospital that is not in your plan, you will be fully liable for the bill.

EMERGENCY ROOM PROCEDURES

When you go to the emergency room, tell the admitting staff about your most serious complaint first, and try not to cloud the issue with vague symptoms that are not associated with the emergency. Give any critical past history that may be important to treatment, such as an ulcer, past stroke or heart attack, or diabetes.

The emergency room staff can help you more efficiently if you carry an identification card that lists all of your medications and allergies. If you are the caregiver for an elderly or dependent person, be sure to carry medication/allergy information for that person as well. If you regularly use herbs or nutritional supplements, add that information to your medication card. You should give these cards to the emergency room personnel immediately—do not wait for them to ask about them.

If you smoke or use illegal drugs in any amount, tell the truth about it. The presence of these drugs in your body can necessitate treatment modifications. Know the date of your last tetanus shot; if you do not have this information, you may routinely be given a tetanus shot as part of your treatment.

Verify all information on any form before you sign it (either for yourself or on behalf of a relative). In particular, be certain that the problem being treated has been identified correctly on the form, noting especially the side of the body on which the injury or problem exists ("right eye" or "left hip").

If at all possible, have your advance medical directive (or the directive of the patient) with you when you go to the emergency room (see p. 26).

APPROPRIATE USE OF THE EMERGENCY ROOM

As many as 90 percent of the people who present themselves at an emergency room (particularly in the evenings and on weekends) use it for problems that are not of an emergency nature, and which could wait for a regular office visit. Such misuse of emergency services is not only expensive (a visit to an emergency room costs three to five times what an ordinary office visit costs), but it ties up medical personnel who need to be available to treat true emergencies.

The following conditions are true emergencies that are appropriately treated in the emergency room:

- lacerations (cuts or tears in the skin)
- significant injury to extremities (hands, arms, feet, legs)
- significant bleeding
- injury from car accident or fall
- suspected fractures
- chest pain
- severe pain in the right upper or lower side of the abdomen
- fainting episodes after strenuous exercise or exertion
- stroke symptoms
- head injury
- loss of consciousness
- breathing difficulties
- seizures
- acute allergic reaction
- poisoning
- total emotional or mental collapse
- suicide attempts
- persistent or severe vomiting
- persistent or severe dizziness
- loss of or dramatic change in vision

If you accompany a patient to the emergency room, remember that efficient patient treatment can be jeopardized if you go into the treatment area with the patient and get in the way of medical staff. However, if the patient is a child, or an adult who cannot communicate, it may be extremely useful for you to be present—particularly if you witnessed the accident or health crisis, since you may be able to provide information that would be helpful for treatment. Once you have given this information, it may be best to go back to the waiting room.

A person who is treated and released from the emergency room should be given written and verbal instructions for any necessary care at home. If medication is indicated, the patient should be given either a prescription or the actual medication needed—with complete instructions for taking it. The patient should also be advised on how and when to return to a regular daily schedule.

Often, additional or follow-up treatment is needed after an emergency room visit. If such treatment is needed, the patient should be told when to see his or her regular physician. To guarantee continuity of treatment, most emergency rooms send a report directly to the patient's regular physician.

Some emergency rooms also double as urgent care centers, which treat minor injuries that require quick medical attention but are not life-threatening. In recent years urgent care centers not affiliated with hospitals or emergency rooms have been established. These centers free emergency rooms to deal with serious and life-threatening emergencies, and prevent the disruption of physicians' busy office schedules.

CHAPTER 5

Surgery

Surgery is defined as the treatment of disease, injury, and deformity by an operative procedure. Surgery has been practiced for centuries, having been mentioned in the earliest records of civilization. Early operations were simple, and often performed without any type of anesthesia. Although the complexity of operations increased over time, it was not until the 14th century that a knowledge of anatomy was considered essential for surgeons.

Today, surgeons are highly skilled professionals and their knowledge of anatomy is superb and detailed. Their technical tools are becoming space age, and their computerized monitoring equipment and elaborate instruments allow intricate surgery and virtual miracles to be performed in the operating room. However, some surgical techniques and instruments can cause stress to the human body. Furthermore, "assembly line" surgery is becoming far too common, particularly in larger hospitals, making people feel like mere numbers rather than patients in need of help. Patients are sometimes referred to by the name of the organ requiring surgery ("the appendix at 8 A.M." or "the gallbladder in room 4"). Communication, touching, and prevention can and do suffer when management, computers, and medication become more important than people.

There is no doubt that surgery is frequently a life-saving procedure. Emergency surgery ac-counts for 20 percent of all surgery, and its necessity and efficacy is not debatable. Reconstructive surgery that repairs birth defects, or repairs and rebuilds damaged bodies should certainly be performed. New techniques that give relief to Parkinson's victims, and cataract surgery that restores vision are surgical victories.

Nevertheless, the efficacy of some surgery is subject to much argument. It should be noted, as well, that there are alternative and preventative healing methods that can make some surgeries either unnecessary or far less serious and extensive than they normally are. However, surgeons seldom know much about (or recommend) alternatives to surgery.

In 1979 a committee of the United States Senate investigated unnecessary operations, and reported that in the United States, 2.4 million unnecessary operations were performed in that year alone, at a cost of $4 billion. More than 50 million surgeries are now performed yearly in the United States, and one has to question how many of these are unnecessary—especially since the rate of surgeries performed varies from location to location, apparently based more on the number of surgeons available than on the prevalence of disease. In the United States, surgeons are paid for each operation they perform, whereas in the United Kingdom surgeons in the National Health Service are not paid on a fee-for-service basis. Even so, some of the surgery performed in the United Kingdom is unnecessary—and the surgery rate in the United Kingdom (on a per capita basis) is half that of the United States!

Dr. Stephen Fulder, in his book *How to Survive Medical Treatment,* lists the following operations as the most commonly performed *unnecessary* surgeries: appendectomy, back surgery, biopsy, circumcision, gallstone removal, heart bypass surgery, hernia repair, hysterectomy, mastectomy, tonsillectomy and adenoidectomy, and tympanostomy. Many hospitals now have committees that review operations to see whether they were necessary or justified; surgeons who perform too many unnecessary operations are subject to censure. Dr. Fulder notes that the existence of these committees has been shown to reduce surgery by two-thirds in the hospitals that use them.

TYPES OF SURGERY

Simple operations (such as the removal of a wart or mole in a physician's office, or a biopsy performed in the hospital) are classified as minor surgery. Minor surgery does not involve serious hazard to life, and usually does not require general anesthesia. Bandaging; application of splints and casts; suturing of lacerations; and excision, incision, and drainage of superficial structures are all classified as minor surgery. However, there may be no such thing as true minor surgery, because all surgery requires special training, and the potential for complications to develop is always there.

Major surgery is usually defined as surgery in which the chest, cranium, or abdominal cavity is opened, or as any surgery that is performed under general anesthesia. It is carried out by a surgical team that usually consists of a chief surgeon, assistant surgeons, surgical nurses, and an anesthesiologist. Major surgery always takes place in an operating room or theater, and requires intensive hospital nursing afterward, so the patient spends several days in the hospital.

Examples of major surgery are: appendectomy, hysterectomy, gallbladder surgery, hip replacement surgery, brain surgery, and transplant surgery.

The majority of operating theaters are located in hospitals. However, in recent years day surgery clinics not affiliated with hospitals have opened in the United States and a few provinces in Canada. A patient reports to such a clinic early in the morning, the surgery is performed, and the patient is dismissed in the afternoon or at the end of the day. These clinics are very successful, but a problem can develop if a patient does not recover completely enough to be safely sent home on the same day. It is prudent for these surgery clinics to be close to a hospital or emergency facility, because problems can occur that cannot be handled at the clinic, in which case patients have to be transported to a hospital. If you use this type of clinic, be certain your insurance approves of the facility. In Canada, Medicare does not cover these private services.

Many hospitals have their own day surgery clinics, where outpatient surgery is performed. A patient has surgery in the hospital operating room in the morning, and is dismissed from hospital before the day is over. Both time and money are saved, because the patient is not spending unnecessary time in the hospital or having extraneous laboratory tests performed. Outpatient surgery is safe for dilatation and curettage (D&C), breast biopsy, hernia repair, cataract extraction, cystoscopy, tubal ligation, tonsillectomy and adenoidectomy, varicose vein removal, and excision of skin or tissue lesions.

Laparoscopy, a technique that came into common use in the late 1980s, has allowed some kinds of operations that were once major surgical procedures to become outpatient procedures, and has made inpatient stays for other operations much shorter. Laparoscopy involves inserting specialized instruments and a miniature TV camera through three very small incisions in the patient's abdomen. The surgeon views the operating field through the camera, and performs the surgery using the specialized instruments. A patient who has a laparoscopy has less post-operative pain and a shorter recovery time than one who has conventional surgery for the same condition. Hysterectomies, appendectomies, tubal ligations, and gallbladder surgery are among the procedures that can be performed via laparoscopy.

Surgery is performed on an emergency basis for life-threatening conditions such as a ruptured appendix or an aneurysm. It is done on a scheduled basis for such non-emergency operations as repair of a deviated septum, or performance of a routine hysterectomy. Elective surgery is done when the operation is to be performed strictly because of the patient's wishes, rather than because of medical necessity. Cosmetic surgery is an example of elective surgery.

RISKS OF SURGERY

Even when surgery is clearly indicated and is genuinely needed, it is not without risk. Surgery is a shock to the body on a physical, mental, and emotional level, and the potential for nosocomial infection always exists. Furthermore, there is the possibility of surgical error: the surgeon may not have mastered the method; the surgeon or anesthesiologist may not be adequately prepared for an emergency; or, in the case of bilateral organs, the operation may be performed on the wrong side.

Drug reactions are possible, both to anesthesia and other medications given. The wrong medication may be given at the wrong time to the wrong patient, and patients' charts and X-rays can be mixed up. Blood transfusions may be necessary, and these, too, are not without risk.

ANESTHESIA

Oliver Wendell Holmes coined the word "anesthesia" in 1846 to describe the effects of ether, an early form of anesthetic. Today the word is used to describe the total or partial loss of sensation induced by an anesthetic. If the anesthetic (administered either by injection or inhalation) causes the loss of sensation by rendering the person unconscious, it is classed as a general anesthetic. If the anesthetic (administered topically or injected into the tissue or nerves) causes loss of sensation in only a small area of the body, it is classed as a local anesthetic.

Eighteenth-century studies on combustion and gases led to the recognition that nitrous oxide had anesthetic powers, and paved the way for the development of modern anesthetics. There was no systematic search for anesthetics, even though surgery without them was filled with pain and terror for the patient. The discovery of substances with anesthetic properties was simply fortuitous.

This century's developments in chemistry and pharmaceuticals has vastly expanded the types of anesthetics available to surgeons. Anesthesia can now be induced and maintained for long periods, which allows surgeons to perform operations that may last as long as 10 to 12 hours.

General Anesthesia

Most general anesthetics are administered by inhalation, and render the patient unconscious as well as unresponsive to pain. There are other compounds that are classified as general anesthetics, but which are administered by injection. Some are used alone, and others are usually administered to patients before they are given inhalation anesthetics.

Even though the anesthetics of today are relatively safe, they are not without problems: reflex coordination can be disturbed, and there can be disturbances of the respiratory system, circulation, the autonomic nervous system, the kidneys, the heart, and the liver. Muscle rigidity and hyperpyrexia (very high fever) can also occur as a response to general anesthesia. This happens mainly in children and young adults when there has been physical exertion just before surgery (for example, a sports accident treated immediately with surgery). There can be allergic reactions to the anesthetics used, and side effects from the muscle relaxants that are often given in preparation for surgery. As well, some anesthetics can produce psychiatric changes (excitement states, delirium, unpleasant dreams). Finally, some people simply detoxify anesthetics slowly, which affects their rate of recovery from surgery.

More rarely, surgery can trigger malignant hyperthermia. This genetic condition occurs in one in 40,000 adults and one in 15,000 pediatric patients, but it is dormant until people with the disease are given potent anesthetics and muscle relaxants. They then develop tachycardia (racing of the heart), breathing irregularities, skeletal muscular rigidity, and high body temperatures. Left untreated, the episode terminates in cardiac arrest and death. Dantrolene, a specialized muscle relaxant, can reverse malignant hyperthermia, but only if administered early enough in the disease process. Malignant hyperthermia attacks should be avoided because even if the attack is stopped, permanent organ damage can result.

If anyone in your family has ever had malignant hyperthermia, the safest procedure is to assume that you may have it too. If you have to undergo surgery, talk to the anesthesiologist before the operation and make it known that you are susceptible.

Local Anesthesia

Local anesthetics are administered topically or by injection (into tissue or directly into a nerve, depending on the amount and degree of anesthesia needed). They provide anesthesia to a particular area of the body by blocking nerve conduction from that area, but allow the patient to remain conscious. Local anesthetics are used for procedures as simple as stitching a laceration, or as complex as performing a Cesarean section.

Epidural anesthetics are injected into the fibrous membrane that forms the outermost covering of the brain and spinal cord. The lower extremities receive the analgesia, the site of the injection and position of the patient determining the extent and location of the pain control. The patient remains conscious, and may also be given mood-altering drugs to control anxiety.

Spinal anesthetics are injected into the cerebrospinal fluid of the vertebral canal, and give the same analgesic effect experienced with an epidural.

Allergic reactions to commonly used local anesthetics have been reported, some of them severe. These reactions include local swelling at the injection site, hives, fainting, hyperventilation, seizures, asthmatic attacks, anaphylaxis, and even death.

Other reactions to local anesthetics can be caused by the epinephrine (adrenalin) that is frequently mixed with the anesthetic (particularly in dentistry). Epinephrine can cause anxiety and a vasovagal reaction (a drop in blood pressure, marked pallor, and sometimes a loss in consciousness and excess sweating). The preservatives used in local anesthetics are sometimes a problem also.

BLOOD TRANSFUSIONS

If blood volume and red blood cell numbers fall below a critical level, a blood transfusion is required to maintain life. Blood transfusions may be necessary when too much blood has been lost (either prior to or during surgery) or when the patient has serious anemia. Some operations (for instance open-heart surgery and transplant surgery) cannot be done without blood transfusions.

Blood used for transfusions may come from a compatible donor, or it may be the patient's own blood that was "banked" before the surgery. If the blood is from a donor, the blood is typed and crossmatched according to the ABO blood groups and the Rh factor. In some cases, additional blood factors may have to be considered to achieve a compatible crossmatch. You should know both your ABO blood group and your Rh factor. If you receive a blood transfusion, either you or your family should check the label on the blood to be certain your name is on the bag and that the indicated blood group and Rh factor are correct.

The administration of blood can be life-saving—and though there may be problems with transfusions, such reactions generally can be treated, whereas people who have bled to death are past help. You should keep this in mind as you read the discussion that follows, which points out some of the difficulties that can arise from receiving a blood transfusion.

Transfusion Reactions

Transfusion reaction is the name given to any unfavorable event or symptom that is caused by a transfusion. These reactions can and do occur for several reasons:

- Although the chances are very slight, it is possible for the wrong blood to be given to the wrong patient, through an error in paperwork or a mix-up in the delivery of the blood. The chances of this happening, though, are only one in 600,000. Knowing your blood group and Rh type will help reduce this possibility still further.
- Most transfusion reactions of antigenic nature are caused by differences in minor antigens. Giving packed red blood cells from which the plasma has been removed reduces some potential antigenic problems, because the antibodies that could damage the red blood cells of the patient are in the donor plasma.
- Hemolytic reactions may be caused by the use of incompatible blood, by bacterial contamination, or by storage of blood at room temperature (or higher).
- Allergic reactions are signaled by the appearance of hives, edema, or tendency to asthma, and may be associated with fever and chills.

- Pulmonary problems can be caused by circulatory overload from rapid infusion.
- Cardiac arrest can occur because of massive transfusions, which can produce citrate intoxication (citrate may be used to preserve blood during storage).
- Immediate post-transfusion jaundice may occur when large quantities of blood nearing its expiration date are administered, releasing amounts of hemoglobin that exceed the body's bilirubin-clearing mechanisms. (As blood cells age, they rupture and release their hemoglobin.)

Immune System Problems

Many studies report multiple immunological impairments following blood transfusion. For example, Dr. Donald Fry, head of surgery at the University of New Mexico Medical School in Albuquerque, reports that it may take the immune system as long as two years to recover from a blood transfusion.

Studies reported in the *American Journal of Surgery* (1988) indicate that cancer patients who received blood transfusions during surgery showed higher rates of cancer recurrence and poorer survival rates than those who received no transfusions.

Transfusion-Related Acute Lung Injury

After surgery, some patients develop difficulty breathing and may require oxygen or even intubation; they are said to have a transfusion-related acute lung injury. This condition can occur with either donor blood or the patient's own stored blood, if it has been stored for three weeks or longer. While the cause of this condition is unknown, it may be that a toxic substance builds up in stored whole blood, packed cells, and possibly platelets.

Transfusion-Transmitted Diseases

AIDS and hepatitis are the best known diseases transmitted by transfusion, but they are not the only ones. Screening tests have greatly increased the safety of the blood supply, but the possibility of transfusion-transmitted diseases still exists. Diseases that may be passed in a blood transfusion include such viral infections as cytomegalovirus (CMV) and Epstein-Barr virus (EBV); bacterial infections such as syphilis, gonorrhea, and Lyme disease (theoretically possible); and parasitic infections (malaria, toxoplasmosis, trypanosomiasis, filariasis, and babesiosis).

Researchers and transfusion specialists continue to work to reduce the risk of receiving an infection from a blood transfusion. According to the American Association of Blood Banks, eight screening tests are used on donor blood, including tests for the syphilis spirochete, HIV-1, HIV-2, human T-cell lymphotrophic virus types 1 and 2, hepatitis B virus, hepatitis C virus, and two surrogate tests for non-A and non-B hepatitis viruses. Testing of donor blood for parasites is not yet practical in North America because of their low incidence. The chance of getting AIDS from donated blood is now one in 450,000 to 660,000.

Other procedures used to increase the safety of transfusions include the use of erythropoietin and other blood growth factors; the recycling of a patient's own blood "lost" during surgery; and more careful surgical techniques to reduce blood loss. Also, in recent years physicians have realized that patients can tolerate a much lower hematocrit level (ratio of red blood cells) than had been thought without having to undergo transfusion. Many transfusions can be avoided just by administering oxygen to the patient to increase the arterial oxygen concentration.

Autotransfusions

In autotransfusions, the patient donates blood several weeks before planned surgery, for use as necessary during the operation. Autotransfusion is the most widely used substitute for donor transfusion; it avoids the possibility of infection as well as immunosuppression. However, even autotransfusions are not without risk, as any blood can become contaminated with bacteria.

Furthermore, Michael Kanter of the Kaiser Permanente Medical Center in Woodland Hills, California, examined medical records of women undergoing hysterectomy and found that the patients who had donated blood were 22 times more likely than others to receive a transfusion—even though they had not lost an abnormal amount of blood. The main reason for this transfusion incidence was the anemia developed by the women as a result of having banked blood before surgery.

Nevertheless, in many cases, particularly in surgeries for which the chance of needing a transfusion is high, the benefits of autotransfusion outweigh the risks.

NEED FOR SURGERY

Your physician should suggest surgery to you only when a problem cannot be corrected by other methods. Some physicians are more prone to using surgical solutions than others, and you must take steps to determine whether the proposed surgery is really necessary and whether your physician has considered all other treatment options.

Ask your physician the following questions:

- Why do I need surgery?
- Is there a less invasive, non-surgical way to correct my problem?
- What could happen to me if I do not have the surgery?
- What are the benefits of having the surgery?
- What are the risks?
- What will be done to me during the surgery?
- How long will the actual operation take?
- Am I likely to need a blood transfusion?
- What are the possible complications and side effects of this particular surgery?
- What is the average hospital stay for this particular surgery?

- How long is the recovery time?
- If I were a member of your family, would you recommend that I have this surgery?

Find out why you developed this disease or condition at this time. You need to know if it is an isolated incident or part of a pattern of recurring disease. Thoroughly research other non-surgical treatment options, including the chances of success and the side effects of each option. Be certain to investigate alternative and non-conventional treatment.

Never agree to surgery without first getting a second opinion. The second opinion may help confirm that you need surgery—or it may cast doubt on the need for an operation. Most health insurance will pay for a second opinion (and some even require it). Good physicians and surgeons do not feel threatened by the prospect of second or even third opinions obtained by their patients.

Do not go to the partners of your physician in seeking a second opinion, as the medical philosophies of partners are probably quite similar. Instead, check with friends, co-workers, relatives, nurses, pharmacists, dentists, physical therapists, or the hospital of your medical plan for the name of a physician to see for a second opinion. Do not tell the second specialist the diagnosis and conclusion of your physician. The specialist should repeat all of the necessary tests (except those that involve significant risk, such as X-rays—you can furnish X-rays from your previous workup), and should reach an independent diagnosis.

CHOOSING A SURGEON

If your personal physician does not perform surgery, you will have to find a surgeon. Your physician will recommend one or several surgeons to you, but you do not have to accept any of these surgeons if you do not feel comfortable with them and their skills. Again, talk to friends, co-workers, relatives, and other health care professionals about their experiences with these and other surgeons. Do research in a medical library regarding the procedure you are to have, and find out who is listed as an expert. Become familiar with all of the techniques that can be used to correct your condition, because sometimes new procedures are safer and gentler. You will need to find a surgeon who is familiar with these techniques and proficient in their use.

Once you narrow down the choices, check the credentials of the surgeons you are considering with the local medical society. Find out which surgeons have finished specialty training and are board certified. Make consultation appointments with the most likely candidates. Be sure to take notes or tape record the conversation (with the doctor's permission) so you can review the information later on, when you will be more detached.

You should ask:

- How many times has the doctor actually *performed* (not watched or just supervised) this particular procedure? For the safest results, the surgeon should have carried out the procedure 10 times or more. The most important factor is the number of times the surgeon has performed your particular procedure, and the success rate achieved.
- What are the possible complications of the procedure (and its aftermath), and what is the mortality rate?
- What particular technique does the surgeon use in this procedure?
- How likely is it that you will need a blood transfusion? (If there is a likelihood that you may need one, investigate the possibility of an autotransfusion, and ask about the possibility of blood recycling—which can be used only for certain types of surgery, such as vascular and orthopedic surgeries.)
- What symptoms should you expect after the anesthesia wears off?
- How long is the usual recovery period?

- What is the surgeon's philosophy regarding pain control? (You do not want to be either overmedicated or undermedicated.)
- What will the surgery cost (including both the surgeon's fees and an estimate of hospital fees)?
- Which hospitals does the surgeon prefer to use?
- Which anesthesiologists does the surgeon prefer to work with?

Ease and clarity of communication with this physician should also be of paramount importance. Be sure to talk to the surgeon again just before the surgery to be certain all aspects of the surgery are defined, agreed upon, and correct. For example, wrong-sided operations do happen, and you want to be certain your surgeon knows the exact area for the surgery. You will also need to confirm that the surgeon is going to perform the surgery personally, rather than merely supervising a less experienced surgeon. (For additional information on selecting a physician, see Choosing a Physician in chapter 1, Overview.)

CHOOSING THE ANESTHESIOLOGIST

Anesthesiologists are physicians who have completed an anesthesiology residency. Nurse anesthetists are registered nurses who have two additional years of specialized training in administration of anesthesia. Nurse anesthetists administer 65 percent of all anesthesia in the United States, and 70 percent in rural areas. In addition to administering anesthesia and muscle relaxants, the anesthesiologist or nurse anesthetist will monitor your blood pressure and blood gases; control your breathing; and observe your brain, heart, and kidney function.

Check the credentials and record of the anesthesiologist or nurse anesthetist your surgeon works with, just as you did for the surgeon. If you wish, you can select your own anesthesiologist. However, you need to discuss your choice with your surgeon early, and the surgeon must also feel comfortable with the anesthesiologist you prefer.

You will always meet with the anesthesiologist when you come in for your pre-operative blood work. However, it is probably better to make an appointment to see this physician much earlier than that, because there are many things you will need to discuss, and that discussion may need to be held earlier than the day before your surgery. It is essential for your safety that you tell the anesthesiologist the absolute truth about your health and drug history, both past and present.

The anesthesiologist will need to know your exact height and weight, as your medication doses are determined by these values. You will also have to talk about your smoking and drinking habits, and any recent drug consumption (both prescription and illegal), including dose and duration of consumption. The anesthesiologist will want to know about any medical conditions you may have (such as asthma, allergy to drugs, diabetes, hepatitis or liver problems, coronary problems, blood pressure problems, or breathing disorders), and as well, about any adverse reactions to anesthesia that you (or your relatives) have had in the past.

You will also want to discuss the following with the anesthesiologist:

- what pre-medications will be used, and their possible side effects;
- what anesthesia will be used, and its possible side effects;
- whether there is a possibility of using a local anesthetic instead of a general anesthetic;
- what medications or substances, if any, will be administered intravenously;
- the possibility of using relaxation and stress reduction methods instead of tranquilizers; and
- the use of hypnosis and/or acupuncture to

help with pain relief and relaxation, in order to reduce the amounts of anesthetic and medications needed.

INVESTIGATING THE HOSPITAL

Once you know which hospital you will be using, it is important to check it out. In the United States, hospitals are not regulated directly by the federal government, but are self-regulated through the Joint Commission on Accreditation of Healthcare Organizations (JCAHO). In Canada, standards are maintained by the Canadian Council on Health Services Accreditation. In the United States, about 90 percent of all hospitals have been accredited, with certain recommendations for improvement. Only 1 percent of hospitals that apply for accreditation are actually turned down—a hospital must be really substandard to be denied accreditation. Make sure the hospital you will be using is on the list of institutions approved by the Joint Commission on Accreditation of Healthcare Organizations or the Canadian Council on Health Services Accreditation (see Sources).

Inquire about the following:

- the hospital's ability and willingness to handle special needs;
- whether there is a patient advocate and counselor on staff;
- whether any type of natural medicine service is available (in addition to traditional medical services);
- whether the hospital has an intensive care or cardiac care unit; and
- the hospital's patient-to-staff ratio.

For additional information about hospitals, see Choosing a Hospital in the preceding chapter.

PREPARING FOR SURGERY

In order to make your surgery and recovery go more smoothly, you will need to prepare yourself for your hospital admission physically, mentally, and emotionally. The following section includes alternative medical suggestions, as well as some that might be recommended by modern medical practitioners.

PHYSICAL PREPARATION

Your body needs to be as strong as possible before you have surgery, for several reasons:

- Your immune system needs to be strong to reduce your risk of acquiring an infection in the hospital.
- Your detoxification pathways should be operating efficiently so that your body can process all of the toxins (anesthesia, medications, and the substances resulting from tissue damage) to which it will be exposed.
- Patients who actively prepare for surgery heal faster, experience less post-operative pain, require fewer pain relievers and other medications, and are released from the hospital earlier.

Your body repairs itself when you rest and sleep, and you want to be rested and energetic when you enter the hospital. Before surgery, you should reduce your toxic load as much as possible, because after the surgery you are going to have many chemicals and medications to detoxify. Simple measures such as detoxification baths (both before and after surgery) are very helpful (see Krohn, *The Whole Way to Natural Detoxification*). Exercise will strengthen your body as well as help you to detoxify.

Be very careful of your diet both before and after surgery. Healthy eating should include good quality, highly nutritious food containing as many vitamins and minerals as possible. Be certain to consume sufficient calories, as your body will need both the calories and a balance of vitamins and minerals to heal from the surgery and to detoxify from exposures encountered during surgery. Eat adequate amounts of fiber and drink at least six to eight, eight-ounce glasses of quality water each day.

Avoid known allergens in order to remove

stress from and strengthen your immune system. Avoid "empty" calories (sugars and other sweets); refined foods; canned, preserved, and overcooked foods; food additives; fatty animal foods and saturated fats of all kinds; and food that is old or outdated. Avoid fluoridated water, as fluorides can delay tissue and bone healing.

To help minimize problems following surgery, take the following nutrients for four weeks before and six weeks after surgery. (*Note:* These are adult doses. Children's doses are one-half these amounts.)

- vitamin C – a minimum of 1,000 mg three times a day, up to bowel tolerance (the level at which you develop diarrhea) (promotes healing of connective tissue). *Caution:* Do not take during the 24 hours preceding surgery in order not to interfere with anesthesia.
- zinc picolinate – 30 mg one or two times a day, taken together with 2 mg of copper (stimulates growth of DNA for new cells and encourages wound healing)
- hydroxyfolate drops – five drops a day (stimulates growth of DNA for new cells). Contains B_{12} and folate liquid; made by Scientific Botanicals (see Sources).
- multiple vitamin/mineral – one to four capsules a day, depending on the brand (a balance of 40 to 45 nutrients is required by the body for maintenance and repair; minerals in particular are required by the detoxification pathways)
- vitamin E – 400 IU a day (taking this vitamin orally as well as applying it topically helps prevent scarring). *Caution:* Because of this vitamin's blood-thinning properties, omit for several days before and after surgery.
- coenzyme Q_{10} – 30 mg a day (increases cellular oxygen utilization that helps healing and detoxification)
- vitamin A – 25,000 IU a day. *Caution:* Do not take more than 8,000 IU a day if you are pregnant or if there is a chance you might be pregnant (essential for wound healing; aids in the production of collagen, and boosts immunity to infection).
- quercetin or other bioflavonoid – 500 mg two times a day (strengthens the integrity of tissue as it heals)

For a few days before and at least a week after surgery, take one of the following. *Avoid for the first 24 hours after surgery because bleeding time can be increased with these preparations.*

- bromelain – three capsules three times per day, one hour before meals or two hours after meals (for 2 days before and 10 days after surgery) (lessens swelling and inflammation, giving shorter healing time)
- Protozyme – one to five tablets three times per day, one hour before meals or two hours after meals (for 2 days before and 10 days after surgery) (lessens swelling and inflammation, giving shorter healing time). This product can be obtained from Marco Pharma (see Sources).

Herbs can also be of help to patients undergoing surgery. *Be sure that you tolerate specific herbs before using them in preparation for surgery.*

- gotu kola – two capsules (250 mg each) two times a day, beginning a few days before surgery and continuing for several weeks afterward (reduces healing time and makes healed tissue stronger; aids in the prevention of scar tissue)
- ginger – 250 mg four times a day, beginning two to three days before surgery, and continuing for two or three days afterward (an anti-inflammatory agent). *Caution:* Ginger can contribute to increased bleeding in people taking a blood thinner.
- garlic, onions, ginger, and turmeric – use as a condiment on your food to augment the drugs that may be prescribed for you. Take a

little shaker of these herbs with you to the hospital (contain blood-thinning agents that can help if your physician prescribes a blood thinner).

MENTAL AND EMOTIONAL PREPARATION

Preparing your body for surgery both mentally and emotionally can enhance your chances for a successful surgery and a smooth and speedy recovery. It can also minimize trauma and discomfort, and reduce or eliminate anxiety.

New York's Columbia-Presbyterian Hospital has a Complementary Care Program that now uses yoga, Tai Chi, guided imagery, massage, hypnosis, and acupressure to relax patients before surgery and to improve response during and after surgery. Dr. Mehmet Oz, a cardiac surgeon and director of the program, has his patients practice various relaxation techniques (including deep breathing and guided imagery) that focus on keeping their incisions free from infection, minimizing bleeding, and reducing pain and discomfort. Patients who have used these techniques before and after open-heart surgery show significantly reduced anxiety, pain, infection, and symptom recovery after surgery, as well as better overall cardiac function. Because of the success of this approach in cardiac patients, the program is now being expanded into the neurology, urology, and pediatric departments.

Being optimistic, feeling relaxed, and feeling reasonably in control are positive indicators for withstanding surgery well. Use the following suggestions to help reduce the stress of surgery.

- Have confidence that your surgery is necessary, and that you have done your homework and made all proper preparations for safe surgery.
- Think positively; consider your surgery as a positive step that will have a positive outcome. Do not think of yourself as a victim, and refuse to entertain negative thoughts.

- Be realistic about your emotions. A little fear is normal when facing surgery; acknowledge your fear and put it in the proper perspective.
- Have realistic expectations. Recognize that there are some risks, and that you may experience some discomfort—but expect that your careful preparation will minimize these.
- Know your coping style. If you cope by taking control, the more details you know about your surgery and the more you prepare for it, the more comfortable you will feel. If you cope by being passive, know the important facts, but trust your surgical team for all the rest.
- Learn to relax. Anxiety, stress, and tension can increase pain, prevent sleep, and slow down healing. Learn a simple relaxation or breathing exercise you can easily do in the hospital to reduce your stress levels, anxiety, and tension. A massage with lavender oil before and after surgery is relaxing.
- Receive healing energy. Arrange to have sessions of Reiki or Therapeutic Touch for two or three days before and after your surgery. A number of studies have documented that these techniques can promote the innate ability of the body to heal.
- Control what you hear. Anesthetized patients do hear speech and sounds, and studies show that hearing soothing music before, during, and after surgery reduces stress hormones and reduces the need for pain-killing medication. This technique is particularly important in an intensive care unit, where there can be a good deal of commotion and the patient is often disoriented.
- Use a guided imagery audiotape to induce a state of focused concentration. This produces a sense of physical and emotional well-being, permits relaxation, and can control depression, anxiety, and stress. It may also enhance healing and strengthen the immune system. Patients who use guided imagery have less pain and anxiety after surgery.

- Give your body healing instructions. Audio-tapes that provide positive verbal suggestions help to reduce complications and restore normal body functions more quickly. Positive affirmations (for example, keep the incision infection-free, minimize bleeding, reduce pain and discomfort, normalize blood pressure) played or read aloud during surgery can reduce the amount of post-operative medication needed.

  You will have to get advance permission to bring an auto-reverse cassette player with earphones into the operating room, if you want to use one to play affirmative or focusing tapes. You will need to discuss this possibility with the surgeon, anesthesiologist, and the proper authorities at the hospital. If you cannot obtain permission, listen to the tapes until the minute you leave for the operating room, and arrange for a member of your support team to put the earphones on you the minute you return to your room from surgery.

- Develop a pain control plan. Pain control is important for recovery, since lessened pain allows you to move about sooner and reduces your chance of complications. It is better not to let pain exceed a certain level—use drugs if you need them, but also try using such non-drug approaches to pain control as imagery, music, massage, heat, ice, distraction, and breathing or relaxation exercises.

- Develop a support network. Reach out to family and friends, and ask them for what you need—whether it is pain medication, information, a blanket, something to drink, or someone to hold your hand or stay with you.

- If you belong to a religious organization, have members of your congregation pray for you. Several studies have shown that patients for whom prayers have been offered have fewer surgical complications and make more rapid recoveries.

RECOVERING FROM SURGERY

Proper preparation prior to surgery can minimize problems and speed recovery, but there are also post-surgery techniques and treatments that are helpful.

Unless you are bed- or room-bound by your condition, move around as much as you are able. Walk in the hospital halls several times a day. Even if you must stay in bed, exercise by contracting your muscles one by one. A few days of inactivity can cause muscles, nerves, and body functions to suffer. Exercise will help prevent the problems that can result, and can help you maintain a better frame of mind.

If you need additional nutrition after surgery, you can use one of the ready-to-mix liquid diets. Both of the diets listed below are 100 percent complete, and can be used as often and for as long as is necessary:

- UltraClear by HealthComm
- NutriClear by Biotics Research

As soon as possible after surgery, start taking the following homeopathic remedies. *(Remember to ask your surgeon to write an order in your chart allowing you to do so.)*

- *Arnica montana* – 1 tsp. of a 30C solution (or four pellets under the tongue) every one to three hours for pain (helps to heal traumatized and bruised tissue). *Caution:* Do not take food or water at the same time.
- *Calendula officinalis* – 1 tsp. of a 30C solution (or four pellets under the tongue) every one to three hours (taken internally, fights infection and dramatically promotes healing; used topically, will often control bleeding and can soothe incision pain).

Several other homeopathic remedies are helpful in recovering from the effects of surgery. Consult a trained homeopath for the best remedy to take. Take a dose of the following remedies every two to four hours, as needed:

- *Acetic acid* – anesthetic poisoning.
- *Arnica montana* – trauma of respiraton; discomfort of bedridden patient.
- *Calendula* – helps people come out of anesthesia and gives painless recovery.
- *China* – post-operative gas.
- *Graphites* – prevents keloids (thick scars) after surgery.
- *Ledum* – hematoma from intravenous sites and bedsores.
- *Phosphorus* – anesthetic poisoning and weakness, emaciation, and vertigo after surgery.
- *Pyrogenium* – fever after surgery.

- *Strontium carbonicum* – surgical shock; post-operative problems; exhaustion after surgery; bone pain; never well since surgery.

Post-surgery trauma can also be helped with herbal therapy. Use any of the herbs listed below, in capsule form or as a tea. Take three times a day.

- red cloves
- licorice root
- Oregon grape root
- stillingia
- prickly ash bark
- kelp
- burdock root
- *Cascara sagrada* bark
- sarsaparilla root
- buckthorn bark

CHAPTER 6

Radiology

Radiology is the branch of medicine that deals with radioactive substances, X-rays, and other ionizing radiation in the diagnosis and treatment of disease. Radiologists are physicians who are certified in both diagnostic and therapeutic radiology.

Diagnostic radiologists specialize in the study of imaging tests: X-rays, ultrasound, mammography, computerized tomography (CT scans), magnetic resonance imaging (MRI), and nuclear medicine. These tests allow physicians to "see" inside the body without opening and invading it. The therapeutic subspecialty trains radiologists to administer radiation treatments that utilize X-rays and radioactive substances. Radiation therapy allows them to treat cancers without opening the body. Many of these techniques, both diagnostic and therapeutic, are extremely expensive.

DIAGNOSTIC RADIOLOGY

Imaging techniques are used to identify healthy or abnormal conditions within the body. They can be used to reveal the condition of organs in the body, to determine the condition of bones, to show relationships between bone and adjacent soft tissue, and to search for foreign bodies. They can be used to detect certain health problems, as well as to check the progress of a disease and the effectiveness of treatment.

X-RAYS

X-rays were discovered in 1895 by Wilhelm Roentgen of Germany, and are the basis of the most commonly used diagnostic imaging technique. According to Dr. Stephen Fulder in *How to Survive Medical Treatment,* 8 out of 10 North Americans have diagnostic X-rays every year. X-rays are very high frequency waves with high energy, that easily pass through living tissue. When ionizing radiation from an X-ray tube passes through the body, the bones and other dense structures leave a "shadow" on the photographic film. The radiologist reads this picture for signs of disease or damage. While the information from X-rays is valuable, repeated exposure can be dangerous.

Modern X-ray equipment is more accurate and uses less total radiation than older equipment did. The film is also more sensitive than films of earlier years, and this allows the visualization of soft tissue as well as bone. There are many different diagnostic X-ray techniques; only the more common ones are discussed below.

Bone X-rays
After an injury, X-rays of the bone are usually taken to determine whether there has been a fracture. Fractures appear on X-ray as lines across the bone, and in cases of severe injury, as fragmented bone.

Bone X-rays can evaluate bone infections and tumors, though they are not accurate for early signs of infection or tumors of the bone. X-rays can also check on the healing of fractures and re-establishment of normal bone.

Chest X-ray

A chest X-ray is a screening tool—that is, one that is used to detect disease for which no symptoms have yet appeared. Chest X-rays can detect lung or heart problems, and high-risk individuals may be asked to have them annually. (Smokers are in this category because of the danger of lung cancer.) However, the American College of Radiology (ACR) has recommended that chest X-rays be eliminated as a routine procedure for hospital admissions, tuberculosis screening, or as part of pre-employment physicals. The ACR has found that these X-rays rarely show problems, and are not worth the cost and risk. Only if a patient's health, medical history, or work exposures warrant it should chest X-rays be part of a routine examination.

A chest X-ray will give an image of the lungs, the air spaces, the blood vessels, the large bronchial tubes, and the spaces and tissues around the lungs. The heart and major blood vessels, the lymph nodes from the center of the chest, the rib cage, and the diaphragm can also be imaged. However, chest X-rays are not sufficiently accurate to diagnose lymph diseases. Because early changes cannot be detected, other tests are more accurate.

GI Series

The upper gastrointestinal tract (the esophagus, stomach, and the duodenum of the small intestine) is examined in a GI series. A contrast medium is necessary for this X-ray. The patient is asked to drink a barium sulfate solution, which allows a greater contrast between the filled organ and surrounding tissues.

Any abnormal shapes or contours of the gastrointestinal tract are visible on the X-ray, and problems and diseases can be identified. An ulcer can be seen in profile as a pit or depression in the normal contours of the esophagus, stomach, or duodenum, while a cancer is usually seen as a mass that protrudes into the affected structure.

Inflammation causes abnormal motion of the organs. Such abnormal motion can also be visualized, using fluoroscopy (a form of "real-time" X-ray; see pp. 49–50 for more information).

A GI series is considered an accurate diagnostic tool for ulcers and cancers. However, endoscopy (a procedure in which a flexible tubing is used to allow direct visualization of the stomach and duodenum) allows a more accurate diagnosis. Biopsies can be performed through an endoscope, and these permit direct diagnosis of disease.

Small Bowel Series

The small bowel series may be performed alone, or in conjunction with the GI series. It is commonly used to detect inflammatory diseases and cancer. Ileitis (an inflammatory disease of the small intestine) can be detected with this series, as can some diseases that cause impaired absorption of nutrients. Rare small intestine tumors and rare conditions caused by parasites can also be detected.

The small bowel series uses barium sulfate as a contrast medium, and is a lengthy procedure. It takes time for the entire small bowel to fill, so films taken at half hour intervals can show each section separately. An examination that takes longer than two to three hours indicates a disease process that is delaying the normal passage of the barium. Fluoroscopy may also be used in conjunction with this series.

Barium Enema

The large intestine is examined with a barium enema. Most patients are, understandably, quite reluctant to undergo this procedure. A barium sulfate solution is introduced into the large intestine through a tube inserted into the rectum. When the bowel is filled, its motion is monitored by fluoroscopy. Not only the large intestine, but also organs adjacent to the bowel (the kidneys, bladder, and reproductive organs) can be visualized using this technique. Diverticulitis (sac-like protrusions), colitis (an inflammatory disease), polyps (mushroom-like growths), and cancers can be diagnosed with a barium enema.

Colonoscopy is a technique that uses a flexible tube to permit direct visualization of the bowel. In some circumstances it is a substitute for the barium enema; in other cases, the two techniques are used in conjunction. A colonoscopy can be used to visualize the entire large intestine or only part of it, and tissue samples can be taken using this procedure. It is an accurate examination that involves no radiation, but it can miss some diseases. There is also potential for injury as the colon can be accidentally perforated during the procedure.

Intravenous Pyelogram

The intravenous pyelogram (IVP) tests kidney function and evaluates the size and shape of the urinary system. An organic iodine compound injected into a vein in the arm is used as the contrast medium. It travels through the bloodstream to the kidneys and then passes to the ureters and into the bladder.

The IVP is the best test available for detecting many kinds of obstructions. It is less accurate for imaging tumors of the kidneys and bladder, and additional techniques must be used if such tumors are suspected. The IVP is of only moderate value for showing sources of bleeding except where stones, tumors, or prostate gland enlargement are visible. The IVP can demonstrate small, poorly functioning kidneys or kidney stones, and films taken after voiding will evaluate bladder function, particularly in males who have enlarged prostates.

Mammogram

A mammogram (an X-ray examination of the breast) is used to screen for, detect, or exclude the presence of breast cancer. It may also be used to evaluate a lumpy or painful breast, and it can detect disease not revealed by manual examination. The newer mammogram equipment is more efficient and much safer than the older equipment, giving improved diagnostic accuracy and reduced radiation dosage. Mammograms can help distinguish between cancer and fibrocystic disease, because breast cancers have specific patterns (they are usually irregularly shaped masses). The tumors produce calcium deposits that are frequently too small to be felt, but modern mammograms can detect cancers the size of the head of a pin.

For a mammogram, the breasts are compressed to make the thickness of the breast tissue as uniform as possible. According to radiologists, the compression is "slight" and causes "moderate" discomfort. However, most women would probably dispute the word "slight" and rate the discomfort considerably higher!

Mammograms can detect breast cancer. However, some cancers do not appear on X-ray because the borders of the cancer blend with the surrounding normal tissue. In those cases, a biopsy may be necessary to rule out cancer. Cysts are usually benign, but can harbor a cancer. If cysts require periodic draining, they should be removed.

Radiologists consider that mammograms provide only a low dosage of radiation, and say that the risk of developing cancer from a mammogram is minimal. Women over 50, who are at the greatest risk for breast cancer, are the least likely to be adversely affected by repeated radiation exposure to the breast because they will not undergo as many radiation procedures as a younger woman might.

Fluoroscopy

Fluoroscopy is an X-ray technique in which the X-ray, instead of being used to make a film, is directed onto a type of fluorescent television screen. It allows real-time examination of internal body structures and their motion.

Fluoroscopy is frequently used in conjunction with other imaging techniques. The amount of radiation received during a fluoroscope procedure is higher than that received in still radiographs.

CT Scans

Computerized Axial Tomography Scanning (commonly called a CAT or CT Scan) is an X-ray procedure in which X-rays are perceived by detectors and analyzed by a computer, which creates a three-dimensional picture. To produce a CT scan, the patient is placed on a scan table that gradually moves through the scanner. The patient may hear the humming of the equipment and feel the slight movement of the table as it progresses though the scanner. The CT scan is painless, but for some scans a contrast agent must be used (see below).

CT scans may be used to visualize many parts of the body:

- Abdomen: Cancers of the liver, lymph nodes, kidneys, pancreas, and bile ducts can be clearly imaged on a CT scan, as can infections in the abdominal area. Frequently, no additional tests are needed in order to identify these conditions.
- Central nervous system: CT scans have replaced many older X-ray tests for neurologic abnormalities, which were dangerous and painful. However, an MRI scan, where available, is more effective in detecting central nervous system cancers, strokes, and herniated discs.
- Spine: CT scans have largely replaced the myelogram (a test in which the spinal column is injected with a contrast agent) although sometimes both a CT scan and a myelogram are employed for greater diagnostic precision. Herniated discs, and injuries to the brain and the spinal cord can be diagnosed with a CT scan.
- Chest: A CT scan of the chest can give more information than a chest X-ray. It can confirm a diagnosis, evaluate lymph nodes, monitor results of treatment for lung cancer, and evaluate trauma to the chest.
- Head and neck: A CT scan is the X-ray technique of choice for evaluating head and neck diseases, particularly those caused by injury or a tumor.

RISKS OF X-RAYS

X-rays do involve some risks to the patient. X-radiation can cause damage to the genetic structures that govern how cells duplicate. This damage can manifest as cancer in the person receiving the radiation, or as cancer and abnormalities in subsequent generations. There may also be hidden risks that are not as yet known. Small doses of radiation involve less risk, but there is no dose below which X-rays are harmless. Each exposure has an effect, and these effects accumulate. It is best not to be exposed to X-rays of any kind unless it is absolutely necessary.

Barium Sulfate Contrast Media

Contrast media can also cause problems for patients. Barium sulfate is commonly used for routine work because it gives good mucosal coating and is inexpensive. However, the National Academy of Sciences has calculated that one examination of the intestines in which barium sulfate is used results in as much cancer risk as would smoking 5 to 20 cigarettes daily for a year. (Even dental X-rays have an equivalent cancer risk to smoking half a cigarette every day for a year.)

Most patients experience bloating from barium sulfate during or after an examination, and though the barium will eventually pass through the intestines, it can solidify as it does so. If the patient has delayed intestinal transit time, the barium may solidify above a bowel obstruction. Patients must drink a large volume of fluids after the examination is completed, and some may need to take a laxative to prevent painful bowel movements.

In the lung and lining of the abdominal cavity, barium sulfate causes an inflammatory reaction that heals by fibrosis. There are water-soluble non-ionic contrast media that are effective and safer in GI diagnosis. If there is a possibility of aspiration, leakage into the abdominal cavity, or bowel obstruction, it is preferable to use these agents rather than barium.

Organic Iodine Compounds

The organic iodine compounds that are used for contrast can trigger moderate to severe allergic reactions within one to three minutes from the time the injection is begun. Although these reactions are supposed to be rare, they may be more common than is acknowledged. The first symptoms are usually mild flushing and the sensation of being hot. Hives, itching, nasal stuffiness, and tearing may also occur. Antihistamines can be used to treat less severe reactions, but if the reaction is severe, emergency procedures may be necessary.

The osmolality (concentration) of these substances, which may be five to eight times that of plasma, is responsible for some reactions. In addition to the symptoms listed above, a decrease in blood pressure and an increase in heart rate can occur. Decreased cardiac output may also occur, and an abnormal electrocardiogram may result from effects on the conductivity system of the heart. Kidney toxicity can occur, as well as bronchospasm, circulatory collapse, and facial and laryngeal edema. If these contrast agents escape into the tissues, irritation, local edema, and cutaneous ulceration with scarring can occur.

Asthmatic patients and patients with allergies are at increased risk of reactions to the contrast media. Those patients who have had previous reactions to contrast media may require pretreatment steroid therapy or treatment with his-

tamine antagonists before undergoing X-ray procedures requiring iodine contrast media.

Non-Ionic Contrast Media

The new non-ionic contrast media are organic, iodine-containing compounds that do not break down into ions (charged particles). They are water soluble. They have equal or better efficacy in imaging when compared to other contrast media, and the incidence of allergic reactions is very minimal. There is no sensation of heat on injection, and nausea and vomiting are extremely rare. Should these substances leak into the tissue, there is much less tissue damage.

The non-ionic agents have many advantages, both when used intravenously and in the GI tract. However, they are 15 to 20 times more expensive than the more common ionic agents. In the United States, complete conversion to these contrast agents would cost from $300 million to $1 billion per year. These increased costs are a result of an effort on the part of the manufacturers to recoup development costs, as well as import taxes on agents manufactured outside the United States.

Attempts have been made to identify high-risk patients who need to use the non-ionic agents. However, many physicians feel they should be used for *all* patients. An Australian study showed a higher rate of adverse reactions in low-risk patients given ionic contrast agents than in high-risk patients given non-ionic contrast agents.

OTHER IMAGING TECHNIQUES

There are other imaging techniques that do not involve the use of X-ray, and that are very accurate and valuable diagnostic tests.

Magnetic Resonance Imaging

Magnetic Resonance Imaging (MRI) is used to detect abnormalities in the bones, joints, or muscles; disorders of the cardiovascular system, brain or nervous system; possible tumors; and problems with major organs. The MRI uses a strong magnetic field in combination with radiofrequency waves. The patient lies on a table, and is carried into the MRI machine, a cave-like structure. Some people experience claustrophobia during MRI exams, and some are startled by the loud noises heard when the magnetic fields are activated. The patient must remain motionless during the scan, and is strapped to prevent movement.

The images from an MRI represent tissue "slices" similar to those of the CT scan, but they appear in more detail. They may also be obtained in many more geometric planes. Contrast dyes are necessary for some scans, to outline less dense, hollow organs and vessels. Patients should drink extra water after an MRI that uses a contrast medium, in order to flush the dye out of the system.

Paramagnetic substances (ions with unpaired outer-shell electrons) can enhance tissue contrast and lesion visibility by affecting the protons of the atoms. A gadolinium (a silvery, metallic element) compound is used in MRIs for this purpose. It does not cross the blood-brain barrier and does not accumulate in the normal brain. If there is a disruption of the blood-brain barrier, gadolinium accumulates and alters the signal intensity, improving the imaging of brain lesions. Gadolinium can cause lowered blood pressure, perspiration, nausea, and headache. Anaphylaxis has occurred, but is rare.

MRI scans and CT scans produce equally accurate images of the abdomen and pelvis, but the CT scan is more frequently used because it is cheaper. As well, MRI scans cannot detect gallstones, calcifications in kidney stones, or certain tumors. They are affected by motion (such as breathing, or the movements of the gastrointestinal tract). The MRI is superior to the CT scan for visualizing strokes, brain tumors, and diseases such as multiple sclerosis. It is also superior for diagnosis of spinal column problems,

and has largely replaced the myelogram for these purposes. (In a myelogram, dye is injected into the spinal canal in order to study the spinal cord and nervous system.) The MRI can visualize small differences in soft tissues, and is ideal for evaluating cancers of the head and neck; it is also the best imaging technique for the diagnosis of joint disease.

Newer MRI systems are built to accommodate very large patients, who did not fit through the older MRI machines. The oversized opening also allows parents to support and comfort children from within the machine, eliminating the need for sedation. The magnets of some MRI systems are designed to allow the patient's head to remain free of the magnet bore.

Some patients are unable to undergo an MRI scan, including patients with pacemakers that could be shut down by the procedure, those who have surgical clips in the head or eyes that could dislodge, or who have metal implants, metal joint replacements, and life-support systems containing metal. Pregnant patients should not undergo an MRI, and patients with claustrophobia may be unable to do so. Because metallics may interfere with the accuracy of the test, patients should not wear jewelry or eye makeup. They may also need to remove their glasses. Metallic objects in the scanning room can become projectiles in the influence of a strong magnetic field. A few patients report side effects (such as nausea) after having an MRI.

Nuclear Scanning

In nuclear scanning, radioactive materials, or isotopes, are given to a patient (by injection or orally). These isotopes cause specific organs to temporarily emit gamma rays, and a pattern of rays is detected by a special camera connected to a computer. A characteristic image representing the organ's shape, size, and function is displayed on a video monitor; the image is transferred to X-ray film.

A few isotopes cause side effects, including

cardiac arrhythmias, dizziness, nausea, pain, and shortness of breath. The scans that use these isotopes include:

- Bone scans, which use technetium labeled phosphorus (injected into an arm vein). Bone scans are nonspecific: that is, they will show an existing problem, but arthritis, fracture, infection, and cancer may all look the same. Other tests must then be used to differentiate among these conditions.
- Whole body scans use gallium isotopes injected intravenously; images are obtained daily for three days. Whole body scans can be used to search for hidden infection, to evaluate suspected bone infection when a routine bone scan is negative, and to evaluate lymph nodes for the presence of cancer. This type of scan is used when CT scans are equivocal, or where they are negative but a tumor or an infection is considered likely.
- Liver scans use technetium-99 labeled sulfur colloid, primarily to detect metastatic cancer and to evaluate for cirrhosis. The isotope also travels to the spleen.
- Lung scans use technetium-99 labeled particles (introduced intravenously) in perfusion scans primarily to evaluate blood flow through the lungs and identify blood clots. Ventilation scans, which use inhaled xenon-133 isotopes, can also be used to evaluate lung function in lung cancer, emphysema, and other chronic pulmonary diseases. The two types of lung scans can be performed one after the other.

Ultrasound

Ultrasound involves no radiation; it uses sound waves to obtain an image of various organs and tissues. A transducer produces inaudible, high-frequency sound waves that are beamed through solid and fluid-filled structures of the body. The echoes bounce off these structures and an anatomical sound image is displayed on a screen. These images can be transferred to X-ray film to create a permanent record.

Ultrasound produces very precise images of soft tissue and reveals internal motion such as blood flow and heartbeat. Normal organs and tissues have specific ultrasound patterns, as do diseased organs. Color imaging is now possible with some ultrasound equipment. Color adds new and independent diagnostic information, and improves imaging of many parts of the body. It can be used for the imaging of deep veins as well as abdominal vessels, and is of value in evaluating the liver. Color ultrasound images are also helpful in vascular surgery, cardiology, urology, obstetrics, and gynecology.

The only sensation patients feel while undergoing ultrasound is the pressure of the transducer. Fasting is necessary for some ultrasounds, and a full bladder for others. Patients having an ultrasound should wear comfortable clothing and avoid wearing jewelry. They should also avoid drinking soft drinks, as the carbonation develops bubbles that may interfere with the image.

Ultrasound can be used to scan many different areas of the body. Ovarian and uterine masses (both cancerous and non-cancerous) and their size, location, and appearance can be accurately detected. The size, shape, and structure of the kidneys can be visualized well, and obstructions, cysts, and cancers can be detected with sufficient accuracy that further testing is usually not necessary. Ultrasound visualization of the pancreas can detect infections of the pancreas as well as blockage of the bile ducts. If used in conjunction with a liver ultrasound, a pancreas ultrasound can evaluate the entire bile duct system. Stones in the gallbladder can be identified. Ultrasound can also be helpful in diagnosing appendicitis.

Ultrasound is frequently used during pregnancy to check fetal growth rate, due date, structure, and heartbeat. However, there are doubts about its safety when used in this way.

Laboratory studies have shown that this test can cause slowed nerve development, low birth weight, and altered emotional behavior in animals. This is difficult to test in humans, but dyslexia is higher in children who have been scanned in the womb. Babies who had multiple exposure to ultrasound in utero have a significantly lowered birth weight, but catch up with their peers by the end of their first year (W. MacDonald et al., August 17, 1996 *Lancet*).

The International Childbirth Education Association believes that a child's immune status and behavioral and neurological development are affected by ultrasound. The American College of Obstetrics and Gynecology and the National Institute of Child Health and Human Development, after summarizing clinical research on ultrasound, have concluded that ultrasound is generally of little benefit. An ultrasound should not be done on pregnant women unless there are clear medical reasons for doing so.

RADIOLOGY TREATMENT

Radiation as therapy is used predominantly for the treatment of cancer. Up to 50 percent of cancer patients are treated with radiotherapy. For some cancers it is the predominant form of therapy, while for other types of cancer it is used in conjunction with surgery or chemotherapy (see Cancer, p. 216). Advances in radiation and computer technology have allowed earlier detection of cancer, and have also resulted in improvements in treatment accuracy and outcomes. Side effects still occur, but they are less frequent and less severe. Radiation treatment does not involve pain or any other sensation. For suggestions to minimize the effects of radiation see chapter 17, Cancer.

Radiation therapy is used for cancers in which there is a selective ability for the radiation to destroy cancer cells while allowing normal cells to survive. Small daily doses given over a long period of time can destroy the cancer cells while largely sparing normal cells, and giving them time to recover. This balancing act is more difficult to achieve when radiation is used in conjunction with chemotherapy, which also harms normal tissue. The sensitivity of cancer cells to radiation is determined by their origin, and sensitivity can also vary within a cancer site, with some cells more sensitive to radiation than others.

Radiotherapy can be effective for cancers in the oral cavity, lip, cheek, or tongue; the larynx and nasal cavity; the skin; the cervix or testicle; for small-cell cancers of the lung; and in early lymphomas and Hodgkin's disease.

Clinical trials have established the optimal values for radiation doses and the length of treatment courses. More rapid treatment can lead to more severe side effects, but lower doses used over a longer course may reduce the effectiveness of radiation therapy. There is no relationship between the severity of side effects and the effectiveness of the treatment. Some people simply are better able to tolerate radiation treatment than are others, and therefore experience fewer side effects.

TREATMENT EQUIPMENT

Radiation treatments are administered with X-ray energies of over one million electron volts, whereas common X-ray tests use energies in the range of thousands of volts. Modern super-voltage treatment units are "skin sparing" and very little radiation affects the skin surface. (Treatments with older machines involved skin damage as a side effect.) Modern equipment also has a minimal scatter of X-rays, which means that most of the energy is focused on the tumor.

There are two main types of supervoltage therapy units, the Cobalt 60 and the Linear Accelerator units. While their construction is different, they both are supervoltage machines and their therapeutic properties are similar. The Cobalt 60 uses an isotope that emits approximately one million electron volts in the form of gamma rays. The Linear Accelerator delivers 6 million to 18 million volts of X-rays, and gives very precise treatment with a sharp beam edge. The Linear Accelerator can also be programmed to treat with electrons, rather than X-rays.

TREATMENTS AND SIDE EFFECTS

Different parts of the body can be treated with radiation therapy, and side effects differ, depending upon the organs being treated. For example, radiation administered to the brain causes temporary swelling of the brain. Cortisone can help relieve the swelling, but some patients report side effects of severe headaches, projectile vomiting, and visual changes. Confusion, disorientation, and sleepiness may persist for a few hours after treatment. Hair loss occurs if treatment lasts longer than three or four weeks.

Radiation to the face and neck area results in a gradual reduction and thickening of saliva, and the sense of taste may be diminished. Radiation to the chest causes swelling of the esophagus, which is experienced as heartburn or a "lump" in the throat or chest. Irritation to the trachea and bronchi causes increased coughing and mucus production.

Radiation to the upper abdomen (above the navel) causes nausea and indigestion. These symptoms result in loss of appetite, and must be treated so the patient's nutrition does not suffer. Radiation to the lower abdomen (below the navel) puts both the large and small intestines in the path of the targeted organ, and causes diarrhea by the second or third week of treatment. Again, this symptom must be treated. Radiation to the rectal area commonly causes irritation to the anal opening, and rectal spasm is also possible. These conditions are treated with cortisone ointment and suppositories. When the bladder undergoes radiation, spasm often occurs, so that even a small amount of urine in the bladder creates an urgent need to urinate.

Other side effects of radiation can include skin inflammation, fatigue, changes in bone marrow cells, sexual dysfunction, reduction in fertility, injuries to the small intestine, bladder damage, scarring of the lung, respiratory symptoms, and immunosuppression. Nutrition is very important in combating this damage and in helping the body to repair itself.

Radiation therapy can also be administered via an implant placed directly into malignant tissue. For example, radium can be implanted into a malignant tumor in the mouth or in the uterine cavity. In cases of cervical cancer, radiation "bullets" are sometimes inserted into the vagina. Liquid radioisotopes are also used to treat cancers; colloidal suspensions of gold or phosphorous can be instilled into the pleural or peritoneal cavity to deliver local irradiation. Other liquid radioactive substances may be used for treatment, on the basis of their affinity for a given organ or location.

Side effects do result from implant radiotherapy. Normal cells close to the cancerous cells may be damaged, and the effects of such damage may show up many years after exposure. Implants can be a hazard to those involved in the care of patients, because the patient with an implant becomes a "radiation hazard" when the gamma rays penetrate beyond the body. Liquid radioactive substances can cause additional biohazards. For example, radioactive iodine is excreted in the patient's sweat, tears, and saliva, and all articles used by the patient must be considered possible radiation hazards.

INTERVENTIONAL RADIOLOGY

Interventional radiology procedures can be used to allow minimally invasive procedures to be substituted for those that formerly required major surgery. Often these radiological procedures can be performed without general anesthesia, have reduced mortality and morbidity, and are lower in cost than more invasive alternatives.

For example, image guidance using ultrasound or contrast-enhanced fluoroscopy is used to locate veins and permits accurate placing of central venous catheters and peripherally inserted central lines. Swallowed objects in the esophagus can be removed using balloon catheterization under fluoroscopic guidance (the balloon is inflated below the object and slowly withdrawn until the foreign body is in the mouth). Tracheobronchial stricture (narrowing) can be treated by placing a balloon catheter at the stricture and inflating it three times, at 60 seconds per inflation. The image on the monitor will actually show the stricture enlarging.

AVOIDING UNNECESSARY RADIATION

While diagnostic or therapeutic radiation can certainly be life-saving, the FDA has calculated that at least one-third of all medical radiation performed in the United States is unnecessary. Whether you are receiving diagnostic radiation or radiation therapy, you must weigh the health cost of the radiation exposure against the seriousness of the problem and the benefits that the radiation could confer. If the X-ray is being used to look for internal injuries or broken bones, or to diagnose a suspected serious disease, then certainly it is necessary. However, some X-rays are of no benefit to you, and you should refuse them. These X-rays include:

- precautionary X-rays to protect the physician against malpractice actions
- routine dental X-rays in the absence of specific problems

- X-ray examinations for jobs, institutions, or the army
- just-in-case procedures to quieten anxiety of the patient or doctor (these may account for 30 percent of all X-rays ordered in the United States)
- routine chest X-rays for hospital admission

There are several things you can do to avoid unnecessary radiation. First, always find out what question the X-ray will answer, and what the consequences of not having the X-ray would likely be. If you have previous X-rays containing the necessary information, make sure to provide them.

If you do need to have an X-ray, ask that a newer, low-dose X-ray machine be used. These machines are easily recognized, because they have rectangular or adjustable apertures. When the X-ray is being taken, make sure you are given a lead apron that covers the thyroid, thymus, ovaries, and testes (the organs most sensitive to X-rays). Follow instructions to the last detail to avoid a retake.

Unless a serious disease is suspected, refuse X-rays if you are pregnant. Females of childbearing age should be X-rayed only during or just after their periods.

Be sure to protect children from unnecessary exposure to X-rays. Young children are more vulnerable to the cancer-causing effects of X-rays than are adults.

CHAPTER 7

Childhood Vaccinations

Most physicians, regardless of their specialty, are firm believers in vaccinations and the benefits they provide. Childhood vaccinations are therefore an established procedure in North American medicine. Their benefits and efficacy are fully presented by most pediatricians to the parents of their patients, while the negative side of vaccination is seldom, if ever, mentioned. As a result, the public has a skewed view of vaccinations. In the information that follows, a more balanced set of facts is presented, in hopes that readers will be better able to formulate an opinion regarding vaccination.

Vaccines are injections or oral solutions of specific weakened or attenuated viruses, dead bacteria, or altered bacterial toxins, which are given to prevent disease. They stimulate the body to produce antibodies against the organism that has been used in the vaccination.

The incidence of infectious disease began to decline in the last part of the 19th century and the early part of the 20th century, largely due to improved housing, better sanitation, and the provision of clean public water supplies. Consequently, many of the "killer diseases" had almost disappeared by the time immunization was introduced on a large scale. Proof that mass immunization programs work is largely based on a decrease in the diseases they target—but the two events may not be causally related.

Today there are numerous vaccines available, including those that protect against diphtheria, pertussis (whooping cough), tetanus, *Hemophilus influenzae,* polio, hepatitis B, chicken pox, measles, mumps, and rubella (German measles). Walene James (author of *Immunization: The Reality Behind the Myth*) notes that four main assumptions underlie the practice of vaccination:

1. Vaccinations are relatively harmless.
2. Vaccinations are effective.
3. Vaccinations are the main cause of the decline in infectious diseases.
4. Vaccinations are the only dependable way to prevent epidemics and the transmission of potentially dangerous diseases.

However, many studies demonstrate that these four assumptions are not valid.

Most viruses and bacteria normally enter our bodies through the respiratory system; the polio virus enters through the gastrointestinal system. Normally, when a protein (like those in bacteria or viruses) enters the body, it goes into the intestine and then passes through the liver. However, when vaccines are used, weakened organisms are injected into the skin or muscle and are absorbed directly into the bloodstream. They do not pass through the liver, and therefore may cause diseases at the cellular level, and in other organs. These diseases are more difficult to recognize and are less likely to resolve spontaneously.

Childhood diseases are experiences that help the immune system to mature. They prepare a child to respond appropriately and promptly to any subsequent infections he or she may develop. The immunity gained from infection with a disease is better than that gained through vaccination, as is evidenced by the epidemics that frequently break out among "immunized" individuals.

Viruses and live viruses used for vaccines contain pure genetic material (DNA and RNA). Live viruses attach their genetic material to the chromosomes of the host cell and replicate with it. They can survive and remain latent for years without causing acute disease. In the 1960s, Dr. Joshua Lederberg, a Nobel Prize winner from the Department of Genetics at Stanford University, stated that, "Live viruses are…genetic messages used for the purpose of programming human cells. We already practice biological engineering on a rather large scale by the use of live viruses in mass immunization campaigns."

According to Dr. Robert Simpson of Rutgers University and Dr. Wendell D. Winters of UCLA, the use of viral genetic material in vaccines could be a precursor to (or could easily provoke) autoimmune diseases such as systemic lupus erythmatosis, multiple sclerosis, rheumatoid arthritis, and Parkinson's disease.

VACCINE CARRIERS

When a person is vaccinated, not only is the virus introduced into the bloodstream, but so are the carriers for the viral material. These may be formaldehyde, thimerosal (a type of mercury), aluminum phosphate, monkey kidney cell culture, chick embryo, calf serum, and antibiotics (including neomycin, a very potent sensitizer).

For example, diphtheria and tetanus toxoids contain formaldehyde, aluminum salts, and thimerosal. The DTP vaccine (which is diphtheria, tetanus, and pertussis combined) contains aluminum salts, which act to promote antibody response. Aluminum-containing vaccines can cause local reactions such as redness, pain, swelling, and abscesses at the site of injection, as well as fever and irritability. Blennow and Granstrom reported in *Pediatrics* (1989) that infants given pertussis vaccine that contained aluminum had more reactions than those who received vaccine that did not contain aluminum.

DTP also contains thimerosal, as do the vaccines for hepatitis B and Hib *(Hemophilus influenzae B)*. Thimerosal (also found in some eyedrops and allergy shots) is a mercury sodium salt used to prevent bacterial overgrowth, and it is a common cause of allergy. Mercury is a strong poison and can also cause neurological and kidney damage. In 1989 Dr. A. Totsi reported in *Contact Dermatitis* that 37 percent of patients receiving allergy shots containing thimerosal developed hypersensitivity to it. Some patients receiving vaccinations containing thimerosal also develop such hypersensitivity.

Formaldehyde (formalin), a known carcinogen, is added to most vaccines to inactivate viruses and detoxify bacterial toxins. Formaldehyde inactivates the polio virus in killed polio vaccines, but it does not inactivate the SV40 virus, a polio vaccine contaminant.

VACCINE CONTAMINANTS

Between 1954 and 1963, millions of people were given polio vaccines that were contaminated with the SV40 virus, derived from monkey organs used to prepare the vaccines. Some of those people developed antibodies to SV40, and SV40 has been isolated from the stool of some persons who received oral polio vaccine. Recent studies have found DNA sequences of SV40 in human brain cancers, bone cancers, and mesothelioma cancers of the pleura (the membrane enveloping the lungs and chest cavity). According to the U.S. Bureau of Biologics, other monkey viruses also contaminated polio vaccines, including one that is closely related to HIV (Human Immunodeficiency Virus).

REACTIONS TO VACCINES

There are two types of adverse effects produced by vaccines: immediate or short-term reactions, and delayed or long-term reactions. Immediate reactions include fevers, allergic reactions, seizures, deafness, paralysis, central nervous system disease, and death. Delayed reactions are less immediately obvious, and may include epilepsy, mental retardation, learning disabilities, and behavior disorders.

In his book *A Shot in the Dark,* noted medical historian Dr. Harris Coulter presents evidence showing that the long-term side effects of vaccinations may be more common than is usually believed. He suspects that autism, dyslexia, learning disabilities, seizures, mental retardation, hyperactivity, and attention deficit disorder may in some cases be related to vaccinations. Autism, for example, was first diagnosed as a rare condition in Japan in 1945; after World War II a mandatory vaccination program was instituted in Japan, and now autism is very common there. Europe received the pertussis vaccine in the 1950s, and autism was first diagnosed there later in that decade.

Vaccine reactions are clearly underreported, for several reasons. Dr. Edward Brandt, former Assistant Secretary for Health in the Department of Health and Human Services, states that since few physicians recognize adverse vaccine reactions, it follows that such reactions will be underreported. If a reaction occurs more than 48 hours after a vaccination, most physicians do not believe that it is related to the vaccine. In fact, the vaccine injury table allows only a three-day window for development of impaired brain function or residual seizure disorders after the

DTP vaccine—but many of those reactions occur one to two weeks after the vaccination.

The seriousness of the problem of vaccine reactions can be gauged by the fact that in 1986, the U.S. Congress passed the National Childhood Vaccine Injury Act. That law requires physicians to provide parents with information about childhood diseases and vaccines prior to vaccination; it also requires physicians to report all vaccine reactions to federal health officials. As well, Congress established a tax on the sale of mandated vaccines, in order to pay compensation for vaccine injuries or deaths occurring after October 1, 1988. This was done largely because vaccine manufacturers threatened to discontinue the production of mandated vaccines in the face of multi-million-dollar damage lawsuits. By the end of October 1990, several thousand compensation claims for injuries or death caused by vaccines had been filed, and by January of 1991 more than $82 million in claims had been awarded.

The Vaccine Safety Committee, established after the enactment of the Vaccine Compensation Amendments of 1987, searched the literature for reports of adverse reactions to vaccines. The Committee established an arbitrary time period of two weeks following vaccination, within which adverse reactions must occur if they are to be considered a result of the vaccine. Guidelines for causation were developed that were so detailed and specific that a causal relationship would be difficult to find. Furthermore, because they compared vaccinated children against vaccinated children—with no true control group—they reported nearly all vaccine reactions as "spontaneous events." Despite these limitations, the Vaccine Safety Committee did find anaphylaxis caused by several vaccines; cases of polio and death caused by polio vaccine; Guillain-Barre syndrome caused by polio vaccine; thrombocytopenia (low blood platelet count) caused by the measles vaccine; death caused by the measles vaccine; and acute arthritis caused by rubella vaccine.

COMMON CHILDHOOD VACCINES

POLIO

Polio is caused by a virus that infects the gastrointestinal tract. It is shed in the oral secretions and stool of infected patients. Natural polio virus produces no symptoms in over 90 percent of the people who are exposed to it, even under epidemic conditions. In those who do become ill from the virus, however, polio can attack the brain and motor nerve cells of the spinal cord, producing permanent paralysis. Symptoms of polio include fever, headache with nausea, malaise, sore throat, diarrhea, abdominal pain, and vomiting. Most studies report that the ratio of asymptomatic infections of polio to symptomatic infections is between 100 to 1 and 1,000 to 1.

Several factors increase the chance of paralysis from a polio infection. These include stress, pregnancy, tonsillectomy, or immunization against whooping cough or diphtheria just prior to polio infection, exercise during the acute stage of infection, and age at onset of less than five years. If the patient develops neurological invasion, he may experience stiffness of the neck and back, weak muscles, pain in the joints, paralysis of an arm or leg, and paralysis of the breathing muscles. Only a small percentage of paralytic cases have residual paralysis. If breathing is affected, a respirator or iron lung is used. Five to ten percent of the cases of paralytic polio lead to death, usually from respiratory paralysis.

From 1923 to 1953, before polio vaccine was introduced, the death rate from polio in England, European countries, and the United States was already declining. In England, before polio vaccinations began in 1956, the incidence of death from polio had decreased by 82 percent.

In his book *How to Raise a Healthy Child in Spite of your Doctor,* Dr. Robert Mendelsohn (former Chairman of the Medical Licensing Committee of the State of Illinois and National Director of Project Head Start's Medical Consultation Service) points out that some European countries did not vaccinate against polio, and polio epidemics ended in those countries too.

The killed polio vaccine (injectable) was developed by Dr. Jonas Salk in 1955. The live-virus vaccine (oral) was developed by Dr. Albert Sabin in 1959. Many states reported more cases of polio in the year ending August 1955—after mass inoculation with the killed-virus vaccine was begun—than in the previous year, before polio vaccine was available.

In 1962, at the Intensive Immunization Hearings, Dr. Bernard Greenberg (head of the Department of Biostatistics at the University of North Carolina School of Public Health) noted that the number of cases of polio increased by 50 percent between 1957 and 1958, and by 80 percent between 1958 and 1959—*after* the introduction of mass immunization.

However, changes in the way statistics were gathered made it look as though the opposite were true. When the polio vaccine was introduced, the definitions for "polio epidemic" and "paralytic polio" were altered, and cases of polio appeared to decline *because* of the changes in definition. For example, illnesses previously classified as polio were now called by other names: what had been identified as "non-paralytic polio" before introduction of the polio vaccine was now classified as "aseptic meningitis."

Since 1961, most cases of polio in the United States have been caused by the Sabin vaccine. Since 1979 all cases of paralytic polio in the United States (except those contracted while traveling in a foreign country) have been caused by the oral vaccine. Dr. Samuel Katz, of Duke University in North Carolina, wrote an article in

Pediatrics in 1996, suggesting that in the United States, use of the polio vaccine should be stopped.

DIPHTHERIA (THE "D" IN DTP)

Diphtheria is caused by a bacterium that infects the throat. The disease is spread through airborne droplets that pass from infected patients (or carriers) to others. Symptoms include a sore throat, difficulty swallowing, fever, and swollen lymph nodes in the neck. A thick membrane develops on the surface of the tonsils, the roof of the mouth, and the throat, and may extend into the windpipe and bronchial tubes. The membrane interferes with breathing and swallowing, and may block breathing altogether. The diphtheria bacterium produces a toxin that allows it to invade more deeply, causing inflammation of the heart muscle and nerves. The toxin also affects the nerves that control the muscles in the throat and eyes, as well as the muscles used for breathing, and can cause paralysis.

Diphtheria is rare in the United States, although there have been recent outbreaks in Russia. Diphtheria cases started to decline before the diphtheria vaccine was produced. However, Dr. Eleanor McBean reported in *Vaccinations Do Not Protect* and *The Poisoned Needle* that when Germany began a compulsory vaccination program in 1939, the number of cases of diphtheria increased from 40,000 in that year to 250,000 in 1945—and almost all cases were found in immunized children. France originally refused to use the vaccine, and when the vaccination program was forced upon it during the Occupation, the number of diphtheria cases in the country increased. In Sweden, which has no immunization program in place, diphtheria has almost disappeared. All in all, about 50 percent of all those who develop diphtheria have been fully vaccinated.

It seems that the vaccine does not protect well against diphtheria. In 1975 the Bureau of Bio-

logics and the FDA found that diphtheria toxoid "is not as effective an immunizing agent as might be anticipated." They noted that diphtheria may occur in vaccinated persons, and stated that "the permanence of immunity induced by the toxoid...is open to question." (Minutes of the 15th meeting of the Panel of Review of Bacterial Vaccine and Toxoids with Standards and Potency, presented by the Bureau of Biologics and the Food and Drug Administration, 1975)

A study carried out in England (1949–50) showed no correlation between the existence of antibodies against diphtheria and protection against the disease. People who had low antibody titers (levels) were often highly resistant to diphtheria, while people with a high antibody count often developed the disease.

TETANUS (THE "T" IN DTP)

Tetanus is caused by a bacteria found in soil and animal feces; any soil that contains manure may transmit the infection. Tetanus symptoms are caused by a toxin secreted by the bacteria. This toxin affects the nervous system, and patients develop tightening of the muscles, stiffness of the neck and jaw muscles (thus the common name for tetanus, "lockjaw"), a change of facial expression, and facial pain. These symptoms can progress to sudden contractions of muscle groups, causing an arching of the back. Spasms of the throat, chest, and diaphragm muscles can lead to breathing failure. The death rate in untreated cases is more than 50 percent; with proper treatment, however, 80 percent of those who contract tetanus will survive.

Tetanus bacteria grow in deep puncture wounds, because the bacteria are anaerobic organisms (organisms that grow in the absence of oxygen). Wounds containing foreign material or injured tissue, crushing injuries, deep second- and third-degree burns, and infected wounds are tetanus-prone. All wounds should be cleaned thoroughly, and kept open until they are healed. Foreign material, as well as dead tissue, should be removed carefully.

More than 90 percent of tetanus cases occur in people 20 years of age or older. Of those, two-thirds are seen in people 50 years of age or above. The mortality rate is higher in the elderly and in newborns (who may get the infection through the umbilical cord). By the age of two, more than 80 percent of all American children have received their primary series of tetanus immunizations—but more than half of all people over 60 years of age do not have protective levels of tetanus antitoxin antibody, even though they may have been vaccinated earlier in their lives. Booster shots are given at age 15 in the U.S. In Canada, 90 percent of school-aged children have been immunized against tetanus, and they receive a booster in the ninth grade.

Even before the vaccine was developed (in the 1930s), the incidence of tetanus had been decreasing. Many people believe this was due to improved wound cleaning and good hygiene. For people who have had at least two doses of tetanus toxoid at any time in their lives, there is a rapid response to a booster of tetanus toxoid, if it is given within 72 hours of the injury. Tetanus toxoid is very effective at preventing the development of tetanus—several large studies carried out during World War II documented its efficacy. For people who have had fewer than two previous injections of tetanus toxoid, human tetanus immune globulin (TIG) is given. It introduces antibodies directly into the bloodstream, and is protective if given within 72 hours of the injury.

Side effects after administration of the vaccine occur in 3 to 13 percent of recipients. They include high fever, pain, recurrent abscess formation, inner ear nerve damage, Guillain-Barre syndrome, nerve damage, arthritis, encephalitis, anaphylaxis, and loss of consciousness. Comparatively speaking, however, in spite of these side effects, tetanus vaccine is more effective and safer than other vaccines.

PERTUSSIS (THE "P" IN DTP)

Pertussis is caused by a bacterium that affects the respiratory system. It is also known as whooping cough, because patients make a high-pitched whooping noise after they cough, as they are trying to catch their breath. Symptoms occur in three stages.

The first stage (catarrhal), during which time patients have a shallow, irritating, non-productive cough and fever lasts one to two weeks.

In the second stage (paroxysmal), which lasts two to three weeks, severe coughing attacks occur. The coughing attacks are often preceded by a feeling of apprehension or anxiety, and tightness in the chest. The cough begins with short explosive expirations, followed immediately by a long crowing inspiration caused by breathing in through a partially constricted throat. During paroxysmal coughing, the child's face often becomes red or blue, the tongue sticks out, and the eyes bulge. The child usually is well and free from cough between paroxysms. Coughing may be brought on by crying, drinking, eating, or physical activity. The paroxysmal coughing is most severe for about one week, and then subsides.

During the third (convalescent) phase of the disease there is sporadic coughing. This phase can be complicated by secondary bacterial infections, such as pneumonia. The active disease lasts for about six weeks in all, and convalescence may take two to three months. Adults, partially immunized people, older children, and infants younger than six months do not have the typical paroxysms. Household contacts of a pertussis patient may have asymptomatic infections.

Pertussis is spread by respiratory droplets and is among the most contagious of diseases. There is no specific treatment for pertussis, though cough suppressants help a little. If a child becomes blue from lack of oxygen during a paroxysmal cough, oxygen is given. Immunity wanes 5 to 10 years after vaccination, and the vaccine is not given to children age seven or older because severe reactions are more common. Of adults who visit the emergency room for a cough that has lasted longer than two weeks, over half are diagnosed as having pertussis.

The major complications of whooping cough are pneumonia, bleeding in the brain, malnutrition, seizures, paralysis, low oxygen levels, and encephalopathy, all of which are most common in younger patients. Fifteen percent of pertussis patients younger than five years are hospitalized, while 60 percent of those younger than six months must be hospitalized. Death following pertussis infection (usually caused by pneumonia) occurs in 0.17 percent of all cases. Children over one year of age rarely die, but permanent lung damage and neurological deficits can occur.

In the United States and Canada, morbidity and mortality rates for pertussis were falling before the introduction of the vaccine in 1936. The vaccine seems to be 40 to 45 percent effective. In most pertussis epidemics, at least half the patients who develop whooping cough have been adequately immunized. The United States has never conducted clinical trials to demonstrate that the pertussis vaccine is safe for children less than one year of age. It relies on data collected in England in the 1950s, which was based on studies of children who were mostly older than 14 months.

In animal studies, pertussis vaccine has been shown to produce anaphylactic shock, and may cause an acute autoimmune encephalomyelitis (allergic encephalitis, an inflammation of the brain). Studies carried out in 1948 demonstrated that the pertussis vaccine sensitized mice to histamine (released in allergic reactions), lowered blood sugar, and increased the virulence of viral infections. Pertussis toxin is one of the most reactive substances in nature.

Many major studies have been carried out to investigate adverse reactions to pertussis vaccine. Unfortunately, a controlled study cannot be undertaken, since most North American children are vaccinated—which means there is no unvaccinated control group available. Fevers, seizures, and Sudden Infant Death Syndrome all occur during the first year of life among vaccinated as well as unvaccinated children, so only careful evaluation of the relative frequency of those events among the two populations can assess the effects of the vaccine.

The pertussis vaccine can cause fever up to 106°F, pain, swelling, diarrhea, projectile vomiting, excessive sleepiness, inconsolable crying, seizures, collapse and a shock-like state, brain damage, thrombocytopenic purpura (a severe bleeding disorder), breathing problems, and death. As well, three studies done in the United States during the 1980s have found a time-linked association between DTP vaccine and the deaths of infants from SIDS—though four other studies found no significant associations between SIDS and pertussis immunization. Encephalopathy can occur, which causes changes in levels of consciousness, confusion, irritability, changes in behavior, screaming attacks, neck stiffness, seizures, visual and auditory disturbances, and motor and sensory deficits. The risk of seizures after DTP vaccination is 5.3 times that following DT immunization alone. Dr Edward Brandt, Jr., Assistant Secretary of Health, reported in 1985 that every year 35,000 children in the United States suffer neurological reactions because of this vaccine.

Immunization with the pertussis vaccine was stopped in Sweden in 1970. Since then pertussis has become endemic in Sweden and has reached incidence rates close to those of the pre-vaccination era. Despite this, no child has died of pertussis since 1970, and the clinical course of pertussis in Sweden is milder than it is in the United States. Similar situations exist in other European countries that have ceased requiring pertussis immunization.

Babies who have eczema, asthma, hay fever, or allergic skin rashes are more likely to react adversely to the pertussis vaccine. In particular, milk allergy may be a warning sign for vaccine reaction. The tendency to react violently to the DTP shot seems to run in families.

In 1981, because of the public outcry about side effects of the whole-cell pertussis vaccine, the Japanese began to use a new pertussis vaccine called acellular pertussis. This vaccine is thought to be less likely to cause side effects than the standard pertussis vaccine.

However, there are conflicting reports on its use. In Japan, use of the acellular vaccine caused a 60 percent reduction in mild reactions (especially febrile seizure) but the rate of severe reactions was no different from that produced by the whole-cell vaccine. Sweden withdrew an application for licensing the acellular vaccine after it proved to cause a higher rate of reactions than the whole-cell vaccine, and after four children had died of bacterial infections shortly after vaccination. The acellular vaccine has been approved in the United States for all five pertussis doses since 1996, and in Canada since 1997.

MEASLES (RUBEOLA)

Measles is a highly contagious disease caused by a virus. It is popularly known as "hard measles" or "six-day measles." Measles is spread through respiratory droplets, in which the virus can survive for at least two hours. The disease is characterized by cough, coryza (inflammation of the upper respiratory system), and conjunctivitis. Patients develop a high fever (102° to 105°F); runny nose; sore, red, and sensitive eyes; and a skin rash. The skin rash begins on the face about two to four days after symptoms of illness appear, and spreads across the body over a period of six days. The fever usually peaks one to three days after the rash begins. Symptoms generally last about 10 to 14 days. Patients are contagious beginning four days before the rash appears, and continue to be contagious for four days after the rash appears.

Children with a mild vitamin A deficiency have an increased mortality rate from measles.

Vitamin A given to children with measles decreases their risk of complications and risk of death. In populations that have not been exposed to measles, adolescents and young adults may develop serious complications from the disease. However, most cases of measles are not serious, especially in areas where the virus is endemic.

Pneumonia following measles is the most common cause of measles-related death. Diarrhea and malnutrition can result from measles infection, especially in the developing world. Measles encephalitis occurs approximately once in every 1,000 cases of measles, although this number is thought to be only one in 10,000 (or even one in 100,000) for patients who are well nourished and not living in poverty. About 15 percent of measles encephalitis patients die; 25 to 35 percent have permanent neurological damage.

A live measles vaccine was introduced in 1967, and mass vaccinations began after 1973. As with other diseases, measles had begun to decline many years before the vaccine was introduced. The death rate from measles was the same in the early 1960s (before availability of the vaccine) as it was in the 1970s (after the vaccine was introduced).

We began to see outbreaks of measles on college campuses in the late 1970s and early 1980s, with people who had been vaccinated more at risk of developing the disease than those who had not been vaccinated. Although natural measles conveys lifelong immunity, it was found that the measles vaccine confers immunity for a maximum of 20 years; consequently, most cases of measles now no longer occur in children, but in adolescents—and the risk of pneumonia is much higher in this older group.

The measles vaccine can cause ataxia (loss of coordination), learning disabilities, aseptic meningitis, seizure disorders, encephalitis, paralysis of eye muscles, vision loss, Guillain-Barre syndrome, subacute sclerosing panencephalitis (a fatal brain disease), deafness, paralysis affecting one side of the body, and death. Other reactions include malaise, allergic reactions, sore throat, headache, fever, rash, tenderness and redness at the site, thrombocytopenia, and hives. Inflammatory bowel disease (including Crohn's disease) has been linked to the measles vaccine.

RUBELLA

Rubella is also known as "German measles" or "three-day measles." It is a mild viral disease, with rash, slight fever (usually not above 100°F), runny nose, malaise, poor appetite, sore throat, nosebleeds, and swollen lymph nodes on the back of the head, behind the ears, under the jaw, and along the neck. Joint pain and swelling may occur in adults. Symptoms usually last about three days.

Rubella is not a dangerous disease to children or adults. Nevertheless, rubella is considered a major health problem because it is the most powerful teratogen (cause of birth defects) known. Approximately 20 to 50 percent of babies born to women who contract rubella during pregnancy will have severe birth defects, including cataracts, hearing loss, limb defects, delayed development, and heart abnormalities. Rubella also causes miscarriages and stillbirths.

Rubella vaccination was begun in 1969 to provide "herd immunity" and thus lower the risk of a pregnant woman contracting the disease—especially since rubella is such a mild disease that it can go undetected in the mother, but can still harm a fetus. As a result of the rubella vaccination campaign, the incidence of rubella and congenital rubella has decreased in the United States—but the rate of rubella susceptibility in the post-pubertal population is now only slightly lower than it was in the pre-vaccination era. In 1989 Dr. James Cherry of UCLA noted in *Hospital Practice* that we have controlled the disease in people 14 years of age or younger, but have given it free rein in those 15 years or older. Pregnant women are now tested

for rubella immunity, and those who are susceptible are revaccinated after delivery.

Protection provided by the rubella vaccine lasts only a short time. About 25 percent of those vaccinated against rubella show no evidence of immunity against the disease five years later. Because the vaccine-induced immunity wears off so readily, recently inoculated children may be prevented from developing this mild disease and thereby acquiring natural, long-lasting immunity—and thus may be at *increased* risk of developing rubella during their childbearing years.

Rubella vaccine has been linked with Chronic Fatigue Syndrome by Dr. Allan Lieberman of the Center for Environmental Medicine in North Charleston, South Carolina. Arthritis is a well-known side effect of the rubella vaccine, and joint pain and arthritis occur in 10 to 40 percent of women after rubella vaccination. As many as 26 percent of children who receive the rubella vaccine develop joint pain or swelling following inoculation. The arthritis may last for weeks, months, or years, and has been diagnosed as rheumatoid arthritis in some patients. Women and adolescent females are most prone to side effects from the vaccine.

Other reactions to the rubella vaccine include malaise, encephalitis-type symptoms, meningitis, Guillain-Barre syndrome, sore throat, headache, fever, rash, tenderness and redness at the injection site, thrombocytopenia, inflammation of the peripheral nerves, and hives.

MUMPS

Mumps is caused by a virus that attacks the salivary glands. The patient develops swelling beneath the ear along the jaw line, fever, loss of appetite, headache, muscle aches, and vomiting. The testicles can also become inflamed (orchitis), as can the ovaries and pancreas. The symptoms last about 10 days, but about 30 percent of mumps cases are asymptomatic. Mumps can also cause aseptic meningitis (an infection of the lining of the brain and spinal cord), encephalitis, and nerve deafness. The encephalitis rate is estimated at five cases per 1,000 reported mumps cases. Deafness occurs in fewer than five of every 100,000 cases of mumps. Death caused by mumps infection is rare, but is more likely to occur in adults. In males above the age of puberty, orchitis occurs in 20 to 30 percent of clinical mumps cases. About 35 percent of those cases develop atrophy of the testicles, but sterility rarely occurs.

The live mumps vaccine was licensed in 1967, and was recommended for routine use in 1977. Mumps cases now appear more frequently in adults, who are more likely to develop complications of the disease. The mumps vaccine can cause parotitis (inflammation of the parotid gland), fever, seizures, unilateral nerve deafness, meningitis, encephalitis, and orchitis. Meningitis has occurred as frequently as once in every 1,000 doses of vaccine delivered. (Encephalitis and meningitis occur in two to four of every 1,000 cases of natural mumps.) Other reactions include malaise, sore throat, headache, fever, rash, tenderness and redness at the site, thrombocytopenia, and hives. Mumps vaccination has been known to stimulate the onset of diabetes (as does natural mumps infection).

Measles, mumps, and rubella are usually given as a combined vaccine (MMR) at 12 to 18 months and a second dose is given at age 5 to 12 years. Thus, unless antibody studies confirm the specific cause of a reaction, it is difficult to separate the vaccine reactions. Symptoms noted for any one of the vaccines may occur with the combination vaccine. In 1993 the Ministry of Health and Welfare in Japan discontinued the use of MMR, based on the risk of encephalitis and the risk of vaccinated children and their unvaccinated contacts contracting mumps from the MMR vaccine.

HEMOPHILUS INFLUENZAE TYPE B (HIB)

Hemophilus influenzae is a bacteria that causes ear infections, deep infections of the skin, infections of the joints and bones, meningitis, pneumonia, and epiglottitis (swelling of the epiglottis—a structure in the back of the throat—which can block breathing). *Hemophilus* occurs more commonly in Inuit, Native American, and Afro-American children.

Meningitis in children often begins with cold-like symptoms: fever, headache, nausea, vomiting, tiredness, and irritability. The children then develop stiffness of the neck, seizures, and a change in alertness. Infants may develop a bulging fontanel (soft spot on the skull), and older children may develop arthritis and pneumonia. Mortality from Hib meningitis ranges from 3 to 8 percent. Hearing loss occurs in 10 percent of cases. Some studies have found learning disabilities, reading problems, and lower IQ scores to be more common in children who have had meningitis than in children who have not. However, recent studies have found no such differences among children with a history of meningitis compared with their sibling controls. The peak incidence of meningitis is found in children six to seven months of age, with half the cases occurring in infants less than one year of age. Only 25 to 30 percent of cases occur in children over 18 months of age, and in those children the mortality rate is about 5 percent. Children in daycare have a higher than average risk of infection.

Children with epiglottitis develop high fever and a sore throat. The throat becomes so sore that affected children refuse to swallow their saliva, and they have difficulty breathing. Children with epiglottitis usually have to have a tube placed in their airway to enable them to breathe. The peak incidence for epiglottitis occurs at two and a half years of age.

In 1988 a new Hib vaccine was approved for use in children at least 18 months of age, and by 1991 its use was extended to babies two months of age or older. Hib vaccination is now mandated in at least 44 states and in three provinces in Canada. A study reported in the *Journal of the American Medical Association* (Osterholm, et al, 1988) showed that 41 percent of Hib cases occurred in vaccinated children. In the beginning, children were more likely to get the disease if they had been vaccinated; the vaccine seemed to lower their resistance. Since then the rate of Hib disease has fallen dramatically.

The Hib vaccine has been found to cause seizures, anaphylactoid allergic reactions, serum sickness-like reactions (joint pain, rashes, and swelling), thrombocytopenia, crying, and high fevers. The most common reaction has been the increased incidence of Hib disease following vaccination. Guillain-Barre syndrome and transverse myelitis (a paralyzing disease of the spinal cord) have also been reported after administration of the Hib vaccine.

The Hib vaccine is usually given at the same time as the DTP vaccine and polio vaccine, so it is often difficult to sort out what has caused a given reaction. This will be all the more true in future, since Hib and DTP are now available in a combined vaccine, while Hib and hepatitis B are also marketed as a single vaccine.

HEPATITIS B

Hepatitis is an infection of the liver and is caused by many different viruses. Hepatitis B is a blood-borne or sexually transmitted disease. Occasionally, hepatitis B can be contracted by a household member with daily exposure to a person who is a hepatitis B carrier. About one-third of all hepatitis B cases have no known source of infection. For more information on all types of hepatitis, see Hepatitis in chapter 22, Socially Transmitted Diseases.

Most cases of hepatitis B recover completely. However, in about 10 percent of cases, patients will develop a chronic form of hepatitis, with liver damage, which can lead to liver cancer. In about 1 to 3 percent of all patients, a sudden and severe case of hepatitis B can occur, with liver failure followed by coma and death. Babies born to mothers who are hepatitis B carriers are at high risk (90 percent) of developing hepatitis

B and becoming carriers themselves. Younger children are at greater risk of becoming hepatitis B carriers than are adults. In the United States, fewer than 1 percent of the population have become carriers, but in Africa, Southeast Asia, the Amazon basin, and Alaska the carrier rate is greater than 8 percent. In areas where hepatitis B is highly endemic, beginning the vaccination series at birth and continuing it thereafter does prevent perinatal infection and the subsequent chronic carrier state. This approach has worked well in Taiwan, Indonesia, China, and Alaska.

In North America, the original use of the hepatitis B vaccine was to protect homosexual men (in whom hepatitis B was rampant) and medical and dental personnel (who have frequent inadvertent exposure to blood and blood products). But by 1991 only 40 percent of health care workers had been vaccinated. The strategy of immunizing high-risk groups failed to lower the incidence of hepatitis B, presumably because of the difficulty of achieving high levels of immunization among high-risk groups.

Although fewer than 1 percent of hepatitis B cases occur in children younger than 15 years of age, many states now mandate the use of hepatitis B vaccines in infants, and the Centers for Disease Control recommends universal vaccination of children beginning at birth. Such recommendations are based on the idea that immunized children will not get hepatitis when they are older. In many states, hepatitis B vaccinations are mandated in the seventh grade. In Canada, grade six children are encouraged to receive the vaccine, and in 1999 it will be given to newborns. However, the long-term effectiveness of hepatitis B vaccine appears to be quite variable. Hepatitis B vaccine is 80 to 95 percent effective, and immunity usually persists for five to nine years after three doses of vaccine. However, some people do not develop antibodies regardless of how many doses they have received. There have been several cases of babies who were born to hepatitis B carriers and who were immunized at birth, but developed hepatitis B by the time they were seven or eight years old.

Dr. George Peter, a former chairman of the American Academy of Pediatrics, gave the following rationale for providing hepatitis B vaccine to infants:

- Hepatitis B is a public health problem that sometimes occurs outside of high-risk groups.
- High-risk groups have not accepted vaccinations or are hard to reach.
- Children are accessible.
- It costs less to vaccinate a child, because a smaller dose is required.

A more logical strategy would be to immunize only high-risk infants and high-risk teenagers. This would provide more immediate protection for those most in need of it, and would be more cost-effective.

Some of the serious side effects of hepatitis B vaccination include Guillain-Barre syndrome, decreased platelet count, arthritis, nervous system diseases, anaphylaxis, neurological tremors, Bell's palsy, hives, and a chronic fatigue–like syndrome. Other side effects include rash, muscle pain, joint pain, hepatitis-like illness, influenza-like syndrome, diarrhea, headaches, fever, nausea, vomiting, fatigue, and dizziness.

CHICKEN POX (VARICELLA)

Chicken pox is caused by the varicella zoster virus, a member of the herpes virus family. It is generally regarded as a mild childhood illness, which has few complications. However, it may be a more serious disease in newborn infants, immuno-compromised children, and all adults (although more than 90 percent of adults have immunity to varicella). Complications include pneumonia and encephalitis, which together represent more than 80 percent of all reported complications of the disease.

The patient with chicken pox often has low-grade fever (usually from 100° to 102°F) and fatigue for one to two days, followed by the appearance of flat, red areas on the skin. These become bumps, which soon become blisters. The blisters become pus-filled, and then crust over. The rash appears in crops, and children have open lesions for about a week. The rash is very itchy and appears most commonly on the central part of the body. About 5 percent of children develop complications, most commonly secondary bacterial infections of the rash. About 16 to 33 percent of adults who contract chicken pox show evidence of pneumonia on X-rays. The incidence of encephalitis (and associated deaths) following chicken pox has been decreasing; the risk of death from chicken pox in healthy children is 0.0014 percent. Adults who develop chicken pox usually have a more prolonged and serious illness, and encephalitis occurs more commonly in adults. Acyclovir, an antiviral agent, is used to modify chicken pox and reduce its severity.

The vaccine seems to be effective 90 percent of the time in producing antibodies to the varicella zoster virus, and it has decreased the rate of varicella seen in vaccinated children. However, Dr. Philip Brunell, the Deputy Director of the Department of Pediatrics at Cedars-Sinai Medical Center in Los Angeles, notes the concern that use of the vaccine may simply postpone chicken pox—which in childhood is a mild disease—to adulthood, at which time side effects are likely to be more severe. Most adults are never revaccinated, and if the varicella vaccine is not protective for long periods of time, reimmunization is not a reliable solution.

Side effects of the varicella vaccine include a rash that resembles that of chicken pox. Shingles, which sometimes occurs after natural chicken pox, also can occur after administration of the vaccine. It is not yet known whether the incidence of shingles after vaccination is higher (or lower) than that of shingles after naturally acquired chicken pox. We do not know what long-term adverse reactions may occur from introducing this live virus vaccine into the body.

MAKING VACCINATION CHOICES

Pediatricians are convinced that vaccines save children's lives. They have been trained to believe that the diseases against which they inoculate their patients present much higher risks than do the vaccines themselves, so naturally they want to continue providing vaccinations. Physicians have a difficult time accepting the fact that a medical procedure designed to save lives can actually *take* lives. They therefore tend to believe that a child who has suffered a severe vaccine reaction must have had an underlying abnormality that was only "brought out" by the vaccine. They sometimes become upset and accusatory if parents do not want to have their children vaccinated.

Parents are generally convinced that vaccines are worthwhile, but they base that opinion on minimal information. If a child is vaccinated and has side effects as a result, parents do not feel guilty—because they did what they were told to do, and they feel any negative reaction was not their fault. However, if parents choose *not* to vaccinate, against a physician's advice, they have to overcome anxiety, and if the child develops a disease, they must deal with guilt. It is easy to understand why parents may be more anxious about a disease than about the vaccination to prevent that disease.

Legally, you have the freedom to choose not to have your child vaccinated. You can choose to accept some vaccines and refuse others, or you may want to have vaccines given later than is generally suggested. Although officials from the Centers for Disease Control have convinced state legislatures to pass mandatory vaccination laws, most states provide for waivers, which permit parents to refuse mandated vaccines on personal, religious, or philosophical grounds. As well, parents in 22 states can exercise a "philosophical objection" to vaccination. A child can also be exempted from vaccination if the parents obtain a written statement from a doctor stating that the vaccine would be harmful to the child's health. If you live in the United States you can request a copy of your state's immunization laws by contacting the State or County Health Department and your State Board of Education or local school district. For information on guidelines in Canada, contact the provincial Ministry of Health.

In order to make your own decisions about vaccinating your children, you need to get information and evaluate the pros and cons of vaccines for yourself. *The Vaccine Guide,* by Randall Neustaaedter; *A Shot in the Dark,* by Harris Coulter and Barbara Loe Fisher; and *Vaccines: Are They Really Safe and Effective?* by Neil Z. Miller are all excellent sources of information. Most parenting magazines present only the traditional view of immunizations. However, *Mothering* magazine also discusses the dangers of vaccinations.

Parents of unvaccinated children may feel some anxiety about exposing their children to playmates who have been vaccinated. While it is true that children who have been vaccinated with oral live polio may shed virus in their stools, it is unlikely that your child will get polio from exposure to a dirty diaper. In any case, it should be remembered that there have been no cases of paralytic polio in North America since 1979, other than those contracted by oral polio recipients or by people traveling abroad.

In the end, you need to make your own choice about vaccinating your child. Parents whose children are unvaccinated may be lectured by friends, grandparents, and physicians. Your physician should be a source of support and should respect your opinions and judgments. If he or she does not, you should find another physician.

If you decide not to have your child immunized, you need to strengthen your child's immune system. Breast-feeding for at least four months (and preferably for a year or longer) is the first step to take. Good nutrition is important, with a diet abundant in natural foods. Avoid excessive fats, refined flour, and sugary foods. Lowering stress helps the immune system. Regular rest and sleep, and schedules that are not too busy, are important for children.

Nutritional preparation for immunizations can help to counteract the side effects of vaccines. From the 1960s to the 1980s, Dr. Lendron Smith, a retired pediatrician from Portland, Oregon, gave 100 mg of vitamin C, 500 mg of calcium, and 50 mg of vitamin B$_6$ the day before, the day of, and the day after vaccinations. This regimen seems to have eliminated the problems that accompany vaccinations, even in the case of DTP immunizations.

Homeopathic Remedies
Homeopathy was useful in protecting children during epidemics in the 1800s and early 1900s, according to the American Institute of Homeopathy's *Special Report of the Homeopathic Yellow Fever Commission* and T. L. Bradford in *The Logic of Figures or Comparative Results of Homeopathic and Other Treatments*.

There are protocols for the administration of homeopathic nosodes (specific remedies) for the short-term prevention of whooping cough, meningitis, diphtheria, tetanus, polio, and other diseases, but there is no evidence to support the use of homeopathic remedies for long-term prevention. However, homeopathic remedies specific to the vaccination, if begun one week before vaccination and continued for two weeks after it, can help to prevent damage and complications from vaccination.

There are also homeopathic remedies that treat acute reactions to vaccinations and help heal the adverse effects of vaccinations. These remedies include:

- *Apis* – swelling at vaccination site or hot hives and welts on the body; symptoms better with cold compress.
- *Antimonium tartaricum* – asthma after vaccination.
- *Belladonna* – whole body reaction, hot, red, throbbing, swelling with high fever.
- *Calcarea carbonicum* – colds and flus following upon immunization.
- *Carcinosum* – worse since vaccination.
- *Diphtherinum* – worse since DTP.
- *Hepar sulph* – failure to heal at injection site; there may be pus, and hypersensitivity to touch.
- *Hypericum* – painful injection site (may be sharp, shooting pains); can be given before vaccination as a preventative for side effects and an acute reaction to vaccination.
- *Ledum* – preventative for side effects of vaccination and acute antidote for vaccination; bruising at injection site.
- *Malandrinum* – ill effects of vaccination.
- *Mezereum* – skin eruptions after vaccination.
- *Pulsatilla* – problems after MMR.
- *Sarsasparilla* – skin eruptions after vaccination.
- *Silicea terra* – backache, convulsions, and nausea since vaccination; worse, lowered resistance to infections since vaccination; children with very low energy and very sleepy.
- *Sulphur* – never well since vaccination.
- *Thuja occidentalis* – asthma and other problems after vaccination.
- *Vaccininum* – antidotes vaccination symptoms.
- *Variolinum* – problems after smallpox vaccination (smallpox vaccination is no longer given in the United States or Canada).

PART 2

Alternative Medicine

CHAPTER 8

Overview

Alternative medicine is usually defined as any medical theory or practice that does not belong to modern medicine. Several other terms are also used to refer to alternative medicine: complementary medicine—implying that alternative medicine complements modern medicine, and indeed it can and does; and integrative medicine, which implies the integration of alternative medicine therapy with modern medicine therapy. While all of these terms are accurate and meaningful, in writing this book we have elected to use the term alternative medicine to emphasize training and treatment approaches that are different from those of modern medicine.

Alternative medicine is not commonly a part of medical school curriculum; it is not generally used in hospitals; and its costs are usually not reimbursed by health insurance providers. However, conventional medicine is beginning to consider and study alternative therapies. Thirty-two medical schools in the United States have added some alternative therapies to their curriculum as elective courses, and there are alternative medicine research centers at Columbia, Harvard, and the University of Maryland, and at Vancouver General Hospital (University of British Columbia) in Canada.

Many enlightened modern medicine practitioners are using alternative therapies to augment their healing techniques. Until recently only individual seminars were available for training medical professionals in these techniques, but since 1997 The Capitol University of Integrated Medicine in Washington, D.C. has been offering a two-year postgraduate program for physicians and professionals with other medical degrees. The ultimate goal is to offer a full four-year medical education program in integrative medicine, and to establish integrated medicine state boards in each state for licensing of graduates.

In addition, insurance companies are beginning to change their attitudes toward alternative medicine, because of its cost-effectiveness. Eighty-five percent of insurance companies in the United States (as well as Medicare in Canada) now cover chiropractic treatment, and many carriers will cover acupuncture and massage therapy when prescribed by a physician.

Despite this progress, the modern medical establishment still presents many and varied claims against alternative medicine, most of which are without merit. These arguments include the following:

- "Alternative treatment delays people from receiving proven modern medical treatment." Many accepted modern medicine therapies have not been proven by double-blind studies (see p. 10 for a discussion of double-blind studies).
- "Alternative treatment takes too long." It is

true that some alternative treatments take longer than some modern medicine treatments. However, the alternative treatment may result in a higher level of "cure" and resulting health.

- "Alternative medicine is a fad that will pass." Chinese medicine and Ayurvedic medicine are both centuries old, and even homeopathy is 200 years old.
- "Alternative therapists do not monitor their patients closely enough." Alternative therapy usually requires more monitoring of the patient than does modern medicine.
- "There may be a perception of improvement early in the treatment that does not last." This view is somewhat of a paradox—alternative practitioners are also criticized because "too many" cures are attributed to them.
- "Non-standard therapy is often based on oversimplified, pseudoscientific theories that claim a single cause and hence a single intervention to cure the problem." In fact, most alternative practitioners utilize far more treatment modalities than do modern medicine practitioners.
- "There are too many theories, points of view, and different types of practice within a given alternative discipline." This is also true in every branch of modern medicine. Differing viewpoints result in different types of treatment for a given problem.
- "Alternative medicine does not do enough research nor does it communicate its studies and information in acceptable medical journals." Research grants to study alternative topics and methods are difficult to obtain. Furthermore, most modern medicine journals will not accept papers on alternative topics.

EVALUATION

In general, alternative medicine treats people—not disease. It works *with* rather than *against* nature, emphasizes the effect of lifestyle on health, and seeks to prevent common recurring health problems. Its focus is on the *causes* of disease and health problems rather than their *symptoms.*

The human body can heal and rejuvenate, given the opportunity and proper circumstances. Alternative medicine attempts to provide both the opportunity and the circumstances for health. It does not use pharmaceuticals, but rather utilizes many different nontoxic and noninvasive modalities to help the body heal. It treats the whole person, and looks at all aspects of a patient's life: physical, social, psychological, and spiritual. In alternative medicine, responsibility for health is shared by the patient and the practitioner.

The term "alternative medicine" refers collectively to a great many different theories and practices, some centuries old, and others which have been developed recently. Some of them are true alternatives to modern medicine, and in fact, may provide more effective treatment for some specific conditions than does modern medicine. Others are meant to be used as adjuncts to modern medicine.

Modern medicine is far better than alternative medicine in handling trauma, illnesses requiring surgery, and those problems requiring emergency treatment. Alternative medicine offers no quick fixes, and is not for the patient who wants to put very little thought or effort into health care. The patient whose attitude is, "Here is my body, fix me!" should stay with modern medicine.

Alternative medicine, on the other hand, is of great help in treating common ailments such as asthma, GI (gastrointestinal) disorders, headaches, or sinusitis. It is more effective than modern medicine in dealing with chronic degenerative diseases such as coronary artery disease, multiple sclerosis, and rheumatoid arthritis. Alternative medicine is better than modern medicine at helping patients learn to handle stress, which has been implicated in a wide range of health challenges (headaches, skin problems, allergy, heart disease, back pain, and gastrointestinal problems). Many health problems are a result of poor lifestyle, and alternative medicine helps people change their health behavior. Prevention and cure are often the same.

Neither modern medicine nor alternative medicine should be abandoned in favor of the other; the best of both disciplines should be utilized. To make this possible, there must be freedom to use whichever discipline is most effective for a particular health condition, as well as the opportunity to learn about what each discipline has to offer. Informed people can make informed choices, and being knowledgeable about health care choices is essential for your health.

ALTERNATIVE PRACTITIONERS

Alternative practitioners vary widely in their skills, training, and the techniques that they use. A practitioner who specializes in only one alternative therapy will have narrower training than a practitioner who practices within the structure of an alternative total health care system. Some alternative practitioners know very little basic science, and a college degree is not required for certification or licensing in many of the alternative disciplines. However, most practitioners who work within an alternative total health care system will have graduated from a professional school that offers comprehensive training in that system. They will certainly have a broader background and more training than a practitioner who offers only one technique—who will likely be quite skilled at that technique, but may not be able to evaluate the total health picture of the patient. (Of course, in some cases such evaluation may not be necessary.)

A practitioner trained in several modalities (many alternative medical disciplines, or a combination of alternative and modern medicine) can usually be most helpful to patients. For example, an allopath, Dr. Robert Atkins of New York, saw his patient success rate jump from 25

percent to 80 percent when he began to practice complementary medicine in the 1970s. His practice uses every valid healing art, including naturopathy, chiropractic, herbal medicine, and other techniques. Dr. Atkins practices these techniques without abandoning his modern medical training, using the best of both worlds.

CHOOSING AN ALTERNATIVE PRACTITIONER

Alternative practitioners and modern medicine practitioners are often reluctant to work together, and some alternative practitioners have been treated badly by modern medicine. You should be aware, however, that some alternative practitioners are just as biased in their ideas and views as are some modern medicine practitioners. Regardless of whether the practitioner you choose to see is trained in modern medicine or alternative medicine, make sure that the practitioner's approach allows the best possible treatment of your particular problem, and that the practitioner is someone with whom you can communicate easily and effectively.

A good alternative practitioner should have good skills and clinical judgment, as well as the intuition gained only through experience. Your examination should be carried out with care, and once all studies have been completed, you should be given a diagnosis and a complete picture of your physical, mental, and emotional state of health. The practitioner should know what treatment will help your health problem, and not simply try out treatments to see what will work. He or she should also have an understanding of modern medical diagnoses, drugs, and treatments for your condition. The practitioner should be able to give you advice on diet and lifestyle while being sensitive to your particular circumstances and needs, and should be ready to refer you to other alternative practitioners (or back to modern medicine) if your problem is beyond or outside the competence of the practitioner.

You should be wary of practitioners who claim to have a secret treatment; if a treatment is safe and reliable, it will not be a secret. Be aware that a lot of professional credentials after a practitioner's name is not a guarantee that the degrees they represent were earned in an accredited school. Find out what each abbreviation represents, and from what school that degree or certification was obtained. Also find out if the practitioner belongs to a professional organization and how many members are in the organization. Remember that the abilities of practitioners vary widely, whether they are alternative or modern medicine practitioners.

Be skeptical of a practitioner who claims to be all things to all people. While there are many practitioners who can help patients with many problems, no health care practitioner can take care of every medical problem. Ask how long a practitioner has been in practice, and if possible talk to other people who have been helped by the practitioner.

Many people apply a different standard of practice to alternative practitioners than they do to practitioners of modern medicine. It is important to allow as much time—or sometimes even more—for an alternative treatment to work as you would for modern medicine treatment. Many people also are reluctant to pay alternative practitioners a reasonable fee for their services, even though these practitioners have undergone extensive training and have office overheads similar to those of allopathic physicians. Some of this reluctance may be due to the fact that people have insurance covering most or all of their medical expenses, except for many alternative therapies.

USES OF ALTERNATIVE MEDICINE

Many seriously ill people are unable to find relief or cure for their medical problems through modern medical treatment. As a result, more and more people are turning to alternative med-icine for help. According to the *New England Journal of Medicine* (January 28, 1993) more than one-third of Americans used an unconventional or alternative therapy in 1990—and 70 percent of these people did not tell their conventional physicians that they had done so. Eighty percent of those interviewed used modern and alternative medical treatments concurrently. The number of people seeking alternative care in Canada has been rising rapidly over the past 10 years.

However, even when modern medicine does not provide the best solution to their health problem, some people are reluctant to see an alternative practitioner. Often, people who are used to giving the control of their health over to an authority figure (their physician) see consulting an alternative practitioner as taking a stance contrary to that authority. The attitude of modern medicine practitioners toward alternative medicine only adds to the difficulty of the decision.

Regardless of whether people seek modern or alternative medicine—they need to know the advantages and disadvantages of the therapy, its risks, side effects, costs, likely results, and how long treatment will take to show results. In general, alternative treatments involve less risk than allopathic treatments, surgery, and drugs. However, if they are not the best treatment for your particular problem, alternative treatments can be expensive and wasteful of money, time, and effort.

Some alternative medical disciplines are unproven and not governed by any state board or professional agency, but many are licensed (licensing laws vary from state to state and province to province) and their practitioners are trained at professional colleges. The real test of any treatment or therapy—alternative or modern medicine—is whether it helps people to heal and regain their health. If it does not, the treatment should not be used, regardless of the school of thought that proposes it.

It is up to each individual to make an informed choice about the treatment modality to use for a given health problem. The following guidelines can be used to help make a wise choice:

- Be wary of therapies that promise to cure a wide range of serious conditions. Unless the proposed therapy is a total health care system, it will not cure or help many different, complicated conditions.
- Be aware that the effectiveness or reliability of a particular therapy or an individual practitioner is by no means guaranteed just because they are advertised in reputable newspapers or magazines, or on TV or radio. Advertisements are granted to those who can pay for them. Beyond some "truth in advertising" regulations, ads are not subjected to tests of accuracy or reliability.
- Be informed. Read as much as possible of the information available regarding your health problem and all suggested treatment or therapy for it. Find access to a full range of current, valid health information, not all of it published by the modern medical world or the pharmaceutical companies. Most libraries contain volumes of information regarding medical problems and treatments. The Internet also contains a wealth of medical and health information, including research data, addresses of support groups, product information, books, and articles. However, you should examine information on the Internet with care; some of it (particularly from web

sites) is "docu-advertising" that may or may not be scientifically valid.
- Be willing to expand your range of choices and take charge of your health. Make a commitment to your recovery and continued good health.

Alternative treatment methods nearly always require more effort and participation on the part of the patient than do modern medicine treatments. In general, people want a "magic bullet" treatment—yesterday. They have become accustomed to the "take this pill for 10 days and all will be well" scenario that drugs foster—even though many drugs are palliative (they control symptoms) rather than curative. Alternative medicine offers many approaches that let the patient make great strides in improving and maintaining health. However, many people are resistant to the diet and lifestyle changes that alternative treatments may require, and they lack the strong commitment necessary to pursue the treatment.

The discussion that follows is intended to educate the reader about the alternative health care choices available. There are many alternative medical disciplines, and it is impossible to cover all of them. Consequently, we have selected those that are usually licensed or certified in North America. These disciplines are total health care systems, and many of them can be employed instead of modern medicine. Certainly all of them can be used together with modern medicine.

CHAPTER 9

Alternative Medical Disciplines

NATUROPATHY

While the use of the term naturopathy dates from late in the 19th century, many of its techniques are centuries old. Naturopathy is a complete health care system that focuses on the causes of disease rather than the disease itself, and treats by utilizing the natural capacity of the body to heal itself.

There are currently four naturopathic medical colleges in the United States, and one in Canada. Admission requirements are comparable to those of conventional medical schools, and a four-year study program is required for graduation with an N.D. degree. Naturopaths treat disease and restore health by using clinical nutrition, homeopathy, herbal medicine, exercise therapy, counseling, lifestyle modification, acupuncture, hydrotherapy, and physical medicine (manipulation therapy). Many naturopathic physicians are trained in minor surgery, and perform laceration repairs, abscess incising and draining, skin biopsies, sclerosing therapy for spider and varicose veins, non-invasive hemorrhoid surgery, and circumcision. They also set fractures.

Several schools in North America offer correspondence-only courses that lead to an N.D. degree. Some health care professionals (dentists, chiropractors, and nurses) use these courses to add to their basic medical knowledge. However, other individuals with no science or health care background can also take these courses and receive a degree. While the latter individuals learn the several health care therapies used in naturopathy, they have not studied basic sciences, nor have they had the clinical training and hands-on experience that those in full-time attendance at naturopathic medical colleges receive. If you seek the help of a naturopath, inquire about the source of the practitioner's training, and consider whether the expertise of the practitioner will be adequate to help you with your particular problem.

Currently, 11 states in the United States and five Canadian provinces license naturopaths, and efforts are being made to secure licensure in additional states. Other states and provinces either have no regulations, or regulate naturopathic practice but do not grant licenses to naturopathic practitioners. In some of these states, naturopathic physicians are able to practice without a license. In states where they are licensed, naturopaths function as primary care physicians and perform physical examinations, gynecological examinations, metabolic analysis, nutritional and dietary assessments, and allergy testing. They also order laboratory tests, X-ray examinations, and other diagnostic tests.

Naturopaths prefer non-invasive treatments that utilize the natural healing mechanisms of the body and minimize the risk of harmful side effects. A naturopathic physician looks for the causes of the presenting disease or health problem, and then treats the whole person—taking into consideration physical, emotional, genetic, environmental, and lifestyle factors.

Naturopaths endeavor to keep minor health problems from turning into serious diseases, and teach their patients the principles of living a healthy life. They also use natural healing methods to treat illnesses such as colds, flu, bronchitis, ear infections, illnesses with fever, digestive problems, childhood illnesses, sinusitis, urinary tract infections, gynecological problems, and many other problems. Naturopathy's greatest strength is in the treatment of chronic degenerative diseases such as arthritis, autoimmune disease, cancer, and all the illnesses for which modern medical physicians use suppressive therapy. Some naturopaths deliver babies, using natural childbirth techniques, and many assist in home deliveries.

Naturopathic physicians do *not* treat acute traumas (such as injuries resulting from a serious car accident), surgical emergencies, conditions requiring major surgery, emergencies of childbirth, or orthopedic conditions requiring surgery. Naturopathic practices can differ greatly; some naturopathic physicians use only a few kinds of therapies, but most utilize many therapies.

CHIROPRACTIC

Chiropractic is a drugless, non-surgical health care system. It is the largest alternative healing system in the United States, and the second largest health care system in North America (following allopathy). After years of controversy, chiropractic now has worldwide acceptance, and indeed there is now new controversy over whether it should continue to be classified as an alternative therapy.

Modern chiropractic was established by Daniel David Palmer of Iowa in 1895, but the origins of chiropractic date from ancient times—many years before the birth of Christ.

Types of spinal manipulation have been practiced through the centuries; at one point chiropractic was known as "bonesetting." Nearly all ancient cultures, including that of Native Americans, have used some form of spinal manipulation as part of their health care practice.

Chiropractic believes that for a person to experience good health, there must be an unobstructed flow of nerve impulses from the brain through the spinal nerves and out to every part of the body. If the vertebrae of the spine become misaligned—because of physical factors (poor muscle tone, poor posture, or injury), mental factors (stress), genetic factors (genetic predisposition), chemical factors (imbalance or toxicity), or thermal factors (extreme changes in temperature)—they block nerve impulses from the brain and can cause impaired bodily function, pain, and illness.

Vertebral misalignment (subluxation) can be corrected by chiropractic adjustment, allowing the body to heal and helping to maintain the overall health of the nervous system and organs. When properly administered, chiropractic adjustmen s are painless and safe, even for pregnant women. However, there have been instances of injuries to patients caused by improper adjustments. As with choosing any medical practitioner, you should carefully evaluate the qualifications of a chiropractor (see Choosing a Physician in chapter 1, Overview).

Chiropractic care can treat many musculoskeletal disorders including low back sprain and strain, neck problems, whiplash injuries, sciatica, arthritic conditions, peripheral joint injuries, sprains, and bursitis. It also treats organic conditions such as high blood pressure, neuritis, headache, migraine headaches, bronchial asthma, respiratory conditions, heart trouble, gastrointestinal disorders, menstrual problems, and nervous disorders of organic origin.

Chiropractors use X-rays to locate subluxations and areas of spinal stress. They also examine the X-rays for evidence of pathology, such as fractures or tumors, which would require referral to a modern medicine practitioner. Some modern medicine practitioners feel that chiropractors use X-rays excessively for diagnosis, and that their patients are therefore exposed to too much radiation. However, with the newer X-ray equipment, overexposure is less of a problem.

Some practitioners of modern medicine also feel that chiropractors miss serious diagnoses, and attempt to treat cases that should be referred to an orthodox physician for care. The reverse is also true. Practitioners of modern medicine often attempt to treat problems that could be treated better with chiropractic.

Most chiropractic colleges require that applicants have completed two years of college prior to admission (including course work in biology, chemistry, and physics). After completing a four-year chiropractic program, chiropractors are granted a D.C. degree by their medical college. To obtain a license to practice, chiropractors must pass written and oral examinations in the state or province in which they wish to work. The license permits them to use spinal manipulation as therapy; they cannot prescribe drugs or perform surgery. Chiropractors are licensed in all 50 states of the United States and throughout Canada, and most insurance companies in both countries allow reimbursement for chiropractic expenses.

Some chiropractors, known as "straight" chiropractors, use only manipulation therapy in their practices. Others, known as "mixers," include applied kinesiology, acupressure, ultrasound, physical therapy, application of heat and cold, electrical stimulation, massage, and nutritional therapy in their practices. Manipulation therapies may be vigorous or may use "nonforce" techniques.

Several hands-on techniques developed by chiropractors are useful for correcting physical problems, and also for dealing with the emotional aspects of illness. The following are two of the techniques being used successfully throughout the United States and Canada by chiropractors and other licensed health care professionals.

- Nambudripad's Allergy Elimination Technique (NAET). NAET treats and eliminates allergies to many substances, including foods, chemicals, pollens, molds, and danders. The originator of the technique, Dr. Devi Nambudripad of California, also treats emotional problems with this method.
- Neuro Emotional Technique (NET). This technique allows the release of "tissue memory" that is acting as an obstacle to healing. Although it is not a substitute for counseling, many emotional problems can be cleared with NET. According to its originator, Dr. Scott Walker of California, it restores the balance between the structural, emotional, and biochemical aspects of the body.

HOMEOPATHY

Homeopathy—developed over 200 years ago by the German physician Samuel Hahnemann—is a complete health care system that can be used to treat almost any health condition or disease except those requiring surgery. Patients needing surgery are referred to allopathic or osteopathic practitioners. Homeopathy cures illnesses by using very small doses of specially prepared minerals and plants to stimulate the defense mechanisms and healing processes of the body.

In homeopathy, symptoms of disease are treated with a remedy that *produces* those same symptoms in a healthy person; this is referred to as "treating like with like." Whereas in modern medicine the higher the potency the greater the effect, in homeopathy the more dilute the remedy, the higher its potency. Homeopathic remedies are prepared by diluting the remedy substance with water and alcohol and succussing it (hitting it against a hard object).

There are various potencies that are commonly used in treating, and these potencies are matched to the severity of the condition. Decimal or X potencies are diluted in a 1 to 9 ratio. When this 1 to 9 ratio is diluted 30 times, it is known as a 30X potency. Common potencies used are 6X, 12X, and 30X. Centesimal or C potencies are diluted 1 to 99. A common C potency is 6C, which has been diluted in a 1 to 99 ratio six times. The more dilute remedies have a higher potency, act deeper and longer, and require fewer doses for a cure. Because the remedies are so dilute, they are very safe to administer, and cause almost no side effects.

Classical homeopaths treat with one remedy only. Today many homeopaths also treat with combination or complex remedies that contain several remedies to cover a broad range of symptoms for a given acute problem. The appropriate remedies in the formula will have a therapeutic effect, and those not needed will be shed by the body, having no effect. This makes these remedies safe and nontoxic.

Homeopathy has been successfully used to treat diabetes, bronchial asthma, skin eruptions, allergic conditions, arthritis, mental or emotional disorders, acute cold and flu-like symptoms, headaches, female and male health problems, fatigue, neck stiffness, low back pain, headache, respiratory infections, diseases of the digestive system, post-operative infections and symptoms, migraines, bronchitis, sinusitis, motion sickness, bloating, dental problems, and many other conditions.

In 1900 there were more than 20 homeopathic medical colleges in the United States; by 1950 these colleges were either closed or no longer teaching homeopathy. In Mexico, India, Britain, Brazil, and Argentina, however, homeopathy is widely practiced, and there are homeopathic colleges in some of these countries. In North America there are now homeopathic academies that offer training, and the naturopathic medical colleges also teach homeopathy.

Homeopathy is used by many health care professionals, including naturopaths, chiropractors, acupuncturists, and some dentists. In addition, many allopaths and osteopaths have added homeopathy to their practices. There are also lay homeopaths who have not had professional health care training, but who have studied homeopathy and become knowledgeable in the field. Both the National Center for Homeopathy and the International Foundation for Homeopathy provide classes and information in this field (see Sources).

Homeopathy treats the whole person, and treats each person as an individual. Homeopathic treatment lasts for months and years rather than hours, but it is inexpensive and cost effective. Patients should avoid coffee, eucalyptus, camphor, menthol, recreational drugs, and electric blankets while taking a homeopathic remedy. Creams containing steroids, antibiotics, and antifungals should also be avoided, and acupuncture should not be used while receiving homeopathic treatment, as it can counteract the treatment.

Homeopathic remedies are available at many health food stores, as well as from homeopathic practitioners and homeopathic pharmacies. Many homeopathic remedies are considered over-the-counter drugs, while others are available by prescription only from licensed health care practitioners. For simple, acute problems people can self-treat with polycrest (most commonly used) homeopathic remedies. The 6X, 12X, or 6C potencies available at health food stores are commonly used for self-treatment. Higher potencies require more skill to administer.

There are many books that teach people how to use homeopathic remedies. However, the help of a trained homeopathic physician is invaluable for more complex, serious problems for which remedy selection is more difficult.

AYURVEDIC MEDICINE

Ayurvedic medicine is an ancient East Indian system of preventative medicine and health care. It is more than 5,000 years old, the oldest medical system known.

The Ayurvedic physician asks, "Who is my

patient?" (that is, what constitutional type is he?) rather than asking, "What disease is present?" In Ayurvedic medicine, treatment is based on the metabolic body types, or *doshas*. There are three basic types of dosha: Vata, Pitta, and Kapha. Though these types influence physique, they are considered to have a greater influence on a person's health and well-being. A dosha is like a blueprint; it maps the innate tendencies in a person's system, including both physical and mental attributes. Body type dictates diet, physical activity, and the correct choice of medical treatment as well as specific prevention techniques.

Ayurvedic medicine teaches that when the doshas are balanced, the person will have vibrant health and energy. When the balance is disturbed, the body will be susceptible to stressors such as bacteria and viruses, overwork, or poor nutrition. Balancing the body not only prevents disease, but can lift the person into a realm of new awareness.

Most people are two-dosha types, with one dosha being more prominent. However, all people need a balance among all three doshas. In everyone, Vata is the most active dosha and causes the majority of problems, especially those related to stress. The body can be balanced in four ways: through diet, exercise, daily routine, and seasonal routine.

Ayurvedic uses medicinal plants for healing, and holds that the taste or essence of an herb indicates its properties. For example, herbs which are pungent, sour, and salty cause heat and increase Pitta, while sweet, bitter, and astringent herbs cool the body and decrease Pitta. All plants are categorized by these properties, and the Ayurvedic herbalist prescribes accordingly.

Ayurvedic has two approaches to treatment, constitutional and clinical. The goal of both treatments is to balance the doshas. Constitutional treatment includes diet, mild herbs, specifically prepared mineral substances, and lifestyle adjustments to balance the body and re-turn it to a state of harmony. Clinical treatment uses strong herbs and medications; purification and cleansing methods (including medicated enemas); purgation; therapeutic vomiting; nasal medication; and therapeutic bloodletting.

Every aspect of life—physical, emotional, mental, and spiritual—is considered by the Ayurvedic physician. This system is successful in preventing and treating chronic illnesses that are connected to lifestyle, but it can also treat acute and traumatic conditions. If a disease is serious and advanced, the help of modern medicine may be needed to allow time to change lifestyle and increase healing ability.

Most Ayurvedic practitioners live in India, where there are 108 medical colleges that grant degrees in the discipline, upon completion of a five-year course and a hospital residency. Ayurvedic medicine is not licensed in the United States or Canada. However, Ayurvedic treatment is now available in North America from physicians who have come to this country from India. As well, some non-Indian practitioners (naturopaths, chiropractors, osteopaths, and allopaths) have added Ayurvedic medicine to their practices after receiving training through Ayurvedic institutes and seminars. There are also a few private Ayurvedic colleges in North America.

CHINESE MEDICINE

Chinese medicine is an ancient system of health maintenance and healing, having been practiced for over 3,000 years. In Chinese medicine, health is considered to result from a balance between *yin* and *yang*, the two complementary qualities that make up all of nature, including the body. Yang is positive, masculine, expansive, big, light, and is associated with wood and fire. Yin is negative, feminine, contractive, small, dark, and is associated with metal and water. All substances, places, and times are classified as yin, yang, or a mixture of the two. Organs of the body are classified as either yin or yang, with the hollow organs being yang and the solid organs yin. The organs work in pairs, yang organs being paired with yin organs.

Chinese medicine also classifies all substances and objects (including foods, drugs, and organs of the body) by five elements: fire, air, earth, water, and metal.

There are 12 organs *(tsang)* in Chinese medicine—although the term used to indicate an "organ" actually means a "sphere of function." When a Chinese physician speaks of the liver, he is considering not only the liver, but functions related to the liver. Two of the twelve Chinese organs have no exact anatomical equivalent. One of these is the "triple warmer," which assimilates and transports energy and maintains body temperature; some people feel it correlates with the endocrine system. The other is the "circulation-sex" or pericardium (the sac around the heart), which is known as the "gate of life."

In Chinese medicine, there is a basic, universal or vital energy called *chi* (spelled many different ways), that flows both into and throughout the human body. Some of our chi we receive from our parents at conception; the rest comes from our food and the air we breathe. Chi must be balanced: each organ must have the optimum amount of chi for the body to function properly. Disease is considered to result from either a deficiency or an excess of chi. Diagnosis involves locating the chi imbalance, and treatment consists of correcting the chi balance in the organs.

Chi flows throughout the body along invisible energy meridians. Each meridian is named for the organ through which it flows. These meridians have several functions: they transport the chi, they regulate the organ systems, they serve as the communications system for the body, and they connect the interior and exterior of the body. The deep, internal flows of energy in the body are mirrored in the surface, exterior flows. Since the deep flows are inaccessible to medical attention, all treatment must be done on the surface flows.

Chinese doctors utilize four techniques to make a diagnosis: looking, listening and smelling (these two words are identical to one another in Chinese), asking, and touching. "Looking" includes the general appearance of the patient, as well as his complexion, manner, "spirit," posture, and facial expression. It also includes an examination of the patient's tongue, since the tongue reflects the condition of the internal organs and gives clues to the nature of any imbalance.

"Listening" involves assessment of breathing and of the voice. "Smelling" can recognize two body odors (foul and pungent) that are indicators of illness. "Asking" encompasses the physician's queries regarding the patient's history, symptoms, and lifestyle. "Touching" means palpating parts of the body (including the acupuncture points) and taking the pulse. Chinese pulse-taking is complex, as the practitioner reads 28 different pulse qualities that are diagnostic of distinct imbalances.

After completing the examination of the patient, the practitioner correlates his information and identifies any existing imbalance, determining whether it represents an excess or a deficiency. A treatment plan is then implemented, which may include acupuncture, herbal remedies, massage, exercise, diet, or a combination of these and other treatments.

Chinese medicine is a total health care system, and treats any condition that does not require surgery. Chinese medicine is best known for treating chronic illnesses such as high blood pressure, allergy, headaches, gallbladder disease, lupus, diabetes, and gynecological disorders. It can also treat acute problems, such as infectious diseases. In North America, as in China, it is sometimes used together with modern medicine, achieving successes that modern medicine alone cannot achieve.

Chinese medicine is widely available in North America. There are over 30 schools of acupuncture in the United States alone. Programs vary in length from two to four years, depending on the school. Graduates of schools that teach only acupuncture techniques receive a degree as licensed acupuncturists (L.Ac.). However, actual licensing laws vary from state to state and from province to province. Some schools teach a curriculum that includes other Chinese medicine, in addition to acupuncture; these schools grant an O.M.D. degree (Oriental Medical Doctor) or a D.O.M. degree (Doctor of Oriental Medicine), depending on the school. The two degrees are equivalent.

ACUPUNCTURE

Acupuncture is one of the main healing techniques of Chinese medicine; its purpose is to restore the free flow of chi. Chi can be accessed at many superficial points located along the meridians. Each point represents a specific organ, and treatment results in specific responses. Classical Chinese medicine describes 365 acupuncture points, but modern-day practitioners claim there are actually some 2,000.

Acupuncture involves inserting a slender needle into the acupuncture points. The needles are left in place for 15 to 20 minutes, and may be twirled, heated, or connected to a weak electric current.

If the points are stimulated by deep finger pressure rather than by needles, the process is known as acupressure. (See p. 86 for more discussion about acupressure.)

Acupuncture is used to treat a variety of physical problems, including asthma, sinusitis, gynecological problems, urogenital problems, tendonitis, joint problems, and many others. It can also produce analgesia, and may be used both for control of chronic pain and for pain prevention during surgery. Some therapists have used acupuncture to treat drug addiction, smoking, and alcoholism.

HERBAL MEDICINE

Although acupuncture is an important part of Chinese medicine, herbal medicine is the major therapy used. Chinese practitioners use 6,000 medicinal substances, the majority of which are botanicals. Chinese herbal medicine is very exacting and complicated, and its practitioners must undertake six years of study in order to learn their profession.

Chinese herbal remedies focus on balancing the yin and yang. The five elements are important to the herbalist, as are the qualities of hot, cold, warm, cool, and neutral that Chinese medicine assigns to herbs.

Tastes are also assigned to the herbs: bitter herbs dry and drain, acrid herbs disperse, sweet herbs improve tone, salty herbs nourish the kidneys, sour herbs are astringent and prevent loss of body fluid. These tastes also indicate to which organ the herb has a natural and therapeutic affinity. Herbs not falling into any of these taste categories are considered bland, and believed to have a diuretic effect.

Chinese herbs are available at some health food stores. However, the safest and best results will likely be achieved if you seek the advice of a practitioner skilled in Chinese herbal medicine. Choose Chinese herbs with care as reports in recent years have questioned the purity of some imported Chinese herbs. Some have been adulterated with pharmaceuticals.

OTHER ASPECTS OF CHINESE MEDICINE

In addition to the treatment approaches outlined above, Chinese medicine also uses food, specific exercises, and breathing techniques to balance yin and yang. Chinese medicine emphasizes the importance of a well-balanced body in resisting disease; the importance attributed to lifestyle and self-care makes the individual a partner in health care.

CHAPTER 10

Alternative Therapies

Therapies are not total health care systems, but techniques that are useful adjuncts to other forms of treatment (including modern medicine treatments). For many individuals, these therapies open new doors to health.

It is impossible to mention all of the many kinds of alternative therapies within the scope of this book. Instead, we have selected some of the major therapies—those that are usually licensed or certified, and which are generally available in most towns and cities of North America.

BODYWORK

Bodywork refers to a group of therapies that are used to the correct the structure and improve the function of the human body. Basically, these therapies all involve the therapeutic use of touch. Touch is the first sense to develop in humans, and may be the last to fade. Touch is a primal need that is as necessary for growth as food, clothing, and shelter.

Bodywork techniques include soft tissue massage, deep tissue restructuring of the body, movement therapies, correction of postural imbalances, manipulative techniques, neuromuscular techniques, meridian bodywork, and energy balance. Many bodywork systems are a combination of these and other modalities, and are thus difficult to classify into any one category.

All forms of bodywork help to soothe sore and injured muscles and reduce pain. They stimulate blood and lymphatic circulation, increase oxygen supply to the cells, increase availability of nutrients, and help eliminate excess fluid from the tissues. They improve liver function, balance the nervous system, assist in elimination of toxic waste from the body, and promote deep relaxation.

SOFT TISSUE MASSAGE

Massage is usually the first technique that comes to mind when people think of bodywork. Massage involves stroking, kneading, vibration, compression, tapping, wringing, and squeezing the skin and soft tissues. Massage therapy can be carried out using only the hands, but it may also include the use of mechanical or electrical devices, oil, and hot and cold packs. People in every age group and every occupational field, active and sedentary, can benefit from massage therapy.

It can help in cases of muscle spasm and pain, headaches, whiplash, soreness related to injury and stress, spinal curvatures (scoliosis and lordosis), temporo-mandibular joint pain, asthma and emphysema, and in treating chronic inflammatory conditions. Massage is the most frequently used therapy for musculoskeletal problems, and can be used as an adjunct in the treatment of cardiovascular disorders and neurological and gynecological problems. It can help to reduce stress, reduce swelling, improve range of motion, correct posture, increase peristalsis, and speed up elimination of toxins from the body. Massage helps to break up scar tissue and adhesions, increase circulation, loosen mucus, and promote drainage. It is particularly useful in controlling pain, and sometimes can either substitute for pharmaceutical drugs, or reduce the amount needed.

DEEP TISSUE RESTRUCTURING

In deep tissue restructuring, balance and poise are re-established by manually manipulating and stretching the fascia—a thin, semi-solid, elastic membrane that covers every muscle, blood vessel, organ, nerve, and bone. It also plays a role in maintaining posture and ease of motion. Age, injury, chronic stress, misuse, and trauma can cause the fascia to become more rigid and adherent. It then restricts the movement of joints and muscles. Applying pressure to the fascia promotes changes in body structure, enhances neurological functioning, and reduces chronic stress.

People who have pain and stiffness related to mechanical and structural imbalances will be helped by these techniques. Conditions caused by injury, emotional trauma, and sustained stress also respond to deep tissue therapy.

Rolfing, Hellerwork, Looyenwork, myofascial release, and Aston-patterning are a few of the better known schools of deep tissue therapy.

MOVEMENT THERAPY

Movement therapies correct postural imbalances, thus promoting more efficient function of the nervous system. Poor or inhibited use of the body can date back to childhood, and becomes worse with time. This can contribute to the development of many diseases, including arthritis, curvatures of the spine, and several gastrointestinal and breathing disorders. People recovering from an accident or injury, those with limitations of movement, and people suffering from a degenerative neurological disorder or from chronic pain also find movement therapy helpful.

Postural imbalances also involve emotions, in that the image we have of ourselves affects the way we move. The therapist helps the person to recognize problem movements, and uses hands-on and verbal instructions to correct movement patterns and stress-related emotional conditions. The therapist may use physiological re-patterning, movement analysis and performance, and psychological/emotional expression to help the patient. Hypnosis and imagery, exercise, tissue manipulation, and techniques to mobilize body systems may also be used.

The Alexander Technique, Touch for Health, and the Feldenkrais Method are movement therapies. The Traeger Approach combines movement sequences with bodywork.

MERIDIAN BODYWORK

Life energy flows in energy pathways or channels called meridians, which travel on the surface of the skin and throughout the body. When these pathways become blocked, pain and disease can result, with physical, mental, and emotional symptoms all being displayed. In meridian bodywork, blockages are removed by placing the hands on particular points.

Acupressure works on the same points as does acupuncture, but utilizes the pressure of the hands and fingers rather than needles. Its focus is relief of pain and discomfort, and attempts to treat toxicity and tension before they cause illness.

Shiatsu is a form of acupressure in which the practitioner uses the balls of the fingers and thumbs, as well as the base of the thumb. Stimulating certain points on the meridians releases contracted tendons and muscle fibers. This technique is useful for migraine and tension headaches, vertigo, stiff neck, nausea, sciatica, and many other complaints.

Reflexology, originally called zone therapy, uses points on the feet that reflex or represent the entire body. The head, ears, eyes, and palms of the hands also have the same map. Treatment involves applying pressure with the thumbs after warming the feet with gentle squeezing. Tender areas indicate where work is needed. Working the reflexes can cleanse the body, relieve headaches, reduce menstrual cramps, clear congested sinuses, ease backaches, and reduce swelling.

ENERGY BALANCE

Several techniques can be classified as energy balance techniques, in which balancing body energy helps bring about healing and enhanced health and well-being. Disease is present when there is imbalance in body energy; the practitioner accelerates healing by giving the patient an energy boost that reinforces recuperative powers. The practitioner also relieves congestion, removes obstructions, and redirects and restores energy. The laying on of hands (or touching techniques) allows the practitioner to determine energy blocks, enhance the clearing of the blocks, and monitor the healing process.

Reiki is a system of healing that touches a person on all levels—body, mind, and spirit. The practitioner passes the hands above the body of the patient with the intent of transferring positive energy, releasing blockages, and bringing the person back into balance.

Therapeutic Touch and Polarity Therapy are other energy balancing techniques. All of these techniques provide relaxation, acceleration of healing, reduction of pain, reduction of anxiety, and easing of problems associated with autonomic nervous system dysfunction. Sports injuries, emotional disorders, burns, internal diseases, and stress-related illnesses can be helped by these techniques.

Tai Chi and Qigong (also called Chi Kung) are two energy balancing and exercise techniques that can be learned, then performed at home. Tai Chi, described as meditation in movement, emphasizes coordination of breath and the internal environment. A series of continuous, slow, fluid, graceful movements brings the body into a harmonious rhythm and increases vitality.

Qigong refers to various forms of energy work based on *chi* (breath, or vital life force). Qigong restores vitality and flexibility, stores physical energy, and massages the organs of the abdominal cavity.

HERBS

Three major medical systems utilize medicinal plants: Chinese medicine, Ayurvedic medicine, and Western medicine. Because Chinese medicine and Ayurvedic medicine have been discussed in the previous chapter, the focus of this section will be on the use of herbs in Western medicine, specifically those used in North America.

At one time, herbs were the major source of medications in North America. With the development of pharmaceuticals, herb use declined. The new drugs were considered to be more effective and faster-acting. Perhaps more importantly, natural substances cannot be patented. Because of this, there was no incentive for drug companies to investigate the benefits of an herb that people could grow for themselves. The use of herbs declined in North America, though they continued to be studied and used successfully in other countries.

Today there is renewed interest in herbs for several reasons. First, we now realize that pharmaceuticals, and even over-the-counter remedies, are not the "magic bullet" they were once thought to be. Sometimes they are not effective, and even when they are, they may have side effects, which can be quite serious. A renewed interest in preventative medicine is another reason for the return to herbs. Herbs promote wellness, and many of them (like vitamins) can be used to help maintain good health.

Herbs are beginning to appear in health food stores, herb shops, and some drug stores—but it can be difficult for the consumer to know their specific uses. It is important for anyone interested in achieving and maintaining good health to learn about the use of herbs. There are many good books about herbs available, and some herbalists teach courses for the layperson.

In this book, the term "herb" is used to mean any plant that is primarily used for medical purposes. Herbs are rich in compounds that are pharmacologically active and can be used to treat, cure, and prevent disease. Herbs can be used to relieve pain, stimulate the body, kill viruses and bacteria, relieve insomnia, activate the immune system, target specific organ systems, and promote general health. (For more information regarding specific uses for herbs, see the treatments listed in Part 3, Common Health Problems.)

FORMS OF HERBS

Herbs are available in many forms:

- as capsules and tablets (capsules probably contain less filler than tablets do);
- in creams and ointments (for external use);
- dried, for making teas (store in airtight glass containers);
- as prepared teas (in teabags);
- as essential oils (for baths, to be used in perfumes, and for aromatherapy);
- as extracts or tinctures (made by soaking the herb in an alcohol solution);
- as juices (strengths vary);
- in personal care products (shampoos, deodorants, mouthwash, toothpaste, facial cleansers, and moisturizers); and
- as combination products (two or more herbs that work well together are combined in a single capsule, tablet, tea, or tincture).

Be very careful in selecting herbs to purchase, as they are not standardized nor are the conditions of their sale governed by any agency. Purity and potency can vary widely. Look for organic or wildcrafted herbs, which are more likely to be quality herbs. Imported herbs may not be pure, and they are frequently fumigated or sprayed with pesticides when they arrive in this country. Whenever possible, obtain literature that describes how the herbs of a given company are procured and processed.

Fresh herbs are more potent than dried or processed herbs. Check the expiration date on any packaged herb you purchase. Unless the package is still sealed, throw out herbs after you have had them for one year.

Always follow the directions given on the packaging of the herb you purchase. The dosage for an herb or botanical supplement will vary, depending on the form in which it is taken. Teas are usually made from 1,000 to 2,000 mg of dried herb. For herbs purchased as a tincture, the dose is commonly 4 to 6 ml of a 1:5 solution. For a fluid extract (1:1), the usual dose is 0.5 to 2 ml. For a powdered solid extract (4:1), the dose is 500 to 750 mg.

The amount of herb needed and the results obtained will also vary from person to person. A heavy person will need a larger dose than a thin person, an older person will need a smaller dose than a young person, and people who are very responsive to drugs will need smaller amounts of herbs. Very sensitive people and people with allergies may develop reactions to herbs.

Even though they are natural substances, herbs should be used with discretion and appropriate caution. Never use an herb unless you know what it does, how to use it, and the recommended dosage; possible side effects or interactions with other substances you are using; and the length of time you should take it.

People taking herbs need to be aware that there can be interactions between herbs and prescription drugs. Some herbs can negate the action of prescription drugs, while others potentiate their action, causing too much of the desired effect. Seek the help of a trained herbalist if you take prescription drugs and wish to begin taking herbs.

DIET

Lifestyle and diet play a major role in the development of a great many diseases including cardiovascular disease, digestive disturbances, infections, skin disorders, diabetes, some cancers, birth defects, high blood pressure, obesity, decreased immune function, food allergies and sensitivities, urinary system diseases, and women's health problems. Some foods are a problem because of the way their natural chemical composition affects our metabolism. Others are a problem because they are high in fat, sugar, preservatives, chemical additives, antibiotics, hormones, dyes, or stabilizers. Still others cause damage because they have been refined or irradiated, are covered with waxes, or contain pesticide or fertilizer residues.

Food has a fundamental effect on our well-being. It supplies the nutrients that allow our bodies to function and repair, gives us energy, and permits us to be free from disease. All food contains macronutrients, which provide the energy for life (proteins, carbohydrates, and fat); micronutrients, which facilitate cellular metabolism (vitamins, minerals, trace elements, amino acids, and essential fatty acids); and water. Lack of macronutrients leads to malnutrition, starvation, and death. Lack of micronutrients leads to deficiency diseases, decline in health, and death. Lack of water leads to dehydration and death. It is obvious that all three components of food are necessary for life and health.

Just as diet plays a major role in the development of disease, it can also play a major role in the treatment and cure of disease. While there are hundreds of diets that may have therapeutic value, the discussion that follows covers several that we have found to be of value in restoring and maintaining health. (See Part 3, Common Health Problems for foods that will help specific health problems.)

(See Part 3, Common Health Problems for foods that will help specific health problems.)

STANDARD AMERICAN DIET

The Standard American Diet is frequently spoken of as being the "SAD" diet. North Americans are well fed, but they are not well nourished. Fast foods, prepared foods, excess sugar and salt, poor-quality food, artificial colors and flavors, and large amounts of additives and preservatives can harm health and lead to disease. However, if certain precautions are taken and a balanced diet of quality food is eaten, the "sadness" can be removed from the Standard American Diet.

It is important to know where the food you eat was raised, as well as how it was raised. For example, were pesticides and herbicides used for weed control? Was the crop fertilized with chemical fertilizer, or was human night soil (feces) used? What are the possibilities of bacterial or parasitic contamination? Many foods are harvested green and ripened artificially on the way to the market. Consequently, in many instances it is uncertain how long the food has been stored, how many nutrients it still contains, and to what chemicals it was exposed while in storage.

The Standard American Diet should provide good-quality fruits, vegetables, grains, and meats or meat substitutes each day. Most people need eight, 8-ounce glasses of pure water a day. Eliminating bad eating habits and replacing them with healthy habits can be healing in itself. Following these guidelines will lead to a healthier diet for most North Americans:

Avoid:

- all refined sugar and mixtures that contain refined sugar, as well as artificial sweeteners
- refined carbohydrates such as white flour and white rice

- foods high in fat, including fried food
- caffeine
- alcohol in all forms
- high salt intake
- chemical additives (including nitrates, nitrites, MSG, BHA, BHT) and artificial colors, flavors, and preservatives
- processed foods and mixes
- produce that has been waxed, sprayed, fumigated, or dyed
- irradiated or genetically altered foods (until more research has been done)
- too much repetition of the same food

Make sure to eat:

- whole grains
- fresh in preference to frozen foods; frozen in preference to canned foods
- whole vegetables and fruits instead of juices; fruit juices instead of soft drinks or fruit-flavored drinks
- foods high in fiber, such as oat bran and all beans
- low-fat meals
- complex carbohydrates
- unprocessed foods grown with a minimum of chemicals, that do not contain preservatives and have not been artificially ripened
- only foods that will spoil, and eat them BEFORE they do
- organically grown fruits and vegetables
- good-quality meat and poultry, organically raised if possible, free of antibiotics and growth hormones
- fresh fish from unpolluted waters
- a variety of foods

MACROBIOTIC DIET

The word macrobiotic comes from the Greek words *macro* (meaning "large" or "great") and *bio* (meaning "life"). The original macrobiotic diet was designed in the Orient, and is several thousand years old. The macrobiotic diet as we know it today, however, was developed in the early 1900s by a Japanese physician, Sagen Ishtzuka. One of his followers, George Ohsawa, who was cured of tuberculosis by using the diet, devoted his whole life to educating the world about macrobiotics.

Macrobiotics is not only a diet, but rather a way of living that considers the biological, physical, emotional, mental, ecological, and spiritual aspects of our daily lives. It has helped many people to recover from serious illnesses and to find peace of mind and better health.

Macrobiotics holds that each person has a unique yin or yang balance, and that this balance constantly changes. Foods help to restore and maintain a proper balance between yin and yang. Cooked grains and cooked or pickled vegetables (which are near the middle of the yin-yang spectrum) are the mainstay of a macrobiotic diet, because they make it easier to achieve a balance between yin and yang. The macrobiotic diet consists of grains (50 to 60 percent of food intake); vegetables (20 to 30 percent of food intake); soups (5 to 10 percent of food intake); and condiments and other foods (5 percent of food intake).

Macrobiotics stresses eating whole foods that are properly cooked to preserve nutrients, as well as foods that are grown in the same conditions as those in which the person lives. Eating foods grown in other areas predisposes people toward imbalances that can lead to disease. Because the macrobiotic diet is balanced (containing the proper vitamins, minerals, amino acids, and essential fatty acids), the body does not have to work at balancing or buffering extreme yin or yang foods and is able to direct energy toward healing.

Macrobiotic diets must be tailored for each person, and although there are many good macrobiotic cookbooks, the assistance of a trained macrobiotic counselor in devising a diet is extremely helpful. A macrobiotic diet results in slow and gentle healing over time. Many disease processes, including chemical sensitivities, arthritis, cancer, heavy metal toxicity, ulcerative colitis, and other conditions, have been eased or cured by following a macrobiotic diet.

In addition to diet, a macrobiotic program includes specific bodywork, breathing exercises, meditation, meridian stretches, walking outside with bare feet, wearing cotton clothes, singing happy songs, thinking calming thoughts, and being thankful for the small things in life.

BODY TYPE DIETS

Most people realize that the right diet is essential for good health and that there is not one diet that is good for everyone. Dietary and nutritional needs vary widely, as do dietary preferences. Even eating whole, healthy foods does not make a diet the best one for a particular person. Finding the correct diet can be a challenge for some people, and most resort to trial and error.

Some alternative practitioners use body type to help their patients determine the best diet for them. Below are three different approaches to body type diets.

Blood Group Diet

The blood in our bodies contains a genetic "fingerprint" that distinguishes us from all other individuals. The two main factors used to identify or type blood are the blood groups (groups O, A, B, and AB) and the Rh factor (positive or negative) which is spoken of as the blood type. Group O is the oldest blood group; Group A evolved with the development of agriculture; Group B appeared during the period of migration into colder, harsher climates; and Group AB emerged when groups intermingled in later times.

In his book *Eat Right 4 Your Type,* Dr. Peter J. D'Adamo presents diet solutions for staying healthy, living longer, and achieving ideal weight. The diet is actually four diets, based on the four blood groups, and presents the funda-

mental relationship between one's blood group and dietary and lifestyle choices.

Dr. D'Adamo says that a chemical reaction occurs between the blood and the food a person eats, and that a food that is harmful to the cells of people in one blood group may be beneficial to the cells of people in another blood group. Foods contain proteins called lectins, which have agglutinating (clumping) properties that affect the blood cells. When a food that is incompatible with the blood group is consumed, the lectins begin to agglutinate red blood cells in a target area.

Dr. D'Adamo states that following the blood group diets will allow a person to have optimum digestion and metabolism, and avoid many common infections. It will also rid the body of toxins, restore natural genetic rhythms and slow down the aging process by eliminating factors that cause rapid cell deterioration. He contends that the blood group diet can combat cardiovascular disease, gastrointestinal problems, hormonal imbalances, diabetes, inflammatory processes, obesity, and many other problems.

For detailed information on allowed foods, beneficial foods, neutral foods, and foods to be avoided, consult Dr. D'Adamo's book. He also makes specific recommendations for nutritional supplementation and medical treatment that is appropriate to each of the blood groups.

GROUP O

Group O is the largest (as well as the oldest) of the blood groups: approximately 43 percent of the population is Group O. People with this blood group are referred to as "hunters." They are meat eaters, have a hearty digestive tract, and an overactive immune system. They are intolerant of dietary and environmental adaptation, and respond to stress by instituting intense physical activity. Grains and legumes contribute to weight gain for people in Group O, and they have a tendency to have hypothyroidism (low thyroid function). Supplements for the Group O people should stabilize the thyroid, prevent inflammation, energize the metabolism, and increase blood-clotting activity.

GROUP A

Approximately 40 percent of the population is blood Group A. These people are the "cultivators" and do well on vegetarian diets. They have sensitive digestive tracts and tolerant immune systems, and they adjust well to dietary and environmental conditions. Group A people feel sluggish when they eat animal foods, and store meat meals as fat. They tend to have low stomach acid and digest dairy products very poorly. They are biologically predisposed to diabetes, cancer, and heart disease. They deal with stress best by using calming techniques such as yoga, meditation, or Tai Chi.

GROUP B

Only 9 to 12 percent of the North American population is Group B (the "nomads" or "travelers"). They have strong immune systems, and are less vulnerable to many diseases than are people in the other blood groups. They have tolerant digestive systems, and have the most flexible dietary choices of all the blood groups. They can eat dairy products with no problems, but must avoid wheat to lose weight. Group B people deal with stress very well, and require a balance between physical and mental activities to stay slim and mentally alert.

GROUP AB

Blood group AB is the newest and rarest of the blood groups, comprising 2 to 5 percent of the population. This group is something of an enigma, as some people with AB blood are more like those in Group A, while others are more like people in Group B. People in Group AB have a sensitive digestive tract, and have greatly varying and changing responses to environmental and dietary conditions. They have a tolerant immune system and respond to stress on a spiritual level. Group AB people are genetically programmed to eat meat, but a tendency to low stomach acid means that meat consumed tends to be stored as fat.

The Body Type System

A body type system has been developed by Dr. Carolyn Mein, a chiropractor in Rancho Santa Fe, California, and author of *Different Bodies, Different Diets*. She has identified 25 specific body types that are based on the dominant gland, organ, or system of the body. They apply to all races, to men and women, and are evident even in children. These body types include adrenal, balanced, blood, brain, eye, gallbladder, gonadal, heart, hypothalamus, intestinal, kidney, liver, lung, lymph, medulla, nervous system, pancreas, pineal, pituitary, skin, spleen, stomach, thalamus, thymus, and thyroid.

The body type determines body shape, structure, appearance, and metabolism. These characteristics of the body type will always be present, regardless of the person's weight. The dominant gland, organ, or system also determines areas of weight gain or loss.

In addition to the physical characteristics of the body, a psychological profile accompanies each body type, determining personal strengths, tendencies, motivations, and concerns. Understanding body type allows self-understanding as well as understanding and compassion for the differences between other body types.

According to Dr. Mein, weight gain or loss signals that the body is stressed and out of balance. Changes in energy levels also accompany these imbalances. Foods should be chosen to support, stimulate, and rebuild the dominant gland, organ, or system of the body, because these foods provide the nutrients that are depleted first. Dr. Mein describes the optimal foods for each body type.

In addition to different food choices, Dr. Mein has found that each body type requires different eating patterns, and she presents complete diets for all of the body types. There are also differences in exercise requirements.

The benefits of identifying and following a body type diet and lifestyle include better overall health, mental clarity, improved mood, decreased fatigue, improved digestion, and weight and appetite control.

Ayurvedic Diet

In Ayurvedic medicine there are three primary body or constitutional types that define a person's individual nature: Vata, Pitta, and Kapha. Each constitutional type has its own likes, dislikes, strengths, and weaknesses, and predisposes the person to certain types of illnesses. Nearly everyone is a combination of all three constitutional types or "doshas," but one type usually predominates. Each dosha has its own special dietary and lifestyle needs.

Vata is the dosha of the mind, emotions, movement, and the respiration, circulatory, and nervous systems. When this type is out of balance, many problems can result, including anxiety, insomnia, constipation, dry skin, aching joints, brittle nails, and high blood pressure.

Vata people must follow a regular routine with set times for meals and sleep. They need large amounts of salads and raw vegetables as well as warm, cooked foods. They should avoid cold foods and drinks, most beans, and sugar. Sweet, sour, and salty tastes balance vata. Sweet tastes can include milk, rice, bread, pasta, grains, and butter. Yogurt, lemon, grapefruit, and aged cheese constitute sour taste.

Pitta is the dosha of metabolism, light, liquid, and heat. Pitta people experience good digestion, strong focus, and contentment when they are balanced. If they are not balanced, anger, impatience, ulcers, burning sensations, sore throats, and skin rashes can result.

Overscheduling and overworking must be avoided by pitta types, and all meals, particularly the noon meal, must be on time. Dairy products, whole grains, high-protein foods, and most beans help to balance pitta people. They must avoid hot spices, tomatoes, vinegar, alcohol, refined sugar, and acidic or pungent foods. Sweet, bitter, and astringent tastes balance pitta. Astringent tastes include dried beans, bean soups, and green leafy vegetables. Spinach, turmeric, and horseradish are among the bitter tastes. They should eat cooling foods in the summer, and a variety of raw foods. In the winter, warm foods are preferable.

Kapha is the dosha of structure and solidarity. Strength, stamina, good immunity, stability, and even temperament are kapha qualities. Food and security are important to the kapha person. If there is an imbalance, dullness, depression, congestion, high cholesterol, allergies, and excess weight and water retention can result.

Kapha people must avoid oversleeping and should exercise regularly. They need vegetables, fruits, and legumes, and should eat few sweets, meat, dairy, and fatty foods. Pungent, bitter, and astringent tastes balance kapha. Pungent tastes include spicy foods and ginger root. Low-protein diets and hot, spicy foods are best for kapha types. In the summer raw foods should be eaten.

VEGETARIAN DIETS

Although vegetarian diets are becoming more mainstream, most health care professionals still consider them to be alternative diets. Vegetarianism is essentially the consumption of a meatless diet. There are several different types of vegetarians: ovo-lacto vegetarians include some animal protein—usually eggs, milk, and cheese—in the diet, but exclude all flesh foods (meat, poultry, or fish). Semi-vegetarians drink milk and eat milk products, eggs, and some fish and poultry, but no red meat or pork, while lacto-vegetarians drink milk, eat cheese and other dairy products, but do not eat eggs, meat, fish, or poultry. Vegans eat no meat or other animal-related foods (no milk, milk products, eggs, or even honey).

It is important that people on a vegetarian diet consume sufficient protein. This is best accomplished by combining plant-based foods that are low in certain amino acids with other foods that are high in them. Nut and seed combinations, and grain and legume combinations, are good protein sources for the vegetarian. Combination eating does not have to be as exact as it was once thought. The body is now known to be capable of storing amino acids until it needs to use them.

Many vegetarians eat flavored meat substitutes made from soy and grains. Burgers and frankfurters are some of the many products that are available. Texturized vegetable protein (TVP) can be substituted for ground meat in casseroles and other dishes. It tends to absorb the flavors of the other ingredients.

Vegetarians who do not eat dairy products will need to take a vitamin B_{12} supplement, since this vitamin is found only in animal products. Vitamin D may also be deficient, and poor food quality can cause a deficiency in trace minerals. It is important that vegetarians choose high-quality food that still contains its vital nutrients. Supplementation with the proper nutrients is essential if there is any doubt.

People who change to a vegetarian diet should consult an alternative practitioner well-versed in vegetarianism to be certain they will be getting all of the nutrients necessary for good health. The many good vegetarian cookbooks and organizations are a further help in planning tasty and nutritious meals.

Vegetarian diets provide several health benefits. Vegetarians have a decreased risk of developing kidney stones and gall stones. They have a much lower risk of developing cardiovascular and heart disease, and cholesterol levels have been successfully lowered with a vegetarian diet. The body is less burdened by toxins with a vegetarian diet and the anti-cancer defenses are supported. The risk of osteoporosis is also less with both a vegan and vegetarian diet.

NUTRITIONAL SUPPLEMENTS

The importance of nutrition in the maintenance of health and prevention of disease is slowly gaining recognition. Medical students are taught that only people with imbalanced diets need nutritional supplementation. However, with the poor nutritional quality of so much of the food available to most people in North America, this is no longer true. Food is raised with chemical fertilizers to make up for soil deficiencies; it may contain residues of herbicides and pesticides used to control weeds; and artificial ripening of crops and long storage of foods further reduces nutritional quality.

Most North Americans do not eat balanced diets or quality foods. There is much emphasis on processed foods that contain artificial colors, flavors, and preservatives; chemicals and sometimes artificial ingredients are added to foods to increase palatability; nutrients are removed during processing, and sometimes fiber is lost. Processed foods are also high in salt, fat, and sugar.

More and more people are eating out, in a variety of restaurants. Fast foods are notoriously high in fat, sugar, and salt, and contain many additives. While the quality of food is higher in the better restaurants, unless a restaurant serves organic food, meals can still be deficient in nutrients.

Almost half of all North Americans have some type of health problem; some studies indicate that as many as one in four North Americans has a degenerative condition (cardiovascular disease, arthritis, cancer, ulcers, or diabetes). Eating better-quality food and treating nutritional deficiencies could dramatically reduce the incidence and severity of these diseases.

Overstressing the body's chemical detoxification pathways produces nutrient loss, and because we are exposed to an unprecedented number of chemicals in our everyday lives, we use up nutrients at an increased pace. Nutrient deficiencies also occur as a side effect of prescription drugs. Because the main therapy offered by modern medicine is the use of pharmaceuticals, unsuspected nutrient deficiencies occur in many people.

For all of the above reasons, many North Americans need nutritional supplementation, including vitamins, minerals, amino acids, and essential fatty acids. The need for nutrients varies from person to person; this is known as biochemical individuality, and was discovered in the 1950s by the late Dr. Roger Williams, a biochemist at the University of Texas. Some people do quite well on the minimum daily requirements (MDR) and recommended dietary allowances (RDA) established by the government. However, for some people the RDA is best interpreted as a "ridiculously deficient allowance," since those people require significantly higher amounts of nutrients either because of a metabolic genetic defect, or because of an ongoing illness.

Balanced amounts of vitamins, minerals, amino acids, and fatty acids are required for optimal health. A deficiency in any of these nutrients can result in poor health and deficiency diseases. Dr. Abram Hoffer states in his book *Orthomolecular Nutrition* that if nutritional deficiencies and biochemical defects are identified and corrected by treating with the proper nutrients, the health of the patient will be restored, and medication will not be needed. In her recent book, *Depression Cured at Last,* Dr. Sherry Rogers writes that "Every place a drug works there is probably a natural or God-given nutrient correction that could be made that would more inexpensively and permanently fix what is broken."

Many physicians are confused about vitamin dosages. They have been led to believe that biochemical reactions that are dependent upon a specific vitamin can take place only at a certain speed and vitamin concentration. There is some evidence that enzyme systems can be accelerated beyond their usual rates by giving larger amounts of vitamins to stimulate metabolic responses. The patient who responds to these larger doses of vitamins is not "vitamin deficient," but the vitamin is behaving as a "drug" that stimulates the response.

Each person needs the right nutrition to meet his or her individual needs—which may be higher or lower than average. The term orthomolecular medicine was coined in 1968 by the late Dr. Linus Pauling, of Stanford University, and refers to a form of nutritional therapy in which nutrients are prescribed in larger amounts than is usual. The term megadose has come into common use to refer to such prescriptions. Dosage is tailored to each person and, for the best results, slightly more than is required is given. Because nutrients do not work alone, but rather in concert with one another, all nutrients must be present in adequate, balanced, optimal amounts. About 45 different nutrients are prescribed in orthomolecular medicine.

Nutrients can be administered in several different, effective ways. They may be taken as a powder, tablet, or capsule. Tablets and capsules may contain fillers and excipients to which some people may react. Nutrients can also be administered intramuscularly as an injection or intravenously. Recently nutrient sprays for oral administration have been developed, as have nutrients that can be administered rectally.

For help in healing with nutrients, consult an orthomolecular medicine physician, or an environmental medicine physician who has had additional training in nutrition. Determining your nutritional supplementation needs can be done with help from the many excellent books on the subject. As well, a trained nutritionist can tailor a program specifically for you. For information on nutrients that can help with specific health problems, see Part 3, Common Health Problems.

VITAMINS

Vitamins are natural organic substances that are found in foods from both plant and animal sources. The amounts of vitamins needed are tiny—doses are usually in mg (1/1,000 of a gram), with doses of a few vitamins measured in micrograms (1/1,000,000 of a gram). Nevertheless, the presence or absence of vitamins in these small amounts can make the difference between very good health and very poor health as certain cellular processes can take place only in the presence of vitamins.

When they were first discovered, the exact chemical structure of vitamins was unknown, and they were given alphabetical designations (vitamins A through U) rather than chemical or scientific names. There are two basic classes of vitamins: water-soluble and fat-soluble. Fat-soluble vitamins (vitamins A, D, E, and K) are stored in the body. Water-soluble vitamins (for example, the B vitamins and vitamin C) are more easily lost by the body, since they dissolve in water and can be eliminated.

MINERALS

There are at least 18 minerals required for body function and maintenance, and these must be supplied to the body in the diet. Minerals are needed for the formation of bone and blood, the maintenance of healthy nerve function, and the regulation of muscle tone. Minerals are integral parts of enzymes, and serve as cofactors and catalysts in many biological reactions that take place in the body. They contribute to the proper composition of body fluids, and are also responsible for maintaining water balance in the body. Minerals operate in concert, just as vitamins do; the function of one mineral affects that of all the others.

Some minerals, classified as macro minerals,

are required in larger amounts than others; these are calcium, chlorine, magnesium, phosphorus, potassium, and sodium. Others, needed in very small amounts, are called trace elements or trace minerals. These include boron, chromium, cobalt, copper, iodine, iron, manganese, molybdenum, selenium, silicon, sulfur, vanadium, and zinc.

Recommended Daily Amounts (RDAs) have been established only for calcium, iodine, iron, magnesium, phosphorus, selenium, and zinc.

AMINO ACIDS

Amino acids are the building blocks of proteins, which are essential components of every living cell. The particular amino acids, and the order in which they are assembled, determines the nature of each protein.

Amino acids that are classed as essential are those that cannot be made by the body and must be derived from foods. Essential amino acids include histidine, isoleucine, leucine, lysine, methionine, phenylalanine, threonine, tryptophan, and valine. If even one essential amino acid is missing or present in inadequate amounts, protein synthesis will stop or fall to a very low level. Non-essential amino acids are a misnomer: they *are* essential for body metabolism, but they can be made by the body from other amino acids. Non-essential amino acids include alanine, arginine, asparagine, aspartic acid, citrulline, cysteine, cystine, gamma-aminobutyric acid, glutamic acid, glutamine, glycine, ornithine, proline, serine, taurine, and tyrosine.

Food is the source material for all amino acids. A given food may or may not contain all the essential amino acids, but the protein requirements of the body can be easily met if a good variety of food is eaten so that all amino acids become available. Meat, fish, poultry, and dairy products are high in protein and thus contain large amounts of the essential amino acids. Vegetables and fruits are low in some amino acids and missing others completely. They must be combined with meats or other vegetables, fruits, grains, legumes, or nuts containing the missing amino acids to permit protein synthesis. Protein and amino acid requirements vary according to the sex, age, and weight of each individual.

FATTY ACIDS

Fatty acids are classified as either essential fatty acids (EFA), which cannot be made by the body and must be supplied in the diet, or non-essential fatty acids, which can be made by the body. The essential fatty acids are long-chain molecules that are necessary for health. They promote healthy skin and hair, influence glandular activity, help burn saturated fats, help build nerve sheaths, store energy, and participate in most body reactions. They also aid in the transmission of nerve impulses and are needed for normal function and development of the brain. Insufficient amounts cause the deficiency diseases of eczema and acne.

The best food sources of essential fatty acids are vegetable oils (flaxseed and flaxseed oils, grape seed oil, hemp oil, and primrose oil), although some are found in fresh deep-water fish. Fatty acids are also available as supplements. No RDA has been established for fatty acids, but it is suggested that at least 10 to 20 percent of total calories should come from essential unsaturated fatty acids (their molecules are not fully paired, or saturated, with hydrogen and they remain liquid at room temperature).

OPPOSITION TO NUTRITIONAL THERAPY

Opposition to nutritional therapy is very strong among physicians, and it is considered an "unscientific" approach by many of its critics. Dr. Abram Hoffer, a Canadian physician who is a pioneer in orthomolecular medicine, states that while many physicians feel strict scientific studies are required to demonstrate that nutritional therapy works, they are willing to accept the flimsiest "proof" that it does *not* work.

Studies demonstrating the efficacy of nutrients are complicated by the fact that nutrients work slowly, because they are not just treating the symptoms, but are correcting the underlying cause of the disease or health problem. In addition, nutrients do not work singly, but in combination; this can make it difficult to pinpoint the action of a given nutrient.

Furthermore, physicians tend to expect treatment substances to help with a specific problem. However, the same nutrient can help with many different diseases. This non-specific action makes it difficult for some physicians to accept nutritional therapy.

Nutritional therapy does not fit into the present training of physicians. Very few hours of nutrition education are offered in the medical schools, and as a result, those doctors who advocate the use of vitamins and minerals as therapeutic agents are often regarded as mavericks. Nevertheless, many physicians who use nutritional therapy have found it works. They therefore consider it unethical to withhold inexpensive and simple nutrients that have been proven empirically, and to give their patients placebos and pharmaceuticals instead.

AROMATHERAPY

It is well known that scents or aromas affect the way people feel. Scents can cause mental, emotional, and physical changes (both good and bad) and some fragrances can counter the negative effects of stress.

Aromatherapy makes use of scents to treat various health problems. The materials used are essential oils extracted from plants, which carry the taste and scent of the original plant. Most essential oils are highly volatile and have a consistency more like water than oil.

Essential oils are very concentrated, and careful and conservative use is suggested. Essential oils and aromatherapy can affect the digestive, cardiovascular, lymphatic, respiratory, urinary, reproductive, endocrine, and nervous systems.

Aromatherapy remedies may be applied either externally or internally. They may be inhaled, applied to the skin, or taken orally as a tea. They can be used in baths and as massage oils. The use of multiple oils to treat a specific condition such as hemorrhoids, rheumatic pain, influenza, or sinus congestion requires the help of an experienced professional.

LIGHT THERAPY

The oldest form of light therapy is exposure to sunlight, which is full-spectrum light, containing all the wavelengths of light. Full-spectrum light triggers the hypothalamus gland to produce neurotransmitters that govern most body functions, such as blood pressure, body temperature, breathing, digestion, sexual function, moods, the immune system, the aging process, and the circadian rhythm.

Today light therapy uses many different wavelengths, including full-spectrum light, to achieve therapeutic benefits. Alternative medicine practitioners as well as some modern physicians use light therapy to treat a number of health problems. Some frequently used treatments are described below. Many of these treatments can be done at home.

Full-spectrum light applied to the skin helps to treat depression, insomnia, hypertension, PMS, and migraines. Full-spectrum lights used in schools and workplaces reduce absenteeism due to illness. School officials also report that when full-spectrum lights are used, reductions in hyperactivity and behavior problems are seen, and academic achievement improves.

Bright light therapy involves the use of high-intensity white light ranging from 2,000 to 5,000 lux. Bright light therapy decreases depression in people with Seasonal Affective Disorder (SAD), is a chronic depression that occurs in winter. People develop symptoms within the same 60-day period each year. In addition to the depression, they crave carbohydrates, and al-though they feel better when they eat them, they gain weight. They also sleep more, but are always tired, have no interest in sex, feel overwhelmed, have difficulty concentrating, avoid family and friends, and have frequent infections and muscle aches. More than 36 million North Americans suffer from SAD. More women than men are affected, and it seems to run in families.

Most modern and alternative physicians agree that this disorder is related to the changes in light that accompany the seasons, and is probably related to melatonin production. Melatonin is a hormone produced by the pineal gland, and the body produces more melatonin during the winter, when the days are shorter and darker. If these people are exposed to a special bright light for a specified amount of time each day, their symptoms of SAD improve.

Bright light therapy also reduces binging in people with bulimia; normalizes sleep hours for people with delayed sleep phase syndrome; and regulates long and irregular menstrual cycles.

In hemo-irradiation therapy, blood is treated with ultraviolet light, which activates oxidation of the blood. The blood is withdrawn from the body, treated, and re-injected. This process kills bacteria, restores chemical balance, improves calcium metabolism, and increases oxygen absorption.

Colored light therapy is used extensively by alternative practitioners. It makes use of the fact that different colors of light have different effects on the body. Some colors can stimulate hormone production, while others inhibit it. A combination of flashing bright lights and colored lights can be used to treat depression and pain. Colored lights applied to certain areas of the tongue and to acupuncture points help to treat a variety of problems.

Monochromatic red light therapy, another type of colored light therapy, can be used to treat a wide range of problems including shoulder pain, tendonitis, arthritis, sore throat, sinus problems, gastrointestinal problems, and depression. The red light is applied to acupressure points, or sites of localized pain.

Cold laser therapy utilizes a low-intensity laser light to begin a series of enzymatic reactions and bio-electric events that stimulate the natural healing process at the cellular level. Cold laser therapy has been used to control pain, and to treat myofascial syndrome, trauma, skin ailments, and neurological diseases. Cold lasers are also useful in dentistry, particularly for treating infections underneath the teeth. They are effective for patients who do not like the needles of traditional acupuncture, as they can stimulate acupuncture points and balance energy flow in meridians. They can be used in conjunction with other therapies, including homeopathy, nutritional supplements, and herbs.

SOUND THERAPY

It has been known for thousands of years that music and sound have the ability to heal. Certain sounds can slow breathing, create a sense of well-being, reduce stress, alleviate pain, lower blood pressure, slow heartbeat, soothe a restless baby, and improve movement and balance. Sound can also alter skin temperature and influence brain wave frequencies. Sound can be used therapeutically to help regulate corticosteroid hormone levels, reduce cancer pain, control severity of muscle tremors, and reduce stress in heart patients.

Sound is used in many different hospital settings, including operating theaters, recovery rooms, and birthing rooms. Sound therapy can reduce the amount of anesthesia surgical patients require, and minimize post-operative disorientation. It is used in hospices, and in the care of cancer, Alzheimer's, and AIDS patients. Sound can also play a vital role in dentistry and psychotherapy, reducing pain and improving mood.

According to researcher Joy Gardner-Gordon, writing in *Natural Health* magazine in 1994, the voice travels on a healing path from the brain throughout all internal organs. Making a single, long, sustained sound, called toning, produces energizing, calming vibrations.

After 21 years of investigation, Sharry Edwards, teacher, lecturer, and researcher in Denver, Colorado, has developed an alternative medicine sound therapy. She has determined that each person has a distinctive "signature sound," which corresponds to their physiological and psychological status. Frequencies missing from the voice are indicators of physical or emotional distress. Emotional states can be categorized from these missing notes and octaves. If the missing frequencies are provided, she claims the body can repair itself, even when it is dealing with supposedly incurable disease. A Self Management Auditory Device (SMAD), developed under the supervision of Edwards, supplies the missing sounds.

BACH FLOWER REMEDIES

Probably inspired by Samuel Hahnemann and homeopathy, Edward Bach (1886–1936) endeavored to find simple, inexpensive herbal remedies that could be used even by people without medical training. The result of his efforts—the Bach Flower Remedy repertoire—contains only 38 simple-to-understand remedies.

Bach felt that the person, rather than the nature of the disease, should be the most important focus in treating illness. In his system, therefore, the mental aspect of the person guides the practitioner to the correct remedy for the body, and treatment can be made more specific by taking the uniqueness of the person being treated into account. Bach believed that the herbs he prescribed comforted, soothed, and relieved cares and anxieties, bringing the person nearer to the divinity within.

The Bach Flower Remedies can be used in

conjunction with any orthodox treatment. They can improve the success of treatment in all types of cases, acute or chronic.

A potpourri of herbs called the Bach Flower Rescue Remedy contains a combination of *Helianthemum, Clematis, Impatiens, Prunus,* and *Ornithogalum.* It is useful for accidents, injuries, allergic reactions, trauma and shock of surgery, and numerous health crises. It can be administered orally, in water, or by simply wiping the lips or skin of the person with the Rescue Remedy. The dose is just a few drops, and it works quickly and effectively.

PART 3

Common Health Problems

CHAPTER 11

Overview

This part of the book deals with common health problems, which many readers may have to deal with at some time in their lives. The discussion is intended to increase your understanding of these health challenges and the various ways in which they can be treated. For each problem discussed, both modern medicine treatments and alternative treatments are presented. Some are self-help methods, while others require the help of health care professionals.

This book is not intended to be a substitute for the skills and insight of a health care professional. Rather, it is meant to guide you in selecting the most *appropriate* help for your particular health needs. Neither is the book designed to persuade you to abandon either modern medicine or alternative medicine in favor of the other. Rather, it is meant as a teaching tool that will increase your knowledge about health and illness. The book is also intended to illustrate the importance of a healthy lifestyle in maintaining health, in the hope that you will choose to make that lifestyle a part of your life.

We discuss many health problems in these chapters—but there are many more that space would not permit us to consider. We describe several treatments for each problem—but again, space does not allow us to list all possible treatments. Most people will not need all of the treatments mentioned in order to regain their health, and, in fact, may not tolerate some of them. Peo-

ple who are quite ill may need most of the treatments, and it may take a long time for health to be restored.

For each health problem we have listed homeopathic treatments, both classical and complex. Because of space limitations we have not been able to list all of the possibilities, but have given some of the major remedies that have been used to successfully treat the condition. Further research may be necessary on your part to determine the best treatment for you. If your health problem is complex, find a competent health practitioner to help you. Some conditions can be self-treated, but many will require the assistance of a trained homeopath. For an explanation of homeopathic potencies and dosages, see pp. 80–81. Some of the complex remedies listed are over-the-counter remedies, and others are available only from health care practitioners.

Patients should avoid coffee, eucalyptus, camphor, menthol, recreational drugs, and electric blankets while taking a homeopathic remedy. Creams containing steroids, antibiotics, and antifungals should also be avoided, and acupuncture should not be used while receiving homeopathic treatment, as it can counteract the treatment.

Herbal or botanical treatments are also listed for each health problem. Herbs may be used alone and in combinations. It was not possible to list the entire herbal pharmacopoeia for each condition. The more common herbal treatments are given, but there are many other possibilities. You may need to research your herbal needs further by consulting a trained herbalist.

Always follow the directions given on the packaging of the herb you purchase. The dosage for an herb or botanical supplement will vary, depending on the form in which it is taken. Teas are usually made from 1,000 to 2,000 mg of dried herb. For herbs purchased as a tincture, the dose is commonly 4 to 6 ml of a 1:5 solution. For a fluid extract (1:1), the usual dose is 0.5 to 2 ml. For a powdered solid extract (4:1), the dose is 500 to 750 mg.

Again, it was not possible to list all of the possible nutrients that might be helpful for each health concern. Only the major nutrients are given, along with their common doses.

All dosages for substances mentioned under treatment protocols are adult doses, and must be adjusted down for children according to the child's weight. (Children 14 years old and older, unless they are small for their ages, can usually take adult dosage.)

Remember to purchase quality vitamins and nutrients that are free of the common allergens such as milk, wheat, yeast, soy, egg, corn, and sugar. If you have difficulty taking nutritional supplements, be tested for tolerance and dose by an alternative practitioner who has that testing capability.

There are many excellent books available that will enable you to learn more about nutrients and how they may help you. If your health problem is severe or complex, seek the help of a person trained in nutritional treatment, such as an environmental medicine or orthomolecular medicine physician.

Ayurvedic medicine and Chinese medicine are very effective total health care systems. Because of their complexity and many treatment modalities, in most cases we have not listed specific treatments. For conditions for which these systems might be helpful, we have suggested that you consult an Ayurvedic or Chinese medicine practitioner.

The more health challenges you have, the more important it is that you find a competent health care practitioner to help you. For complex problems, always seek the help of a qualified practitioner.

CHAPTER 12

Headaches

Headaches are the most common health complaint in North America. They occur even more frequently than the common cold, and were mentioned in ancient literature as early as 3000 BC. Everyone has a headache from time to time, but 12.5 million Americans have a headache every day. It is estimated that at least 90 percent of men and 95 percent of women have at least one headache during each calendar year. More than 70 percent of North Americans take painkillers at least once a month for relief from headaches. Headaches are responsible for 80 million office visits to physicians each year in North America and are an expensive health problem. The annual cost attributable to headaches (including the cost of absenteeism and medical bills) is estimated to be $50 billion.

A headache is a symptom rather than a disorder in itself, and accompanies many diseases and conditions, including emotional distress. For this reason, headaches should not be ignored as they can signal a serious health problem. However, headaches are a complicated and often misunderstood problem. There are many types of headaches, and just as many factors that contribute to creating them. The frequency, severity, and duration of headaches varies widely, ranging from slight headaches of short duration to chronic, incapacitating headaches that last for days. At least 50 million North Americans suffer from chronic headaches, but only 7 percent seek medical help for them, probably because of the dismal record of modern medicine in effectively treating headaches.

TRIGGERS FOR HEADACHES

There are many different factors that can trigger headaches:

- autoimmune disturbances – blood clotting disorders
- dental problems – jaw clenching, teeth grinding, TMJ (temporomandibular joint) syndrome, abscessed teeth, jaw infections, and misaligned or crooked teeth
- dietary sensitivities – reactions to foods and chemicals in foods such as MSG, aspartame, dyes and colorings, artificial ingredients, flavorings, preservatives, and contaminants
- digestive disturbances – leaky gut syndrome, candidiasis, and constipation
- environmental sensitivities – sun glare, bright or flickering light; chemical pollutants, both indoor and outdoor; pollen, mold, and dust; noise; weather changes; altitude changes
- hormonal imbalances – excess estrogen levels, low progesterone levels, hyperinsulinemia, hypoglycemia, and thyroid problems
- infection – viral, bacterial, fungal and parasitic
- lifestyle factors – sleep problems; smoking; fatigue or overwork; inadequate or poor-

quality diet; changed meal patterns; nutritional deficiencies; overuse of the computer, TV, or VCR; lack of exercise
- medications – birth control pills, diuretics, painkillers, antihistamines, hormonal supplements, diet pills, and medication for asthma, blood pressure, and heart disease
- psychological stress – depression, stress, anxiety, anger, boredom, and repressed emotions
- structural disturbances – head trauma, muscle trauma, musculoskeletal misalignments, poor posture
- vascular problems – hypertension, vascular spasms, and vascular blockage

The following headache symptoms are a signal that medical help is necessary:

- headaches that occur so frequently it is difficult to carry out your normal activities;
- headaches that are constant and unrelenting;
- headaches that cause you to take more than 16 aspirin or acetaminophen tablets a week;
- severe headaches that begin suddenly;
- headaches that are new to you;
- headaches that occur after a head injury;
- headaches accompanied by fever or a stiff neck;
- headaches associated with pain in the eye, ear, or elsewhere in your head;
- headaches accompanied by hearing loss, trouble with speech, blurred vision, seizures, loss of alertness or consciousness, or loss of body function;
- headaches accompanied by disturbances of thought processes (loss of memory, poor concentration, confusion, or inability to think clearly); or
- headaches associated with sleep disturbances (wakefulness in the middle of the night or insomnia).

When you make an appointment with your physician to discuss your headaches, ask for enough time for a thorough examination. When you go for your appointment, take with you a list of all medications (prescription and over-the-counter) that you are taking, as well as a list of all the chemicals to which you are routinely exposed. Also take along a written record of all symptoms that accompany your headache (including a description of the location, type, and duration of the pain), any triggers associated with your headaches, and a note on when headaches tend to occur.

TYPES OF HEADACHES

Headaches are more effectively treated if the cause of the headache can be identified. Most headache pain is probably generated by three mechanisms: irritation of nerve endings in the head and neck as a result of tense muscles; irritation of nerve endings as a result of the swelling of blood vessels; and inflammation of the lining of certain tissues.

The type of pain is important for identifying the cause of a headache: the pain can be aching, boring, crushing, piercing, throbbing, burning, pressing, squeezing, or dull. The location of the pain can help to determine the origin of the headache. Although localized in the head, the pain may actually be referred pain from arteries, veins, sinuses, or the upper spine.

Accompanying symptoms such as dizziness, visual disturbances, vomiting, ear ringing, numbness, constipation, and other symptoms are also important in identifying the type and cause of a headache.

Headaches are classified according to their symptoms (though these may vary widely among individual sufferers with the same type of headache).

ORGANIC

Organic headaches include headaches with very serious, sometimes life-threatening causes. A medical professional should be contacted immediately if an organic headache is suspected. There are over 300 conditions that can cause organic headaches, but the following are the more common ones: brain tumors, meningitis, ruptured aneurysm (rupture of a sac formed in the wall of an artery), trigeminal and occipital neuralgia (nerve disorders), temporal arteritis (inflammation of the temporal arteries), glaucoma, reactions to a spinal tap, subdural hematoma (accumulation of blood under the skull), and hypertension. Hypertension headaches are not caused by continuous high blood pressure, but by a sudden rise in blood pressure that may cause swelling and tiny hemorrhages in the brain.

The pain of organic headaches is usually excruciating, and appears suddenly with little or no warning. Organic headaches can on occasion mimic other types of headaches. Signs of a dangerous headache include:

- headaches with neurological symptoms such as slurred speech, memory loss, mental confusion, sensory disturbance, double vision, seizures, or loss of motor control;
- headaches accompanied by numbness or weakness on one side;
- headaches accompanied by nausea, vomiting, and/or high fever;
- headaches accompanied by blood or clear fluid coming out of the nose or ears;
- headaches associated with head injury;
- sudden headaches (especially when there is no history of headaches);
- headaches that affect breathing;
- headaches that start early in childhood or in old age;
- headaches with no recognizable pattern of pain and symptoms;
- headaches that become more intense, are of longer duration, and become more frequent with time; or
- headaches that prevent performance of daily activities.

TENSION

Tension headaches are associated with cycles of pain caused by muscle tension. Any kind of stress can cause muscle tension, which brings on pain, which then brings about more stress and more muscle tension. This is an overused category, because any headache that is not identifiable as an organic, migraine, or cluster headache is considered a tension headache. However, many of these headaches have nothing to do with tension. "Stress" headaches might be a more accurate designation. Anything that affects the balance of the body is considered to be a stress, and can be a precipitating cause of a headache.

True tension headaches are muscle-contraction headaches and have a gradual onset. They are usually mild, accompanied by dull aching, and generally do not throb. People describe the pain as a viselike squeezing or heavy pressure around the head. There may be a knotted, clenched, and uncomfortable feeling in the back, neck, and shoulders, and there may be a feeling of stress and anxiety that can be accompanied by mood swings and depression. These headaches may be episodic, usually occurring once or twice a week, once a month, or even less frequently. They may also be chronic and occur almost daily.

The pain of a tension headache is attributed to two mechanisms involved in muscle contractions; nerve compression within the muscle that can be caused by poor posture or structural misalignment, or nerve irritation that is generated by a buildup of metabolic wastes. The pain comes from the tensing and stretching of the scalp and neck. Many researchers believe that tension headaches are probably related to vascular headaches, because they too are accompanied by alterations in muscle tension, changes in serotonin levels, pressure in the nerves of the neck and head, and contraction and dilation of blood vessels.

MIGRAINE

There are two types of migraine: common and classical migraines. Both are typically experienced as a one-sided vascular headache accompanied by visual disturbances (called an aura), fatigue, disorientation, throbbing pain, nausea, and vomiting. The pain is related to vascular changes. In the prodromal (onset) stages the veins in the scalp constrict, and once the headache starts they dilate. For migraines caused by food allergies, the pain is sometimes relieved or lessened when the person vomits. Migraines are on the rise in North America; one out of every five individuals will experience at least one migraine during a lifetime.

Eighty percent of all migraines are common migraines, also known as a sick headache. With this type of migraine there are no prodromal symptoms, though they can be preceded by a feeling of unease. There can also be nausea, vomiting, food cravings (especially for sweets), depression or exhilaration, and either hypo- or hyperactivity. Although there can be brief jolts, the pain is usually throbbing and steady and may be synchronized with the pulse. Activity aggravates the pain, which is generally one-sided and centered above or behind one eye. It can begin at the back of the head and spread to affect one side of the head. Sometimes the neck is stiff and the scalp is tender and sore.

As many as 90 percent of common migraines are thought to be triggered by dietary or environmental sensitivities. Food allergy plays a major role in setting off these headaches, and even the smell of a food allergen can trigger a headache in an overloaded, sensitive individual. Common foods that trigger migraines include milk, eggs, chocolate, corn, wheat, oranges, tomatoes, pork, beef, soy, oats, coffee, peanuts, bacon, potatoes, apples, peaches, grapes, chicken, bananas, strawberries, melon, and carrots. Additives to food (such as MSG) can also trigger migraines, as can artificial sweeteners containing aspartame (such as NutraSweet).

Foods and beverages containing tyramine (an amino acid that reduces the levels of the neurotransmitter, serotonin) are known triggers for many migraines. Tyramine is found in bananas, cheese, chicken and beef livers, eggplant, meat tenderizers, pickled herring, cured meats such as hot dogs and salami, sour cream, yogurt, soy sauce, yeast, dark beer, red wine, gin, bourbon, vodka, and alcohol in general. Chocolate contains a relative of tyramine and it, too, can trigger migraines.

Chemical sensitivities can also trigger migraines. An exposure to tobacco smoke, gasoline, or fresh paint can cause a headache for some people. Perfumes, fabric softener, and various scented products are also powerful triggers for individuals sensitive to those substances. Several types of pharmaceuticals (both prescription medications and over-the-counter drugs) can also precipitate migraines. In some cases it is the drug itself that is the offender, but the excipients, fillers, binders, and even the capsule can also cause the headache.

Infections (particularly viral infections and yeast infections) trigger migraines. Loud noises, strong smells, weather changes, changes in time zones, travel, alterations of sleep-wake cycles or meal schedules, structural misalignments, and emotional factors such as stress, anxiety, and anger are also triggers for migraines.

One in seven women who have migraines have headaches associated with hormonal imbalances that coincide with menstrual periods. Oral contraceptives and hormone replacement drugs can play a role in migraines.

Twenty percent of migraines are classical migraines, which have the same triggers as common migraines. These headaches have a prodromal stage of about 30 minutes before the headache begins. There is a warning aura during this stage that consists of visual disturbances (zigzag lines, blind spots, hallucinations, or light flashes). There may be shimmering, sparkling, or flickering spots with a geometric design around the edge. It is thought that the aura is caused by electrical and chemical changes in the brain and a reduction in blood flow to some parts of the brain. There may also be sensory motor disturbances such as yawning, smelling strange odors that may or may not actually be present, or numbness or tingling in an arm or leg. Mental function disturbances can include confusion, difficulty talking, speech impairment, and disorientation.

Other symptoms of classical migraine can include weakness, nervousness, anxiety, and depression; an increased need to urinate and an urge to move the bowels; dizziness, lightheadedness, faintness, or loss of balance; cold and clammy hands and feet; hot flashes alternating with chills; reddened or teary eyes; stomach pain; nausea or vomiting; intolerance for light, noise, and smells; water retention; hyperventilation; and nasal and sinus congestion.

These headaches can last from three hours to as long as three days. A headache that lasts longer than that is called a status migrainosus and requires immediate medical attention. Classical migraines may occur infrequently, or can happen as often as several times a week. Average frequency is one to three headaches per month.

The International Headache Society, based in Cheshire, England, has set criteria for diagnosing migraines: if a headache patient has at least two of the symptoms in Group A and at least one of the symptoms in Group B, the headache is considered to be a migraine.

Group A:
• The pain is located on one side of the head.
• The pain is throbbing or pulsating.
• The pain is severe enough to interfere with or keep the person from normal daily activity.
• The pain is worsened by exertion.

Group B:
• The pain is accompanied by nausea or vomiting.
• The pain is accompanied by sensitivity to light and noise.

Migraine seems to run in families, though nutritional deficiencies, such as deficiencies of cop-per and magnesium, can make people more prone to migraines. Some people wake up with a migraine even though they felt well when they went to sleep; migraines develop during the phase of REM (Rapid Eye Movement) sleep more frequently than at any other time of the day or night. Some migraines that develop during the night are triggered by a food allergy to something that was consumed at the evening meal.

Stress plays a role in migraines and some people are described as having a "migraine personality." They are compulsive workers and perfectionists. Some migraine sufferers may have difficulty managing anger—they either blow up over everything, or are unable to express anger at all. Repressing intense emotions overstresses the body.

Migraines usually appear first when people are in their 20s and 30s, and sometimes they go into remission after age 50. However, children can have migraines, and if they do, there will frequently be other people in the family who have headaches. Headache symptoms in children are not as well defined as those of adults, and tend to fit the personality of the particular child. They may have vague rather than localized pain, and sometimes they have no pain at all. Instead they may have stomach pain, nausea, confusion, and dizziness. These children nearly always have allergies and digestive problems, and are highly sensitive. Fifty percent of children with migraines appear to outgrow them. People who have motion sickness as children are prone to develop migraines as adults.

CLUSTER

Cluster headaches are vascular headaches that begin with a sense of fullness in one ear; progress to a stab of unilateral pain near the eye, forehead, or cheek; then, in minutes, become a full-blown headache. The pain of a cluster headache is one of the worst pains known, exceeding that of childbirth. It is so severe that sufferers often inflict pain on other areas of their body to distract their attention from the head pain.

These headaches tend to develop during sleep, two to three hours after retiring, or in the early hours of the morning. They can last from fifteen minutes to three hours. Cluster headache may be accompanied by a red and teary eye; a drooping eyelid; stuffy nose and drainage of clear fluid from one nostril; sweating on the forehead, abdomen, and trunk; flushed face; and exhaustion when the pain subsides.

Cluster headaches affect 1 in 250 men and 1 in 1,000 women. Sufferers tend to be men who are 20 to 50 years old, taller than usual, active, ambitious, and hard-working. These men rarely express emotions, and drink and smoke heavily. If the male is Caucasian, he tends to have hazel eyes and a red complexion with thick skin and deep, coarse lines around the forehead, mouth, and chin. There is no familial tendency to cluster headaches.

Cluster headaches are frequently mistaken for other types of headaches, particularly temporomandibular joint syndrome (TMJ) headaches, because they radiate around the jaw. They may also be mistaken for organic headaches because of the pain intensity, or for allergy or sinus headaches because of the eye and nose involvement.

The causes and triggers of cluster headaches are difficult to identify. Most researchers and health care practitioners agree that cluster headaches are related to abnormal expansion and contraction of blood vessels, but the actual cause (or perhaps multiple causes) of these changes is not known.

Alcohol consumption, smoking, and drug consumption are the most common triggers for cluster headaches. Ninety-one percent of cluster sufferers drink regularly, with two-thirds of them professing to be heavy drinkers. Ninety-four percent are smokers, but there is no evidence that cluster headaches improve if they stop smoking. Many cluster headache sufferers take an assortment of medications in an effort to reduce the pain.

TRAUMA

Trauma headaches occur after an injury to the head, neck, or spine. They may begin within 24 hours after the injury, but can occur for the first time years after the accident. A minor bump can cause chronic headaches, even though a neurological exam fails to demonstrate injury. Headaches caused by trauma can mimic migraine or tension headaches, as well as vascular headaches. The pain can be aching, stabbing, excruciating, dull, or sharp at the site of the injury.

Other accompanying symptoms can include runny or stuffy nose, postnasal drip, and sneezing; diarrhea; fever; sweating on forehead, abdomen, and trunk; drooping, red, and tearing eye; visual and sensory disturbances; insomnia; anxiety; limited attention span; weakness, shakiness, and blacking out; irritability; intolerance for noise and light; or nausea and vomiting. These headaches may come in clusters, they may be continuous, they may occur daily, or they may be rare. They can last from 20 minutes to all day long.

If the headache is related to a forgotten trauma, it can be difficult to diagnose. The trauma may be as simple as bumping the head of a playmate, or physical trauma from a fall as a toddler. It may even be related to the use of forceps or complications at birth. Whiplash injury can cause headaches even if there was no actual blow. The force of being jerked can exert pressure on the muscles, ligaments, and tendons of the neck, head, and spine that can damage nerves and bruise blood vessels in the brain. Closed head injuries cause excessive pain because the brain takes the force of the blow, whereas in a fracture the blow is absorbed by the bone. The vibration from the blow may bruise the brain and interfere with neurotransmitters and nerve connections. The inner ear can also be damaged, which can result in vertigo and ringing in the ear.

The delay that sometimes accompanies the onset of trauma headaches is difficult to understand. A buildup of scar tissue is a possible explanation for the delay. Other existing problems can also make it difficult for the body to sustain enough energy to heal the wound and maintain other systems. Among these problems are food, chemical, and environmental allergies and sensitivities; candidiasis and other infections; digestive disturbances; nutritional disturbances; structural imbalances; changes in weather and altitude; dental problems, blood clotting problems; and emotional or psychological factors.

ALLERGY/SENSITIVITY

Seventy percent of all headaches may be allergy/sensitivity headaches that are triggered by reactions to foods, chemicals, inhalants, and other substances. In allergy/sensitivity headaches the temporal arteries in the skull expand, the vessel walls are thinned, and fluid leaks into surrounding tissues. This causes the brain to swell, and pain occurs as the tissues stretch and the brain presses against the skull. Allergy/sensitivity headaches usually begin within 4 to 12 hours after exposure to the substance (although for some people the onset may be more rapid). Generalized head pain can be aching, throbbing, or dull, and may be felt continuously or in brief jolts. It is worsened by activity.

Other symptoms accompanying this type of headache include:

- nasal congestion, sneezing, or watery eyes;
- weakness, nervousness, anxiety, or depression;
- increased need to urinate and an urge to move the bowels;
- dizziness, lightheadedness, and faintness;
- cold, clammy hands and feet;
- stomach pain and diarrhea;
- nausea and vomiting;
- hot flashes followed by chills;
- intolerance to noise and light; and
- symptoms that resemble an alcoholic hangover.

These headaches are easily confused with other types of headaches, both because the symptoms may be similar to those of other types, and because allergy headaches are frequently caused by a combination of factors. As well, the reaction is often delayed—making it difficult to connect the headache with the causative factor(s).

Allergy/sensitivity headaches can be caused by many substances, including:

- airborne pollutants;
- foods and food preservatives;
- the consumption of cold foods or of too much sugar, coffee, or junk food;
- overindulgence in either food or alcohol (hangover);
- nutritional deficiencies that result from a poor diet (vitamin and mineral deficiencies);
- low blood sugar (hypoglycemia) after skipped or irregular meals;
- constipation, which allows toxins in the stool to be absorbed back into the bloodstream;
- hormonal imbalances;
- nutritional and enzyme deficiencies;
- leaky gut and other digestive disturbances;
- circulation problems;
- a compromised immune system;
- physical trauma;
- drugs;
- heavy metals; and
- water that is not tolerated.

SINUS

Sinus headaches represent fewer than 2 percent of all headaches. Sinus headaches begin as pressure between the eyebrows, above or below the eye sockets, or in the eyes, forehead, bridge of the nose, and cheekbones. The pressure increases and results in a gnawing, dull, aching pain, tenderness, and swelling. There may also be pressure in the back of the head and neck and/or in the top of the head, and the headache intensifies as the day progresses. A sinus headache may last for as little as one hour, or it can last all day. It can be accompanied by a runny nose, postnasal drip, red and teary eyes, and fever; bending over will increase the throbbing in the face and forehead. Fifteen to twenty percent of people who have migraines also have sinus headaches.

Sinus headaches are caused when there is an infection or mucus buildup in the sinus tissues. This creates pressure against the sinus linings, which swell, push against nerve endings, and cause pain.

The most common causes of sinus headaches are:

- colds (because they cause mucus production and can lead to infection);
- sinusitis (the medical term for a sinus infection);
- allergies that bring on heavy secretion of phlegm and mucus;
- an anatomical deformity (either inherited or resulting from an injury);
- a deviated septum (a misalignment of the wall that divides the two nostrils);
- nasal polyps (non-cancerous growths in the nasal passages);
- muscle tension and structural misalignments that produce vascular changes in the face;
- pain referred from another location but felt in the sinuses; and
- stress, which can cause excess mucus secretion.

TMJ/DENTAL

The American Dental Association estimates that as many as 60 million Americans may have temporomandibular joint (TMJ) syndrome. Dental problems such as tooth decay, crooked teeth,

impacted wisdom teeth, gum disease, jaw misalignment, ill-fitting dentures, muscle spasms, and low-grade infections can irritate the nerves in the jaw and cause a headache. The stress that all these conditions bring to the lower jaw causes muscular and structural compensations in the jaw, and triggers symptoms that include a sore jaw joint, difficulty chewing or talking—and headaches.

The junction of the temporal bone of the skull and the side of the lower jaw (the mandible)—just in front of each ear—is known as the temporomandibular joint. It is this joint that is active in opening and closing the mouth, and if that action is not balanced on each side, a sensation of pressure and pain will result.

A TMJ/dental headache is characterized by dull, steady pain, usually felt as pressure on top of the head. Chronic TMJ occurs daily, but most TMJ headaches occur from twice a week to once a month or even more infrequently. TMJ headaches last from one hour to all day long. With TMJ, there is a tendency to chew on only one side. Chewing is painful and tiring, and there may be a clicking sound when chewing. People with TMJ may grind and clench their teeth; their smile may be strained; and they may have bleeding gums; pain in the face, neck, and/or shoulder; and sometimes an earache.

In addition to the conditions already mentioned, triggers of a TMJ/dental headache include:

- a faulty or uneven bite;
- dental infections;
- trauma to the mouth or head (which can throw the entire jaw out of alignment);
- muscular imbalances;
- gait and postural problems;
- mercury amalgam fillings (which are highly toxic and can cause headaches and other symptoms);
- constriction of blood vessels in the head brought on by stresses in the mouth and jaw;

- hormonal imbalances;
- diet and allergy (which may interfere with the development of the teeth and upper jaw); and
- stress (which can lead to teeth grinding, clenching of the jaw, and nail biting—which in turn can worsen muscle spasm and contribute to the pain cycle).

Some apparently harmless habits can cause stress on the teeth and jaw and contribute to head pain and headaches. Whether or not you have headaches, it is best to avoid the following activities: yawning excessively or widely; chewing gum, candy, ice, and hard crunchy foods; playing with your jaw; resting your chin or cheek in your palm; cradling the telephone receiver between your jaw and neck; reading, eating, or watching TV while lying down; licking your teeth; clenching your teeth; biting or licking your lips; biting or sucking your cheeks; sucking or chewing on pens and pencils; and chewing only on one side of the mouth. According to Dr. Michael Gello, director of the TMJ and Facial Pain Program at the New York University College of Dentistry, wearing improperly fitting shoes can also cause headaches because there is a definite and important relationship between the mouth and the feet.

EYESTRAIN

Eyestrain headaches result from referred pain initiated in the muscles around the eyes. Squinting, straining, blinking, and carrying out visually stressful tasks put pressure on the muscles across the face and scalp, and eventually result in frontal pain that is felt behind the eyes. Eyestrain headaches are often triggered by presbyopia (a progressive decrease in the ability to focus at close range); refractive disorders (which cause blurred vision or an inability to see objects that are either too near or too far away); or astigmatism (an irregularity in the curvature of the lens of the eye that results in blurred vision).

Eyestrain headaches can also be caused by an inability of the two eyes to work together; by postural problems (sitting bent over a desk while reading or doing close work for long periods of time); wearing improperly fitted contact lenses or glasses (or wearing lenses for too long); by uncorrected vision; by poor lighting; and by prolonged exposure to computer screens, video monitors, or television screens.

The pain of an eyestrain headache resembles that of a tension headache; it is a steady pain that may be felt as pressure on the top of the head. The eyes may be teary or reddened and may hurt. The duration of these headaches may be as short as one hour, or they may last all day. They usually begin while a person is reading or doing close work, and often happen in the afternoons or on weekends.

REBOUND

Rebound headaches are caused by the very medications people take to relieve the pain of their original headache. Rebound headaches occur as soon as the medication wears off, forcing the person to take more medication and thus starting the cycle again. It is the consumption and withdrawal of the stimulants that are added to these medications, as well as the medications themselves, that cause the roller-coaster effect. After a year or two on such a cycle, the headaches are constant, and the patient does not know why. Eighty percent of all headache sufferers experience rebound headaches.

Rebound headaches begin 12 to 24 hours after the last dose of medication has been taken. They begin with a feeling of fullness in the head, and symptoms and pain peak in 20 to 48 hours; headache intensity then decreases over the next five to six days. Rebound headaches are generalized, with throbbing and steady jolts of pain. There may also be anxiety; nervousness; restlessness; irritability; depression; fatigue; nausea; intolerance of movement, noise, or light; a tender scalp; stiff neck; and insomnia. Some people may experience flu-like symptoms.

There are several types of rebound headaches, including analgesic (painkiller) rebound headaches and caffeine withdrawal headaches. People can develop rebound headaches even from such painkillers as Tylenol and aspirin. Weekend, holiday, and travel headaches are rebound headaches, but are usually experienced by people who change their coffee, tea, or soda consumption patterns during those periods. Post-surgery headaches are also rebound headaches. They were originally attributed to the affects of general anesthetic, but it is now becoming evident that they may be related to caffeine withdrawal resulting from the requirement that patients eat and drink nothing for 12 to 24 hours before surgery.

A positive response to three or more of the following questions indicates that a headache is probably a rebound headache:

- Do the headaches occur daily or almost daily?
- Are caffeinated products, over-the-counter medications, or prescription drugs consumed daily?
- Is the person suffering headaches anxious, irritable, or depressed?
- Does the person have difficulty sleeping?
- Are there periodic attacks of more serious headaches (migraines or cluster headaches)?
- Do headaches run in the family?

EXERTION

Exertion headaches are usually harmless, short-lived headaches. They occur with equal frequency in men and women, and are typically seen in people over the age of 40. They usually last for about 20 minutes, but can continue for the entire day. The pain is sharp and throbbing and can be either generalized or localized. Although their sudden appearance can be frightening, exertion headaches are rarely a sign of a more serious condition.

There are three types of exertion headaches.

Exercise headaches are seen in people 40 and older who are out of shape and rarely push their bodies, and occurs when they begin an exercise program or take part in strenuous exercise. Sexual headaches are triggered by the exertion of lovemaking or masturbation. They are more common in men and usually begin just before or during orgasm. Coughing headaches begin during or after coughing, sneezing, crying, laughing, or straining the bowels.

Exertion headaches can also be triggered by the Valsalva maneuver—in which a person automatically holds the breath and bears down in order to clear the ears after steep ascents or descents, or preparatory to exertion or having a bowel movement. This backs up the blood and rushes pressure into the head, stretching the blood vessels. Hormonal changes, structural abnormalities, poor cardiovascular fitness, hyperventilation (panting breaths), unexpressed or hidden emotions, and abrupt movements that throw the body out of alignment can also play a role in exertion headaches. People with other headache conditions seem prone to exertion headaches as well.

MODERN MEDICAL TREATMENT

Diet

Dietary recommendations for headache are mainly confined to migraine. Physicians tell their patients to avoid tyramine-containing foods such as alcoholic beverages, bananas, broad beans, aged cheese, cultured dairy products, eggplant, hot dogs, bologna, meat tenderizers, nuts, soy sauce, yeast, and yeast extracts. Chocolate contains a chemical relative of tyramine that can contribute to headaches.

Exercise and Lifestyle

Exercise may help reduce the frequency and severity of some migraines, as well as some cluster headaches. However, most physicians do not routinely suggest exercise as treatment for head-ache, as patients report that both migraine and cluster headaches can also be triggered by exercise.

Biofeedback techniques are recommended for all types of headaches, and relaxation techniques can help with tension headaches. It is sometimes suggested that people modify aspects of their behavior in order to control headaches—for instance, that they avoid sleeping late, maintain a regular sleeping pattern, and that they stop smoking.

Simple techniques often help to relieve headache pain: cold compresses to the head and neck, rest in a quiet dark room with the head higher than the rest of the body, pressure to the temples, and cold water to the hands or the whole body can be soothing.

Drug Therapy

Modern medicine's primary approach to pain control for most types of headache is the use of pharmaceuticals. For pain control in simple headaches, physicians may prescribe over-the-counter drugs such as acetylsalicylic acid (Anacin, Empirin, Genuine Bayer aspirin) and acetaminophen (Tylenol, Maximum Strength Panadol). Non-steroidal medications work much as aspirin does, but offer more pain control. They include ibuprofen (Advil, Motrin, Nuprin), naproxen (Aleve, Anaprox, Naprosyn), diclofenac (Voltaren), and mefenamic acid (Ponstel). If more pain control appears to be needed, physicians can prescribe painkillers such as butalbital (Fiorinal, Fioricet), codeine sulfate or phosphate (Tylenol #3, Fiorinal #3), hydrocodone (Lortab, Vicodin), meperidine (Demerol), morphine (Duramorph), oxycodone (Percocet), pentazocine (Talwin), or propoxyphene (Darvon).

Muscle relaxants may be prescribed for tension headaches. For a discussion of these medications and their side effects, see Back Pain in chapter 14, Musculoskeletal Problems.

Methysergide maleate (Sansert) prevents or reduces the intensity or frequency of migraine and cluster headaches. Side effects include fibrotic changes in tissues (a thickening of cardiac, pulmonary, and peritoneal tissues). The drug can also cause nausea, vomiting, diarrhea, heartburn, abdominal pain, insomnia, drowsiness, dizziness, flushing, edema of the extremities, weight gain, neutropenia (a decrease in the normal number of neutrophils, a type of white blood cell), and eosinophilia (a increase above the normal number of eosinophils, a type of white blood cell), weakness, and joint and muscle pain.

Sumatriptan (Imitrex) is used for migraine, and may be given by injection, tablet, nose spray, or suppository. This drug mimics serotonin, which is in short supply before and during migraines. Although many people achieve relief with this drug, for some it works less well each time it is used. Side effects include gastroesophageal reflux, diarrhea, burping, gas, joint pain, mental confusion, chills, rashes, tingling, sensation of warmth, and cardiovascular events.

Like Imitrex, zolmitriptan (Zomig) has an affinity for serotonin receptors on blood vessels. It does not have a prophylactic action, but is used for management of migraines. Its effectiveness has not been established for cluster headaches. All adverse side effects are described as infrequent and include allergic reactions, chills, facial edema, arrhythmias, hypertension, increased appetite, thirst, back pain, leg cramps, bronchitis and bronchospasms, itching, rashes, dry eyes, and eye and ear pain. There have been rare serious cardiac events.

Ergot alkaloids are used in the early stages of migraine headaches. They work by narrowing the dilated blood vessels that cause the headache pain. These drugs can cause nausea, vomiting, and muscle weakness, and may also cause blood circulation problems because they constrict the blood vessels. Doses must be closely monitored.

Other side effects include leg cramps, numbness and tingling of the fingers and toes, chest pain, abnormal heart rate, and itching and swelling of the extremities. If taken frequently, rebound dilation of the blood vessels develops when the effects of the medication wear off. Ergotamine (Ergomar, Ergostat, Cafergot, Wigraine) may be used as a tablet, an inhaler, suppository, or an injection, depending on the medication. Dihydroergotamine (DHE) is given intravenously, and dihydroergotamine mesylate (Migranal) is given in a nasal spray.

Midrin (a combination tablet containing a vasoactive to constrict blood vessels, an analgesic, and a sedative substance) is used to abort migraines. Its side effects include dizziness and rash. Midrin cannot be used by patients with high blood pressure, glaucoma, or those on MAO inhibitors (see pp. 409–10).

Adrenergic blocking agents (beta blockers) are used to block migraines with uncommonly severe pain, or those that occur very frequently. Beta blockers include propanolol (Inderal), timolol (Blocadren), and nadolol (Corgard). They are taken orally, and prevent the dilation of blood vessels. These drugs can cause slowing of the heart rate, which in turn can cause fatigue, depression, and anxiety. People with asthma who take beta blockers may experience more difficulty in breathing. (For more discussion of beta blockers see p. 190.)

Calcium channel blockers, which decrease spasms of the arteries, can be useful for people with migraines who cannot take beta blockers. Verapamil (Calan, Isoptin, Verelan) and nifedipine (Adalat, Procardia) are among these drugs, which are taken orally. They may cause constipation, dizziness, and weight gain. (For more discussion of calcium channel blockers, see pp. 189–90.)

Antidepressants are also used, at times, to prevent migraines. Taken orally in low doses, amitriptyline (Elavil, Endep) and doxepin (Sinequan) can prevent migraine attacks for some people. However, these drugs can cause drowsiness, and they also interact with other drugs. (See pp. 409–11 for more discussion of antidepressants.)

ALTERNATIVE TREATMENT

Diet

To help reduce the causes of headaches, practice good dietary habits and do not skip meals. Because food allergy plays a major role in migraines, identify and avoid food allergens, or receive treatment for food allergies (see Food Allergy, p. 382).

Exercise and Lifestyle

Exercising for 20 to 30 minutes three times a week can help to reduce the severity and frequency of headaches. Exercise reduces stress, eliminates constipation, stabilizes hormones and blood pressure, strengthens internal organs, promotes vascular and muscle tone, and produces natural painkilling endorphins.

Try a yoga exercise called the "neck roll." To do the neck roll, kneel on the floor and place your forehead on the floor (or on a folded towel). Position your hands under your shoulders; breathe out slowly and roll your head forward, gently, to stretch the back of the neck, then return to the starting position. Repeat 20 times. It is best to learn yoga exercises from a professional. Do *not* use this exercise if you have neck problems.

Do an environmental cleanup to help eliminate headaches triggered by chemical sensitivities (see Chemical Sensitivities, p. 388).

Reducing stress in your life will also help remove some headache triggers:

- Assess and modify your schedule to reduce the stressful components of your life.
- Use biofeedback techniques, sound or music therapy, breathing exercises, and meditation or guided imagery, both to relax and to help you handle headache pain.

- Try self-hypnosis, while sitting in a comfortable chair with no distractions. Close your eyes and relax all of your muscles, one at a time; then focus on a pleasant image or visualize the cause of your headache vanishing.

Correct your sleeping habits:

- Be sure to get enough sleep.
- Be sure your sleeping position is relaxed and use a pillow of the proper height.
- Get up at the same time each day and do not sleep late.
- If you grind your teeth at night, see a dentist about a bite plate.

Nutrient Therapy
Useful nutritional supplements are:

- vitamin B-complex – 50 mg of most of the B vitamins, three times a day (balances extra B_6)
- vitamin B_2 – up to 400 mg a day (in total when combined with the amount in the B-complex) (prevents migraine headache)
- vitamin B_3 – up to 300 mg a day (in total when combined with the amount in the B-complex) (vasodilation; improves circulation)
- vitamin B_5 – up to 200 mg a day (in total when combined with the amount in the B-complex) (anti-stress vitamin)
- vitamin B_6 – 50 mg three times a day, over and above the amount in the B-complex (acts as a mild diuretic)
- vitamin C – 2,000 to 8,000 mg a day in divided doses (antihistamine action; anti-inflammatory)
- vitamin E – 400 IU a day initially, gradually working up to 1,200 IU a day (improves circulation)
- calcium – 1,500 mg a day (dilates blood vessels; relaxes muscles)
- chromium – 150 mcg a day (in picolinate or nicotinate form) (helps maintain blood sugar levels)

- copper – 3 mg a day (needed for healthy nerves)
- magnesium – 1,000 mg a day (increase dose if muscles are tense) (alleviates muscle tension)
- potassium – 100 mg a day (prevents water retention)
- zinc – 30 to 50 mg a day (needed to balance copper)
- bioflavonoids – 500 to 1,500 mg a day (stabilizes blood vessels; inhibits inflammation)
- choline – 500 to 1,000 mg a day (necessary for proper transmission of nerve impulses)
- coenzyme Q_{10} – 30 mg twice a day (improves oxygenation of tissues)
- evening primrose oil – 500 mg three to four times a day (essential for transmission of nerve impulses)
- L-glutamine – 500 mg twice a day (for relief of cluster headaches)
- L-tyrosine – as directed on your product (for relief of cluster headaches)
- quercetin – 500 mg twice a day (anti-inflammatory action). *Caution:* Do not take if taking an MAO inhibitor drug.

Herbal Therapy
Herbal preparations are helpful in treating headaches. Those listed below are but a few of the many possibilities. If you have frequent, serious headaches, seek professional help.

- bilberry – eyestrain headaches
- cayenne pepper – cluster and vascular headaches
- chamomile – allergy headaches
- coriander – trauma headaches
- feverfew – migraine preventative, tension headaches
- goldenseal – dental headaches. *Caution:* Do not take if you are pregnant.
- meadowsweet – rebound and general headaches
- peppermint – tension and sinus headaches
- skullcap – stress headaches
- valerian – headache prevention

Homeopathic Remedies

Numerous homeopathic remedies will help with many different types of headaches. Only a few are listed below. If you do not experience relief with these remedies, seek the help of a homeopathic practitioner.

- *Arsenicum album* – headache associated with eating foods that are too cold or fatty; pain alternates between head or stomach; scalp itches intolerably; walks with head thrown backwards; worse after midnight, right side.
- *Belladonna* – sudden and violent, throbbing pain; bursting headache in temples; eyes bloodshot and red; restlessness, congestion, red-flushed face; right-sided migraine; burning sinuses and temples; light and sound intolerance; sun headache with full pounding pulse.
- *Bryonia* – acute head, eye, or forehead pain, especially on the left side; worse motion; nausea, constipation, and irritability; headache after injury; headache when stooping, as if brain would burst through forehead; headache brought on by playing or watching others play.
- *Glonoinum* – throbbing pain; worse sun exposure or heat; blurred vision with dizziness; intolerance to heat and motion; sunstroke and headache without unconsciousness; better cold application, keeping head high, or long sleep; short nap sometimes aggravates; violent headache.
- *Iris versicolor* – right-sided migraine; vomit is bitter and relieves pain; burning and acidity; throbbing and severe pain causes disturbance of vision; worse rest; sick headaches with diarrhea; worse coughing, cold air; better gentle motion.
- *Natrum muriaticum* – headaches associated with menstruation, before, during, and after; pain comes after reading; headache develops after intense mental work; disturbance in vi-

sion; ambitious, driving, and eager to achieve; headache increases with rise of the sun and stops at sunset; sweating; fiery zigzag before headache; hammering as if hammers knocking in the head; bursting, compressing as if in a vise, as if the skull would be crushed; general migraine.

- *Nux vomica* – splitting pain upon waking or after overeating or drinking; nausea, vomiting, irritability, and oversensitivity; intense, ambitious personality; irritability and anxiety; overwork; too little sleep; aching pain as if beaten; headache better in the evening.
- *Silicea* – migraine-like pain that travels from neck to one eye; sometimes vomiting; pain in the nape of the neck; associated with nervous exhaustion; headache relieved by wrapping and covering; worse in dark and better in light.
- *Sulphur* – vascular type headaches; hot head, cold feet; constant heat on top of head; heaviness and fullness; beating headache, worse stooping and with vertigo; sick headaches; better open air; worse standing.

Other Therapeutic Measures

The following substances can be used for relief of headache pain:

- White willow bark is a mild pain remedy containing salicin, which is similar to aspirin. Use one to two capsules (500 mg each) up to three times a day. White willow bark is available at health food stores and has no cornstarch filler, so is suitable for corn-sensitive patients.
- DL-Phenlyalanine (DLPA) causes the endorphins of the body (and painkillers) to be metabolized more slowly. DLPA can be taken alone or with a pain reliever.
- Bi-carb Formula (from Klaire Laboratories—see Sources) will reduce acidity, and correcting body pH will help relieve headache pain. There is a pH shift with all headaches and al-

lergic reactions. Take four to six capsules initially, followed by two to four capsules every 15 to 30 minutes.

- "Magic Brew" will relieve headache pain by reducing acidity and correcting pH imbalance. Mix 1 tsp. of salt and 1 tsp. of baking soda in 1 quart of water and chill. Slowly sip 1 cup of this mixture.
- Vitamin C (either buffered C or ascorbic acid) will help relieve headache pain. Take 2,000 to 4,000 mg of vitamin C every 15 to 30 minutes (alternating buffered C and ascorbic acid, as bowel tolerance permits).
- Organic germanium improves tissue oxygenation. Two to three capsules will help relieve a headache. Repeat if needed.

Use hydrotherapy to relieve headache pain. Placing the hands in ice water relieves headaches for some people. For others, several repetitions of the following treatment will reduce headache pain significantly. Take a bath in water as hot as you can stand it, submerged as deeply as you can be. Soak until the water cools off, then drain the tub, refill with hot water, and repeat the soak.

You can also soak your feet and ankles in hot water while using an ice pack or cold cloth at your forehead and temples. (Limit the cold treatment to 20 minutes to avoid damage to the skin.) Try applying ice packs to the neck and upper back for tension headache, and to the area of pain for other headaches. Take alternating hot and cold showers, or use alternating hot and cold water on your wrists.

Try aromatherapy to ease headaches: add one drop of peppermint essential oil to an unscented lotion and apply the lotion under the nose and behind the ears. To reduce the intensity of headache pain, inhale the vapors directly from the bottle of peppermint oil. Or rub eucalyptus oil on the temples and forehead to relieve headache pain.

You can also use Ayurvedic headache remedies:

- Sip a mixture of 1 Tbsp. of sugar, ¼ tsp. of salt, and the juice of half a lime in 1 pint of water for a "vata" headache (one caused by constipation and frequently accompanied by dehydration; aggravated by high altitude).
- Mix 1 tsp. of sandalwood powder with enough water to make a paste, and apply to the forehead and temples for a "pitta" headache (shooting, burning, piercing pain that is worsened by bright light and associated with nausea; these headaches are related to stomach problems).
- Mix ½ tsp. of ginger powder, 1 tsp. of cinnamon, and a pinch of clove powder into a cup of boiling water for a "kapha" headache (occurs in the winter and spring, generally strikes in the morning and evening, and is worse when bending down). Steep for a few minutes, then strain and drink.

An enema can help with headaches by removing toxins from the body. Use a plain water cleansing enema, or a coffee retention enema using caffeinated organic coffee. For the latter, take two small enemas, one after the other, not exceeding two cups volume per enema. Make the coffee using 2 Tbsp. of coffee per quart of water; allow the coffee to cool before using. Hang the enema bag low to prevent the enema from going up too high in the colon. If the correct low volume is used, the caffeine in the coffee will not cause a "buzz" response.

Consider having your mercury amalgam fillings removed. If possible, consult a biological dentist for advice and help (see Sources).

Use Five Flower Remedy, or Bach Flower Rescue remedy to help clear a headache.

Headaches also respond to bodywork. Use reflexology to relax the body, working the solar plexus, eye, ear, and head points on the hands as well as the face points on the hands and lower back points on the feet. Have massage done by a professional, or you can use a simple routine yourself. Use fingertips to massage the scalp, temples, forehead, and back of the neck. Finish with a shoulder rub.

Use Feldenkrais work, Trager work, or shiatsu to help in easing or preventing headaches (see Bodywork, p. 85) or you might want to consult a chiropractor (see Chiropractic, p. 79) or an osteopath.

Use acupuncture both to clear and to prevent headaches. Press on the following acupressure points:

- Press the center of the webbing of your hand with your thumb slightly toward the bone that connects with the index finger. Hold for one minute, then switch hands. *Caution:* Pregnant women should not try this technique as it may cause uterine contractions.
- Press the hollow areas at the base of the skull, two to three inches apart. Close your eyes and tilt your head slowly back. Hold for one to two minutes and take deep, long breaths.

- Press the center hollow at the base of the skull with your right thumb. With your left thumb and index finger, press the hollows of your eye sockets near the bridge of your nose. Tilt your head back and breathe deeply for one to two minutes while holding these points.

Have biofeedback training, which can be effective in dealing with several different types of headaches. In biofeedback training, a monitor helps patients gain control over body function such as blood pressure, circulation, digestion, heart rate, and perspiration. This allows the patient to become aware of problem areas and to learn voluntary control of physiological responses. Once the control has been learned, the monitor is no longer necessary.

CHAPTER 13

Respiratory System Problems

The respiratory system consists of the nose, nasal cavity, pharynx, larynx, trachea, bronchi, and lungs. Oxygen is supplied to the cells and carbon dioxide removed by the respiratory system, along with the circulatory system. The respiratory system also makes it possible for us to speak, sing, and laugh by varying the tension of the vocal cords as exhaled air passes over them. The upper respiratory passages extend from the nose to the level of the vocal cords. The bronchial tube system (lower respiratory tract) extends from the vocal cords through the lungs.

UPPER RESPIRATORY TRACT INFECTIONS

Upper respiratory tract infections (URIs) affect the nose, sinuses, and throat, and can ultimately affect the ears. They are the most common infectious diseases seen in North America. URIs cause more than 250 million days of work to be lost each year in the U.S., are the reason for over 100 million physician office visits, and instigate the expenditure of over $500 million on non-prescription cold remedies. Upper respiratory infections include the common cold, influenza (flu), otitis media (ear infections), sinusitis, and pharyngitis (sore throat, strep throat, and mononucleosis). Although some of these diseases are caused by bacteria, most are caused by viruses.

COLDS AND FLU

Colds are the most common URI in the world, and they cause more acute illness than any other disease. The common cold can be caused by any of over 200 viruses, from five different families of viruses, which is why it is possible for us to catch colds again and again. The average adult has two to four colds a year, while children generally have six to eight. Nearly half the United States population will catch a cold during a given year, with 40 percent of the cases developing into flu.

The most common cold virus is a rhinovirus, but parainfluenza virus, respiratory syncytial virus (RSV), adenovirus, and coronavirus can all cause colds. Because a different virus affects us each time we catch a cold, and viruses also mutate and change, it has been impossible to develop an effective vaccine against colds. To be effective, the vaccine would have to stimulate the immune system to make antibodies against all 200 cold viruses and their mutations. Several years ago the molecular receptor that enables rhinoviruses to infect human nasal passage cells was discovered, and this may increase the possibilities of developing an effective vaccine. However, there are at least seven other types of viruses that also cause colds and probably have different receptor sites.

Cold Symptoms

A cold is an infection of the membrane lining the upper respiratory tract, including the nose, the sinuses, and the throat. The membrane swells, and in an attempt to trap the viruses, increases its rate of mucus formation. This results in congestion, stuffiness, and nose blowing. The increased mucus formation also leads to a postnasal drip, which is irritating and causes the scratchy throat and cough of a cold. A change in voice quality occurs because the blocked nasal cavity is no longer available as a resonating chamber. In addition, laryngitis (pain and hoarseness caused by inflammation of the voice box and lower throat) can develop.

The sinuses usually become blocked because of the excessive swelling of the membranes, resulting in sinus pressure and a headache. Swelling in the upper throat can block the Eustachian tubes that lead to the ears. This blockage can cause accumulation of fluid and pressure in the middle ear, which can be painful and can affect the patient's hearing.

A cold is a self-limiting infection that usually runs its course in a week to 10 days. If a cold has not gone away within that time period, it is possible that the patient has developed a secondary infection: perhaps an acute sinusitis, a middle ear infection, acute bronchitis, or pneumonia. Secondary infections require additional treatment. Sometimes a cold will clear, the patient will enjoy a few days of good health, and then the sore throat and nasal symptoms will start again. In that case, there is either an allergy, or a new cold caused by a different virus. It is possible to have cold after cold, each caused by a different virus.

Although a cold can develop at any time of year, cold viruses usually circulate during cold weather. Twenty percent of rhinovirus cases present in September, seventy-five percent of parainfluenza cases occur between October and January, and approximately fifty percent of respiratory syncytial virus (RSV) colds appear between December and February. It is unfortunate that the term "cold" has been given to this type of infection, because it implies that the cold weather, walking in the rain, sitting in a draft, or getting chilled causes a cold. There is no evidence to support this; a cold or the flu is always caused by an infecting organism. The increased incidence of colds in the winter reflects the fact that people spend more time indoors in bad weather, making the transfer of viruses from person to person that much easier.

Many physicians prescribe antibiotics for a cold, even though antibiotics are not effective against viruses. The usual justification for this practice is that the antibiotic will guard against or treat any secondary infection. This practice has led to the overuse of antibiotics, and has contributed to the problem of bacterial resistance to antibiotics.

Flu Symptoms

Sometimes it is difficult to tell whether an infection is a cold or the flu, as they begin in a similar fashion, and many of the symptoms are the same for both conditions. Although influenza is caused by the same viruses that cause colds (as well as the influenza virus) it develops more quickly, it is more debilitating, and the person with flu will often say, "I feel as if I've been hit by a truck." Both the upper and lower respiratory tracts are affected by the flu, and it can be accompanied by diarrhea, vomiting, and acute fatigue. In susceptible individuals, the flu can lead to pneumonia. Colds seldom cause a fever of over 101°F, as flu does, and influenza victims may also experience chills and coughing spasms. People with colds can usually go about their daily activities while they are sick, whereas people with the flu cannot.

December and January are the months during which flu epidemics hit. While flu is generally not considered to be a serious disease, it contributes to 20,000 deaths each year in the United States. World-wide epidemics of new, virulent strains of influenza also appear from time to time, causing many more deaths. In susceptible people, the flu can develop into a secondary bacterial pneumonia, and some flu viruses can themselves cause pneumonia. If pneumonia develops, the cough will be deeper, there can be chest pain with the cough, and there may be shortness of breath. These complications can require hospitalization and/or time off work spent at home in bed (see Pneumonia, below).

Catching Colds or the Flu

We catch colds and the flu from other people when they sneeze or cough, or even when we shake hands (40 percent of people with a rhinovirus cold have the virus on their hands). It is now known that cold viruses can survive for up to three hours outside the body. During that time they can live on the skin, as well as on hard, nonporous surfaces such as telephones, doorknobs, and countertops. RSV can survive on the skin for 15 minutes, and for hours in droplets and on environmental surfaces. An influenza virus survives for up to three days on a nonporous surface, but for only 10 minutes on the skin.

You can literally pick up viruses from these surfaces, and if you touch your eyes, nose, or mouth, the virus enters your body. It is estimated that 40 percent of colds are contracted in this manner. However, the main route of transmission for both cold and flu viruses is the air, where they arrive via sneezing, coughing, and nose blowing.

Around 25 percent of the people infected with rhinovirus do not develop cold symptoms. Their immune systems are strong enough to fight off the infection. Studies suggest that stress, allergic disorders, and other factors that burden the immune system can lower resistance to infection. The result of an exposure to any kind of infection depends on the ability of the body to resist it. Maintaining a healthy immune system is the best defense against colds and the flu—or any other infection.

The chances of developing a viral infection are directly related to the amount of stress a person is under. The stress causes the release of hormones that shrink the thymus, reducing its immune activity. Studies done by Cohen, Tyrell, and Smith, and reported in the August 1991 *New England Journal of Medicine,* showed that people who experienced high degrees of anger and tension were four times more likely to develop a cold than those who did not experience those emotions.

Allergies also play a role in infection by decreasing resistance to infection. Dairy products are mucus producers and cause congestion, which increases susceptibility. Airborne allergens (dust, pollen, mold, and animal danders) may decrease resistance and permit viral infections to get a foothold in the respiratory tract. Congested, swollen membranes in the nose, sinuses, and throat are vulnerable to attack by infecting organisms, both viral and bacterial.

MODERN MEDICAL PREVENTION

Diet

Patients are advised to eat a well-balanced diet.

Exercise and Lifestyle

Regular exercise programs should be stopped during acute colds and flu. Patients are advised to stop smoking and to avoid getting chilled.

Flu Vaccines

Modern medicine considers the influenza vaccine to be 90 percent effective in preventing influenza in adults. Because the influenza virus strains (A and B) mutate rapidly, flu vaccines are manufactured with viral strains from Asia, where the flu season is six months ahead of ours and mutations that will later affect us have already taken place. Patients may be advised to have a flu shot unless they are allergic to eggs or thimerosal (a preservative); have had a bad reaction to a previous flu shot; or are pregnant or plan to become pregnant within the next three months.

Older people and high-risk individuals should probably take the vaccine between October 15 and November 15. However, many people hesitate to have a flu shot because there are frequent reports of flu-like symptoms following the inoculation. Manufacturers of the vaccine claim that the only common side effect of the vaccine is soreness at the vaccination site, and that fewer than 5 percent of those vaccinated experience fever, muscle soreness, and general achiness for one to two days afterward.

Other Therapeutic Measures

A very important part of prevention is hand-washing after being exposed to someone who has a cold or the flu. Patients are advised to avoid touching their eyes or nose until they have washed their hands with soap and warm water. They are told to wash for at least 30 seconds and to scrub fingernails and creases between the fingers. Increasing the frequency of hand-washing can significantly cut down on winter colds and flus.

Patients who have colds and flu are told to cover their nose and mouth when they sneeze or cough. People are advised to avoid a cold by covering their nose and mouth when they are around people who have colds and flus. They should refrain from kissing people who have an upper respiratory infection, particularly during the first three days of the infection. They are also advised against sharing food, drinking glasses, eating utensils, or eyeglasses with the sick person. They are also told to disinfect contaminated articles and equipment that is shared with others, and to cover all open wounds.

ALTERNATIVE PREVENTION

Diet

Reduce sweets in your diet, as they impair the infection-fighting ability of white blood cells. Eat less fat, in order to prevent the immune system having to work overtime to prevent a cold, as well as heart disease and cancer. Eat more fresh fruits and vegetables. Drink more water, juices, and herbal teas. Limit or stop alcohol intake.

Exercise and Lifestyle

Strengthen your immune system by managing and reducing your stress. Get regular exercise, but be careful not to overdo. Overtraining can cause an increase in the number of respiratory infections.

Nutrient Therapy

Take the following nutrients to help prevent colds and flus.

- vitamin C – to bowel tolerance every day (strengthens immune system)
- Monolaurin – 500 to 1,500 mg a day (prevents viral attachment to cells) (Cardiovascular Research—see Sources)
- L-lysine – 500 to 1,500 mg a day (prevents viral replication)

Herbal Therapy

Take the following herbs on the indicated schedules as a preventative measure.

- echinacea – take two weeks on and two weeks off throughout the fall and winter season (powerful immune system enhancer)
- goldenseal – take two weeks on and two weeks off (natural antibiotic; immune system stimulator). *Caution:* Do not take if you are pregnant.

Homeopathic Remedies

Take the following homeopathic remedy as a preventative.

- Oscillococcinum – one dose per week throughout the fall and winter flu season (available at health food stores)

Other Therapeutic Measures

Increase ventilation in your home and at your workplace. Also observe the preventative therapeutic measures from modern medicine.

MODERN MEDICAL TREATMENT

Diet

A light diet and extra fluids are suggested for patients with a cold or the flu.

Exercise and Lifestyle

Patients are told not to exercise during an acute infection and to stop smoking. They are also advised to rest and not to go to work, to avoid infecting their co-workers.

Drug Therapy

Treatment for viral diseases (including colds and flus) is largely symptomatic and palliative. To control symptoms, patients are given cough syrups, throat sprays, decongestants, expectorants, and antihistamines. They are also told to take acetaminophen to ease aches and pains.

They may be given rimantidine hydrochloride (Flumadine), or amantidine hydrochloride (Symmetrel), which are antiviral medications for the flu and must be taken within 48 hours of the onset of symptoms. Side effects of these medications include nausea, dizziness, and insomnia.

An antibiotic may be prescribed if bacterial involvement is suspected.

ALTERNATIVE TREATMENT

Diet

Drink extra fluids—at least eight glasses a day. Some of the fluids can be diluted vegetable juices, soups, and herb teas. Fluids moisten the mucus in the throat, which traps the viruses and sends them into the stomach where they are destroyed.

Eat hot spicy soups (including the proverbial chicken soup), which make the nose run and shortens the amount of time cold germs stay in your nose. Also eat garlic, which boosts the immune system's production of antibodies.

Avoid dairy foods—these products are all big mucus producers—and sugar, since both refined and natural sugars depress the immune system.

Exercise and Lifestyle

Do not exercise during an acute infection.

Nutrient Therapy

Take the following antiviral nutrients. If taken early enough, they will abort viral infections, and in any case will shorten the duration and severity of the infection. They must be taken at reduced doses for two weeks after the infection appears to be over.

- L-lysine – 1,500 to 3,000 mg a day in divided doses (prevents the replication of viruses)
- Monolaurin – one to six capsules a day in divided doses (prevents the virus from attaching to the cell) (Cardiovascular Research—see Sources)

Take the following nutrients:

- vitamin A – 25,000 IU a day. *Caution:* Do not take more than 8,000 IU a day if you are pregnant or might be pregnant (Strengthens immune system; helps support mucus membranes).
- vitamin C – 500 to 1,000 mg (or to bowel tolerance) every two hours, or daily from the first throat tickle until the cold or flu has completely cleared up (strengthens immune system)
- beta carotene – 200,000 IU a day (strengthens the immune system)
- bioflavonoids – 1,000 mg a day (anti-inflammatory)
- zinc lozenges – 180 mg zinc gluconate, containing 23 mg of elemental zinc. Suck on one lozenge for at least 10 minutes every two waking hours for one week. *Caution:* Do not use for longer than one week. Zinc has antiviral activity against several viruses

that cause colds, and will reduce the severity and duration of the infection.

Herbal Therapy

Use the following botanical medicines.

- astragalus – increases interferon production and secretion; enhances the immune system; stimulates synthesis of proteins that prevent viral infections
- echinacea – enhances the immune system, neutralizes viruses, destroys bacteria, and increases the migration of white blood cells to areas of infection
- elderberry – stimulates the immune system; anti-inflammatory; good all-purpose herb for the flu and common cold
- elecampane – soothing, relaxing, and stimulating expectorant for irritating coughs and bronchial irritations
- eyebright – antimucus and anti-inflammatory; useful in respiratory conditions, especially those of the nasopharynx and the sinuses
- goldenseal – enhances the immune system; activates white cells. *Caution:* Do not use if you are pregnant.
- licorice – enhances the immune system and induces interferon production, which causes significant antiviral activity; is particularly effective in treating respiratory tract infections
- yarrow – calms an upset digestive tract and is anti-inflammatory; helps with infections such as the flu where there is fever, malaise, and decreased appetite

For a scratchy or sore throat, try the following teas. Drink them hot.

- lemon tea – use two lemons to a pot of tea, steep, and add 1 Tbsp. of honey per cup
- vinegar and honey – use equal parts of honey and vinegar, in hot water

Homeopathic Remedies

Take a homeopathic remedy for a cold or the flu. If you do not receive relief of your symptoms, seek the help of a homeopathic physician. The following remedies are but a few of the many possibilities.

- *Aconitum napellus* – for sudden cold or flu; symptoms begin after exposure to cold; better in open air and worse after midnight; may have anxiety and extreme thirst.
- *Allium cepa* – eyes and nose stream with watery, burning discharge; frequent sneezing; thirst; worse with warmth; better in fresh air; aborts colds that begin with sneezing.
- *Arsenicum album* – exhaustion; burning nasal discharge; sneezing; area under nose is red and burns; patient is cold; thirst for sips of water; restlessness; desire for company.
- *Eupatorium perfoliatum* – deep bone ache; thirsty; cough with chest soreness; worse in cold air.
- *Euphrasia* – common cold; pronounced sneezing and watering of the eyes.
- *Gelsemium* – general feeling of weakness, tiredness, and aching; symptoms start with chills "running up the spine"; runny nose, heavy eyes, headache, and sore throat.
- *Pulsatilla* – "ripe" head cold; thick and creamy mucus; better with gentle movement and fresh air; nose stuffy inside and unstuffs outside.
- *Rhus toxicondendron* – general cold; no well-defined symptoms; glands swollen; restlessness; bright red tip of tongue.

At the first sign of feeling sick, take the homeopathic remedy sold as either *Oscillococcinum* or Flu Solution, which contains *Anas barbariae hepatis et cordis.* This remedy has been proven effective against Influenza A in double-blind clinical studies. It reduces symptoms of colds and flu in 80 percent of the people who use it. Take in three doses, six hours apart.

Many patients respond to complex homeopathic remedies. You may want to try one of the following (see Sources section at back of book).

- BHI Cold or BHI Flu – tablets for colds and flu.
- Engystol N from BHI – tablets and injectable. Stimulates the immune system and if taken early can abort the infection. Helps to shorten duration and severity of infection.
- Viral Colds from CompliMed – for viral colds, runny nose, sneezing, cough, sore throat.
- Influenza CM from CompliMed – flu, fever, chills, body aches, nausea, vomiting.
- Flu Symptom Drops I from PHP – relief of flu and fever-like symptoms.
- Flu Symptom II Drops from PHP – relief of intestinal flu symptoms.
- Cold and Flu from PHP – temporary relief of fever-like flu and intestinal symptoms.

Other Therapeutic Measures

If you are getting a cold, take a very hot bath and go to bed in a warm bed. Get plenty of rest; bed rest may be required for the flu.

Retire cloth handkerchiefs and use disposable tissues to blow your nose and cover your mouth, unless you wash the handkerchiefs in very hot water.

Do not use over-the-counter cold formulas, cough syrups, decongestants, expectorants, or antihistamines, as they overdry mucus membranes.

Steam the nasal passages (in the shower, with a commercial steam inhaler, or over a pot of boiling water) for 15 minutes, three times a day.

Have acupuncture treatments. Consult an Ayurvedic or Chinese medicine physician. Try an appropriate aromatherapy treatment.

Take allergy extracts for any microorganisms to which you test positive (see Allergy chapter).

Have NAET treatments for your particular infection (see Chiropractic section in chapter 9, Alternative Medical Disciplines).

EAR INFECTIONS

Otitis media (an ear infection or earache) is the number-one reason parents take their children to see the doctor. Each year more than one-fourth of the prescriptions written for antibiotics are for the treatment of otitis media. More than 80 percent of all children have one or more episodes of otitis media by the age of six, with the highest incidence occurring between the ages of two and six. Repeated infections can lead to a hearing loss, and deficiencies in learning and language development. Apart from colds, ear infections are the most commonly diagnosed childhood ailment.

Despite a huge increase in the use of antibiotics, the incidence of otitis media in children has grown exponentially. Since 1975, the annual rate of ear infections has doubled, and the incidence of otitis media in children under two has increased 224 percent. Although this increase in otitis media has been attributed to improved diagnostic ability and/or increased doctor awareness, many experts suspect it is caused partly by the widespread use of antibiotics.

Redness of the eardrum is the most common sign used to diagnose ear infections, but the eardrum can be red for many reasons other than infection—including allergy, crying, high fever, and inflammation. Ear infections are typically diagnosed in children with fever and who are crying while being examined. Crying in itself causes the eardrum to look red. Pneumatic otoscopy is a more accurate means of making a diagnosis, but it is not used by most pediatricians. In this procedure, air is pumped into the ear chamber to see if the eardrum moves. The eardrum does not move if the middle ear space has fluid inside it, which indicates the possibility of infection.

Eustachian tubes lead from the back of the throat to the middle ear space of each ear. They become swollen and blocked due to colds, sinus infections, or allergies. When Eustachian tubes become blocked, they secrete fluid into the middle ear space behind the eardrum. Bacteria can then migrate from the nose up the Eustachian tube and into the middle ear space, where they begin growing. The Eustachian tubes of children are shorter and straighter, and lead in a more direct path to the middle ear space, which is why they get ear infections more frequently than adults do. The congestion in the middle ear space causes painful pressure on the eardrum and other sensitive structures near the middle ear area. The pressure sometimes ruptures the eardrum. The fluid then drains out, reducing the pressure and relieving the pain. However, rupturing leads to scarring of the eardrum.

During the day, when the head is held up, the Eustachian tubes drain into the back of the throat. Chewing and swallowing pull the tubes open and allow air into the middle ear space. During sleep, however, people do not swallow as often, and the tubes no longer drain naturally. The air in the middle ear becomes absorbed, a vacuum occurs, and the eardrum is pulled inward. This is why earaches are more common in children at night, and why children with ear infections are more comfortable when they sleep sitting upright.

An acute ear infection presents with sharp, stabbing, dull, or throbbing pain in the ear. Young children may pull at their ear, or be irritable. There may be fever, drainage from the ears, sleeplessness, changes in eating habits, dizziness, changes in hearing, and nasal obstruction or discharge.

Chronic ear infections are known as otitis media with effusion, serous otitis media, or secretory otitis media. In this case, the middle ear space is chronically filled with fluid, the eardrum is retracted, and hearing is diminished. The fluid may be thin and watery; thick, sticky, and mucus-like; or glue-like. Again, the child will be irritable and pull at his ear, but will usually not have a fever. Chronic ear infections can permanently damage hearing.

CAUSES OF EAR INFECTIONS

The four main causes of ear infections are allergy and sensitivity, infection, mechanical obstructions, and nutrient insufficiency.

Allergy and Sensitivity

Allergy can cause swollen tonsils, swelling of the Eustachian tubes, nasal and sinus congestion, excessive mucus production, inhibition of the white blood cells' ability to attack bacteria, and fluid behind the eardrum. Children with untreated allergies are prone to recurrent ear infections, and one-third of allergic children have poor Eustachian tube function. Numerous studies have shown the connection between recurrent ear infections and allergies, including allergies to foods, pollens, and indoor air allergens, such as mold and dust mites.

In a 1994 study Dr. Talal M. Nsouli of Georgetown University School of Medicine tested 104 children with recurrent middle ear problems for food allergy. Eighty percent of the group proved to have food allergies, and most children were allergic to more than one food. Of these children, 86 percent improved after eliminating the offending foods for 16 weeks. When the offending foods were re-introduced, 94 percent of the children again developed fluid in the middle ear. The most common food allergens were cow's milk products, wheat, egg white, peanut, and soy.

Despite the many studies showing a connection between allergies and recurrent ear infections, many pediatricians still do not want to consider allergy in their treatment of chronic otitis media, even when parents raise the issue.

Indoor air pollutants can also cause recurrent ear infections by inducing swelling of the Eustachian tube, which predisposes to infection.

House dust mites, volatile organic compounds, and cigarette smoke all contribute to ear infections. Cigarette smoke causes paralysis of cilia in the respiratory tract and depletion of antioxidants. More than 80 percent of volatile organic compounds in the smoke are known mucus membrane irritants.

Infection

The most common bacterial causes of ear infections are *Streptococcus pneumonia* and *Haemophilus influenzae*. Bacteria in the nose and throat area can migrate up the Eustachian tube to the middle ear space. However, almost half the children with an ear infection have a viral respiratory tract infection for which antibiotics are not effective.

Children attending daycare are at higher risk for ear infections because they are exposed to more people with upper respiratory infections.

Mechanical Obstructions

The Eustachian tubes can be blocked by swollen tonsils or adenoids, or other structural components. The bones of the skull, the bones of the cervical spine (neck), or the tempero-mandibular joint can all cause blockage of the Eustachian tube. Mechanical obstruction can be caused by traction of the neck at birth, causing separation and dislocation of the vertebra, and/or soft tissue injury to the area around the spinal cord. Toddlers fall frequently, and may have mild strains of the upper neck.

Dr. Joan Fallon, a chiropractor from New Rochelle, New York, has treated 400 children with otitis media, and has demonstrated that tympanogram readings (which indicate the pressure in the middle ear and the presence or absence of fluid) improve after spinal manipulation. Almost 80 percent of the children in her study had no further cases of otitis media within the six-month period following their first chiropractic visit.

Nutrient Insufficiency

Children who are malnourished have impaired immune function. Even children with only one or two trace element deficiencies have increased susceptibility to infection. Most North American children do not eat the proper nutrients. They consume a high percentage of processed and fast foods, which have lower nutritional content than unprocessed foods and whole foods, and they also eat large amounts of sugar. Sugar can decrease immune function for up to four hours, which explains why many children become sick after a birthday party.

Many children diagnosed with recurrent ear infections have no bacteria in their middle ear space, but only inflammatory substances that the body produces to help fight infections. These children would benefit from dietary and nutritional intervention.

MODERN MEDICAL PREVENTION

Patients are given antihistamines and decongestants when they have a cold, in the hope of preventing ear infections. Prophylactic antibiotics are often given to children who get recurrent ear infections, sometimes for several months at a time.

ALTERNATIVE PREVENTION

Diet

Breast-feed your baby. Early bottle feeding is a risk factor for recurrent ear infections. If you bottle-feed, avoid propping the bottle. Because the Eustachian tubes are straight in children, fluids can back up in them. Do not allow your child to suck on a pacifier frequently, especially after the age of one year.

Use the following dietary guidelines. Avoid the introduction of solid foods until the child is at least six months old. After that, use whole foods as much as possible, and avoid foods with non-essential fatty acids or food with partially hydrogenated oil (cookies, pastries, doughnuts, candy bars, some crackers, French fries, chicken nuggets, deep-fried fish, margarine, vegetable shortening, corn chips, potato chips, and chocolate or carob malt balls). Replace peanut butter in the diet with walnut butter, which is higher in essential fatty acids that help fight infection.

Offer no fruit juice until the child is at least six to nine months old, and then give no more than four ounces of fruit juice a day in the first year of life. Give no more than 8 to 12 ounces a day after the first year, and no more than 12 ounces a day for children aged three to five.

Avoid using foods to which the child is allergic. RAST testing or intradermal testing can identify food allergies (see Allergy chapter).

Exercise and Lifestyle

Keep to a regular exercise program, and try to get some outdoor exercise. Parents must quit smoking and not use a fireplace or wood-burning stove.

Nutrient Therapy

Use the following nutritional supplements. These oils help prevent infection and inflammation.

- Give one perle of flaxseed oil a day (open up the perle and put the oil on the child's food).
- Give one perle of evening primrose oil or borage oil every other day (open up the perle and put the oil on the child's food).

Herbal Therapy

Give the following botanical supplement: echinacea – five drops of tincture in a glass of water, three times a day for a child over two years, and three drops three times a day for a child under two years. Use for two weeks on, then two weeks off throughout the fall and winter.

Use an herbal tea to reduce congestion and build up energy in a weakened child (*Do not use for child less than one year of age*). Make a tea with ⅛ tsp. raw honey, and fresh ground ginger root, cinnamon, or cayenne.

Homeopathic Remedies

Use a homeopathic remedy for the following symptoms to prevent ear infections.

- *Allium cepa* – much sneezing associated with watery eyes and a runny nose; nasal discharge tends to be clear, watery, and offensive; irritating to the upper lip and increases when entering a warm room; eyes frequently burn from the profuse tearing; hoarseness and tickling sensation in the throat; hay fever.
- *Antimonium tartaricum* – cough comes on gradually and is associated with rattling of mucus with little expectoration; children drowsy and weak; face is cold, blue, and pale; often quivering of chin; latter stages of respiratory problems that do not improve.
- *Belladonna* – used in early stage of a cold; comes on rapidly with little warning; hot red skin, flushed face, glaring eyes, restless sleep, and hypersensitivity; throat is hot and dry with swollen tonsils; skin is dry; commonly no thirst; child almost unaware of what is going on around him; fears of imaginary things.
- *Hepar sulphuricum* – used in the latter stages of a cold when the nasal discharge has become thick, yellowish, and offensive; children are easily irritated and hypersensitive; cough is loose, rattling, and commonly worse in the morning.
- *Kali bichromicum* – sinus congestion; pain around the root of the nose; nasal discharge is thick, ropy, and greenish-yellow; violent sneezing.
- *Natrum muriaticum* – awakens with much sneezing; heavy nasal discharge, like raw egg white; small eruptions from around the lips; lips and corners of the mouth are dry, ulcerated, and cracked; crack in the middle of the lower lip; children are irritable, weepy, and wish to be alone; symptoms worse with consolation.
- *Pulsatilla* – thick, bland, yellowish-green discharge, sometimes accompanied by a dry or

loose cough; dry cough in the evening and at night; in the morning there is a loose cough with copious expectoration of mucus; nose often stuffed at night; child weepy, easily discouraged, and melancholy; symptoms improve when the child is outdoors; child likes the head held high and desires to sleep with more than one pillow.

- *Spongia* – coughs that are dry, barking, and croupy; cough usually improves after eating or drinking, especially warm drinks; profuse nasal discharge alternating with blockage; children are anxious and fearful; excitement aggravates their cough; may awaken in the middle of the night with a fearful suffocating sensation.

Other Therapeutic Measures

Avoid large daycare centers (those that care for more than four children) in the first two years of your child's life. Have caregivers wash their hands frequently. Teach children not to share food or utensils.

Install an electrostatic filter on the furnace (especially if there is a family history of allergy or the patient has allergies).

Avoid using products that contain volatile organic vapors, such as cleaning solutions, mothballs, new carpets, and particleboard products.

Use a water-filter vacuum or HEPA filter vacuum.

Test for pollen, mold, and inhalant allergies, and treat for them if they are present.

Use acupressure for colds and nasal congestion. Treat each point for about 45 seconds, using the pads of your fingers. Press:

- on the back of the neck, beneath the base of the skull on either side where the spine meets the skull
- at the flare of the outer nostrils where they join the cheek (on the cheek rather than on the nostrils)
- on the back of the skull, the width of one

hand above the base of the skull in line with the top of the ears
- on the top of the head, midway between the ears. *Caution:* Do not use on a small child whose fontanel (soft spot) is still open.
- one and a half thumbs' width above the most prominent crease of the wrist (toward the shoulder), in line with the thumbnail, along the top of the wrist, deep in a small hollow
- the width of one thumb to either side of the spine, slightly below a bone between the tips of the shoulders.

MODERN MEDICAL TREATMENT

Diet

Patients are advised to eat a well-balanced diet.

Exercise and Lifestyle

Regular exercise programs are encouraged, and parents and older patients are advised not to smoke.

Children should not be placed in daycare.

Drug Therapy

In addition to antihistamines and decongestants, antibiotics are prescribed for 10 days for an acute ear infection. Antibiotics are used because of the risk of ear infection spreading to the mastoid area behind the ear and to the brain. However, children are now developing recurrent ear infections caused by bacteria that are resistant to all commonly used antibiotics, and so the treatment of ear infections is beginning to change. A number of studies reported in the 1980s have shown that at least 85 percent of ear infections will clear by themselves, without the use of antibiotics. Many studies have also shown that there is no difference in the clinical course of otitis media, or the rate of complications, under different treatment regimens: the use of antibiotics, the use of antibiotics with ear tubes, the use of ear tubes alone, or the use of neither ear tubes nor antibiotics.

Children who receive no antibiotics have

fewer recurrences of ear infection than those receiving antibiotics. In Canada, antibiotics are used aggressively for ear infections, while in the Netherlands antibiotics are used less frequently, yet there is no difference between the two countries in the occurrence of mastoiditis (infection of the mastoid area). In Denmark, where antibiotics are not commonly used, there were only six cases of mastoiditis in 1994.

We do not really know how antibiotics work in ear infections. It is common, for instance, for a child with an ear infection to improve within half an hour to 45 minutes after the first dose of antibiotic. Such improvement cannot have been caused by a reduction in the number of bacteria, because levels of antibiotic in the middle ear are not yet high enough to have had an effect on the organisms. Antibiotics may have some other effect, totally unrelated to their ability to kill bacteria, that resolves symptoms quickly. If this is so, perhaps one dose of antibiotic could be used to decrease pain.

Surgery

Chronic and recurrent ear infections are often treated surgically by the insertion of a myringotomy tube (or PE tube), which is placed through the eardrum to assist in the drainage of fluid out of the middle ear space. Insertion of the tube does not cure the underlying problem (blockage of the Eustachian tube). Children with tubes in their ears have an increased likelihood of further problems with ear infections. Over 40 percent of children who have had tubes inserted have eardrum scarring and thickening of the tympanic membrane. The treatment of recurrent ear infections remains an unsolved problem.

Sometimes the Eustachian tube is blocked by enlarged adenoids. Children with this problem often have a characteristic appearance, with a flat face, pinched nose, and narrow nostrils. They breathe through their mouths, and have a chronically blocked nose. They may benefit from removal of their adenoids. However, in 1988 Dr. Jack Paradise of the University of Pittsburgh carried out a two-year study of 281 children who had recurrent ear infections. The outcomes for children who had surgery (adenoidectomy with or without tonsillectomy) were no different from outcomes for children in the non-surgical group.

A study reported in 1994 in the *Journal of the American Medical Association* by Charles Kleinmen of New Haven, Connecticut analyzed over 6,000 cases of children who had surgery for tube placement. Almost 60 percent of the operations were considered to have been done on the basis of equivocal or inappropriate indications.

ALTERNATIVE TREATMENT

Diet

Avoid all milk and milk products in the diet for at least three months, as well as sugar in any form (including fruit juice). Avoid all food allergens. To avoid developing new food allergies, follow a rotation diet so that you do not repeat foods too frequently.

Exercise and Lifestyle

Stop smoking and do not allow anyone to smoke around your child.

Nutrient Therapy

Take the following nutritional supplements.

- beta carotene – (age in years × 20,000) IU a day up to 200,000 IU maximum (strengthens immune system)
- B-complex – one capsule a day (25 mg of each B vitamin) (strengthens immune system)
- vitamin C – (age in years × 500) mg a day or to bowel tolerance (strengthens immune system)
- bioflavonoids – (age in years × 50) mg a day up to 250 mg maximum (anti-inflammatory)
- zinc picolinate – (age in years × 2.5) mg a day up to 15 mg maximum (strenghtens immune system; aids in reducing infection)

- evening primrose oil – (age in years) capsules a day up to six capsules maximum (anti-inflammatory)
- borage oil – one perle a day for a child under four, two perles a day for children four and older (anti-inflammatory)
- flax oil – 1 tsp. a day for a child under four, 1 to 1½ tsp. a day for children four and older (anti-inflammatory)
- thymus extract – (age in years × 50) mg a day (strengthens immune system)
- *Lactobacillus acidophilus* – 1 to 2 tsp. a day (normalizes intestinal flora)

Herbal Therapy
Give the following botanical supplements.

- echinacea – 10 to 15 drops three times a day (strengthens immune system)
- goldenseal – 10 to 15 drops three times a day (strengthens immune system). *Caution:* Do not use during pregnancy.
- licorice root – 10 to 15 drops three times a day (strengthens immune system)

Homeopathic Remedies
Consult a homeopathic physician to determine the homeopathic remedy that best describes your child's symptoms.

- *Belladonna* – earache comes on suddenly; hot, red skin with flushed face; restless sleep, glaring eyes, and hypersensitivity of all senses; throat hot and dry; not thirsty; ear and eardrum often bright red; high fever sets in abruptly with little warning; child delirious and unaware of surroundings, pupils dilated; intense pain.
- *Chamomilla* – children are irritable and cross; want something, but throw it back when given it; not easily consoled, but may feel better if carried around; impatient and are intolerant of being spoken to, interrupted, or looked at; not mentally calm;

bright red cheeks; acute, stabbing ear pain that may drive the child frantic; discomfort associated with teething.

- *Hepar sulphuricum* – not used in early stages of an earache; used when symptoms have progressed and pus has formed in the middle ear; nasal discharge that is first watery and then becomes thick, yellow, and offensive; intense throbbing pain in the ear, accompanied by diminished hearing; child irritable and sensitive, cross and easily angered; oversensitivity to touch, cold, and pain.
- *Lycopodium* – symptoms are on or begin on the right side; humming and roaring sensation in the ear with diminished hearing; thick, yellow, offensive discharge is common; nose stopped up; digestive complaints such as gas and bloating; children are thin and weak; fearful, apprehensive, and afraid to be alone; adverse to taking on new things; headstrong and scornful when sick.
- *Mercurius* – pus formation; chronic cases of ear infections; nasal discharge is yellow-green and offensive; profuse, offensive perspiration; lymph nodes swollen; great thirst; skin almost constantly moist; increased salivation, bad breath, puffiness of tongue; acutely sensitive to heat, cold, and most environmental influences; weak and may tire at slightest exertion; sometimes muscle trembling; loss of willpower.
- *Pulsatilla* – one of the most frequently used remedies for ear infections; children gentle, weepy, sensitive, and love to be held; children want attention and are easily consoled by a sympathetic response; moody, feel sorry for themselves and lament their plight during illness; cheeks are pale; feel better when in open, fresh air; thick, bland, yellowish-green nasal discharge; ear is swollen, red, and hot, with itching deep in it; pain often goes through the whole side of the face; stopped-up sensation in the ear; dry or loose cough; symptoms often come on gradually and

frequently follow a cold; child feverish but not thirsty.

- *Silica* – discharge from the ear; cold or bronchial condition is slow to respond or long-standing; roaring in the ears; child sensitive to noise; child is cold, chilly, and wants plenty of warm clothing; hates drafts, and hands and feet are icy cold; offensive sweat on the hands, feet, and armpits; pain behind the ear on the mastoid process; children are yielding, faint-hearted, and anxious; nervous, excitable, and sensitive, but can be obstinate; children tend to be weak and easily exhausted.

Your child may respond to a complex homeopathic remedy. You may want to try one of the following (see Sources section at back of book).

- BHI Ear is a prescription remedy for ear infections.
- PHP Mucus Dissolver dissolves excess mucus.
- Warm several drops of liquid Traumeel by BHI on a teaspoon, then place three drops in the affected ear and cover with cotton. *Caution:* Do not use if there is drainage from the ear, or if the eardrum is ruptured.

Other Therapeutic Measures
Use these simple treatment techniques to stop pain.

- Use a hair dryer on a low, warm setting to put warm air into an aching ear.
- Place one to two drops of warm (body temperature) baby oil, sweet oil, mullein oil, plantago major tincture, olive oil, or mineral oil in the ear. *Caution:* Do not use if you think the eardrum is ruptured or punctured, or if there is drainage from the ear. Cover with cotton. Repeat three times a day.
- Apply a warm pack or a warm water bottle to the ear.
- Keep the head up.
- Swallow some clear liquid to open the Eustachian tubes, every 15 to 30 minutes.

Use acupressure for earaches. Press the following points with the pads of your fingers (in the order listed) for 45 seconds two to three times a day:

- on the outside of the foot, the width of three thumbs away from the crown of the outer ankle, in a line drawn between the crown (bony protuberance) of the outer ankle and the nail of the smallest toe
- on the inside of the leg, the width of two thumbs above the crown of the inner ankle, still on the inner side of the leg, but almost to the rear of the leg
- on the inside of the leg, between the crown of the inner ankle and the tip of the heel (this may be a large point)
- between the thumb and index finger, where a mound forms when the thumb is placed next to the finger
- on the back of the arm, two thumbs' width above the most prominent crease of the upper wrist, in line with the middle finger
- on the back of the neck, beneath the base of the skull on either side where the spine meets the skull
- on the lower fleshy part of the ear (gently)
- in front of the ear, one-half thumb's width below the area between the upper cartilage and lower cartilage.

Do this lymphatic flush to drain fluid away from the Eustachian tube and tonsillar area, and decrease congestion:

- Lay the child on his back. Apply unscented oil or hand lotion to your hands and rub it up and down the front and sides of the child's neck. Stroke the muscle on the affected side from the mastoid bone behind the ear, to the collarbone.
- With one hand on each side and broad hand contact, beginning about one inch up from the collarbone, stroke downward in the direction of the collarbone. Repeat with moderate pressure five to six times.

- Place your hands one inch higher and stroke downward five to six times. Repeat this until hands are up at the angle of the jawbone.

For recurrent ear infections, have craniosacral manipulation performed by a trained practitioner such as a massage therapist, physical therapist, osteopath, or chiropractor.

Have chiropractic or osteopathic treatment.

In addition, follow the recommendations for prevention, above.

Chew xylitol gum or use xylitol candies. The xylitol is a sugar alcohol that does not support bacterial growth. Chewing will help keep the Eustachian tube open.

SINUSITIS

Sinus disease is our most common chronic ailment, affecting more than 33 million North Americans. The number of cases of acute and chronic sinusitis has been rising over the past 20 years. Adult visits to physicians for sinusitis have tripled over that time, while children's visits have doubled. Ten percent of all prescriptions for antibiotics written in 1992 were for sinusitis.

The sinuses are membrane-lined cavities in the bones of the face that drain into the nose. The ethmoid sinuses are adjacent to the nose, the maxillary sinuses are under the cheekbones, the frontal sinuses are under the eyebrow area, and the sphenoid sinus is behind the nose next to the brain. Bacteria become trapped and filtered out by mucus and hair in the nose (called cilia), and the sinuses around the nose help remove inhaled bacteria and impurities, and also moisten, purify, and warm the air before it goes into the lungs.

Sinus disease can occur when there is:

- something that reduces the effectiveness of the cilia (cigarette smoke or air pollution)
- swelling from a cold (upper respiratory infection)
- blockage from a polyp or foreign body
- hypertrophy (enlargement) of the adenoids

- crooked middle part of the nose (deviated septum)
- an allergen that causes blockage of the sinus openings or linings
- an adjacent dental infection
- exposure to dry or cold air
- an underlying immune deficiency

Irritants, allergies, and viral infections cause swelling of the mucus membranes of the sinuses, increase mucus production, and damage the cilia. The sinus openings become blocked, mucus stagnates, and bacteria overgrow. *Streptococci, Pneumococci, Staphylococci, Moraxella catarrhalis,* and *Haemophilus influenzae* are the most common bacteria found in sinus infections.

Emotional stress, recurrent use of antibiotics, and environmental pollution weaken the immune system and make the body less able to fight off infection. Nutrient insufficiency is often a contributing factor. A few people have abnormal cilia or abnormal mucus (as in cystic fibrosis). Some medications (such as birth control pills) or a sensitivity to a medication can cause nasal congestion. Simple trauma (from such activities as swimming and diving) can also cause sinusitis by forcing water into the sinuses.

Chronic sinusitis is associated with allergy, and treatment consists of treating the food and/or pollen allergies that are the underlying cause. Many people who think they have chronic sinus infections probably have severe allergic reactions, with blockage of the sinus openings. If patients continue to have chronic allergic sinusitis or sinus infections, they may eventually develop blockage and thickening of the opening of the sinuses—at which point, surgery may be necessary.

SYMPTOMS OF SINUSITIS

A person with sinus disease develops nasal congestion, a purulent discharge, postnasal drip, sore throat from drainage, sometimes fever and chills, cough, bad breath, and local tenderness over the sinuses. Sinus pain is typically dull and aching, and the sinuses may throb or feel full. When the maxillary sinuses are involved, the pain is over the teeth, and sometimes people see the dentist because they think they have a toothache. In infections of the ethmoid or sphenoid sinuses, the pain is around the eye socket or over the head, while in infected frontal sinuses the pain is localized in the region over the eyes.

Pain is worse when the person awakens and improves during the day (because they are standing up). It is worsened by shaking the head, holding the head lower than the rest of the body, straining, or wearing a tight collar, and it can be increased by exposure to cold air, alcohol, emotional excitement, or tension. Fever over 102°F suggests more than simple sinusitis, as does any alteration in mental status. These symptoms should be investigated further by a physician.

In adults, chronic sinus infections often produce no symptoms other than postnasal drainage or a non-productive cough. In 25 percent of adult patients with chronic maxillary sinusitis, there is an underlying dental infection. In children, however, sinus disease can be associated with unremitting asthma and cough, and many children with asthma improve only after sinus infections are treated. As many as 70 percent of allergic children presenting with chronic rhinitis have abnormal findings when their sinuses are X-rayed. Children with chronic sinusitis often suffer from fatigue.

MODERN MEDICAL PREVENTION

Drug Therapy
Modern medicine uses antihistamines and decongestants as preventative medications for sinusitis.

ALTERNATIVE PREVENTION

Diet
Avoid sugar and food allergens in your diet. Common food allergens affecting sinuses are eggs, milk, chocolate, citrus, peanuts, wheat, corn, food additives, tomato, and caffeine.

Exercise and Lifestyle
If you are prone to sinus infections, prevention works better than treating symptoms. Get adequate rest and reduce stress.

Exercise regularly, but avoid exercising near busy streets.

Do not smoke, and avoid the cigarette smoke of other people.

Drink 8 to 10 glasses of pure water a day.

Nutrient Therapy
Take the following nutritional supplements.

- vitamin A – up to 25,000 IU a day. *Caution:* Do not take more than 8,000 IU a day if you are or might be pregnant (protects mucus membranes).
- beta carotene – 25,000 IU one to two times a day (strengthens immune system)
- vitamin C – 1,000 to 2,000 mg three times a day (strengthens immune system; aids in preventing infection; decreases mucus)
- bioflavonoids – 1,000 to 2,000 mg a day (strengthen immune system)
- vitamin E – 400 IU a day (antioxidant; helps prevent infection)
- copper – 1 to 2 mg a day (to balance zinc)
- selenium – 100 to 200 mcg a day (antioxidant; protects immune system)
- zinc picolinate – 20 to 40 mg a day (antiviral agent; boosts immunity)
- pycnogenol or grape seed extract – 100 mg one to two times a day (antioxidant; reduces inflammation)
- N-acetyl cysteine – 500 mg a day (antioxidant)
- flaxseed oil – 2 Tbsp. a day (anti-inflammatory)

Herbal Therapy
Take a botanical supplement.

- echinacea – boosts the immune system; fights bacterial and viral infections
- garlic – helps fight infection
- licorice root – increases fluidity of mucus; stimulates production of interferon. *Caution:* Do not take for longer than four to six weeks, as it causes potassium loss and water retention. Do not take if you are pregnant or have high blood pressure.

Other Therapeutic Measures

Damp-dust bedrooms twice a week. Remove dust-catchers such as rugs and stuffed animals. Use a HEPA air filter for the bedroom or house, and humidify the indoor air. Vacuum regularly with a central system, a water-trap vacuum, or a HEPA vacuum. Change filters in the heating system regularly, and have a professional clean the ducts.

Use the following procedures both as a preventative and as treatment when you are ill.

- Steam the sinuses (in the shower, with a commercial steam inhaler, or over a pot of boiling water) for 15 minutes once a day. Use an essential oil such as eucalyptus, sage, thyme, or tea tree in the steam unit (terpene-sensitive people may not tolerate this).
- Follow steam inhalation with nasal irrigation using saltwater (¼ tsp. of salt in 1 cup of water; you may also add ¼ tsp. of baking soda). Use a spray bottle, ear syringe, the palms of your hand, a neti pot (a pot with a spout developed in India to clear the sinuses—see Sources), or an attachment to your Water Pik (see Sources). Incline your head forward over a sink, putting your right side up. Keep the nose higher than the mouth. Pour water into your right nostril and allow it to drain out the left nostril. Some water may also come out of your mouth.
- Carry out the same procedure on the left nostril. Repeat two to three times.

If possible, avoid living in large cities. If you cannot manage that, do not live near freeways, major roadways, or industrial parks. Pollution causes inflammation of sinuses and adversely affects the function of the cilia.

In your home and workplace, also avoid plastics and synthetic materials which release substances that can irritate the sinuses.

MODERN MEDICAL TREATMENT

Diet

A well-balanced diet is recommended for patients with sinusitis.

Exercise and Lifestyle

Patients are encouraged to continue their regular exercise program. They are advised not to smoke, and to avoid the smoke of others.

Drug Therapy

Antihistamines, decongestants, and antibiotics are prescribed for sinusitis. Topical nasal steroids are used for chronic sinusitis. These steroids can irritate the nose and cause perforation of the nasal septum.

Antihistamines can cause drying of the nasal lining and delay clearing of the sinuses, and they have not been shown to be effective for treating sinusitis. Decongestants inhibit movement of the cilia and decrease local blood flow, and their value for sinusitis has not been proven by clinical trials. In 1992, Dr. Ann Dohlman of the University of Alabama School of Medicine reviewed sinusitis treatment, and found no evidence that antibiotics are effective for the condition.

Antibiotics kill the beneficial nasal bacteria (which help prevent harmful bacteria from taking over) and overuse of antibiotics leads to the development of antibiotic-resistant bacteria. Antibiotics also impair immune function, and can delay recovery if the infection is viral rather than bacterial.

Surgery

For chronic sinusitis, surgery is performed to remove polyps.

Other Therapeutic Measures

Patients are told to take a shower with water hot enough to fog the mirror, or to lean over a pan full of steaming water with a towel draped over the head, inhaling the vapors as they come up toward the nose. Patients are also advised to run a vaporizer in the bedroom. The vaporizer should be cleaned once a week so that it does not become moldy.

ALTERNATIVE TREATMENT

Diet

Limit sugars (including fruit sugars) to less than 50 grams a day. Eliminate the common food allergens (milk, corn, wheat, eggs, peanut butter, citrus, soy, and yeast). Also avoid chocolate, caffeine, tomatoes, and food additives.

Eat garlic, which helps make the mucus less sticky; horseradish, to help drain mucus (bottled will work); and cayenne peppers, which may act as a natural decongestant.

Drink plenty of fluids.

Exercise and Lifestyle

Walk or exercise. This releases adrenaline, which constricts the blood vessels in the nose. Exercise also helps to open up sinus openings.

Do not smoke or use tobacco in any form, including smokeless (chewing) tobacco. Avoid secondhand smoke.

Nutrient Therapy

Take the following nutritional supplements.

- vitamin A – 25,000 IU a day. *Caution:* Do not take more than 8,000 IU a day if you are pregnant or may be pregnant (protects mucus membranes; helps heal mucosa).
- beta carotene – 200,000 IU a day (precursor of vitamin A)

- vitamin C – 500 mg every two hours to bowel tolerance (strengthens immune system; aids in preventing infection; decreases mucus)
- bioflavonoids – 1,000 mg a day (strengthen immune system)
- vitamin E – 400 IU twice a day (antioxidant; helps prevent infection)
- selenium – 200 mcg a day (antioxidant; protects immune system)
- zinc lozenges (23 mg in each lozenge) – take one every two waking hours for one week. *Caution:* Do not take this dose for longer than one week, as it can cause immuno-suppression (antiviral agent; boosts immunity).
- bromelain – two capsules between meals three times a day (enhances effectiveness of quercetin)
- quercetin – as directed on label of your product (increases immunity)
- thymus extract – 500 mg twice a day (protects immune function and health of mucus membranes)
- pycnogenol or grape seed extract – 100 mg three times a day (antioxidant; reduces inflammation)

Herbal Therapy

Take the following botanical supplements.

- echinacea – boosts the immune system; fights bacterial and viral infections
- goldenseal (antibiotic) – its effectiveness is improved by taking it with 250 to 500 mg of bromelain. *Caution:* Do not take if you are pregnant.
- *Yerba mansa* or Oregon grape root – can be substituted for goldenseal

Take an herbal formula: two parts of echinacea, two parts of wild indigo, and one part of poke root. This formula is available commercially, or can be mixed at an herbal store.

Inhale the vapors from a bottle of eucalyptus essential oils.

Homeopathic Remedies

Take the homeopathic remedy that best fits your symptoms every two hours (for intense symptoms) or every four hours (for mild symptoms).

- *Hepar sulphuris calcareum* – rarely needed at the beginning of a sinus condition; sneezing followed by sinusitis from the least exposure to cold air; nasal discharge is thick and yellow; nostrils sore from the acrid discharge; nasal passages become sensitive to cold; sensation of a nail or plug being thrust into the head and boring or bursting pain; headache above the nose is made worse shaking the head, moving, riding in a car, stooping, moving the eyes, or the weight of a hat; relieved by the firm pressure of a tight bandage; combing the hair can be painful.
- *Kali bichromicum* – nasal discharge is thick and stringy; extreme pain at the root of the nose lessens by applying pressure; bones and scalp feel sore; dizzy and nauseated when rising from sitting; severe pain may lead to dimmed vision; pain worse by cold, cold damp air, light, noise, walking, stooping; pain is worse in the morning upon awakening, at 9 A.M., or at night; prefers to lie down in a darkened room; better with warmth, warm drinks, and overeating; foul smell in sinuses or loss of smell; frontal sinuses are chronically congested, with constant postnasal drip and nasal obstruction.
- *Mercurius solubilis* – feels as though head is in a vise; pain aggravated by open air, sleep, eating and drinking, and extremes of hot or cold temperature; scalp and nose very sensitive to the touch; teeth feel long and painful, and the person may salivate excessively; nasal discharge is usually green and too thick to run; it may be tinged with blood, offensive smelling and acrid, causing rawness and ulceration of the nostrils; worse at night; perspire easily, which aggravates the condition.
- *Pulsatilla* – head pain worse when lying down, in a warm room, but better in cool air; infection may begin after overheating; worse when stooping, sitting, rising from lying down, and eating; pain often in front of the head and accompanied by digestive problems; some relief from walking slowly in open air or by wrapping the head tightly in a bandage; nasal discharge thick and yellow or green.
- *Spigelia anthelmia* – sinusitis with a sharp pain that is worse on the left side; sinusitis after exposure to cold, or cold, wet weather; pain from warmth or when stooping or bending the head forward; relief from cold compresses or from washing with cold water.

Many patients respond to complex homeopathic remedies. You may want to try one of the following (see Sources).

- BHI Sinus – alleviates congestion.
- Euphorbium Compositum Nasal Spray from BHI – drains sinuses and alleviates sinus congestion.
- Sinutarrh from CompliMed – relieves sinus pain and pressure, sinus headache, runny nose, sneezing.
- Sinustat from CompliMed – for sinusitis, rhinitis, inflamed sinus passages and nasal membranes.
- PHP Sinusitis Drops – provide temporary relief of sinus congestion and irritation.

Other Therapeutic Measures

Use the procedures for steaming the sinuses under prevention, above.

Follow the saltwater nasal irrigation with irrigation with an herbal solution (goldenseal, *Yerba mansa*, or Oregon grape root). Use a tea or 5 to 10 drops of a glycerin-based tincture to 1 Tbsp. of saltwater; dilute further if this is irritating.

Inhale the vapors from a bottle of menthol or eucalyptus essential oils.

Place menthol or eucalyptus packs over the sinuses (terpene-sensitive people may not tolerate this). Place wet hotpacks over the sinuses for three minutes, followed by a cold compress for 30 seconds. Repeat at least three times.

Take hot footbaths with a cold compress held over the sinuses.

Avoid using medicated nose sprays. These work well for three to four days, but after that each time the medication wears off, the nasal mucosa swells even more than it had previously, creating a vicious cycle of use and rebound.

Use saltwater nose drops (¼ tsp. of salt in 1 cup of water). Or place in a small glass, tilt your head back, close one nostril, and sniff the solution with the open nostril. Then blow your nose.

Blow one nostril at a time. This helps prevent pressure building up in the Eustachian tubes and bacteria traveling up them.

Sniffle frequently, and spit out or swallow mucus. This drains the sinuses and removes old mucus.

Rest and sleep propped up to increase the size of the openings of the sinuses.

Use acupressure:

- Press both thumbs half a finger's width to the side of the lower end of the nose on both sides, and hold for 15 to 30 seconds.
- Press the point between the nail and the first joint of the thumb, just behind the nail on the side farthest from the fingers.
- Press the point four fingers up from the inner ankle joint, just behind the tibia bone.

PHARYNGITIS AND TONSILLITIS

The throat includes the pharynx and larynx, which are the passageways that connect the nose and mouth with the respiratory and digestive systems. The pharynx includes the back of the throat and the tonsils, and pharyngitis is the medical term for sore throat. Tonsillitis refers to an infection of the tonsils, and is included in the term pharyngitis.

Sore throats are rarely serious problems in themselves, but they may be the first symptoms of many other health problems. When you have a sore throat, the throat hurts when speaking and may feel raw. It may also feel as if the throat needs to be cleared constantly. There may be fever, and attempting to swallow saliva, food, or drink can be quite painful. The throat pain is often referred to the ears, and both children and adults will sometimes complain of an earache when they really have a sore throat.

CAUSES OF SORE THROATS

Whenever there is an infection near the throat, the surrounding blood vessels dilate to increase blood flow to the area and bring blood cells to act as scavengers. The increased blood flow causes the mucus membranes to become red and the underlying tissues to swell. The swelling is primarily responsible for the pain, but in severe sore throats, spasms of the throat muscles can increase discomfort. With any kind of sore throat, the lymph glands (or nodes) under the jaw swell and become tender, because white blood cells come to the lymph nodes to help fight infection. People often complain of swollen or sore glands along with the throat pain.

Only 10 to 20 percent of sore throats in children are caused by streptococci (a bacteria); the rest are caused by viruses. In adults, over 90 percent of sore throats are caused by viruses. It is estimated that 10 to 25 percent of the population are carriers of group A streptococci (which causes strep throat), but do not become ill from it. Staphylococcus (another bacteria) can be cultured from the throats of some people, but it does not usually cause an infection. Some physicians erroneously choose to treat these situations with antibiotics. Viral sore throats can be more difficult to identify than sore throats caused by bacteria, because culture techniques that detect viruses are complicated, expensive, and not practical.

Sore throats can also be caused by dryness of the air, irritating substances (cigarette smoke or smoke from wood-burning stoves), allergies, or overuse of the voice. Some sore throats are caused by postnasal drip. In this case the throat is sore in the morning but improves as the day goes on. A sore throat upon awakening can also be caused by sleeping with the mouth open, and some people have a morning sore throat from the backup of stomach acid into the throat at night.

Many people with recurrent or chronic sore throats have food sensitivities, often to wheat and milk. Anger or grief can cause the sensation of a lump in the throat, which may feel like a sore throat. However, a continued sensation of a lump in the throat, accompanied by persistent hoarseness, should be checked by a physician as these can be symptoms of cancer of the larynx.

STREP THROAT

Most bacterial infections of the throat are caused by strep infections. Strep throat can be associated with abscesses around the tonsils, infection of the lymph nodes of the neck, or ear infections.

Strep throat is usually a benign infection in itself, but its consequences can be dangerous. The body produces antibodies against strep, but these may attack the heart or kidneys, damaging the heart valves (rheumatic heart disease) or inflaming the kidneys (glomerulonephritis).

Rheumatic fever can appear in the aftermath of a strep infection, occurring two to three weeks after the sore throat is gone. It presents with symptoms such as joint tenderness, heat, swelling, and redness; fever; inflammation of the heart; changes on the EKG; or Sydenham's chorea, a movement disorder. Treatment of strep throat with antibiotics reduces the risk of rheumatic fever by a factor of 10. However, if a patient is treated within nine days of the appearance of the first sore throat symptoms, rheumatic fever can still be prevented.

Scarlet fever is a strep infection accompanied by a rash. Today it is not a serious infection, and does not cause the severe side effects of deafness and blindness that it used to. Scarlet fever is rare in children less than three years of age, and very rare in adults. A scarlet fever rash feels like sandpaper, is felt more than it is seen, and blanches with pressure. It first appears on the upper chest about 24 hours after the onset of symptoms: red lines appear in the inside of the elbow, the face is red but the area around the mouth is pale, and the tongue appears red. A week later the rash may begin to peel, especially on the hands.

Strep throat is most commonly seen in children between the ages of 5 and 15. In temperate climates, it usually occurs in the winter and early spring. A history of contact with a person with strep throat makes the diagnosis more likely. People with strep throat generally present with a sore throat of sudden onset, pain on swallowing, and fever. Some people will develop headache, nausea, vomiting, and abdominal pain. The tonsils are generally very red, and sometimes have a coating of pus. There is redness and swelling of the uvula, petechia (small broken blood vessels) on the roof of the mouth, and tender, enlarged, lymph nodes under the jaw. The taste buds of the tongue may be red and swollen; this is known as strawberry tongue. Younger children occasionally have chronic, low-grade fever; swollen lymph glands; a runny nose with crusting beneath the nostrils; and a throat that is not red. However, this is not a common presentation.

Use of a scoring system, developed by Dr. Warren J. McIsaac of the Department of Family Medicine at the Toronto Faculty of Medicine, can improve the accuracy of strep throat diagnoses and reduce the inappropriate use of antibiotics. The scoring system awards one point for each of the following findings:

- a history of fever above 100.4°F (38°C)
- no cough
- swollen tonsils
- swollen or tender neck glands
- patient younger than age 15

Deduct a point for patients older than 45. Patients whose score is less than two points probably have a viral infection. Patients with two or three points are borderline cases and should have a throat culture. Patients with a score of four or higher have about a 50 percent risk of a group A streptococci infection and should have their throats cultured. Patients with sore throats whose findings do not suggest strep throat usually should *not* be cultured because even if the culture is positive, the person is more likely to be a carrier than to be truly infected.

To culture a sore throat, a Q-tip is swabbed on the tonsils and the back of the throat. The swab is then rubbed on a culture plate of sheep blood agar. The plate is incubated for 24 hours at body temperature, and then read for the presence of strep colonies. Strep throat is often hard to detect early in the illness (the first 24 hours) because there may not be enough bacteria present to be detectable. Rapid strep detection kits are now available and test for the strep bacteria itself. These tests take 5 to 15 minutes to obtain results.

VIRAL INFECTIONS

Summer sore throats are typically caused by adenovirus. The throat becomes very painful and there may be an associated eye infection. Preschoolers are most commonly affected. Coxsackie virus (hand-foot-mouth disease) is another cause of sore throat. With this virus, tiny blisters or red spots appear on the palms of the hands, soles of the feet, and throat. *Herpes simplex* type I virus (the cold sore virus) can also cause blisters in the mouth and throat.

Infectious mononucleosis is caused by the Epstein-Barr virus and is most commonly seen in teenagers. They develop fever, fatigue, severe sore throat, and swollen lymph glands. Some patients may also develop swelling of the liver, jaundice, or elevation of the liver enzymes. A few may also develop swelling of the spleen, which may not be noticeable on clinical exam, but can put patients at high risk of a ruptured

spleen if they are injured. Patients with "mono" have enlarged tonsils covered with white pus. They usually feel fatigued for several weeks or even months, although the mono itself lasts only about two weeks.

MODERN MEDICAL TREATMENT
Diet
Patients are advised to eat a well-balanced diet.

Exercise and Lifestyle
Patients should not exercise when acutely ill.

Drug Therapy
For patients with strep throat, antibiotics are prescribed. However, patients with uncomplicated strep throat who are not treated with antibiotics recover as rapidly as those treated with antibiotics. By the sixth day of illness, symptoms have resolved in almost all patients.

Antibiotics vary widely in the numbers and types of bacteria they will kill. Those that are effective for many different bacteria are known as broad-spectrum antibiotics. Sensitivity tests performed in the laboratory allow the physician to prescribe the most effective antibiotic for a particular bacteria. A major problem in the use of antibiotics is resistance to the antibiotics, caused by both overprescribing for humans and the increased use of antibiotics for animals being raised for human consumption. There is concern that widespread resistance of bacteria will result in there being no effective antibiotics left to treat infections.

Antibiotics have the potential for causing allergic reactions, and side effects range from mild to serious, depending on the antibiotic and the sensitivity of the individual taking it (some sensitive individuals are unable to tolerate any antibiotics). Side effects may include rashes, hives, fatigue, headache, diarrhea/loose stools, nausea, vomiting, vaginitis, liver dysfunction, abdominal pain, anemia, depression, fever, anaphylaxis, and photosensitivity.

Other medications are also recommended for strep throat and sore throat. Antacids or an antacid and liquid Benadryl combination are used to soothe the throat. Patients are told to take acetaminophen, aspirin, or ibuprofen for pain. Throat sprays (which may contain phenol) and throat lozenges may also be suggested.

The organisms causing sore throats are found deep in the throat tissues, and only an agent that can deliver adequate amounts of medication to these tissues will be effective in treatment. Use of antiseptic gargles, mouthwashes, or medicated lozenges does little to cure or prevent sore throats, though they may provide temporary relief of dryness and minor irritations of the mouth and throat. Some gargles may provide relief from inflammatory pain by providing a temporary anesthetic effect, and some lozenges contain a topical anesthetic that will give short-lived pain relief.

Other Therapeutic Measures

Patients are told to use humidifiers in their bedrooms if they breathe through their mouths when they sleep.

They are told to sip lemon juice mixed with honey in hot tea or water throughout the day. Gargles with warm saltwater (1 tsp. salt in 2 cups warm water) are also suggested.

For sore throats caused by a backup of stomach acid, patients are advised to tilt the bed frame so the head is four to six inches higher than the foot. Do not just pile more pillows under the head, as this causes increased pressure on the esophagus and makes the problem worse.

ALTERNATIVE TREATMENT

Diet

Increase fluid intake. Avoid milk, orange juice, and caffeine. Drink diluted vegetable juices, soups, and herb teas.

Limit simple sugar consumption (including fruit sugar) to less than 50 grams a day.

Exercise and Lifestyle

Do not exercise when you are acutely ill. Rest when you have a sore throat.

Do not smoke, and avoid secondhand smoke.

Nutrient Therapy

Take the following nutritional supplements.

- vitamin A – 25,000 IU a day. *Caution:* Do not take more than 8,000 IU a day if you are or might be pregnant (protects mucus membranes; helps heal mucosa).
- beta carotene – 200,000 IU a day (precursor of vitamin A)
- vitamin C – 500 mg every two hours to bowel tolerance (strengthens immune system)
- bioflavonoids – 1,000 mg a day (strengthen immune system)
- zinc gluconate lozenges (23 mg) – one lozenge every two hours. *Caution:* Do not use for longer than seven days (boosts immunity).
- thymus extract – 500 mg two times a day (protects immune function and health of mucus membranes)
- L-lysine – 500 mg three to four times a day (for viral sore throats); continue for a week after the sore throat is gone (prevents viral replication)
- Monolaurin – three capsules a day (for an acute viral sore throat), then decrease to one a day for several weeks after the sore throat is gone (prevents attachment of viruses to cells) (Cardiovascular Research—see Sources)

Herbal Therapy

Use a botanical supplement.

- Gargle with warm chamomile tea (soothing to the throat).
- Gargle with a mixture of hot water, ¼ tsp. of turmeric powder, and a pinch of salt (soothing to the throat).
- Apply a warm chamomile poultice to the throat (soothing to the throat). To make the

poultice, add 1 Tbsp. of dried chamomile flowers to 1 or 2 cups of boiling water. Allow to steep for five minutes and then strain. Soak a towel in the tea, wring out the excess, and apply to the neck. Leave on until the cloth is cold.

- Eat garlic or take garlic extract for sore throat (antimicrobial).
- Mix 1 Tbsp. of pure horseradish, 1 tsp. honey, and 1 tsp. of ground cloves in a glass of warm water and sip (stir periodically, as it tends to settle) (soothing to the throat).
- Take goldenseal – *Caution:* Do not take if you are pregnant (an anti-inflammatory that soothes mucus membranes).
- Take echinacea (does not kill strep effectively or prevent rheumatic fever, but stimulates the immune system).
- Suck on horehound or slippery elm bark lozenges or cough drops (soothing to the throat).
- Drink licorice-root tea, mullein tea, or slippery elm bark tea (soothing to the throat).

Homeopathic Remedies
Take the homeopathic remedy that best fits your symptoms. If you do not obtain relief, seek the help of a homeopathic practitioner. The remedies listed below are a few of the many possibilities.

- *Aconite* – use at the beginning of the illness, within the first 24 to 48 hours; caused by fright, shock, exposure to cold, dry wind; thirst; sudden onset of symptoms, that are worse at night with intolerable pains; the throat is burning, red, and dry.
- *Arsenicum* – burning pains, ulcers in throat, better with hot drinks, worse with cold drinks, worse when swallowing.
- *Belladonna* – throat constricted, irritated, raw; swollen glands, pain severe, stitching, worse on right side; neck is tender to touch; talking is difficult; constant desire to swallow despite extreme pain; sips drinks with head held bent forward; tongue may be red, coated with white dots; throat reddens and throbs painfully, radiates heat; aversion to drinks; sleep is restless and delirium may occur.

- *Gelsemium* – intensely weary; arms and legs feel as if weighted down with lead, trembly with exhaustion; comes on gradually, takes days to develop; pain extends to the ears and the throat feels rough.
- *Mercurius solublilis* – pain spreading up to ears and neck, stitching feeling; tonsils swollen and dark-red, ulcerated, worse at night; on right side of body; dryness and soreness with a constant desire to swallow, which is painful; intense inflammation, rawness, and smarting; offensive breath; thick, tenacious saliva and foul breath; rarely needed at onset of the illness.
- *Phytolacca* – a dark red discoloration and inflammation of the tonsils, pharynx, or root of the tongue, worse on the right side; hot-feeling throat with pain on swallowing that may radiate to the ear; throat pain better with cold drinks and worse with warm drinks; pain in throat as from a "burning hot ball"; neck pain and stiffness, worse at night, worse on right side; hard, painful swelling of the cervical glands; intense dryness, smarting, and burning in the throat; tonsils may be large and dark blue.

Many patients respond to complex homeopathic remedies. You may want to try BHI Throat or CompliMed Sore Throat, for sore throat, hoarseness, laryngitis, or inflammation caused by smoke or pollution (see Sources).

Other Therapeutic Measures
Use a facial sauna (a device that produces steam and has a plastic shield to fit around the face) or place your face over a pot of boiling water with a towel covering your head.

Inhale saltwater nose mist from a commercial saline spray.

Throw away your toothbrush when you start to feel ill. Use another while you are ill and replace it when you begin to feel better.

Treat strep throat with nutrients and herbs for immune support for a week to see if there is response. If there is no response, use antibiotics.

LUNG PROBLEMS

Many people visualize lungs as two empty sacks. They actually consist of several lobes and are made up of many parts. The trachea, or windpipe, branches into two bronchi, or bronchial tubes, one of which enters each lung. Within the lungs, the bronchi branch many times into bronchioles, which branch further to end in air sacs, or alveoli. There are approximately 300 million alveoli in addition to tubes, blood vessels, and elastic connective tissues. The alveoli are the site of gas exchange with the blood. Fresh air comes into the alveoli, and the oxygen diffuses into the blood, where it combines with hemoglobin that carries it throughout the body.

Unless a person is ill, the lower respiratory tract (vocal cords through the lungs) is usually sterile. It contains a number of protective mechanisms, including a continuous coating of mucus within the bronchi. This mucus captures particles, bacteria, and viruses, and with the help of cilia (microscopic, hair-like projections) moves it to the mouth for removal. Coughing also aids the removal of particles from the lungs. Other defense mechanisms include antibodies, white blood cells, and a lymph drainage network.

Asthma and bronchitis typically affect the bronchial tube system. Emphysema and pneumonia affect the alveoli.

RESPIRATORY INFECTIONS

Respiratory infections are an acute condition that can be caused by viruses, bacteria, fungi, or a combination of organisms. These infections can affect the lungs and air sacs, as in the case of pneumonia, or the airways and bronchi, as in the case of acute bronchitis.

ACUTE BRONCHITIS

Acute bronchitis is typically a viral infection of the bronchial tubes that often occurs after a cold. In bronchitis, the airways are inflamed and filled with mucus, pus, and debris from cells. The cough accompanying bronchitis can last for weeks, causing loss of sleep and appetite. Studies have demonstrated that treatment of acute bronchitis with antibiotics does not change the outcome. If the cough lasts longer than four to six weeks, or if there are other symptoms (night sweats, weight loss, or chest pain), it is important to see a physician.

PNEUMONIA

Pneumonia is the fifth leading cause of death in the United States. It is a respiratory condition in which the air sacs become inflamed and filled with mucus, pus and dead cells. It is most often seen in winter. Patients develop a cough that produces yellow, green, brown, or rust-colored mucus that is often bad-tasting. Patients typically have fever, and will often have an abrupt onset of shaking chills, difficulty in breathing, and sometimes pain in the chest. However, symptoms may be mild, with a low-grade fever, cough, and some mucus; this is known as "walking pneumonia," because the patient is able to be up and about. The term "double pneumonia" is sometimes used when both lungs are involved. It takes a patient two to three weeks to recover from pneumonia.

Pneumonia tends to occur when the defense mechanisms are depressed; for instance, after a viral infection (especially influenza), with cancer, when a person has been exposed to cigarette smoke, and after aspiration of stomach acid. It can be caused by a viral, bacterial, or fungal infection of the lung. Pneumonia can also be caused by toxic fumes or aspiration of food or liquid, and can occur in a person who is unconscious because of a seizure or from alcohol intoxication. The elderly, drug and alcohol abusers, and patients whose immune systems are suppressed by disease or chemotherapy are all prone to pneumonia. Chronic lung disease such as asthma or emphysema can predispose a patient to pneumonia.

MODERN MEDICAL PREVENTION

Pneumococcal and flu vaccines are recommended for people over 60 or those with chronic lung disease.

ALTERNATIVE PREVENTION

Get plenty of rest and avoid body stress and fatigue, particularly after being outdoors for long periods during the winter. Avoid exposures to toxic fumes and pesticides.

Wash your hands frequently and avoid crowds during cold and flu season. Take bowel tolerance vitamin C and immune-system strengthening nutrients (see nutrients listed under treatment below).

Control your allergies, particularly if you are prone to lung symptoms.

MODERN MEDICAL TREATMENT

Diet
For acute bronchitis and pneumonia, modern medicine suggests a well-balanced diet.

Exercise and Lifestyle
Because people with pneumonia and acute bronchitis are acutely ill, exercise is not recommended.

Drug Therapy
Patients are given antibiotics if a chest X-ray or clinical exam demonstrates pneumonia. In some patients, a sputum sample is obtained to look for white blood cells and bacteria and for a culture. If the exam shows bacteria in the sputum, antibiotics are begun. The full course of antibiotics should be completed, and they can be life-

saving if the person is very ill. People with acute bronchitis who do not have a bacterial infection are often given antibiotics even though they do not affect the outcome.

ALTERNATIVE TREATMENT

Diet
For acute bronchitis and pneumonia, eat hot, spicy foods (including garlic, onion, chili peppers, horseradish, and mustard) to open the air passages.

Avoid dairy products, as they tend to thicken mucus. Avoid sugar, white flour, processed foods, coffee, and all teas except herbal teas. Also avoid alcohol and any known food allergens.

Drink plenty of fluids and fresh juices, including vegetable juices. To allow the lungs to heal easily, eat a diet high in vegetable protein and low in meat and animal fats. Include cultured foods, such as kefir and yogurt.

Exercise and Lifestyle
Do not exercise when you are ill, but afterward begin with small amounts and increase as you begin to get well.

Avoid temperature extremes. Do not smoke and avoid being around anyone who smokes.

Use disposable tissues and discard them properly.

Nutrient Therapy
Take the following nutrients for acute bronchitis and pneumonia.

- vitamin A – 25,000 IU a day. *Caution:* Do not take more than 8,000 IU a day if you are pregnant or might be pregnant (heals and protects tissue).
- beta carotene – 200,000 IU a day (protects lung tissue)
- vitamin C – approximately 1,000 mg every hour, to bowel tolerance (see p. 372). This is

most effective when used in the first one to two days of illness (strengthens the immune system; reduces inflammation).

- bioflavonoids – 1,000 mg a day (stimulate the immune system)
- vitamin E – 400 to 800 IU a day (protects lung tissue and increases oxygen utilization)
- zinc lozenges – 23 mg every two hours while awake. *Caution:* Do not take for more than one week (strengthens immune system).
- pycnogenol or grape seed extract – as directed on the product label (boosts the immune system; protects lung tissue)
- thymus extract – 500 mg twice a day (strengthens immune system)

Herbal Therapy
Take a botanical supplement under the direction of a trained herbalist.

- astragalus – further boosts immunity
- echinacea – strengthens the immune system
- goldenseal – soothes irritated mucus membranes. *Caution:* Do not take if you are pregnant.
- licorice – acts as an expectorant; supports the immune system
- lobelia, grindelia, wild cherry bark, white horehound, coltsfoot, and sundew – all are herbal expectorants
- mullein – every four hours to soothe irritation in the bronchial passages

Homeopathic Remedies
Consult a homeopathic physician for the best remedy to treat acute bronchitis and pneumonia. The following remedies are a few of the many possibilities.

- *Antimonium tartaricum* – late-stage pneumonia with collapse, especially in infants and older people; miserable, irritable, and peevish; lips cyanotic; sunken or gaunt features;

cold sweat on face; neck muscles strain with each inhalation; tongue coated, thick, and white; pulse weak and thready; chilly but aggravated by heat and desires to be fanned; better sitting propped; loathing of food and nausea; rattling chest; weak, unproductive, wet-sounding cough; suffocating sensations; expectorate is whitish, purulent mucus.

- *Arsenicum album* – restless and anxious with fear of death and desire for company; collapsed, cold, and prostrated; tight chest that burns with each cough; must sit up, feels suffocated if lying flat; scant expectoration with frothy sputum; offensive breath and sputum; burning tongue, coated white; rigors with slight draft; chilly and desires warmth; worse 12 to 1 A.M. burning pains through whole respiratory tract.
- *Bryonia* – cold starts with a nasal discharge and then moves down into the chest; cough is dry and made worse by motion or by breathing in; person tends to hold the chest with breathing in order to limit the motion of the chest and to control the pain; sensitive to drafts and always catches cold; tickling in the larynx that irritates the cough; dry cough seems to start in the stomach and is worse after eating.
- *Ferrum phosphoricum* – pneumonia develops slowly, over one or two days; high fever, almost always over 103°F; prefers to be left alone; rapid pulse; flushed with pallor around the mouth; extreme thirst for cold drinks; incessant cough with irritation behind the sternum; worse in cold and drafts; blood-streaked sputum in bright, red streaks.
- *Phosphorus* – in delicate, slender tall patients; dry, hard cough, sometimes with a persistent tickly feeling; tearing pain under the breastbone, aggravated by lying down, especially on the left side; wakes up at night, needing to sit up and cough; aggravated by talking, moving, going from a warm room to

cold air or by strong odors; tightness in chest relieved by the warmth of a bed; craves ice drinks; illness is exhausting; nasal discharge may have some blood streaked in it; sputum contains mucus and pus, may be blood-streaked, and has a salty-sweet taste.

- *Pulsatilla* – cough symptoms are aggravated in a warm room or warm weather, by lying down to sleep, and at night; walking in the cool air provides some relief; child must sit up in bed to breathe better, dry cough in the day; productive cough with yellow or green-ish expectoration at night and upon waking.

Many patients respond to complex homeo-pathic remedies. You may want to try BHI Bron-chitis, or PHP Lung Liquescence, which provides potentized nutrients for lung function and regeneration.

Engystol N stimulates your immune system, and is available in both oral and injectable forms.

Other Therapeutic Measures
Use the following foods to relieve cough in cases of acute bronchitis and pneumonia.

- Eat raw garlic at the first sign of a cold.
- Put six chopped white onions in a double boiler and add ½ cup of honey. Cook slowly over low heat for two hours and strain. Take 1 tsp. every four to six hours.
- Drink ginger root tea. Use a one-inch piece of ginger root in 2 cups of water; bring to a boil and simmer for five minutes. Add ½ tsp. cayenne pepper, and simmer one more minute. Remove from heat. Add 2 Tbsp. of fresh lemon juice, honey to taste, and one or two cloves of mashed garlic.
- Drink hot lemon and honey with water every morning.
- Eat horseradish, hot mustard, or wasabi to help liquefy sputum (phlegm).

If you have pneumonia or acute bronchitis, you may have to take an antibiotic. Use the mea-sures below in addition to taking the antibiotic to help speed your recovery. Be certain to take an acidophilus preparation if you take an antibi-otic. Take it at a different time from your antibi-otic dose. Use up to 3 tsp. of acidophilus powder a day in divided doses.

Use a hot cayenne and ginger poultice on your chest. Mix ½ tsp. cayenne powder, 1 Tbsp. lobelia powder, 3 Tbsp. slippery elm, 2 Tbsp. ginger, and enough water to make a paste. Leave in place for an hour.

Apply a heating pad or hot water bottle to the chest and back for 30 minutes a day.

Inhale steam, as follows: boil water on a stove, and stand over it with a towel over your head, forming a "tent" over the pot to trap steam. Breathe the steam through your mouth, with pursed lips. Add sage and/or eucalyptus (ter-pene-sensitive people may not tolerate these).

Take a cough medication that contains potas-sium iodide (Pima syrup), and drink four to six glasses of fluid a day.

Press the following acupressure points:

- one and a half thumbs' width to each side of the center of the spine, at the level of the third thoracic vertebra
- in the depression at the center of the front of the chest on a line joining both nipples
- mid-point from the knee to the ankle, three fingers' width back toward the fibula from the ridge on the front of the shin (on the out-side of the lower leg)
- one hand's width (four fingers) up from the inner ankle point, just behind the tibia bone
- ear point at the base of the piece of cartilage called the tragus at the external opening of the ear.

Get plenty of rest. Be sure to wash your hands frequently and thoroughly.

CHRONIC LUNG DISEASE

Chronic lung disease, also called chronic obstructive pulmonary disease, is caused by loss of lung tissue and in some cases is irreversible. It usually results from frequent irritation of the lungs, such as from cigarette smoke or toxic fumes, rather than an infection. Allergies may play a role, as well as climatic and environmental factors, such as dampness, cold, or dust.

ASTHMA

Asthma has become epidemic in North America, with at least 20 million people—more than 3 percent of the population—affected by this lung condition. The number of asthma cases doubled between 1982 and 1994, with the greatest increase appearing in people between the ages of 18 and 44. Women account for 60 percent of adult asthmatics, but asthma is most common in children under 10 years old. It is the leading chronic illness among children. In the United States one child in ten has asthma, in England one child in seven has asthma, and in Japan one child in five has asthma. Twice as many boys as girls are affected by the condition.

Asthma is defined as "recurrent episodes of inflammation causing reversible spasms of the bronchial tubes." Repeated infections or exposure to allergens or irritants cause chronic inflammation of the bronchial tubes. Once these airways are inflamed, they become irritable or twitchy, and too narrow when they are exposed to substances to which they are very sensitive. People with asthma develop shortness of breath, wheezing, tightness of the chest, and coughing. Asthma can be experienced in many different ways, ranging from occasional wheezing to severe attacks. An attack that lasts for days and cannot be reversed is called status asthmaticus, and it can be fatal.

Indoor air pollution seems to bear the most responsibility for the increase in asthma. In inner cities, cockroaches are a major trigger. Volatile organic compounds emitted by furniture, paint, glues, cleaning products, and many other substances are also suspected triggers. Asthma attacks can be brought on by exercise; weather changes; aspirin; medications such as beta blockers; viral infections; cigarette smoke; irritants such as chemical fumes, cleaning agents, and perfume; foods and food additives; pollens; drugs; molds; dust mites; feathers; and animal danders. Asthma can also be triggered by a reflux of stomach acid into the airway.

Despite what most physicians believe, many studies have documented that food allergies can trigger asthma. Eliminating allergenic foods produces significant improvement in three-fourths of asthmatic children and in one-third of asthmatic adults. In children, the most common acute triggers of asthma are eggs, shellfish, nuts, and peanuts. Foods associated with delayed onset of asthma include milk, chocolate, wheat, citrus, and food colorings. Food additives such as tartrazine, benzoate, sulfites, and sulfur dioxide can also trigger asthma.

There are thought to be two types of asthma: extrinsic and intrinsic. Extrinsic asthma is thought to be caused by allergies with an increased serum immunoglobulin IgE (see Allergy chapter), and accounts for over half the asthma cases in children and young adults. The allergens causing extrinsic asthma are usually airborne, and may include pollen, smoke, dust, animal danders, and automobile exhaust. Intrinsic asthma is thought to be caused by other factors such as cold air and exercise (although many studies show that allergy plays a role in intrinsic asthma as well). Intrinsic asthma can also be secondary to chronic or recurrent infections of the sinuses, bronchi, or tonsils and adenoids. Hypersensitivity to the bacteria causing the infection may be the cause of this type of intrinsic asthma.

Researchers are now finding that hormonal

fluctuations can trigger asthma in women. When estrogen levels are lowest (from three days before a period begins through the fourth day of the period) the lungs are more sensitive to allergens and other triggers.

Asthma patients usually have a family and a personal history of allergy and asthma. If both parents have asthma, at least one in three of their children is likely to develop symptoms at some time. Asthma in mothers is a stronger determinant of early onset asthma in a child than paternal asthma.

Almost half of all asthmatics develop asthmalike symptoms by the end of their first year, and 90 percent do so before the age of five. Seventy-five percent of the children who develop asthma within the first three years of life still have active symptoms by age 11. Children who have eczema, hay fever, or food allergies at a very young age, and toddlers who have frequent bouts of respiratory infections, are at high risk of developing asthma. Dr. George Bray, a physician at the Hospital for Sick Children in London, demonstrated in 1931 that 80 percent of 200 asthmatic children had low levels of hydrochloric acid in their stomachs.

Prevention of asthma attacks is the most important factor in the management of asthma. Emphasizing prevention—even if it means using preventative medication—will reduce the likelihood of dependence on a multiple-drug regimen to control asthma. Taking preventative measures gives the patients a feeling of some control over their disease and reduces their feelings of helplessness, and most patients are eager to learn ways to control environmental and emotional events that can precipitate an attack.

MODERN MEDICAL PREVENTION

Patients are advised to keep the home (particularly the bedroom) and workplace as dust-free as possible. Carpet should be removed from the bedroom and the room should be damp-dusted every other day. Unnecessary clothing and clutter should be cleaned from closets, and washable curtains or window coverings should be hung.

Children's stuffed animals should either be removed or washed as often as possible, and if the children are allergy prone, encase their pillows, mattresses, and box springs in airtight covers to prevent proliferation of dust mites.

Ventilation in the kitchen and bathroom should be optimal to combat mold, and a humidifier should be used in damp areas.

Reduction of exposure to triggers such as tobacco and wood smoke, perfumes, car exhaust, animal dander, and molds is advised. Patients who are allergic to pollens should use an air cleaner (HEPA) in the house during pollen season. In cases of allergy to cats and dogs, other indoor pets or no pets should be considered.

Patients are cautioned not to go to sleep on a full stomach. Those who have acid reflux are told to prop up the bedposts to elevate the head of the bed to prevent reflux into the airway.

If the patient exercises or goes outside in cold weather, a scarf or mask should be used to cover the nose and mouth.

If possible, parents should choose a small-group setting for daycare, and make sure caregivers wash their hands frequently. Parents should not smoke, particularly around their children, and should ensure that others do not smoke in the children's presence.

Modern medicine makes no special recommendations for diet for asthmatics except to encourage overweight patients to lose weight. The extra pounds make it more difficult to breathe.

ALTERNATIVE PREVENTION

Use methods suggested in modern medical prevention. As well, hang some plants (spider plants, Boston fern, English ivy, or striped dracaena) to help absorb toxic gases. If possible, do not use wood-burning stoves or fireplaces.

Use posture and deep breathing exercises to

maintain good air exchange. Drink large quantities of fluid to replace that lost through respiratory distress and coughing. Fluids will also thin bronchial secretions so that they are more easily removed by coughing.

Patients should be aware of the hazards of extremes in eating, exercise, and emotions (for instance, prolonged crying or laughing). Modification and moderation will help avoid overstimulation and an overtaxing of the body systems, which can lead to an attack.

Relaxation techniques that reduce stress may be helpful for many patients.

Be aware of the early signs of an asthma attack so that you can initiate proper treatment.

Take the botanical supplement Reishi (acts as anti-inflammatory) in tea or tablet form, for two months.

Breast-feed babies to minimize respiratory infections, which can help protect them from developing asthma. Delay the introduction of solid foods until after the baby is six months old.

MODERN MEDICAL TREATMENT

Diet
Overweight patients are encouraged to lose weight.

Exercise and Lifestyle
Exercise can help some people with asthma, if they choose an exercise that they can carry out without exacerbating their asthma. Regardless of the type of exercise chosen, patients should breathe through the nose instead of the mouth. They are advised to use a peak flow meter to monitor their asthma while exercising.

Drug Therapy
Modern medical treatment of asthma now focuses on the inflammation of the bronchial tubes that underlies all asthma. Two anti-inflammatory drugs, Nedocromil (Tilade) or Cromolyn (Intal)—both non-steroidal medica-

tions—are used to treat chronic asthma and to prevent asthma. Tilade tastes bad, and side effects of these medications include throat irritation or dryness, coughing, wheezing, and sometimes severe bronchospasm. There may also be dizziness, allergic reaction, pain with urination, tearing, joint swelling, nausea, headache, and burning pain beneath the breast bone.

Steroids, in inhaled or oral forms, are also used in treating asthma. These are powerful anti-inflammatory drugs. Long-term use of oral steroids has been linked to growth impairment in children, weight gain, osteoporosis, high blood pressure, ulcers, susceptibility to other infections, muscle weakness, fracture of the vertebrae, impaired wound healing, thin fragile skin, increased pressure in the brain, irregular periods, manifestations of latent diabetes, glaucoma, and cataracts. A person who has been on steroids for a long time and suddenly stops taking them can become very ill, with signs of adrenal failure, if stressed with surgery or illness. Children who have been on oral steroids (or even inhaled steroids) have developed fatal cases of chicken pox. Inhaled steroids can cause fungal or yeast infections in the mouth, glaucoma, and an increased risk of cataracts later in life.

Albuterol (Ventolin, Proventil) is a beta 2 agonist medication, which works by relaxing the muscles around the bronchial tubes. It comes in a tablet form, as an aerosol or a powder that is aerosolized, or as a liquid that is used in a nebulizer (an air compressor) that produces a mist of particles that can be inhaled into the lungs. Albuterol increases the heart rate and causes a feeling that the heart is beating rapidly and strongly. It may also cause headaches, nausea or vomiting, throat irritation, discolored teeth, nosebleeds, increased blood pressure, tremor, dizziness, and nervousness. When overused by a patient during an acute asthma attack, it can make the patient more resistant to treatment.

An inhaler must be used properly, with activation of the spray at the time of a deep inhalation. Children and some older adults are not able to do this properly, and will need a holding chamber to avoid having to coordinate their activation of the inhaler with inhalation. To use an inhaler, hold it about an inch away from your open mouth, or in your mouth, take a slow deep breath, and just after you start breathing in, activate the inhaler. Continue to breathe in and hold your breath for about 10 seconds. If you see mist coming out of your mouth, you are using the inhaler incorrectly. Take the second puff two to five minutes after the first.

Theophylline, an oral medication related to caffeine, is not as popular a medication for asthma as it used to be, but it has newly identified anti-inflammatory effects. Theophylline helps prevent the airways from becoming hyperreactive, and it also reduces bronchoconstriction. Sustained-release theophylline medication helps maintain therapeutic levels of theophylline without creating wide swings in blood levels of the drug. There is a narrow range between therapeutic levels of theophylline and toxic levels. Becuse it is a stimulant, patients taking theophylline must be careful of caffeine intake. Heart arrhythmias, convulsions, or even death may occur without warning as the first sign of toxicity. Erythromycin and Tagamet can interact with theophylline, increasing blood levels of theophylline. Side effects of theophylline can include nausea, headaches, irritability, sleep problems, muscle twitching, low blood pressure, rapid breathing, and high blood sugar levels.

Ipratropium (Atrovent) is another medication used for asthma, but it is not a first-line drug because it does not open up airways as well as Albuterol. Atrovent can make glaucoma worse, but it does not have the intestinal and cardiac side effects associated with other asthma medications. Side effects can include dryness of the throat, cough, worsening of symptoms, headaches, dizziness, blurred vision, and drying of secretions. Atrovent can cause acute urinary tract obstruction in patients with enlarged prostates.

ALTERNATIVE TREATMENT

Diet

Several foods are helpful for asthma. Chili peppers loosen congestion. Onions, chives, scallions, leeks, shallots, and garlic contain anti-inflammatory substances that help control asthma attacks. Orange juice, grapefruit juice, sweet potatoes, cantaloupe, strawberries, and tomatoes, all of which are rich in vitamin C, make people less likely to develop bronchitis or asthma.

Avoid sugar, eggs, starches, dairy products, food allergens, and the odor of food allergens.

Use a special vegan diet if the asthma does not improve. This diet has no meat, fish, eggs, dairy products, apples, or citrus fruit, and restricts the amount of grain used; this eliminates common food allergens and alters fatty acid metabolism.

For exercise-induced asthma, try a hyperinsulinemic diet (see p. 235).

Drink 8 to 10 glasses of water a day.

Chewing is difficult when you have shortness of breath. Try to eat soft foods, which are easier to chew. Avoid foods that are difficult to swallow, such as dry crackers and nuts. Eat foods of moderate temperature, as very hot or very cold foods can precipitate a coughing attack.

Exercise and Lifestyle

If you have asthma, do aerobic exercise three to four times a week for 20 minutes a session. Avoid exercising in heavy traffic areas. During pollen season, avoid heavy pollen areas.

Some asthmatics have problems with sports. Be aware that swimmers are more likely to have asthma.

Perform Tai Chi or Qigong daily.

Get plenty of rest. Drink at least 2 quarts of liquid (the majority of it water) a day, which will help dilute the mucus, making it easier to expel.

Do regular breathing exercises. See p. 421.

Nutrient Therapy
Take the following nutrients for asthma.

- vitamin B5 (pantothenic acid) – 250 mg a day (supports adrenal glands)
- vitamin B$_6$ – 25 to 50 mg a day for children. (Children with asthma often have a defect in tryptophan metabolism, which can be corrected with B$_6$ or by using a low-tryptophan diet.) Adults can take 50 mg a day (decreases frequency and severity of asthma attacks).
- vitamin B$_{12}$ – 1 mg intramuscular injections weekly for six weeks (particularly helps with asthmatic children) (relieves asthma)
- vitamin C – 1,000 to 2,000 mg two to three times a day (antihistamine; blocks tendency of bronchial tubes to go into spasm). For exercised-induced asthma, take 500 to 1,000 mg one hour before exercise.
- carotenes – 50,000 IU a day (increase integrity of epithelial lining of the respiratory tract; decrease inflammation)
- vitamin E – 400 IU a day (inhibits formation of inflammatory compounds)
- calcium – 500 mg a day (relieves spasms)
- magnesium – 400 mg a day (promotes relaxation of bronchial muscles)
- molybdenum – 30 mcg a day (detoxifies sulfites)
- selenium – 200 to 250 mcg a day (anti-inflammatory)
- cod liver oil – 3,000 mg a day (anti-inflammatory effect)
- betaine hydrochloride, glutamic hydrochloride, or apple cider vinegar before meals (some asthmatics have a stomach acid deficiency).

Use the following nutrients intravenously.

- vitamin B$_{12}$ intravenously (protects against sulfite-induced asthma)
- intravenous magnesium for acute asthma (promotes relaxation of bronchial muscles; stops asthma attack)
- intravenous (IV) vitamins, combining vitamin C, B$_6$, B$_{12}$, magnesium, and calcium (promote relaxation of bronchial muscles; relieve asthma)

Herbal Therapy
Take a botanical supplement. Consult a trained herbalist for the best results.

- angelica – inhibits production of IgE, and allergic antibodies
- Chinese skullcap – anti-inflammatory
- ephedra – take with thyme, an antispasmodic (anti-inflammatory; anti-allergy)
- ginger root – expectorant
- green tea – antioxidant; contains compound similar to theophylline
- Indian tobacco – typically combined with capsicum (pepper) (expectorant; relaxes bronchial muscles)
- licorice – anti-inflammatory; anti-allergy. *Caution:* Do not use over a long period of time.
- marshmallow – for cough
- mullein tea – can be combined with marshmallow and slippery elm (expectorant)
- onions/garlic – inhibits formation of inflammatory chemicals
- slippery elm – anti-inflammatory

Homeopathic Remedies
Consult a homeopathic physician to help determine the remedy that best fits your symptoms. Remedies for asthma may have to be taken every 15 minutes to 2 hours as needed. The remedies listed below are but a few of the many possibilities.

- *Arsenicum album* – restlessness and anxiety occur, and worsen as the asthma continues; the patient fears death by suffocation; symptoms worse from midnight until 2 A.M.; tosses and turns in bed, breathing best when sitting erect and leaning forward; feels weak and tired; chilly and feels better with warmth applied to the chest wall and from warm drinks; thirsty for sips of water only.
- *Cuprum metallicum* – asthma in the elderly alternating with vomiting; suffocative attacks, worse around 3 A.M., face goes blue with coughing; may require medical help.
- *Ipecac* – sudden onset of wheezing made worse by moving about; patients feel as if a weight on the chest is causing suffocation; persistent nausea with loose cough and rattling in chest, but an inability to expectorate; brings up sticky mucus that is blood-streaked; vomiting helps because it gets rid of some of the mucus; symptoms are worse in hot, humid weather and worsened by the least motion; cold sweat on the extremities, difficulty sleeping; tend to salivate excessively.
- *Lobelia* – asthma with nausea and vomiting; prickling sensation all over, even on the fingers and toes, preceding the asthma; asthma aggravated by exposure to cold; weakness in the pit of the stomach and a sensation of a lump above the sternum (breast bone); emphysema.
- *Nux vomica* – feels full in the stomach, especially in the morning or after eating; asthma accompanied by choking, anxiety, pressure in the pit of the stomach, humming in the ears; quick pulse, and sweating; attack can be started by hay fever; relieved by belching and loosening the clothing; constricted feeling in the lower part of the chest.
- *Spongia* – dry, barking, croupy cough; air passages dry, sputum is absent, and voice is hoarse; asthma exacerbated by cold air, warm rooms, tobacco smoke, talking, lying with head low, drinking cold fluids, or eating sweets; symptoms worse in early part of the night; warm food or drinks provide some relief, as does sitting up and leaning forward.

Many patients respond to complex homeopathic remedies. You may want to try BHI Asthma or PHP Lung Liquescence, which provides potentized nutrients for lung function and regeneration.

Other Therapeutic Measures
For acute asthma attacks:

- Perform a Heimlich maneuver to push up the diaphragm, helping to expel trapped air and clear mucus plugs.
- Take ½ tsp. sea salt with ½ tsp. baking soda in 8 ounces of water or juice.
- Drink 1 to 2 cups of caffeinated coffee (adults) or a Coke (children) if you are away from home without your inhaler and have an asthma attack.

For acute attacks, press the following acupressure points for 30 to 60 seconds once or twice a day:

- one and a half thumbs' width to each side of the center of the spine, at the level of the third thoracic vertebra
- in the depression at the center of the front of the chest on a line joining both nipples
- in the hollow directly over the front of the larynx in the center of the lower part of the neck at the "V" of the collarbone.

Press these additional acupressure points for long-term replacement of drugs:

- two thumbs' width above the bone from the inner ankle joint
- three thumbs' width below the joint, under the kneecap, lying on the outer side of the knee and one finger's width back from the sharp edge of the shin bone

- one hand's width (four fingers) up from the inner ankle joint, just behind the tibia bone
- ear point at the base of the piece of cartilage called the tragus at the external opening of the ear.

Receive osteopathic or chiropractic manipulation for the chest and diaphragm.

Consult an Ayurvedic or traditional Chinese medicine physician.

Do visualization techniques and/or have hypnosis treatment.

Have tests performed to determine the acidity of the stomach (see Peptic Ulcer Disease, p. 258). Some asthmatics have low stomach acid and taking an acid supplement can help their asthma.

Do breathing exercises (see p. 421), or learn meditation techniques that help control breath.

If you are overweight, lose weight to make your breathing easier. See Obesity in chapter 18, Metabolic Disorders, for an appropriate diet.

CHRONIC BRONCHITIS

Chronic bronchitis occurs when the airways are always inflamed; people with chronic bronchitis have chronic coughs and shortness of breath. A person who has a cough that lasts for at least three months out of a year for two consecutive years or more, and who is short of breath after minimal exercise, has chronic bronchitis—one of the chronic obstructive pulmonary diseases.

Chronic bronchitis is a slow, progressive disease that typically occurs in cigarette smokers older than 50 years.

EMPHYSEMA

Emphysema is often preceded by chronic bronchitis and is a form of chronic obstructive pulmonary disease (COPD). Over two million North Americans have emphysema, half of them over 65 years old. In emphysema the elasticity of the walls of the air sacs is lost, and air becomes trapped in the lungs. The patient is unable to move air in and out of the lungs effectively, and the lungs remain expanded. The patient's chest becomes barrel-shaped and the restricted breathing often raises fears of suffocation. Because the lungs do not regenerate tissue that has been destroyed, the damage in emphysema is irreversible and it is considered incurable.

The most common symptoms of emphysema are shortness of breath, followed by coughing of large amounts of sputum (mucus from the lungs), even with mild exertion. These symptoms may not occur until middle age when the ability to exercise or do heavy work declines. Patients with emphysema have low levels of oxygen and high levels of carbon dioxide in their blood, and eventually most of them require continuous oxygen treatment.

The most common cause of emphysema is cigarette smoking, directly related to the total amount of cigarettes smoked, but some people lack alpha-1-antitrypsin, an enzyme that is necessary to protect the lungs from self-destruction. Cadmium fumes, from the smelting of lead and zinc ores, can also lead to emphysema.

MODERN MEDICAL AND ALTERNATIVE PREVENTION

Do not smoke.

MODERN MEDICAL TREATMENT

Diet

If the patient has chronic bronchitis and is underweight, high-calorie foods and milkshakes are suggested. Overweight patients with chronic bronchitis or emphysema are encouraged to lose weight. The extra pounds make it more difficult to breathe.

Exercise and Lifestyle

The first step in the treatment of chronic bronchitis and emphysema is to have a patient stop smoking.

For patients who have chronic bronchitis and emphysema, some hospitals are now offering pulmonary rehabilitation programs in which patients perform special exercises under medical supervision.

Drug Therapy

Patients are given an antibiotic at the first sign of a respiratory infection, and are advised to have an annual vaccination against flu as well as a one-time vaccination against pneumonia.

Medications prescribed for patients with chronic bronchitis and emphysema include Albuterol (a beta 2 agonist) and Atrovent (an anti-cholinergic), oral theophylline, and steroid inhalers. Side effects for these medications are discussed under asthma. Dextromethorphan is used to suppress a chronic cough and can have side effects of drowsiness, dizziness, and gastrointestinal disturbances.

Emphysema patients who have an alpha-1-antitrypsin deficiency are given replacement enzyme therapy.

Surgery

Some medical centers are removing the most damaged parts of the lungs in patients with emphysema. Not all patients are candidates for this procedure.

Other Therapeutic Measures

Oxygen is used when blood oxygen levels become low. If oxygen is always required, a trans-tracheal tube (permanent throat tube) is often inserted.

ALTERNATIVE TREATMENT

Diet

For chronic bronchitis and emphysema, eat a low-carbohydrate diet, which lowers the oxygen required by digestion. Metabolizing carbohydrates requires more oxygen consumption than does fat or protein metabolism, and it generates carbon dioxide production. The dietary recommendations for asthma, above, are also helpful.

Exercise and Lifestyle

For chronic bronchitis or emphysema, perform graded exercise training on a stationary bike. Use heart rate as an index to assess fitness. Participate in a pulmonary rehabilitation program.

Perform Tai Chi or Qigong daily.

Get plenty of rest. Drink at least 2 quarts of liquid (the majority of it water) a day, which will help dilute the mucus, making it easier to expel.

If you have bronchitis or emphysema, stop smoking, and avoid other people's smoke. If there is a persistent cough, have a sputum culture performed to determine whether an infection is present.

Do regular breathing exercises. See p. 421.

Nutrient Therapy

Take the following nutrients for chronic bronchitis and emphysema.

- vitamin A – 15,000 to 30,000 IU a day. *Caution:* Do not take more than 8,000 IU of vitamin A a day if you are or might be pregnant (improves lung function).
- beta carotene (natural) – 25,000 to 50,000 IU a day (antioxidant; neutralizes harm from smoking and air pollution)
- vitamin C – 3,000 to 6,000 mg a day (antioxidant; neutralizes harm from smoking and air pollution)
- vitamin E – 400 to 800 IU a day (antioxidant; neutralizes harm from smoking and air pollution)
- magnesium – 400 to 800 mg a day (relaxes muscle spasm; opens bronchial tubes)
- selenium – 200 mcg a day (anti-cancer; antioxidant)
- coenzyme Q_{10} – 50 to 100 mg a day (for increased work of breathing)
- N-acetyl cysteine – 500 to 1,000 mg a day (antioxidant)
- omega-3 fatty acids – 6,000 to 12,000 mg a day (anti-inflammatory)

- pantethine – 300 to 900 mg a day (supports adrenal glands)
- quercetin – 500 to 1,000 mg a day (strengthens blood vessels; works with vitamin C; anti-inflammatory)
- thymus extract – as directed on your product (strengthens immune system)

Herbal Therapy

Take a botanical supplement under the direction of a trained herbalist.

- astragalus – further boosts immunity
- echinacea – strengthens the immune system
- goldenseal – soothes irritated mucus membranes. *Caution:* Do not take if you are pregnant.
- licorice – acts as an expectorant; supports the immune system
- lobelia, grindelia, wild cherry bark, white horehound, coltsfoot, and sundew – all are herbal expectorants
- mullein – every four hours to soothe irritation in the bronchial passages

Homeopathic Remedies

Consult a homeopathic physician to help determine the remedy that best fits your symptoms. The remedies listed below are but a few of the many possibilities.

- *Ammonium carbonicum* – emphysema; increasing difficulty in breathing; better in cool air; chest feels tired; worse after any effort and entering a warm room or climbing a few steps; slow, labored breathing, bubbling sound; rattling in chest, but expectorates little; may expectorate blood after cough; cough every morning about 3 A.M.; burning in chest.
- *Drosera* – bouts of continuous, dry, barking cough; spasmodic, tickling cough that is accompanied by choking, cold sweats, and vomiting; cough aggravated by lying down and is worse after midnight, especially at 2 A.M.; cough irritated by talking, eating, or drinking cold fluids; holds onto the chest during the coughing spells because of the pain.
- *Ipecac* – much mucus, with a spasmodic cough that ends in choking and gagging; face is pale and there is great shortage of breath; blood-stained mucus, constriction of the chest, and a tickling of the throat, causing a cough; coughs with every breath and salivates excessively, cough worse in hot, humid weather or in changing weather; common medicine for infants.
- *Phosphorus* – in delicate, slender tall patients; dry, hard cough, sometimes with a persistent tickly feeling, tearing pain under the breastbone, aggravated by lying down, especially on the left side; wakes up at night, needing to sit up and cough; aggravated by talking, moving, going from a warm room to cold air or by strong odors; tightness in chest relieved by the warmth of a bed; craves ice drinks; illness is exhausting; nasal discharge may have some blood streaked in it; sputum contains mucus and pus, may be blood-streaked and has a salty-sweet taste.
- *Pulsatilla* – cough symptoms are aggravated in a warm room or warm weather, by lying down to sleep, and at night walking in the cool air provides some relief; child must sit up in bed to breathe better, dry cough in the day; productive cough with yellow or greenish expectoration at night and upon waking.
- *Sulphur* – long-standing chronic bronchitis; respirations worse in the evenings; sleep apnea, jumps from sleep with a suffocating sensation; cough worse at night in bed.

Many patients respond to complex homeopathic remedies. You may want to try BHI Bronchitis, or PHP Lung Liquescence, which provides potentized nutrients for lung function and regeneration.

Other Therapeutic Measures

Use the onion, ginger root tea, or horseradish and mustard preparations listed for acute bronchitis and pneumonia.

Press these additional acupressure points for long-term replacement of drugs:

- two thumbs' width above the bone from the inner ankle joint
- three thumbs' width below the joint, under the kneecap, lying on the outer side of the knee and one finger's width back from the sharp edge of the shin bone.
- one hand's width (four fingers) up from the inner ankle joint, just behind the tibia bone
- ear point at the base of the piece of cartilage called the tragus at the external opening of the ear

- mid-point from the knee to the ankle, three fingers' width back toward the fibula from the ridge on the front of the shin (on the outside of the lower leg).

Consult an Ayurvedic or traditional Chinese medicine physician.

Do visualization techniques and/or have hypnosis treatment.

Take a cough medication that contains potassium iodide (Pima syrup), and drink four to six glasses of fluid a day.

Do breathing exercises (see p. 421), or learn meditation techniques that help control breath.

If you are overweight, lose weight to make your breathing easier. See Obesity in chapter 18, Metabolic Disorders, for an appropriate diet.

CHAPTER 14

Musculoskeletal Problems

The musculoskeletal system is composed of bone, cartilage, ligaments, tendons, joints, and skeletal muscle. Its function is to support and protect the body, as well as to enable it to move. The skeleton, composed of 206 bones, provides rigid support for the body. It also protects vital internal organs from injury, and serves as a mineral reservoir for the body. Bone tissue is made up of mineral components, mostly inorganic calcium and phosphate salts, which impart rigidity, and an organic framework, which gives it elasticity. The organic framework, in which the minerals are embedded, is formed by collagen fibers, which give the bones great strength without their being brittle.

There are over 600 different skeletal muscles that account for 40 to 45 percent of body weight. These muscles are attached to the bones by tendons, bands of dense fibrous tissue that form the end of the muscle and make the actual attachment to the bone. The bones are articulated or linked together at the joints and are moved by the action of muscles attached to them.

Joints are classified according to the material that connects them, and the movement allowed by the joints. Fibrous joints are linked by ligaments, a band of sheet-like fibrous tissue that strengthens the joint and allows very little movement. Cartilage, a fibrous connective tissue, holds the bones together in cartilaginous joints, which are capable of slight movement. The articulating surfaces of bones are covered by a type of cartilage, and a fibrocartilaginous pad between the bones serves as a shock absorber.

Most of the joints of the body are freely movable synovial joints, which are further classified according to the movement they permit. Synovial joints contain a fluid-filled cavity between the surfaces of the bones where they join. A capsule, which is a double-layered membrane, surrounds and encloses the joint. The outer layer of this membrane is composed of fibrous connective tissue, which strengthens the joint. The inner layer is called the synovial membrane. It produces a thick substance called synovial fluid, which lubricates the joint surfaces and provides nourishment for the cartilage.

Synovial membranes also form bursae, which are not part of the synovial joints, but are often associated with them. Bursae are small sacs lined with synovial membranes that act as cushions between the structures they separate. Most bursae are located between the tendons and the bone and prevent friction between these structures.

OSTEOPOROSIS

Osteoporosis, or "porous bone," is the loss of bone mass associated with aging. It can also occur in paralyzed or immobilized limbs. Osteoporosis is believed to occur when the rate of bone formation slows, while the rate of bone absorption remains normal. The organic portion of the bone is not replaced as rapidly as it is broken down, and as a result, the bone gradually comes to contain a greater proportion of inorganic salts. Bones then become porous, fragile, brittle, and relatively easily broken.

Osteoporosis can occur in both men and women, but men have more bone mass than women and do not begin to lose calcium until after the age of 60. As a result, osteoporosis occurs much later in men, and with less severity. Women tend to lose 2 to 5 percent of their bone mass each year for the first five years following menopause, after which bone mass loss levels out. If women enter menopause with low bone mass, or if it becomes low during menopause, bone density may reach the fracture threshold. However, osteoporosis can also begin earlier in women, and is not strictly a postmenopausal problem.

Bone loss often begins before menopause. Rates of hip fracture in women begin to rise between the ages of 40 and 44—well before menopause. From age 50 to age 90, the risk of hip fracture in white women increases 50 times, and the risk of spinal fracture increases 15 to 30 times. It is estimated that about 40 percent of 50-year-old women will sustain one or more osteoporosis-related fractures of the spine, hip, or wrist during their remaining lifetime. Of women who fracture a hip from osteoporosis, 50 percent will never walk on their own again, and 25 percent will die within a year.

Bone loss is most commonly seen in the spine, hips, and ribs. Bone loss in the vertebrae causes them to be subject to compression fractures that can result in a slight loss in height, or even a dowager's hump.

Early warning signs of osteoporosis include chronic back and leg pain, bone pain in the spine affecting cranial nerves, unusual dental problems that involve bone loss in the jaw and tooth sockets, and bone fractures from trivial injuries. Some women are unaware of having osteoporosis until a minor accident causes a broken bone.

In Canada 1.4 million people over 50 are affected by osteoporosis, and in the United States it affects over 25 million people. Risk factors for osteoporosis include lack of exercise; thinness; high-protein diets; smoking; excess alcohol intake; estrogen deficiency; progesterone deficiency; calcium, magnesium, and vitamin deficiencies; genetic tendency; and never having had a child. Estrogen helps to prevent bone loss, and progesterone stimulates bone formation. Synthetic progesterones are not as effective as natural progesterone in building bone.

A diagnosis of osteoporosis is confirmed by the finding of low bone mass, evidence of fracture on X-ray, a history of osteoporotic fracture, or kyphosis (height loss) indicative of spinal fracture. Bone density is tested by bone densitometry, a low-dose X-ray technique. This test is useful for establishing a baseline. Many alternative physicians perform a urine test to examine the breakdown products of bones to determine if bone is being lost.

MODERN MEDICAL TREATMENT

Drug Therapy

Hormone replacement therapy (HRT) is widely used to prevent loss of bone density. Hormone therapy to prevent osteoporosis is usually started during menopause, and often stopped within a few years. Estrogen therapy may preserve mineral density during the time it is used, but it does not protect against fractures that occur once it has been stopped. On the other hand, beginning hormone therapy later in life may provide almost as much protection against osteroporotic fractures as starting HRT at menopause—and using that approach can cut exposure to hormones in half.

The FDA has recently approved 0.3 mg Estratab (esterified estrogen) as an adequate protection against osteoporosis. (Previously, the standard dose had always been 0.625 mg, which is also the recommended dose for menopausal symptoms.) Estratab causes less breast tenderness, fewer headaches, and less nausea than the higher estrogen doses.

A recent study in the *Journal of the American Medical Association* noted the outcome of HRT in preventing osteoporosis. Women who took various estrogen or combined hormone protocols for three years had hip bone density readings that were only 3.4 percent better than women who did not take hormones.

Patients are also given biphosphonates—pamidronate disodium (Aredia) and tiludronate (Skelid)—or alendronate (Fosamax) for the treatment and prevention of osteoporosis. Biphosphonates are drugs containing phosphons that bind to bone crystals, inhibiting bone reabsorption. These expensive drugs have to be taken in the morning with water, at least 30 minutes before breakfast. Patients have to remain upright; lying down can cause esophageal irriation.

Alendronate is the most commonly used biphosphonate for the prevention and treatment of osteoporosis. Biphosphonates can cause local irritation of the upper gastrointestinal mucosa, inflammation of the esophagus, esophageal ulcers and bleeding, abdominal pain, nausea, constipation, diarrhea, gas, difficulty swallowing, abdominal distention, bone, muscle, or joint pain, muscle cramps, headache, dizziness, and taste perversion.

Exercise and Lifestyle

Patients are urged to do weight-bearing exercise for 20 to 30 minutes three times a week and to take calcium (1,000 to 1,500 mg a day).

Patients are also advised to stop smoking as it can cause bone loss.

ALTERNATIVE TREATMENT

Diet

Avoid cola and root beer drinks, as these are high in phosphate and will leach calcium from the bones. Eliminate sugar, caffeine, and alcohol. Minimize salt in your diet. Avoid red meats, and reduce animal protein. A diet high in animal protein, salt, and sugar causes the body to excrete increased amounts of calcium and the body then takes calcium from the bones to maintain a normal level of calcium in the blood. Limit foods high in oxalic acid, which inhibits calcium absorption. These foods include almonds, asparagus, beet greens, cashews, chard, rhubarb, and spinach. Limit citrus fruits and tomatoes, as they also inhibit calcium absorption. Avoid yeast products; they are high in phosphorous, which competes with calcium for absorption by the body.

Eat foods high in complex carbohydrates (unless you have hyperinsulinemia) and low in fat. Include whole grains, vegetables, sea vegetables, and lean meats such as turkey. Eat flavonoid-rich foods such as blueberries, blackberries, citrus rind, and red, yellow, and green fruits. Also eat foods that are high in calcium and vitamin D such as broccoli, chestnuts, dandelion greens, most dark green leafy vegetables, hazelnuts, kale, kelp, molasses, oats, sea vegetables, sesame seeds, soybeans, tahini, tofu, turnip greens, wheat germ, clams, flounder, oysters, salmon, sardines, and shrimp. Sulfur is needed for healthy bones and is found in eggs, garlic, asparagus, and onions.

Exercise and Lifestyle

Exercise in a weight-bearing sport for 20 to 30 minutes three times a week. Walking may be the best exercise for maintaining bone mass, and duration is more important than intensity. Get early morning sunlight for vitamin D.

Do not smoke, as it depletes many vital nutrients.

Do not take cortisone over long periods of time, as it leaches potassium and weakens bones.

Nutrient Therapy

Take the following nutritional supplements (divide the doses into three portions and take with meals):

- vitamin A – 50,000 IU a day for one month then reduce to 25,000 IU a day. *Caution:* Do not take more than 8,000 IU a day if you are or might be pregnant (helps retard the aging process).
- beta carotene – 25,000 IU (15 mg) a day (important in the formation of bone)
- vitamin B_6 – 50 to 100 mg a day (reduces homocysteine, which may contribute to osteoporosis)
- vitamin B_{12} – 1,000 to 3,000 mcg a day (promotes normal growth; reduces homocysteine)
- folic acid – 5 to 20 mg a day (reduces homocysteine)
- vitamin C – 500 to 1,500 mg a day (important for collagen and connective tissue formation)
- vitamin D – 400 to 1,000 IU a day (plays a role in calcium uptake)
- vitamin E – 400 to 800 IU a day (important in retarding the aging process)
- vitamin K – 1 to 2 mg a day (necessary for synthesis of the protein in bone tissue on which calcium crystallizes)
- boron – 2 to 3 mg a day. *Caution:* Do not exceed this amount (improves calcium uptake).
- calcium (hydroxyapatite or citrate) – 800 to 1,500 mg a day (necessary for maintaining strong bones)
- copper – 1 to 2 mg a day (balances zinc; aids in the formation of bone)
- magnesium – 400 to 800 mg a day (important in calcium uptake)
- strontium – 3 to 6 mg a day (contributes to bone strength)
- zinc – 30 to 50 mg a day (important in calcium uptake)
- DHEA – 10 to 25 mg a day (precursor for hormones that stimulate bone formation)
- pregnenolone – 25 to 50 mg a day (precursor for hormones that help stimulate bone formation)

Herbal Therapy

Take a botanical supplement.

- black cohosh – has estrogenic activity
- dong quai – increases the effects of ovarian and testicular hormones
- false unicorn root – has estrogenic activity
- fennel – has estrogenic activity
- horsetail – high in silicon, a vital component for bone and cartilage formation; helps the body absorb and use calcium
- licorice – has estrogen- and progesterone-like effects
- parsley – high in boron, which improves calcium uptake

Homeopathic Remedies

Take the following homeopathic remedy that best fits your symptoms. These remedies cannot reverse bone loss, but they have an affinity for and affect the nutrition of the bones.

- *Calcarea carbonica* – faulty development of bones; rickets; curvatures; bone growths; growing pains; neck stiff and rigid, weakness in small of back.
- *Calcarea phosphorica* – delicate and easily breakable bones; bones of extremities are weak and fragile; predisposition to glandular and bone diseases; speeds knitting of broken bones.
- *Silica* – diseases of the bone and cartilage; decay, necrosis, and softening of bones; frac-

tures; ankles weak; diseases of bones of the spine; hip-joint disease.

- *Strontium carbonica* – easily sprained ankles, suffer bone pain that comes and goes; problems with bones, especially the femur.

Other Therapeutic Measures

Avoid aluminum cookware, non-filtered computer screens, electric blankets, and fluorescent lighting, all of which tend to leach calcium from the body.

Have thyroid function checked, as too much thyroid hormone can cause bone loss. In addition, have a urine test to look at the breakdown products of bones. This test can be both diagnostic and a way of determining whether a particular treatment is working.

ARTHRITIS

Many people consider arthritis to be synonymous with rheumatism. However, in the medical world "rheumatic disease" is a broader term referring to conditions in which there are changes to any connective tissue (muscle, tendons, joints, fibrous tissue, and bursae). "Arthritis" refers only to the type of rheumatic diseases in which there is an inflammatory condition involving the joints.

Arthritis and other rheumatic diseases are a major cause of chronic disability in North America. The National Institutes of Health estimates that in the United States at least 15 percent of the population has arthritis. It affects people of all ages, including over 2,000 children who have some form of the disease. Arthritis is more prevalent in women who are over 45, and in men who are below this age. By age 65, at least 75 percent of the population has X-ray evidence of the disease in the hand, foot, knee, or hip. In the United States over one million new cases of arthritis are diagnosed each year. Despite the fact that arthritis can be a crippling disease, however, the majority of arthritis cases are not crippling.

RHEUMATOID ARTHRITIS

The two main types of arthritis are rheumatoid arthritis and osteoarthritis. Rheumatoid arthritis (RA) is the less common of the two, which is fortunate because it is the most virulent and disabling of the rheumatic diseases. It is estimated that 1 to 2 percent of the world population suffers from rheumatoid arthritis. Symptoms generally begin between the ages of 20 and 50, and though RA affects equal numbers of men and women, women are more likely to have symptoms severe enough to require medication. In children, rheumatoid arthritis can begin before the age of seven, but 75 percent of children with the disease are said to grow out of it.

Rheumatoid arthritis affects all of the synovial joints of the body. It incapacitates, damages, and destroys the synovial tissue that lines the joints and secretes the lubricant that allows bones to move painlessly against other bones. Bone surfaces can be destroyed, and joints affected by rheumatoid arthritis make a sound like crinkling cellophane when moved. The joints swell and fluid accumulates in them, causing pressure on the nerves and resulting in muscle stiffness, pain, and difficulty moving. Joints are tender, swollen, and fused. Eventually they become deformed and are destroyed. Around 35 percent of rheumatoid patients suffer serious disability with impaired movement, and as many as 10 percent progress to almost complete disability. However, 60 percent of RA patients have only mild disability and can continue with active lives.

The onset of rheumatoid arthritis can be gradual, with mild or no symptoms in the beginning; but the symptoms can become severe in a matter of weeks. The symptoms of rheumatoid arthritis include fatigue, weakness, low-grade fever, joint stiffness, and vague joint pain. Depression, lethargy, and night sweats also occur, and in some cases patients will experience inflammation of the eyes, muscles, and lining of the heart, as well as fibrosis of the lungs.

Symptoms can come and go, with attacks followed by remissions of varying lengths. For most people, attacks become more frequent and severe, and result in disability and deformity. However, in 10 to 20 percent of cases rheumatoid arthritis goes away on its own and never returns.

Causes of Rheumatoid Arthritis

The cause of rheumatoid arthritis is unknown, and probably there is more than one causative factor. It is considered an autoimmune disease, and in some cases it appears to be the result of the immune system attacking the joints, producing abnormal antibodies against its own cells and tissues. There is evidence that hormones such as DHEA (dehydroepiandrosterone, the precursor of steroid hormones) and progesterone protect against autoimmune diseases, and some women with these diseases have abnormally low levels of those hormones.

Infection is also a prime candidate as a cause for rheumatoid arthritis, and some researchers think that an undefined virus or another microorganism such as *Mycoplasma* may play a role in the disease. Stress, both physical and emotional, may be a trigger, particularly in juvenile rheumatoid arthritis. Some researchers feel that stress can initiate rheumatoid arthritis in a susceptible person, and can make established disease worse.

A 1981 study by Drs. Charles Lucas and Lawrence Powers at Wayne State University in Detroit shows that fat content of the diet may affect rheumatoid arthritis. Rheumatoid patients eating a low-fat diet had significant reduction in swelling and stiffness, which returned within 72 hours of eating fat-containing foods again. Food allergy may also play a role. Several studies have shown that symptoms of rheumatoid arthritis improve within about 10 days when allergenic foods are removed from the diet. When the offending foods are returned to the diet, symptoms can worsen in as little as two hours.

Other allergens are also implicated: the late Dr. Theron Randolph, father of environmental medicine and discoverer of chemical sensitivity, has demonstrated that chemical substances ranging from natural gas to tobacco are a causative factor in arthritis. Dr. Marshall Mandell, of the New England Foundation for Allergic and Environmental diseases, found that foods, chemicals, pollens, molds, and other airborne substances caused allergic reactions in the joints of 85 percent of the arthritic patients he has tested.

OSTEOARTHRITIS

Half of the adult population over 30 years old has some degree of osteoarthritis, and everyone over 55 years of age has some degenerative joint disease. Over one-third of office visits to primary care physicians are to receive treatment for arthritic symptoms.

Osteoarthritis (OA) is a degenerative disease in which there is progressive deterioration of the joints caused by the "wear and tear" of daily use. The deterioration is found in the cartilage that lies between the surfaces of joint bones, providing a cushion between the bones of the joint and acting as a shock absorber. The ability of the cartilage to self-repair does not keep up with normal degeneration from daily use. It becomes pitted and worn away, leaving the two bones to grate on each other. The cartilage and bone at the margins of the joints become enlarged and deformed, and the synovial membrane thickens. An increase in synovial fluid then develops in the joint, causing swelling and inflammation. These joint changes cause the discomfort and pain of osteoarthritis. In addition to the joint deterioration, small bony growths, calcium spurs, and soft cysts can appear on bones and the joints.

Osteoarthritis is often associated with age, so much so that some physicians consider it a part of the normal aging process. It can range from being a nuisance to being a painful, crippling condition. Symptoms include stiffness (both in the early morning and following periods of rest), pain that worsens with joint use, local tenderness, swelling of soft tissue, loss of joint function, bony swelling, and restricted mobility. Osteoarthritis can affect only one joint, or eventually can involve all joints of the body. Any joint can be affected, but those most often involved are the joints of the fingers and thumbs, the neck and lumbar vertebrae of the spine, the knees, and the hips. Osteoarthritis causes the bones to become brittle, and fractures become an increasing risk.

Pain is usually the first symptom noticed—usually after movement or exercise, particularly toward the end of the day. In addition to being painful, the joints may be stiff and difficult to move, and can be warm, tender, and red. Motion becomes more and more limited as arthritis progresses. Osteoarthritis at the base of the thumb will limit the use of the thumb. The last joint in each finger is commonly affected as well. As these joints deteriorate, use of the hands becomes very painful. Osteoarthritis in the knee causes pain, swelling, and unsteadiness. In the hip it causes pain, a limp, and difficulty lying in bed on the side of the affected hip. The presence of osteoarthritis in the spine may not be as apparent, but it commonly affects the lower back and mid-neck.

Causes of Osteoarthritis

Osteoarthritis can be caused by injury. Athletes frequently develop osteoarthritis in joints they have injured repeatedly. It can also be caused by a defect in the protein that makes up cartilage. In addition to the "wear and tear" discussed above, age-related changes, hormonal changes, altered biochemistry, joint instability, and skeletal defects play a role in osteoarthritis. Genetic predisposition is a factor, and arthritis tends to run in families. Psychological and environmental components can cause and exacerbate the disease.

Allergies play a role in osteoarthritis also, and eliminating allergens can result in remission or improvement of symptoms. Food allergies are important factors in osteoarthritis, with sugar, wheat, citrus, pork, and eggs being major offenders. The nightshade family (potatoes, tomatoes, eggplant, pimentos, peppers, and tobacco) contain an alkaloid that contributes to arthritis in some people; it takes six to nine months to clear the body of this alkaloid after nightshades are removed from the diet. Sensitivity to chemicals can affect arthritis, as can allergies to pollens, molds, and other airborne substances. Microorganisms such as bacteria, protozoa, yeast, and fungi can also trigger or aggravate symptoms of arthritis.

Stress plays a role in osteoarthritis, as it does in rheumatoid arthritis. Stress disrupts the hormone system of the body, affecting progesterone and thyroid production. Many women develop osteoarthritis after menopause because of hormonal changes and deficiencies; osteoarthritis affects three times as many women as men.

Other Types of Rheumatic Diseases

More than one million Americans have gout, which is the third most common form of arthritis. People with gout also tend to have a higher than normal risk of kidney and heart problems. In gout there is a buildup of uric acid, either because uric acid production is out of balance, or because there is inadequate elimination of uric acid from the body. When uric acid levels get too high, the acid crystallizes in the joint cartilage and synovial fluid and tissue, causing sharp, needle-like pain in the joints.

In half of all gout cases, the first attack affects the first joint of the big toe, and is signaled by intense pain. The affected joint is usually red or purple, hot and tender, and the skin stretched over it is usually shiny and tense. Fever and chills then develop, and loss of mobility due to inflammation of the joint can occur. The ankle, knee, and occasionally the wrists and elbow are involved. Gout can also be accompanied by indigestion, constipation, headache, depression, eczema, and hives.

Gout tends to strike at night, and attacks are usually preceded by a triggering event such as excessive consumption of rich food or alcohol, consumption of certain drugs, or surgery. Most patients will suffer a second attack within a year of the first attack; only 7 percent of people with gout experience just one attack. Gout occurs mainly in adult men, and 95 percent of its victims are over 30 years of age. Only 5 percent of women will develop gout, and usually after menopause. Obesity, diabetes, high blood pressure, coronary artery disease, hypothyroidism, psoriasis, and parathyroid hormone imbalance can lead to increased uric acid levels, as well as affecting the ability of the kidney to excrete uric acid. Thiazide diuretics predispose a person to gout, as does ingesting low levels of salicylates, such as aspirin.

There are a number of other rheumatic diseases, but the following are four of the more common ones.

Spondyloarthropathies are a group of disorders that usually affect the spine, causing pain, inflammation, stiffness, and changes in body position.

Systemic lupus erythematosus is a condition in which there is fever, weakness, upper body and facial pain, and joint pain (see chapter 28, Fatigue).

Infectious arthritis is characterized by body aches, chills, and fever; low blood pressure, pneumonia, and shock; dizziness and confusion; and affected joints in which there is redness, swelling, tenderness, and throbbing pain. The pain can spread to other joints, and movement is worse with motion.

Kawasaki syndrome occurs in children and has symptoms of joint pain, prolonged fever, red rash on soles and palms, and heart complications.

WARNING SIGNS OF ARTHRITIS

If you have any of the following warning signs of arthritis, you should consult a health care practitioner:

- joints are stiff in the morning but loosen up as the day goes by

- stiffness that lasts for more than six weeks
- joint pain or swelling that does not respond to aspirin, heat, or ice packs
- joints are hot, red, swollen, and very painful
- stiffness occurs after a joint injury
- chills or fever accompany swollen joints

There is much that can be done to alleviate symptoms and restore function once the type and causes of arthritis have been identified. Of course, treatment must begin before the joints have suffered extensive damage and destruction.

MODERN MEDICAL TREATMENT

Drug Therapy

Pharmaceuticals are the primary treatment for rheumatoid arthritis, but all of the drugs that appear to be effective in treating this disease can produce serious side effects. The main debate is how long to use the drugs used for initial treatment, and when to add the secondary drugs that tend to be more toxic. If the patient is not getting better, most physicians try more aggressive drugs.

Recent studies have shown that antibiotics, if used early, can help decrease the inflammation and joint pain of RA.

NSAIDs (non-steroidal anti-inflammatory drugs) are the usual starting place for rheumatoid arthritis therapy. They include naproxen (Aleve, Naprosyn), ibuprofen (Motrin), nabumetone (Relafen), oxaprozin (Daypro), fluribuprofen (Ansaid), indomethacin (Indocin), and others. NSAIDs have many side effects, and if one drug is producing troublesome symptoms, physicians will switch the patient to another NSAID. Side effects of NSAIDs can be severe. The drugs can erode the stomach lining and cause bleeding ulcers and kidney problems, and they also can cause headaches, dizziness, itching, edema, hearing and visual disturbances, and thirst. People with ulcers, kidney disease, diabetes, heart disease, high blood pressure, nasal polyps, bleeding disorders, and those who are taking multiple medications must use extreme care when taking NSAIDs.

For some patients with RA, NSAIDs will effectively relieve pain and may improve joints. Other patients do not get better on NSAIDs and have to be started on the secondary drugs. Known as DMARDs (disease-modifying antirheumatic drugs), these drugs slow the progression of the disease. Methotrexate (Rheumatrex) is used when NSAIDs are not working and the RA becomes more aggressive. Low doses, taken once a week, minimize the side effects of nausea, abdominal pain, diarrhea, vomiting, skin rashes, hives, headaches, dizziness, and itching. Liver failure can occur in patients who have taken the drug for long periods of time.

Hydroxychloroquine (Plaquenil), which is also used to treat malaria, is used as a secondary drug for people with RA that is progressing slowly. Side effects of Plaquenil include irritability, nervousness, headache, nightmares, muscle weakness, changes in vision, bleaching of hair, hair loss, skin eruptions, nausea, blood count problems, weight loss, diarrhea, and vomiting. Eye problems are a serious side effect of Plaquenil therapy, as it can affect the ciliary body, cornea, and retina. Problems with the retina can persist even after the drug is discontinued.

Corticosteroids are used for RA to reduce inflammation and swelling and decrease joint pain. They have numerous side effects when used for long periods, including weight gain, cataracts, bone wasting, elevation of blood pressure, ulcers, bleeding, skin changes, and risk of infection because of immunosuppression.

Penicillamine (Depen) is a chelating agent usually used for Wilson's disease, but which has beneficial effects in rheumatoid arthritis as well. Its mode of action in RA is unknown, but it suppresses disease activity, lowering the IgM rheumatoid factor. Side effects include itching, rashes, altered taste, nausea, vomiting, bone marrow depression, protein in the urine, tinnitus, blood count problems, and numbness in the extremities.

Several chemotherapy drugs, including azathioprine (Imuran), chlorambucil (Leukeran), and cyclopyhosphamide (Cytoxan), are used to treat RA when other drugs have failed to give relief. These medications can be helpful in autoimmune disease, but the mechanism by which they work is not known. Side effects include immune system compromise, an increased risk of infection, and certain cancers. Imuran can also cause liver problems.

Gold injections are frequently used for RA, but can have toxic effects on the kidneys. Gold sodium thiomalate (Myochrysine) and aurothioglucose (Solganal) are the injection substances used, and are most effective when given in the early stages of the disease. Once cartilage and bone damage have occurred, these medications can only prevent progression of the disease; they cannot repair damage. Auranofin (Ridaura), a gold-containing oral medication, can also be used in treating RA. Gold is less toxic if taken orally, but is not as effective.

Rashes and itching are common side effects of both oral and injectable gold, and these reactions may be worsened by exposure to sun. Irritation and ulcers of the mucus membranes of the mouth are also a common side effect of the medication, and there are often allergic symptoms of flushing, fainting, dizziness, and sweating. Other symptoms include nausea, vomiting, malaise, headache, and weakness. The CBC (complete blood count) must be carefully monitored when either oral or injectable gold is used. Side effects can occur at any time during treatment, and for many months after treatment has been discontinued.

If patients have moderately to severely active RA with an inadequate response to one or more DMARDs, a new drug, etanercept (Enbrel) may be prescribed. It does not reverse joint deformities but can significantly reduce disease activity and allow the patient to lead a more active life. Many patients experience a reduction in swollen joints, tender joints, duration of morning stiffness, and pain levels when taking Enbrel. The most frequently reported adverse reaction in clinical trials has been mild to moderate injection site reactions. Fifteen percent of patients in the clinical trial did not respond to Enbrel. Long-term effects of this medication on serious infection, malignancy, and autoimmune disease are unknown. Patients with a serious infection should not take Enbrel.

Treatment for osteoarthritis is a balancing act between achieving pain relief and avoiding the side effects of the medications used. Drugs are used to decrease inflammation, relieve pain, and prevent bone wasting. Because OA is a chronic condition, and treatment will necessarily be long-term, it is important to find an inexpensive and safe medication.

Aspirin and salicylates are usually the first line of treatment for osteoarthritis. However, the high dosage of these medications required to treat arthritis can lead to stomach ulcers. Even the coated and buffered aspirins can cause ulcers, and in addition aspirin can interact with other medications. For this reason, many physicians prefer to use acetaminophen (Tylenol), though it does have a small risk of producing kidney problems if used at high doses for many years. Extra-Strength Tylenol, and intermittent use of Tylenol #3 (containing codeine), are effective in reducing pain for some patients, but they have no anti-inflammatory properties.

If neither aspirin nor Tylenol is effective, other NSAIDs are usually the next drug of choice. Meclofenamate (Mecloman), ibuprofen (Advil, Motrin, Nuprin, or Rufen), indomethacin (Indocin), naproxen (Naprosyn, Aleve, or Anaprox), nabumetone (Relafen), fenoprofen (Nalfon), tolmetin (Tolectin), sulindac (Clinoril), and other NSAIDs are frequently used. Side effects of these medications are listed above under RA treatment. In addition to those side effects, NSAIDs inhibit cartilage formation and accelerate cartilage destruction. While they suppress the symptoms, they accelerate the progression of osteoarthritis.

Propoxyphene hydrochloride (Darvon) is effective for some people and relieves moderate pain. Adverse reactions include constipation, abdominal pain, skin rashes, lightheadedness, headache, weakness, euphoria and dysphoria, hallucinations, visual disturbances, and addiction.

For severe pain hydrocodone plus acetaminophen (Vicodin) and tramedol hydrochloride (Ultram) are frequently used. Vicodin is a semisynthetic narcotic, and side effects include lightheadedness, dizziness, sedation, nausea, and vomiting. Addiction is also a problem. Ultram causes malaise, dizziness, sleepiness, nausea, constipation, sweating, and itching.

Celecoxib (Celebrex) is a new prescription drug that can be used to treat both OA and RA. It is designed to relieve pain, inflammation, and stiffness, which can help patients walk and bend more easily. The most common side effects are indigestion, diarrhea, and abdominal pain. People who are allergic to sulfonamides or who have had asthma, hives, or allergic reactions after taking aspirin or other NSAIDs cannot take Celebrex. There is an increased risk of ulcers if Celebrex is taken with aspirin.

The NSAIDs indomethacin, ibuprofen, and naproxen are used for gout. Their side effects are listed above. These drugs should be taken with meals or milk to prevent upset stomach. Indomethacin can cause central nervous system symptoms in some people, and most physicians feel that Indocin causes fewer side effects than generic indomethacin.

Colchicine is also used for gout. It must be taken immediately after meals to reduce stomach upset. Colchicine has anti-inflammatory properties but is not an analgesic. However, it does reduce pain in acute attacks of gout. Side effects include muscular weakness, nausea, vomiting, abdominal pain, hives, and skin eruptions.

Allopurinol (Zylopurinol) reduces the production of uric acid by the body, and probenecid (Benemid) and sulfinpyrazone (Anturane) increase the excretion of uric acid. These medications should be taken immediately after meals to reduce the chances of stomach upset. Patients must drink plenty of fluids, and for allopurinol, increase consumption of foods rich in iron. Skin rashes and gastrointestinal disturbances are common side effects of these drugs.

Exercise and Lifestyle

Patients are told to do isometric exercises, working up gradually to 15 to 30 minutes a day. They are also told to avoid stress.

Other Therapeutic Measures

Heat application, such as hot packs, heating pads, hot water bottles, or warm soaks, are used on painful areas. To help arthritis of the hands, paraffin baths are used. The hands are immersed in warm paraffin that is kept soft with an external heat source.

ALTERNATIVE TREATMENT

Diet

Observe the following dietary guidelines. Eat a balanced diet, but include more fruits and vegetables and cut down on meat, milk, and dairy products. Eat more deep-water fish (salmon, mackerel, and herring), which can reduce the inflammatory response of arthritis. Eat fresh pineapple, as it contains the enzyme bromelain, which is helpful in reducing inflammation. Eat sulfur-containing foods such as garlic, onions, eggs, and asparagus. Sulfur is essential for repair and rebuilding of bone, cartilage, and connective tissue.

Avoid the nightshade family and grains. If you do eat grains, select them with care as they can adversely affect joints. Avoid caffeine, alcohol, citrus fruits, paprika, salt, and sugar. Eliminate any food allergens you may have.

If you have gout, maintain a low-purine diet, avoiding herring, sardines, mackerel, and anchovies, as well as organ meat, meats, shellfish, and yeast. Keep refined carbohydrates and satu-

rated fats to a minimum. During a gout attack eat only raw fruits and vegetables for two weeks. Eat both cherries and strawberries, as they neutralize uric acid.

Use juice therapy, which is a source of concentrated nutrients that can enhance the natural healing capacity of the body. (If you have hypoglycemia or diabetes, use juice therapy under the supervision of a physician.) Drink the juices immediately after preparing them, as the nutrients will quickly deteriorate with standing. The following juices are helpful for reducing inflammation and pain.

- celery juice
- carrot, celery, and cabbage juice with a little parsley
- carrot, beet, and cucumber juice
- cherry juice
- watermelon juice
- pineapple juice

Caution: Do not drink tomato, potato, peppers, or eggplant juice. These contain an alkaloid that adversely affects osteoarthritis. Do not drink citrus fruit juices. They promote swelling in osteoarthritis.

Exercise and Lifestyle

Exercise regularly, focusing on "range of motion" exercises to reduce pain and keep joints mobile. Move the joint just to the point where you start to feel pain. Use strengthening exercise to improve muscle strength and endurance. Use isometric (use the muscle without moving the joint) and isotonic (use the muscle and move the joint fully) exercises.

Work on endurance exercises, including swimming, walking, and stationary bicycling. Balance periods of activity with rest.

If you have OA of the hip joints, swim and cycle. If you walk, wear shoes with good shock-absorbing properties and use a walking stick if you have a painful hip. Hold the walking stick on the side opposite the hip that hurts.

Exercise in water to remove the weight-bearing aspects of exercise.

Participate in Tai Chi or Qigong.

Plan your day and do things in order of importance so the most important things will be done should you get tired early.

Plan your moves to eliminate or reduce stress on your joints. Keep all of your tools and supplies nearby. Arrange furniture or use a tall stool so you can sit instead of standing while doing your daily activities. Sit in chairs that let you sit down and get up easily.

Install larger handles on household tools and objects to avoid having to grasp tightly.

Utilize your strongest muscles to do a task. Use good posture to avoid placing a strain on your body, and change positions frequently so you do not get stiff.

Nutrient Therapy
Take the following nutritional supplements:

- cetyl myristoleate – as directed on label. Cetyl myristoleate is derived from a naturally occurring fatty ester, and was first isolated and developed 30 years ago by a chemist at the National Institutes of Health in Bethesda, Maryland. It protects certain mammals from developing arthritis, and relieves some humans who are suffering from arthritis. It helps the majority of people who take it and there have been no reported negative side effects or unpleasant interactions with other medications (relieves all symptoms of arthritis in some people) (see Sources).
- glucosamine sulfate or N-acetylglucosamine sulfate – as directed on the label of your product (repairs cartilage)
- chondroitin sulfate – as directed on the label of your product (repairs cartilage)
- boron – 3 mg a day. *Caution:* Do not exceed this amount (helps retain calcium; makes bones healthy).
- proteolytic enzymes – take the amount indi-

cated on the label of your product, either one hour before or two hours after a meal (anti-inflammatory)
- evening primrose oil, borage oil, or black currant seed oil – twice a day as directed on the label of your product (anti-inflammatory)
- sea cucumber – as directed on the label of your product (anti-inflammatory)
- silica – as directed on the label of your product (important for rebuilding connective tissue and the formation of bone)
- superoxide dismutase (SOD) – as directed on the label of your product (anti-oxidant; protects synovial fluid)
- multivitamin (all nutrients needed to aid in repairing tissues and cartilage)
- vitamin A – 10,000 IU a day. *Caution:* Do not exceed 8,000 IU a day if you are or might be pregnant (required for synthesis of normal collagen and maintenance of cartilage).
- vitamin B-complex with PABA (para-aminobenzoic acid) – 50 mg, three times a day (helps with swelling)
- vitamin B_3 in the niacin form – 100 mg three times a day. *Caution:* Do not exceed this total amount, and do not take niacin if you have a liver disorder (increases blood flow).
- vitamin B_5 – 500 to 1,000 mg a day (vital for production of steroids in the adrenal gland; essential for rheumatoid arthritis)
- niacinamide – 250 mg every three hours for six doses (specifically helps with osteoarthritis; decreases pain and inflammation)
- vitamin B_6 – 50 mg a day (reduces tissue swelling)
- vitamin C – 3,000 to 10,000 mg a day in divided doses (anti-inflammatory; antioxidant)
- vitamin E – 400 IU a day (retards erosion of cartilage)
- calcium – 2,000 mg a day (needed to prevent bone loss)
- magnesium – 1,000 mg a day (needed to balance calcium; prevents spasms)

- manganese – 2 mg a day (needed for bone growth)
- selenium – 200 mcg a day (powerful anti-oxidant)
- coenzyme Q_{10} – 60 mg a day (increases tissue oxygenation and helps in repair of connective tissue)
- dimethylglycine – 125 mg three times a day (helps prevent further damage to joints)
- free-form amino acid complex – as directed on the label of your product (supplies protein needed for tissue repair)
- DL-phenylalanine – 500 mg a day every other week (for pain relief)
- cysteine – 500 mg twice a day (component of cartilagenous tissue)
- methionine – 250 mg four times a day (needed for cartilage)
- pycnogenol or grape seed extract – as directed on the label of your product (anti-inflammatory; strengthens connective tissue)
- shark cartilage – 1,000 mg per 15 pounds of body weight, divided into three daily doses. When relief is achieved, reduce the dose to 1,000 mg per 40 pounds of body weight a day (helps with pain and inflammation).
- organic germanium – 150 mg with each meal (powerful antioxidant that also relieves pain)

Herbal Therapy
Take a botanical supplement.

- alfalfa – contains minerals that aid in bone formation
- cat's claw – for relieving arthritis pain; anti-inflammatory
- cayenne – helps with pain
- cherries, hawthorn berries, and blueberries – enhance collagen structure
- feverfew and ginger – for pain and soreness
- garlic – inhibits free radicals that can damage the joints
- white willow bark – for pain

- yucca – helps indirectly to promote synthesis of cartilage

Homeopathic Remedies
Take the homeopathic remedy that best describes your symptoms. If you do not obtain relief, or if your arthritis is severe, seek the help of a homeopathic physician. The following remedies are but a few of the many possibilities.

- *Aconitum napellus* – sudden inflammatory arthritis, especially after exposure; worse at night; red, shining, swollen, very sensitive joints; hip joint and thigh feel lame, especially after lying down; knees unsteady; painless cracking of all joints.
- *Apis mellifica* – inflammation of joints with stinging and burning pains that are worse in warm room and by warm applications; better by cold application and cold air; parts look red and are hot to touch; edema.
- *Belladonna* – acute arthritis; markedly inflamed, red, swollen joint with red streaks radiating; worse from motion or jar; ameliorated by cold applications; shifting arthritic pains.
- *Benzoicum acidum* – arthritic nodules of the fingers or wrists; gouty deposits especially of the knee or big toe; tearing pain in great toe; joint pains; joints crack on motion; nodules very painful; pain, swelling, cracking in knees; strong, offensive odor from urine, which is concentrated, brownish, often with sediment; joint pains alternate with offensive urine.
- *Calcarea carbonicum* – faulty development of bones; pains relieved by constant walking; aggravated by lying or at rest; arthritic swelling or nodular gout of hands and finger joints or knees in fleshy and sweaty persons; worse cold.
- *Causticum* – rheumatoid arthritis; better in damp and warm weather; worse in cold and dry weather; contraction and stiffness of

tendons with weakness and trembling; joints are stiff and tendons shortened, drawing the limbs out of shape; deformity of joints; comfortable when it rains; paralytic trembling, weakness of limbs.

- *Colchicum* – remedy for gout; aversion to food, which smells offensive as soon as served; swelling of joints that may be red or pale; abdomen bloated with gas; albumin in urine that becomes black; scanty urine with edema; marked irritability from pains or odors; worse by motion, touch, or mental effort; better warmth, rest, or sitting; gout or rheumatism in smokers.
- *Kali carbonicum* – pains stitching, stabbing, and burning character; relieved temporarily by cold application and not by rest or motion; shrieks on account of pain; backache accompanied by great weakness and profuse sweating; covering painful part sends pain to uncovered part; aggravation after eating and uncovering.
- *Ledum* – specific in gout and rheumatism; symptoms travel upwards; deposit of chalk stones in finger joints, wrists, and toes; inflammation of joints; chilly, but pains are better by cold application; irritable, desires to be alone; worse by warm application.
- *Medorrhinum* – especially indicated in rheumatoid arthritis that rouses patient from sleep; scanty, high-colored, strong-smelling urine; sensitive to cold with tenderness of the soles; lying with legs drawn up gives relief; pain in heels; weakness of memory; irritable temperament.
- *Natrum sulphuricum* – rheumatism from uric acid in urine; accompanied with gastric troubles; arthritis worse in damp, cold weather; pain in limbs causing frequent change in position; pain in hip joint worse rising or sitting down; gout; stiffness of knees, cracking of joints.
- *Rhus toxicodendrum* – recurring attacks from getting chilled when hot; symptoms caused by damp weather and worse in damp

climate; restlessness; pain worse in the morning and on first motion; better by continued motion; cracking joints.
- *Staphysagria* – rheumatoid arthritis; stiffness and sense of fatigue in all joints; arthritic nodules on joints; worse slightest touch.

Many people respond to a complex homeopathic remedy. You may want to try one of the following complex remedies (see Sources at back of book).

- Zeel by BHI – for temporary relief of arthritis symptoms (tablets and ointment).
- Traumeel by BHI – anti-inflammatory and analgesic effects (tablets and ointment).
- Joint Pain Drops (Large) by PHP – for relief of large joint discomfort in knees, low back, elbows, and shoulders.
- Joint Pain Drops (Small) by PHP – for relief of small joint pain in fingers and toes.

Other Therapeutic Measures

Lose weight; added weight puts more stress on your joints and can make arthritis worse (see chapter 18, Metabolic Disorders).

Be tested for food, pollen, mold, and chemical allergies, and get treatment for any allergies found.

Use a stress management program, breathing exercises, and relaxation techniques. Meditate, and try using guided imagery.

Have bodywork to help relieve symptoms. Consider rolfing, reflexology, acupuncture, yoga, or massage.

Apply heat to the painful areas or keep them warm; use an electric heating pad or hot water bottle. Sleep in a sleeping bag to keep the whole body warm and reduce pain. Wear gloves for painful hands, even at night.

Get chiropractic treatments. Consult an Ayurvedic physician.

Use hydrotherapy, alternating the application of cold gel packs and heat to inflamed joints.

Use aromatherapy: try rosemary and chamomile essential oils. Use six drops of each in four ounces of a carrier oil (almond, avocado, soy, or sesame oils); or put 10 drops of each in a warm bath, and soak in it for 10 minutes.

Use acupressure:

- Press in the fleshy webbing between the thumb and index finger. *Caution:* Pregnant women should not stimulate this point—it may cause uterine contractions.
- Hold your arm out, palm down. Press on top of the forearm 2½ fingers' width above the wrist crease, between the two arm bones.
- Press four fingers' width below the kneecap on the outside of the upper leg.
- Hold your arm out, palm down, and press on the outer elbow crease.
- Press at the base of the skull, in the hollow above the two large vertical neck muscles.

BACK PAIN

Back pain is one of the most common health complaints in our society, and is the leading cause of disability for people under the age of 45. More than 80 percent of North Americans have back pain at some point in their lives, and back pain is second only to childbirth as a reason for hospitalization. Physicians are unable to identify the cause of 85 percent of back pain, but at least two-thirds of patients with low back pain get better within 30 days, regardless of treatment, and 90 percent get better within 90 days, regardless of treatment. Women have more back and spinal injuries requiring bed rest than men do.

The backbone protects the spinal cord and is made of 24 individual bones (vertebrae), separated by flexible discs, ligaments and muscles, and numerous joints. Nerves branch off the spinal cord between the vertebrae, carrying signals between the brain and the rest of the body. Ligaments function to hold the joint together and stabilize joints, limiting the direction and range of bone mobility. The discs are soft cartilage that act as shock absorbers for the back; they begin to wear by our twenties. As the discs

wear, the spaces between the vertebrae become smaller. The bones then begin to wear, and this can cause pain, numbness, and muscle weakness.

Our upright posture makes us susceptible to back pain. The spine is well-balanced, but high-heeled shoes, long periods of time spent sitting, lack of physical activity, and stress all combine to damage the back. In cultures where people squat rather than sit, back pain is rare.

Back pain can be either acute or chronic. Acute pain develops quickly, over a period of hours. It can be caused by a sudden motion, sneezing, or lifting a heavy object. Occasionally it is caused by a fall, or by a chronic imbalance in posture. Acute back pain can become chronic. Chronic back pain comes on slowly, and lasts for months or years. It comes and goes, but is never gone long enough for the sufferer not to be thinking about it.

At least 70 to 90 percent of back pain is caused by muscle or ligament problems related to weakness in the lower back, and the pain typically returns if the underlying weakness is not corrected. Fewer than 5 percent of back injuries are caused by a herniated (ruptured) disc or "slipped disc" (the bulging or rupturing of a disc's soft cartilage, with expelled material pressing on nerve roots). Most discs improve over six weeks of rest, and fit in their normal space again. Very few persons with herniated discs require surgery. In fact, with increased use of CT and MRI scans, physicians have found that many people have abnormalities and herniation of their discs that do not contribute to back pain. Up to 52 percent of asymptomatic people have a bulge of their discs at one or more levels, and 27 percent show disc protrusions on MRI scans.

Low back pain is usually caused by spasm of the large supportive muscles next to the spine. These muscles can bunch themselves into painful, powerful contractions called spasms. Low back pain is a vicious cycle, with injury causing muscle spasms, which causes pain, which causes more muscle spasms.

Severe muscle pain usually lasts from 48 to 72 hours, with days or weeks of less acute pain afterward. Any injury to the back can cause spasms. Consult your doctor if back pain continues for more than three days, you feel numbness in your legs, pain shoots down your leg to your knee or foot, or back pain is accompanied by stomach cramps, fever, or chest pain.

Low back pain affects up to 30 percent of children, with the highest incidence after age 13. The cause is more likely to be serious if the pain occurs spontaneously at night; lasts for several weeks in children less than 11; if it is accompanied by stiffness in the legs or fever; if there are neurological problems; or if it interferes with sports, play, or school attendance. Possible causes of low back pain in children can be infection, trauma, cancer, neurological disease, developmental problems, congenital problems, and psychogenic causes.

Dr. Mary Pullig Schatz (President of the medical staff of Centennial Medical Center, Nashville, Tennessee) states that poor posture and movement can affect the proper function of the spine, leading to back pain. Other factors in the development of low back pain include foot and knee alignment; muscle strength in legs, buttocks, back, and abdominal wall; pregnancy; hip flexibility; the position of the pelvis; the position of the neck; shoulder position; and the shape and flexibility of the entire back. A difference in the length of the legs can cause a curvature of the spine (scoliosis), leading to back pain. Tight muscles in the legs, buttocks, back, and abdomen can cause twisting in the pelvis and leg length discrepancy. Back pain is frequently caused by stress, because during stress the muscles of the back tense and go into spasm.

People with chronic back pain often have symptoms of emotional distress: anxiety, depression, or high blood pressure. They seem to react to life stresses in a maladaptive way, and to overreact to any pain-producing stimulus.

People who are depressed are more likely to suffer from an injury, and to have delayed recovery from an injury. People who do not like their jobs are more likely to hurt their backs than people who are happy with their jobs.

Kidney infections can also cause back pain, a diagnosis that is often overlooked. Painful menstrual periods can cause pain in the back, as can the flu. Gallstones, kidney stones, infections, fibroid tumors of the uterus, and ovarian cysts can cause referred pain. Back pain can be also be due to infection in the back, cancer, abdominal pathology, and blood vessel disease. Dr. Doug Lewis, Chairman of the Physical Medicine Department of Bastyr College in Seattle, Washington, has found that smokers have frequent back pain, which he feels is related to the deficiency in vitamin C that smoking causes.

Pain that extends down the leg to below the knee is called sciatica, and is usually caused by a herniated lumbar disc compressing one of the roots of the sciatic nerve. True sciatica's main symptom is pain radiating from the buttock down into the leg and foot. It is not initiated by a specific trauma or action, such as bending over, and the pain can wax and wane. If you have sciatic pain and loss of bladder or bowel control or weakness of the leg or ankle, see a physician immediately. These symptoms suggest pressure on the sciatic nerve, perhaps from a bulging herniated disc, which needs to be surgically corrected as soon as possible to avoid permanent damage to the nerve.

However, most people with sciatica recover spontaneously, even those with large herniations of the disc(s). Indications for surgery, and its effectiveness, are controversial. At least one in five cases of sciatica is caused not by a herniated disc but by a muscle, the piriformis, found deep in the buttock, which puts pressure on the sciatic nerve. A history and physical can diagnose piriformis syndrome, which is treated with stretching exercises and sometimes deep heat, ultrasound, and deep massage.

Dr. John Sarno, Professor of Clinical Rehabilitation at New York University School of Medicine, believes that most patients with back pain suffer from tension myositis syndrome (TMS), in which the pain is caused by unacceptable repressed emotions, such as anger and anxiety. He notes that TMS affects hard-working, conscientious perfectionists who worry a lot and are self-critical. It typically affects people in their 40s and 50s, while degenerative disease affects patients in their 60s or older. He feels the key to recovery is to realize that the cause of the pain is emotional, and that the back is essentially normal.

PREVENTING BACK PAIN

Prevention is the most effective solution for back pain. Being physically fit, with strong abdominal muscles and strong extensor muscles of the back, helps prevent back pain. When the extensor muscles of the back or the abdominal muscles are weak, the pelvis tips forward, and the hamstring muscle (at the back of the thigh) and hip muscles have to take over the load of the low back. These muscles become tight, and the low back becomes weak.

Some back clinics are using MedX back machines, which work only the lower back, to help build back strength. The isolation of the low back muscles prevents the hamstring and gluteal muscles (the large muscle of the buttocks) from taking over. Dr. Michael Pollock, director of the Center for Exercise Science at the University of Florida, has had an 80 percent success rate by having patients work on such a machine for one session a week, with 10 to 12 repetitions per session.

MODERN MEDICAL TREATMENT

Drug Therapy

Narcotics are frequently prescribed for severe back pain. All of the narcotic analgesics are prescription drugs, and all of them are addictive, some more than others. They act through the central nervous system and will give complete relief from pain for four to five hours. Butalbital (Fiorinal, Fioricet), codeine phosphate or sulfate (Tylenol #3, Fiorinal #3), hydrocodone bitartrate (Lortab, Lorcet, Vicodin, Vanex), meperidine hydrochloride (Demerol), oxycodone (Percocet, Percodan), pentazocine (Talwin), and propoxyphene hydrochloride (Darvon) are among the narcotics prescribed. Side effects include respiratory depression, urinary retention, itching, constipation, headaches, dizziness, nausea, vomiting, lightheadedness, sedation, and sweating. Early indications of addiction are ineffective pain relief and reliance on higher dosages.

Acetaminophen, aspirin, ibuprofen, or naproxen are also prescribed for pain. These drugs are available over-the-counter and are effective for temporary relief of mild to moderately severe pain. One potentially serious problem with taking these analgesics is that people tend to go beyond the recommended dose if they are not receiving the desired pain relief. They feel that because the drug is non-prescription there is little danger in taking more. This is not true, particularly with acetaminophen. It has a narrow window of safety and can cause liver damage. Patients who have just consumed an alcoholic beverage should take half the maximum recommended dose. (See Arthritis, above, for side effects of these medications.)

Tricyclic antidepressants in low doses will help control pain and may also be prescribed. (See Depression section in chapter 27, Mood Disorders, for more information on these drugs.)

Muscle relaxants such as cyclobenzaprine (Flexeril), methocarbamol (Robaxin), and carisoprodol (Soma) are also prescribed.

Flexeril can cause drowsiness, dry mouth, dizziness, and impairment of mental and/or physical abilities required for performance of tasks such as driving a car or operating machinery. It is closely related to the tricyclic antidepressants. It must be used with caution by patients with a history of urinary retention or glaucoma, or by patients taking similar medication.

Robaxin can be given as an injection or as an oral medication. It can cause dizziness, drowsiness, fainting, allergic rashes, blurred vision, headache, and fever. Soma can cause drowsiness, allergic reactions, nausea, vomiting, low white blood count, and a rapid heart beat.

Surgery

Patients are advised to have surgery for back problems that fall into four categories. Surgery is suggested for disc replacement (protruded or "slipped disc"), painful and abnormal motion of one vertebra in relation to another, narrowing of the spine around the spinal cord from overgrowth of bone (spinal stenosis), and misalignment of one vertebra with another (spondylolisthesis).

Only about 1 percent of people with back pain need surgery; 96 percent of all back injuries heal with rest and corrective exercise. Many physicians feel that 80 percent of back surgery is inappropriate. Fewer than half the people who have surgery for chronic back pain receive substantial relief, although good results occur about 67 percent of the time when the surgery is for a herniated disc.

According to United States government data, only 1 percent of patients receiving back surgery appear to benefit from it. There is risk with back surgery that includes the chance of impaired mobility or permanent damage. However, it must be considered if pain is unremitting or getting worse, or if there are signs of rapidly progressive nerve damage such as weakness in a leg, or loss of bladder or bowel function.

At Baylor College of Medicine in Houston, Texas, external spinal skeleton fixation is used to help patients decide whether back surgery will be helpful. Steel rods and screws are temporarily inserted through the skin to simulate spinal fusion. If the patient has complete relief from pain, the same result is likely from permanent fusion. Fusion is a surgical procedure in which the injured disc is removed and the adjoining vertebrae are consolidated so that they cannot move and damage each other. This is done by adding bone chips from the pelvis that grow and literally "fuse" the vertebrae together.

Patients without demonstrable back disease report greater intensity of pain than patients with proven physical abnormalities, and psychological tests are more accurate than physical examinations in predicting whether and when a patient will return to work following a back injury. Psychological testing should be done before surgery is considered, because surgical outcomes are more accurately predicted when psychological testing is combined with a history and physical exam.

Radiology

Diagnosis of back problems is often made with radiology techniques. However, very few back problems show up on X-ray. Many back problems, such as herniated disc or muscle strain, cannot be diagnosed with X-ray because they are a soft tissue (discs, muscles, and ligaments) problem that is not visible on X-ray. Discs can be seen with CT scans and MRIs (see chapter 6, Radiology). Even these tests may not be definitive, as patients can have herniated discs that are not the cause of their back pain. In these cases, surgery to repair the problem disc does not stop the pain.

Exercise and Lifestyle

Exercise after back injuries prevents re-injury. Aerobic exercises, stretches, and modified sit-ups are suggested. Recent studies have shown that moderate activity after the initial acute period is more likely to improve healing than resting in bed for two to three weeks, which can weaken muscles. When the spasms subside, the muscles are likely to be tighter than before the injury and may need to be stretched with exercise, physical therapy, or bodywork. Two months after being seen for a back injury, most patients have quit exercising—and their pain has returned.

Sleep habits should be examined. Most physicians recommend sleeping on a firm mattress. If the mattress is not firm enough, a board can be used under it. Some physicians recommend sleeping on a waterbed, but other physicians feel this does not support the back well enough. Sleeping on the floor on a mattress or futon is also a possibility.

Sleep posture may have to be changed to help the back. A folded towel under the knees will raise them slightly. Patients should not sleep on their stomachs, but on their backs or sides. A small pillow placed underneath the hips to prop the back into its normal curve, or one foot forward to tilt the pelvis, may help. One small pillow that fits in the curve of the neck, rather than large ones that cause the head to jut forward, is preferable.

Daytime posture is also important. Patients are told to stand up straight in proper posture for at least 30 seconds in order to train the body to improve posture. When people stand correctly, the tip of the earlobe lines up with the shoulder and the shoulder is in line with the hip. Both shoulders and both hips should be level. Patients may need help in achieving this.

Unless they have varicose veins, patients are also told to sit with one leg crossed over the other or to prop their feet up on a small stool in front of them, raising the knees a little higher than the hip. A lumbar cushion, a rolled-up towel, or a little pillow can be used for the lower back area when sitting. When riding in a car, patients should stop and stretch every 20 to 30 minutes.

Working posture is also important for the back. Patients should stretch forward, backward, and side to side for 5 to 10 minutes before starting to work. Sedentary workers should change positions every 30 minutes by standing up; walking around; and stretching forward, backward, and side to side. They can prop one foot for 20 minutes and then the other. Patients who stand when they work should stretch and walk around at regular intervals.

While working or reading, patients should keep material at a comfortable distance to avoid putting undue stress on the back. Forearms should be level with the elbows.

When lifting a heavy object, patients are told to get into the squatting position near the object. They should lift by straightening the legs and raising the upper part of the body. They should not lift a heavy load higher than the waist and should not twist and lift at the same time.

Other Therapeutic Measures

Back injuries are treated with ice for the first 24 to 48 hours. It is applied for five to seven minutes at a time with a gentle circular motion. Moist heat is applied after 48 hours.

For acute or subacute back pain, patients are told to go to "back school" provided by the physical therapy department of most hospitals, and to return to work as soon as possible. It is also recommended that they keep their weight down and wear low-heeled shoes.

ALTERNATIVE TREATMENT

Diet

Avoid animal fat in the diet; this decreases the production of substances that cause inflammation. Eat more fatty fish, such as mackerel, herring, and salmon; this also decreases the production of substances that cause inflammation. Avoid coffee, which blocks endorphin receptors (our body's natural narcotic) in the brain.

Avoid pasteurized dairy, caffeine, and red meats in order to reduce uric acid, which can aggravate back pain. Do not eat oils, fats, sugar, gravy, or highly processed food.

Eat foods that are high in minerals, as well as vegetable protein, to help increase bone density.

Be sure to drink at least six to eight glasses of

water a day. Many symptoms of back pain are caused by chronic dehydration, which allows acidic wastes to build up in muscles and other tissues.

Exercise and Lifestyle

Practice stretching exercises daily. Learn the following exercises under the supervision of a physician or physical therapist. With back pain, muscle groups are asymmetrically tight or imbalanced. Hold the stretch for 5 to 10 seconds, then relax for 5 to 10 seconds, and repeat the stretch. The muscle has to be relaxed to be capable of being stretched. (Many of these stretches are taken from *The Back Power Program*, by Dr. David Imrie, director of the Back Care Center in Toronto, Ontario.)

- Pelvic tilt. Lie on your back on the floor with your knees bent and your feet flat on the floor. Put your palm down between the small of your back and the floor. Flatten your back against your hand by tightening your stomach muscles and rotating your hips backward, and exhale deeply. Try to maintain the pelvic tilt position in all the other exercises.
- Sling stretch. Lie on your back, legs straight out. Using both hands, bring one knee as far as possible toward your chest without pain. Stop, and relax the stretch a little. Breathe in deeply, then exhale completely. Relax and pull the knee toward your chest again. Return to starting position. Do three to five times for each leg.
- Mad cat. Get on your hands and knees. Hold your back in a level position and breathe in slowly. Round or arch your back like a dome as you breathe out slowly. Begin with a slight arch only. Return to level, breathing in, then arch your back downward in the sway position, breathing out slowly. Do three to five repetitions.
- Sit-down. Sit on the floor with both knees

bent, feet flat on the floor, and your arms extended in from of you. Holding a pelvic tilt position, curl your trunk down to the floor while counting to seven, then return to the starting position. Do 5 to 10 repetitions.
- Lateral lift. Lie on your side, legs straight out. Cushion your head with one hand and use your other hand for balance. Raise both legs two to four inches off the ground and hold, then slowly raise and lower the upper leg in a scissors movement. Repeat 5 to 10 times on both sides.
- Hamstring stretch. Sit on the floor with one leg bent so that the sole of that foot rests against the knee of the other leg. Curl your upper body toward the knee of the straight leg, while breathing out slowly. Stop when you feel mild tension. Hold the stretch and exhale completely, then gently bend a little farther forward. Repeat three to five times on each side.
- Side stretch. Stand with your feet apart and both hands on top of your head. Bend sideways and slightly forward until you feel tension along the side of the body you are bending away from. Inhale deeply, then exhale. Do three to five repetitions on each side.
- Rectus femoris stretch. (The rectus femoris is the muscle that runs from above the hip down through the kneecap and into the front of the tibia, the inside lower leg bone.) Stand and put one knee on the seat of a chair, and hold the back of the chair with the opposite hand for balance. Pull the heel toward the buttocks and push forward with the pubic bone.
- Pelvic rock. Sit up straight, with your back against the chair. Move your pelvis back as if you are going to slouch. Hold it for a few seconds and then sit up straight.

Perform non-jarring exercise to treat and prevent back pain. Regular exercise such as walk-

ing, swimming, cycling, rowing, and cross-coun-
try skiing helps to build back strength.

Stop smoking; smoking reduces blood flow,
which means greater risk of injury. As well,
smoker's cough can strain back muscles.

Also observe the exercise and lifestyle suggestions in modern medical treatment.

Nutrient Therapy
Take the following nutritional supplements.

- vitamin B_1 – 50 mg plus 1,000 mcg vitamin
  B_{12}, *intramuscularly* once a day for one to
  two weeks (aids in calcium absorption and
  formation of spine cells)
- vitamin B_1 – 100 to 300 mg a day *orally*, together with a B-complex with 50 mg of each
  B vitamin (needed for repair and to relieve
  stress in back muscles)
- vitamin C – 2,000 to 3,000 mg a day (relieves
  pain in back area; essential for formation of
  collagen, which holds tissues together;
  needed for repair of tissues)
- multivitamin and mineral – as directed on the
  label of your product (supplies a balance of
  nutrients important in formation and metabolism of bone and connective tissue)
- boron – 3 mg daily. *Caution:* Do not exceed
  this amount. If you are under 50, take only
  until your back heals (improves calcium uptake).
- calcium – 1,500 to 2,000 mg a day (needed
  for strong bones)
- magnesium – 800 to 1,000 mg a day (for
  spasms; works with calcium)
- coenzyme Q_{10} – 30 mg three times a day
  (helps to oxygenate all cells)
- essential fatty acids – as directed on the label
  of your product (anti-inflammatory; needed
  for repair and flexibility of muscles)
- DL-phenylalanine (DLPA) – 375 to 500 mg
  three times a day, taken 15 minutes before
  meals. Some people require this every day;
  others, every other week (relieves pain).

- tryptophan – 500 mg three times a day
  (reduces pain levels)
- free-form amino acids – as directed on the
  label of your product (essential in bone and
  tissue repair)
- proteolytic enzymes – as directed on the label
  of your product, between meals (reduces inflammation and swelling)

Herbal Therapy
Take a botanical supplement.

- German chamomile – anti-inflammatory
- hops – helps with pain
- horsetail – good source of silica, which is
  necessary for bones and connective tissue
- hot pepper – (use topically) relieves pain
- white willow bark – helps relieve pain
- wintergreen oil – (use topically; this contains
  methyl salicylate, a relative of aspirin) relieves pain

Homeopathic Remedies
Take the homeopathic remedy that best describes your symptoms. If you do not receive relief, seek the help of a homeopathic physician.
The remedies below are but a few of the many
possibilities.

- *Aconite* – the back feels numb, stiff, and painful, particularly in the neck region; bruised
  sensation between the shoulder blades.
- *Aesculus* – severe, continuous, dull ache in
  the lower back region, worse when walking
  or stooping; back pain in pregnancy.
- *Bryonia* – painful stiffness in the neck and the
  small of the back brought on by sudden
  changes of weather; much worse movement,
  but better pressure.
- *Calcarea fluorica* – burning pain in the lower
  part of the back; back pain worse on beginning to move but relieved by continued
  movement; back pain from a strained back;
  curvatures of the spine, may be very severe.

- *Hydrastis* – dull, heavy, dragging pain with stiffness; pain mainly in the lumbar region; help is needed to get up from sitting.
- *Kali carbonicum* – the back feels stiff and weak, especially in the small of the back; back pain with sudden sharp pains; pain shoots up and down the back and into the thighs; back pain drives the person out of bed at night, must rise in order to turn over; worse sitting and walking, better pressure; curvature of spine.
- *Rhus toxicodendron* – low back pain and sciatica; back pain, worse after muscle strains as in car accidents or overlifting; back pain worse sitting still, causes stiffness; back pain better heat or hot baths or showers; back pain better motion and forces the person to get up and move about; back pain better from hard pressure and massage; stiff neck from being in a draft.

Some people respond well to complex homeopathic remedies. You may want to try one of the following complex remedies made by PHP (see Sources).

- Low Back Pain Drops – for temporary relief of back pain or organic or structural abnormalities.
- Low Back Pain Drops II – for temporary relief of back pain or organic or structural abnormalities, but it is a different formulation and contains more remedies.
- Lumbar Drops – provides specific homeopathic support for the lumbar spine.

Other Therapeutic Measures

If possible, rest flat on your back for the first 24 to 48 hours after back pain begins, and be careful not to reinjure the back.

Have your back X-rayed only if a fall or blow to the back caused your back injury. Routine X-rays of the back are the largest source of gonadal irradiation in North America, the added oblique view doubling the dose of radiation. If a physical exam indicates nerve damage, then a CT scan or MRI may be indicated. If there is pressure on the nerves, hospitalization, traction, or surgery may be considered.

Have prolotherapy treatments. Prolotherapy is an alternative medicine treatment that uses an injection of irritant to stimulate injured ligaments or other damaged tissue. Characteristic symptoms from ligament injury are pain from staying in one position for a long time, temporary relief of pain with manipulative therapy such as chiropractic or osteopathic treatment, and numbness (typically in the arm or leg) which is referred pain from a weakened ligament elsewhere.

The irritant used in prolotherapy causes inflammation, which induces healing. Glucose, glycerine, and phenol are the commonly used irritants. This treatment is useful for chronic low back pain, sacroiliac joint pain, chronic neck and back pain from whiplash injury, unstable knee injuries, and recurrent ankle sprain.

Receive colchicine from a physician. Colchicine is an anti-inflammatory agent that has been known for hundreds of years; it is presently used for gout. Dr. Michael Rask of Las Vegas, Nevada, past chairman of the American Academy of Neurologic and Orthopaedic Surgery, developed a protocol for using intravenous colchicine (and later, oral colchicine) for disc disease and back pain resistant to other therapy. He has treated over 6,000 patients with a 92 percent success rate. Colchicine helps back, neck, and limb pain. The main side effects are an occasional burn from extravasation of the solution outside the vein or pain from irritation of the vein. Colchicine decreases inflammation of the spinal nerve roots and discs and washes out crystals of uric acid and calcium pyrophospate dihydrate that may be deposited in the disc.

Chiropractic care has been found to be useful for back pain, and the benefits can last for three years after the chiropractic maneuvers are carried out. Dr. Kelly Jarvis (a chiropractor in private practice in Heber City, Utah) and Dr. Reed Phillips (of the Research Department of Los Angeles College of Chiropractic, Whittier, California) have reported in a 1991 *Journal of Occupational Medicine* that patients treated with chiropractic lost almost 10 times fewer work days than patients treated under medical care. Costs for chiropractic care averaged $468.38 per patient, compared with $668.39 for patients treated with standard, non-surgical treatment.

Dr. F. Batmanghelidj, author of *How to Deal Simply with Back Pain and Rheumatoid Joint Pain* and *Your Body's Many Cries for Water*, has found that back pain is caused by chronic dehydration. Strain, injury, or overwork of the back muscles causes a buildup of acid, and water is needed to flush out the acid. If it is not washed out, inflammatory mediators build up, and cause pain. Dr. Batmanghelidj suggests that drinking at least 2 quarts of water a day (eight 8-ounce glasses) helps back pain. It takes several weeks of increased water intake to get relief. He also recommends specific back exercises in which you lie on your stomach with pillows under your chest and pelvis to gradually bend the spine inward, which causes the anterior spinal bodies to separate, creating a vacuum that pulls the discs away from the nerves and relieves pain. The vacuum pulls water into the disc, separating the facet joints of the spine, which are another source of pain.

Practice acupressure to open a pathway for energy to flow out of the back:

- Lie on your back with your knees bent. Place fingers in the center of the crease behind the knee.
- Hold the point and gently rock the legs back and forth for one minute, breathing deeply as you do so.
- Afterward, rest with knees bent and feet flat.
- Repeat three times a day.

Practice meditation or the relaxation response (see Anxiety section in chapter 27, Mood Disorders).

Receive biofeedback training. Use acupuncture. It has been used successfully to treat herniated discs and avoid surgery.

Get massage, neuromuscular releasing, rolfing, Feldenkrais, or other forms of bodywork (see Bodywork in chapter 10, Alternative Therapies). Be aware that these will help relieve pain, but will not strengthen muscles.

Get osteopathic treatment.

Consider the mind-body connection. Just being aware that back pain can be caused by stress is helpful for some people.

Receive ultrasound. It helps break up local edemas and fibrosis (scar tissue in muscles).

Have NET treatments to release tissue memory that may be contributing to the pain (see Chiropractic section in chapter 9, Alternative Medical Disciplines).

CHAPTER 15

Heart Disease

The heart is a cone-shaped organ, about the size of a fist, that is located between the lungs and under the sternum (breast bone), which protects it. The wall of the heart is made up almost entirely of muscle; it is responsible for the pumping action that initiates the circulation of your blood.

The heart receives blood from the veins at low pressure and sends it to the lungs, where it takes on oxygen. The heart then pumps the oxygenated blood into the arteries at a pressure sufficient to send it through the entire circulatory system and back again to the heart. The heart pumps 100,000 times a day with a split second of rest between beats, moving 4,300 gallons of oxygenated blood through 60,000 miles of blood vessels and arteries.

Arteries carry oxygenated blood away from the heart. They are made up of three layers: the inside layer (the intima) is coated with endothelial cells (endothelium), with a layer of connective tissue underneath. The middle layer (the media) is mostly made up of smooth muscle cells. The third layer (the adventitia) is made up of connective tissue, and provides structural support and elasticity to the artery.

DISEASES OF THE HEART

ATHEROSCLEROSIS

Atherosclerosis is a form of arteriosclerosis, a degenerative process in which cells of the artery walls proliferate so that the arteries become thick and lose their elasticity. This condition is commonly known as "hardening of the arteries."

In atherosclerosis, lipids (fats) build up on the inside layer of medium-sized and large arteries. The aorta (the large artery that leads directly from the heart) and the coronary and cerebral vascular systems (blood vessels to the heart and head) are most commonly involved. The first step in the development of atherosclerosis is damage to the endothelium, by physical, mechanical, viral, chemical, drug, or immune factors. Deficiencies of vitamin C, vitamin E, and magnesium make the lining more susceptible to damage.

Once the endothelium is damaged, white cells and blood platelets begin to stick to the damaged area. When platelets aggregate (clump), they release potent growth factors that cause smooth muscle cells to migrate from the media to the intima, dumping cellular debris into the area. Collagen and elastin (fibrous proteins found in connective tissue) begin to form a fibrous cap, and more fat and cholesterol deposits accumulate. In this way, a lesion called "plaque" is gradually built up.

This area of damage develops an increased affinity for cholesterol, which is deposited there and becomes a part of the lesion. Calcium is then attracted to the area, causing the plaque to become solid. As the atheroma (plaque lesion) increases in size, its bulk narrows the interior diameter of the artery (the lumen). Blood flow is therefore decreased, which can lead to the formation of blood clots. Symptoms do not usually develop until about 90 percent of the arterial diameter is blocked. If the plaque continues to enlarge it will eventually cause the artery to close completely.

An inherited defect that creates high levels of the amino acid homocysteine (homocysteinemia) causes atherosclerosis in over 20 percent of patients with heart disease. Methionine, which is found in red meat, milk, and milk products, is converted to homocysteine during the breakdown of protein. With the help of pyridoxine (B_6), folic acid, and vitamin B_{12}, homocysteine is then further converted to a nontoxic derivative. However, when stress depletes the body of vitamin B_6 and vitamin C, their deficiency causes an accumulation of homocysteine. That accumulation produces free radicals (highly reactive atoms with one or more unpaired electrons). They can damage the endothelial cells and start the atherosclerosis cycle.

Men with high homocysteine levels have three times the risk of heart attack as men with low levels of homocysteine. Elevated homocysteine has also been associated with stroke, miscarriage, neural tube defects in fetal development, multiple sclerosis, neuropsychiatric diseases, and certain cancers. Eighty percent of patients with homocysteinemia respond to treatment with folic acid; about 15 percent require treatment with vitamin B_6; and 5 percent require treatment with both folic acid and vitamin B_6. Vitamin B_{12} helps to secure the full responsiveness of folic acid.

Risk Factors for Atherosclerosis
Atherosclerosis (and its complications) is the major cause of death in North America. Twenty percent of all deaths—550,000 deaths per year in the United States alone—are caused by heart attacks. In Canada heart attacks claim 23,000

people a year. In 1988 nearly one million Americans died of all forms of cardiovascular disease, making it the number one killer in the United States. More than 60 million Americans are now living with cardiovascular disease. According to the Heart and Stroke Foundation of Canada, 77,000 Canadians die yearly of cardiovascular disease.

Atherosclerosis causes strokes, heart attacks, angina, blockage of blood vessels in the legs (which often leads to gangrene), and in some cases, high blood pressure caused by the narrowing of an artery to the kidneys. Atherosclerosis begins early in life: one-year-old infants show fatty streaks in the aorta (the major artery of the body) and by age 23, three out of four men have at least one major blockage in the arteries to the heart. However, atherosclerosis is a gradual process, and is not usually diagnosed until a serious (often lethal) condition develops.

The major risk factors for atherosclerosis are elevated blood cholesterol levels, high blood pressure, cigarette smoking, a family history of heart disease occurring before age 60, being a male over 45 years old, and diabetes. Other risk factors are obesity, stress, physical inactivity, and personality type. Females are not exempt from heart disease, especially after menopause. Heart disease is the number one cause of death in women over 60, and heart disease kills six times as many women as does breast cancer. Women tend to have atypical symptoms that do not fit the "classic" heart attack profile developed from observations on men, and stress tests may miss a woman's unique heart symptoms.

Blood Fats and Heart Disease
Cholesterol and triglycerides are lipids (fats) normally found in the bloodstream. In excess amounts, however, they indicate that a patient is at risk of coronary heart disease.

People with cholesterol levels of 256 mg/dl or over are five times as likely to develop coronary heart disease as are those with levels below 220

mg/dl. The National Heart, Lung and Blood Institute, the American Medical Association, and
the American Heart Association have taken the
official position that too much cholesterol in the
blood does contribute to hardening of the arteries, and that lowering cholesterol levels not only
helps prevent arteriosclerosis, but can result in
its regression. However, high cholesterol is only
one of several factors that are responsible for arteriosclerosis.

It should be remembered that cholesterol at
normal levels is essential to the structure of the
cells of the body. It plays an important role in
the production of bile secretions, and is used by
the body to make such steroid hormones as the
sex and adrenal hormones. The liver makes the
majority of the cholesterol needed by the body,
and most of the rest comes from the intestines.
Only a small amount—5 percent of the cholesterol in the blood—comes from the foods we
eat.

Cholesterol levels in the body are determined
by measuring the lipoproteins in the blood.
Lipoproteins are the proteins that carry fat in
the bloodstream, as the fat is not water soluble
and cannot travel alone. These serum lipoproteins are known collectively as cholesterol and
include the following types:

- Low-density lipoproteins (LDL) transport
  cholesterol to the tissues. LDLs may stick to
  the blood vessel walls, and are thus related to
  the risk of atherosclerosis. However, they are
  harmful only after being oxidized by free radicals (such as unstable oxygen molecules, homocysteine, or chlorine).
- Very low-density lipoproteins (VLDL) are
  made in the liver to carry fats to other parts
  of the body. When they shed their fat they become LDLs. VLDL levels reflect triglyceride
  levels, and are high when the diet includes a
  lot of sugar and pastry.
- High-density lipoproteins (HDL) return cho-

lesterol to the liver to be metabolized into
VLDLs and waste products. HDLs protect
against atherosclerosis.

- Lipoprotein (a) contributes significantly to
  atherosclerotic lesions, although its exact
  function is not well understood. Lipoprotein
  (a) is a strong indicator of cardiovascular disease. In a person under 55 years of age who
  has had a heart attack, lipoprotein (a) is the
  substance that is most likely to be elevated. A
  tendency to have high levels of lipoprotein (a)
  is inherited, and this is a risk factor that is independent of the other lipoproteins. A high
  level of lipoprotein (a) is associated with
  long-term chronic deficiency of vitamin C,
  and the ingestion of vitamin C can decrease
  an elevated lipoprotein (a) level.

Nevertheless, no study has definitively shown
that reducing cholesterol by changes in diet, the
use of drugs, or other methods decreases death
rates from heart disease. Project Monica, a study
of heart disease in Europe, found that the level of
serum cholesterol could account for only 4 percent of the total risk of getting heart disease, and
more than half of all heart attacks occur in people whose cholesterol is lower than 200 mg/dl.
Further, although cholesterol levels in Japan
have increased in the past 10 years, heart disease
rates have dropped. In France, where the diet includes high levels of fat, heart disease is one-
third less prevalent than it is in the United States.
This is thought to be due to the protective qualities of red wine, widely drunk in France.

If your cholesterol levels are high, make sure
the laboratory reading is accurate before starting any type of dietary intervention. Try to obtain at least two readings of your levels of total
cholesterol, HDL, and LDL. If the cholesterol
level is high but the cholesterol/HDL ratio is less
than 4.5, this is probably acceptable. If you are
at high risk of heart disease, lowering your cholesterol by any method will extend your life span

(on average) by about twelve months; if you are at low risk, it will extend your life span (on average) by about three months.

Triglycerides (the chemical form in which fats exist as food in the body) are in part ingested in the diet and in part manufactured by the liver. Lipoprotein molecules called chylomicrons and VLDLs transport ingested triglycerides from the intestine, as well as triglycerides manufactured in the liver, through the bloodstream to the tissues of the body, where they are either used as food or stored in fatty tissue.

High triglyceride levels are almost always associated with low HDL levels, which is an indicator of lowered protection against coronary heart disease. As well, when triglyceride levels are high, LDL molecules tend to be smaller than normal, and these smaller molecules may pose a greater risk of atherosclerosis than normal-sized LDL molecules. Triglycerides themselves thicken the blood and make it less capable of carrying oxygen, also increasing the risk of heart attack. Triglycerides are now considered just as important as cholesterol as a risk factor for coronary artery disease.

Triglycerides are produced mainly from carbohydrates and alcohol. High sugar intake and stress elevate triglycerides, while eating a diet which is more than 65 percent carbohydrates (even if the carbohydrates are from all-vegetable sources) can increase triglyceride levels. Obesity is a major contributor to high triglyceride levels, and weight loss will lower those levels.

At a 1997 meeting of the American Heart Association, Dr. Michael Miller of the University of Maryland Medical Center in Baltimore reported on a recent study that found that people with triglycerides as low as 100 mg per deciliter (mg/dl) were twice as likely to develop heart disease as people with even lower levels. A 12-year study in Gothenburg, Sweden, published in 1985, showed that women with high triglyceride levels have a higher incidence of heart attacks, stroke, and other diseases than women with normal triglyceride levels.

LIPIDS AND DIET

Modern medicine attempts to control cholesterol and triglyceride levels through diet—but while diet is important, it may not be the main factor in controlling triglycerides. Stress plays a major role in triglyceride levels.

Dietary factors affecting cholesterol and triglycerides include not only the total calories ingested, but also the percent of calories from carbohydrates, protein, and fat; the type of fat (saturated, polyunsaturated, or monounsaturated); the ratio of polyunsaturated to saturated fat; the amount of sugar, starch, and carbohydrates consumed; and the amount of alcohol consumed. (See insulin control diets on p. 247, and hyperinsulinemia, pp. 235–236.)

Fats contribute significantly to the calories in food; 60 percent of the calories in a trimmed roast derive from fat, while almost half the calories in ice cream and two-thirds of the calories in some hard cheeses are from fat. Foods from fast-food restaurants provide the most concentrated sources of fat.

However, it is the type of fat you eat that is most important. Saturated fats are found in butter, coconut and palm oils, and hydrogenated oils. Monounsaturated fats include olive and canola oils. Polyunsaturated fats include safflower, sunflower, and corn oils. Lowering the intake of saturated fats does lower cholesterol levels in most individuals, and is strongly recommended. Consumption of polyunsaturated fats can reduce the tendency to form blood clots, which sometimes play a role in initiating heart attacks and strokes.

In addition to affecting cholesterol and triglyceride levels, fats cause the cell membranes to become too rigid, so that the cell cannot function properly. This leads to insulin resistance and hyperinsulinemia, which are major contributors to the development of heart disease. Eating some fat, however, causes the release of the hormone cholecystokinin, which signals the brain to stop eating, and thus helps to reduce obesity caused by overeating.

Only 5 percent of the body's cholesterol level comes from the diet. Dietary cholesterol may have an influence on blood cholesterol levels, but research at the Veterans Administration Hospital in Albany, New York, indicates that cholesterol-containing foods such as eggs, dairy products, and meats may increase the risk of heart disease *only* when they are not fresh—and therefore contaminated with oxidation products. And although many cardiologists still tell their patients to substitute margarine for butter, it is now widely recognized that the consumption of trans-fatty acids, found in margarine, substantially increases the risk of heart disease.

The relationship between fat and heart disease is apparent, but Dr. John Yudkin, a British physician, nutritionist, and biochemist, found an even stronger correlation between sugar consumption and coronary deaths, and identified sugar as the primary cause of heart disease. The combination of high fat and high sugar in the diet creates a particularly high risk of heart disease.

HEART ATTACK

Ischemia refers to a blockage of the blood supply. Coronary artery disease is ischemic heart disease in which there is blockage to the arteries that supply the heart. The blockage may be caused by plaque, a blood clot, or a spasm of the artery. When the blood supply to the heart is blocked, chest pain will result. The pain has been variously described as a squeezing, tightening, or crushing sensation; as being like a vise, or like a heavy weight in the chest. The patient may grimace or show other signs of distress, and may be apprehensive and restless.

The pain may be located in the area beneath the ribs, or may radiate to the left shoulder and down the left arm. Sometimes the pain radiates to both sides of the neck and down both arms, and occasionally pain will be felt in the back or abdomen. Pain can be accompanied by nausea. This pain is known as angina, and it occurs periodically whenever the heart muscles (myocardia) need more blood than they are receiving. Angina may precede a heart attack (known medically as a myocardial infarction), or it may resolve without further incident.

In a heart attack, the blockage of the artery does not reverse, and the area of the heart muscle supplied by that artery dies. If a large part of the heart is affected, the person can develop congestive heart failure, in which the heart is not able to pump adequate amounts of blood. Shock (low blood pressure, because the heart is not pumping well), arrhythmia (abnormal rhythms of the heart), and blood clots can result. Over 90 percent of heart attacks are secondary to atherosclerotic changes in the coronary arteries, and in half of all patients with coronary heart disease, the first sign of the disease is sudden death.

DIAGNOSING HEART DISEASE

One of modern medicine's greatest strengths is its ability to diagnose angina, and to reverse heart attacks in their early stages. Medicines are available that will dissolve clots: the so-called "clot busters"—streptokinase, Eminase, and Tissue-type Plasminogen Activator (TPA) open up coronary arteries blocked by clots, restoring blood flow if the heart attack is caught in its early stages. These drugs prevent permanent heart muscle damage. Therefore, at the first sign of chest pain (especially chest pain as described above), go immediately to an emergency room. Giving the clot buster medication quickly reduces the chance that a heart attack will cause permanent damage.

However, these drugs do not dissolve the plaque deposits that narrowed the artery in the first place, making the blockage by a clot possible. In modern medicine, after the heart attack is over, the patient will usually have bypass surgery, angioplasty, or more drug treatment to reduce the amount of plaque in the artery.

Once a person is diagnosed with coronary artery disease, an angiogram will almost invariably be done. In this procedure, dye is placed by a catheter (a small tube) into the blood vessels of the heart so that they can be visualized, and a radiologist can tell where they are narrowed or blocked. This is an invasive procedure, because an instrument is actually placed in the heart. The catheter causes some spasm of the coronary arteries, and some people are allergic to the dye. The angiogram itself can cause a heart attack, and one person in 1,000 dies from the procedure.

If the angina that led to the diagnosis of coronary heart disease was in fact caused by spasm of the coronary arteries rather than blockage, nothing useful will show up in the angiogram. Collateral circulation (new blood vessels that grow to replace a major artery that has been blocked) also may not show up on the angiogram. These facts do not mean that angiograms should not be used—only that you should be aware of the pros and cons of this procedure before agreeing to it.

There are several non-invasive techniques that are also used to diagnose heart disease. Ordinary X-rays, for example, will show whether any of the chambers or large blood vessels of the heart are grossly larger or smaller than they should be. But perhaps the most commonly used non-invasive test for heart status is the electrocardiogram (ECG; formerly called an EKG). It is used in two ways; the first is the "resting" electrocardiogram, in which the patient is tested while lying down. External electrical sensors are secured on the chest, arms, and legs with a special paste and tape; the sensors detect the electrical activity of the heart, and record the information as a graph on paper strips. The rise or fall in the vertical direction represents a rise

or fall in the electrical potential of the heart, while movement in the horizontal direction shows the amount of time it takes the electrical activity to travel through the heart. There are five "waves" that make up the cardiac cycle. Deviations from the normal cycle are diagnostic for particular conditions.

The electrocardiogram is also used in the "stress test," which measures how the heart functions when it is subjected to extra work. The electrocardiogram is begun as the patient is "strolling" on a treadmill, heading slightly uphill. At the end of 10 minutes, the patient is walking or trotting on the treadmill at the rate of five and one-half miles an hour (many patients with heart problems are unable to complete the test). The interpretation of ECGs has made great progress, and there are physicians who feel they can use ECG results to predict which patients will have a heart attack within the next five years. On the other hand, there are physicians who feel that ECGs are unreliable and that ECG results have led to many misdiagnoses.

There are also new non-invasive tests available, in which a radiotracer is used to assess the adequacy of blood supply to various areas of the heart. These tests include thallium scans, radionuclide cineangiogram (RNCA, first pass), and gated pool (multi-gated radionucleotide ventriculography, or MUGA, a technique used in imaging the heart). The Ultrafast CT scan (computerized axial tomography) is an improved type of CT scan that allows physicians to look at the coronary arteries for evidence of calcification. This is useful because a person of 50 or 60 who does not have coronary artery calcification is at very low risk of having a heart attack or angina. In fact, Ultrafast CT is a better predictor of future events than is an angiogram.

MODERN MEDICAL PREVENTION

Cardiologists agree that prevention of heart disease is far preferable to treating heart disease once it is symptomatic, and they agree that the best prevention can be achieved by diet and lifestyle modification.

The lifestyle approach to prevention of heart disease begins with eliminating smoking. Smoking lowers HDL and increases the risk of heart attack. Next, patients are urged to decrease stress in their lives, since stress management will help lower triglycerides and blood pressure. Regular exercise is also recommended, since exercise can help raise HDL, help a patient lose weight, and lower other heart risks.

Diet is considered an important element in prevention; the standard cardiac diet asks patients to eat little fat, decrease dietary cholesterol, eat more starches and fiber, and drink alcohol only in moderation.

Controlling blood pressure, cholesterol levels, and body weight are central goals of heart attack prevention. If lifestyle changes are not sufficient, drugs are often used to help achieve those goals.

ALTERNATIVE PREVENTION

Alternative and nutritional therapy has been shown to reduce heart disease mortality more effectively than drug treatment. The following measures will help prevent heart disease in both men and women, although in women it appears to be hormone-dependent since most women do not develop heart disease until after menopause.

Diet

Diet plays a major role in alternative prevention. If you are overweight, make appropriate dietary and lifestyle changes to lose weight. In addition, use the following dietary guidelines.

Eat potassium- and magnesium-rich foods such as brown rice and whole grains, fresh greens, garlic and onion, green tea, seafood, tofu, and pitted fruits. Eliminate or reduce consumption of red meats, prepared meats, refined sugar, soft drinks, fried foods, high-salt foods, and caffeine and caffeine-containing foods. Eat no more than 10 percent of total calorie intake as fats, and limit hydrogenated oils and animal fats. Eat fresh eggs, butter, low-fat milk, cheese, and yogurt in limited amounts.

Eat 20 percent of calories as low-fat protein and 70 percent as complex carbohydrates (unless you are hyperinsulinemic). Drink eight glasses of pure water daily.

Exercise and Lifestyle

Alter your lifestyle to include regular, mild daily exercise along with deep breathing exercises to increase oxygenation in your body. Take alternating hot and cold showers to increase your circulation. If your life is stressful, add relaxation techniques to your schedule. Stop smoking, and avoid alcohol in all forms.

Nutrient Therapy

Take the following nutrients:

- vitamin B_6 – 50 mg a day (for synergistic action with folic acid)
- vitamin B_{12} – 300 mcg a day (for synergistic action with folic acid)
- folic acid – 800 mcg a day (to reduce homocysteine levels)
- vitamin C – up to 5,000 mg a day (to help interstitial tissue elasticity and arterial integrity)
- vitamin E – 600 IU a day (synergistic action with vitamin C; strengthens heart muscle; improves circulation)
- chromium picolinate – 150 mcg a day (for insulin resistance and arterial plaque)
- magnesium – 800 mg a day (helps with nerve and muscle transmission)
- potassium – 90 mg a day (for electrolyte balance)
- selenium – 200 mcg a day (synergistic action with vitamin C; deficiency of selenium linked with heart disease)
- coenzyme Q_{10} – 60 mg three times a day (increases oxygenation of the heart)
- L-carnitine – 500 mg a day (reduces fat and triglyceride levels in blood)
- omega-3 fish or flax oils – as directed on your

product three times a day (prevents hardening of the arteries)

- proteolytic enzymes – as directed on your product (increases fibrinolysis; inhibits platelet aggregation)

Herbal Therapy
Use the following herbs daily. See page oo for dosage:

- cayenne pepper – improves circulation
- ginkgo – improves blood flow to the heart
- hawthorn – preventative support; strengthens and clears cardiovascular system

Homeopathic Remedies
Use the following homeopathic remedies as prevention:

- *Cactus* – acts on heart, arteries, and circulation.
- *Crataegus* – excellent heart tonic; acts on heart muscle, lowers pulse, and reduces blood pressure.

MODERN MEDICAL TREATMENT
The modern medical approach to treatment of heart disease involves diet, exercise, medications, and sometimes surgery.

Diet
In modern medical care, patients are advised to eat less fat by avoiding saturated fats, and reducing the percentage of calories that come from fats. Low-fat or non-fat dairy products are recommended. The consumption of eggs and fatty meats should be limited, and alcohol consumption should be limited to no more than two drinks a day. Patients are advised to eat more fiber, fresh fruits, and vegetables.

Exercise and Lifestyle
Exercise improves cardiovascular fitness and may reduce the possibility of heart attack. The Framingham Study (a long-term study conducted in Framingham, Massachusetts) showed that exercise has an ameliorating effect on the clinical course of coronary heart disease.

Aerobic exercise, in which continuous, rhythmic activity of large muscle groups is carried on for extended periods of time, is the recommended type of exercise (swimming, jogging, bicycling, or hard physical work). This type of exercise increases the transport of oxygen, and its utilization by the cardiovascular, pulmonary, and musculoskeletal systems of the body.

Drug Therapy
There are many medications available to treat coronary artery disease: medications that lower blood pressure, lower cholesterol, decrease the work done by the heart, dilate blood vessels, decrease the risk of blood clots, and decrease the heart rate. However, none of these medications changes the underlying medical condition—atherosclerosis.

A recent study reported in 1997 in the *Journal of the American Medical Association* looked at 12,866 men at high risk for heart disease, and found that at the end of seven years there was no difference in the death rate between men who had been given various types of drug treatment and men who had not been medicated. The researchers suspect that reactions to the drugs given (for high blood pressure) caused the higher-than-expected death rate in the intervention group.

Some of the drugs used for heart disease are the same as those used for high blood pressure (beta blockers, diuretics, and calcium channel blockers). Other drugs are used specifically for heart disease (digoxin, aspirin, dipyridamole, nitrates, and lipid-lowering drugs).

CALCIUM CHANNEL BLOCKERS
Calcium channel blockers prevent calcium from entering the cells, decreasing spasm of the coronary arteries and preventing rhythm disturbances of the heart.

Calcium channel blockers are effective in acute heart attacks, but patients on long-term use of calcium channel blockers experience a 60 percent increase in heart attacks compared to patients on diuretics or beta blockers. Calcium channel blockers can cause headaches, flushing, swelling of the feet, excessive drop in blood pressure, and dizziness.

BETA BLOCKERS

Beta blockers are drugs that interfere with the effect of epinephrine (adrenaline) at the cell level. They slow the heart rate, decrease arrhythmias, decrease blood pressure, and decrease the force of heart contractions. They may prevent heart damage caused by lack of oxygen, and they have decreased the mortality by 25 percent in some groups of patients after heart attacks. However, long-term use can cause heart failure, since the beta blockers depress the heart tissue itself.

Side effects of beta blockers include profound fatigue, loss of desire and capability for sex in men, bad dreams, cramps in calves for those with blockage of leg arteries, decrease in sharpness of memory, depression, stomach upset, and constricted breathing. Beta blockers should not be used by patients who have asthma.

NITRATES

Nitrates come in two main forms: as nitroglycerin, and as long-acting nitrates. Nitroglycerin in pill form is used to prevent or relieve the pain of angina, and long-acting nitrates are used to widen the coronary arteries.

Nitroglycerin in pill form has been available for over 60 years, and it has been used intravenously since the 1980s. Nitroglycerin controls high blood pressure during a heart attack and decreases spasm of the injured blood vessels.

Nitroglycerin is a vasodilator, and can cause severe headaches that recur with each dose, light-headedness, low blood pressure, fainting, and rebound hypertension. Occasionally it will increase angina.

Note: If chest pain persists or recurs after you take nitroglycerin for angina, and you break out in a cold sweat, you should quickly seek medical assistance as you may be having a heart attack.

BILE ACID BINDING RESINS

Bile acid binding resins (for example, cholestyramine, colestipol, and gemfibrozil) lower cholesterol by binding with the cholesterol-rich bile acids in the intestine. The cholesterol and resin are then excreted in the stool. The liver removes cholesterol from the blood to make up for what is lost in the stool, and this causes a lowering of total cholesterol and LDL cholesterol.

The bile acid binding resins do not taste good and have the consistency of sand. They also cause (occasionally severe) constipation, abdominal pain, heartburn, belching, nausea, and bloating. When you take a bile acid resin, you need to take a vitamin supplement that contains the fat-soluble vitamins (A, D, E, and K) and folic acid, all of which can be bound by the resin and lost in the stool. The resins have to be taken four hours before or one hour after any other drug to prevent binding to the drug. Pregnant or lactating women, and children, should not take this medication because of the effect on nutrition. Bile acid binding resins can be given with niacin (see Nutrient Therapy, below).

CHOLESTEROL-LOWERING DRUGS

Another category of drugs used to treat heart disease are the statins, which interfere with the manufacture of cholesterol by the liver and thus lower cholesterol and LDL. They can cause liver damage (which resolves when the medication is stopped), accelerated cataract formation, and painful muscles. These drugs also increase the risk of cancer, depression, and suicide.

ASPIRIN

A baby aspirin (80 mg) a day helps to prevent blood clots and keep the blood flowing within the coronary arteries. Aspirin can cause ulcers, but does not usually do so at this low dose.

Surgery

If medications do not improve the patient's condition, surgery is often performed. The most common types of surgery used to treat heart disease are coronary artery bypass surgery and angioplasty (in which a balloon is inserted to widen a narrow or blocked coronary artery). Balloon angioplasty does not require major surgery, hospital stay is short, and recovery is quick. However, in 30 percent of cases, the blockage reappears within six months.

In the United States each year nearly 300,000 bypass surgeries and 250,000 angioplasties are performed. Yet Dr. Nortin Hadler, professor of medicine at the University of North Carolina School of Medicine, wrote in 1992 that none of the balloon angioplasties performed the previous year at the school could be justified, and that only 3 to 5 percent of the coronary artery bypass surgeries done the same year were actually indicated.

In heart bypass surgery, the patient is put on a heart-lung machine, and veins from the legs are sewn onto the coronary arteries to bypass the area of obstruction. (New techniques utilize one of the two arteries from the arm for bypass surgery. These arteries are stronger than the leg veins, and may allow bypass surgery to last longer.) Several major studies have reported that patients who have undergone heart bypass operations have done no better in the long run than patients who have been treated with non-surgical techniques.

Patients who refuse heart surgery are often given fear-inspiring warnings, which Dr. Andrew Weil of Tucson, Arizona, calls "medical hexes." Phrases such as, "You're a walking time bomb," "You are living on borrowed time," and "You could go any minute," from an authority figure such as a physician are damaging words.

Of course, bypass surgery does not address the issue of why the patient developed heart disease in the first place; nor does it affect the ongoing process of atherosclerosis.

Diet

If you opt to follow alternative treatment protocols for heart disease, make the following dietary changes. Buy organic foods, and avoid irradiated foods to reduce accumulation of free radicals. Avoid any food to which you are allergic or sensitive; in some people, angina is triggered by allergenic foods. If you have a tendency to hypoglycemia or hyperinsulinemia, eat a low-carbohydrate diet and eliminate refined sugar from the diet. Watch grain intake if you are hyperinsulinemic. The body responds to high levels of carbohydrates by secreting extra amounts of adrenaline, which can trigger angina in susceptible patients. If you are *not* hypoglycemic or hyperinsulinemic, increase your consumption of complex carbohydrates (grains, fruits, green leafy vegetables, and legumes).

Eat foods high in beta carotene such as carrots, sweet potatoes, spinach, and cantaloupe (it helps prevent free radical damage to arteries). Eat celery, which can help lower blood cholesterol, and contains 3-n-butylphthalide, which seems to lower the stress hormones that cause blood vessels to constrict. Eat apples, pears, prunes, apricots, carrots, and bananas (they contain pectin, which can help lower cholesterol). Eat garlic and onions (both help lower cholesterol, and garlic also helps prevent blood clotting).

Reduce fat intake—especially fried foods, animal fats, and partially hydrogenated oils Use monounsaturated oils (such as olive oil), flaxseed oil, fish oils, borage oil, black currant oil, and evening primrose oil. Oils must be fresh and cold-pressed. Eat fish, which is high in omega-3 fatty acids.

Decrease your consumption of meat. (Those with hyperinsulinemia may have to eat their normal intake of meat.) Eat fresh eggs, butter, low-fat milk, cheese, and yogurt in limited amounts. Eat soluble fiber foods (oat bran, barley, and all beans) or take a soluble fiber supplement (psyllium).

Dr. Dean Ornish, at the Preventive Medicine Research Institute in Sausalito, California, has used a low-fat vegetarian diet (in which only 10 percent of calories come from fat), exercise, smoking cessation, and stress reduction to reverse coronary artery disease. Coronary artery blockages were reversed in more than 80 percent of the patients on this diet, and the program is now covered by some insurance companies.

Exercise and Lifestyle
Stop smoking, and avoid all forms of tobacco. Decrease your alcohol consumption. Better still, avoid alcohol—with the possible exception of red wine, which increases HDL cholesterol.

Regular aerobic exercise is important to maintain a healthy heart. Yoga and meditation are effective ways to help alleviate stress.

Nutrient Therapy
Take the following minerals:

- magnesium orotate or aspartate – 125 mg six times a day (important in functioning of cardiac muscle). Nearly all cardiac patients are low in magnesium. Some people get intravenous or intramuscular injections of magnesium (1,000 mg once a week for six weeks, then less often).
- zinc and copper – must be balanced at the ratio of 30 mg a day (zinc) and 2 mg a day (copper) (aid in cleansing and healing)
- manganese – 15 to 20 mg a day (deficiency leads to atherosclerosis, high cholesterol, heart disease; needed for proper fat metabolism)
- selenium – 100 mcg a day (eliminates free radicals; decreases platelet clumping)
- chromium – 600 to 800 mcg a day (lowers blood sugar and lipids)
- calcium – 800 to 1,000 mg a day (dilates blood vessels; decreases cholesterol)
- potassium – 900 to 3,500 mg a day *Caution:*

This size dose must be taken under the supervision of a physician (needed for electrolyte balance).

Take the following vitamins:

- B vitamins – vitamin B_6, 50 to 250 mg a day; folic acid, 800 to 4,000 mcg a day; vitamin B_{12}, 500 to 2,000 mcg a day; vitamin B_{15} – 50 to 150 mg a day; vitamin B_1 – 50 to 100 mg a day (use higher dosages if you have high homocysteine levels) (deficiency leads to heart disease)
- vitamin B_3 (niacin) – 1,500 to 3,000 mg a day—but note that high doses can cause "niacin flush" (flushing, itching, and burning of the skin). Use the short-acting forms, not the delayed-release forms. Liver tests should be performed periodically (lowers cholesterol and improves circulation).
- pantethine – 900 to 1,800 mg a day (lowers lipids)
- vitamin E – 800 IU a day (powerful antioxidant; protects against free radicals; strengthens heart muscle; improves circulation)
- vitamin C – 3,000 to 10,000 mg a day (extremely important in treating cardiovascular disease)
- beta carotene – 25,000 IU a day (antioxidant; protects against free radicals)

Take the following supplements:

- lecithin – 2 Tbsp. of granules a day (fat emulsifier; aids in the removal of cholesterol from tissue)
- coenzyme Q_{10} – 50 to 100 mg three times a day (increases oxygenation of heart tissue; prevents reoccurence of heart attacks)
- L-carnitine – 500 mg twice a day (reduces fat and triglyceride levels; increases oxygen uptake and stress tolerance)
- cod liver oil – 1 Tbsp. twice a day (decreases platelet clumping)

- bromelain – two tablets three times a day, one hour before or two hours after meals (aids disgestion; reduces inflammation; helps to dissolve plaque; decreases platelet clumping)
- hydrochloric acid and pepsin in tablet or capsule form – take with meals; dosage depends on results of tests for acidity levels (aids digestion if stomach acid is shown to be low)

If you have elevated lipoprotein (a), be certain that you take these minimum amounts of the following nutrients:

- L-lysine – 2,000 to 3,000 mg a day (lowers triglycerides)
- L-proline – 2,000 to 3,000 mg a day (heals heart muscle)
- vitamin C – 3,000 mg a day (reduces lipoprotein [a])
- niacin – 1,500 mg a day (lowers cholesterol; improves circulation). Liver function tests should be monitored regularly.

Take Bios Life 2 by Rexall, a very effective natural product that lowers cholesterol. It provides the proper balance of soluble and insoluble fiber, as well as chromium, which helps stabilize blood sugar (see Sources).

Herbal Therapy
Take a botanical supplement.

- alfalfa – reduces blood cholesterol levels and plaque deposits on artery walls
- cayenne – reduces blood lipids
- garlic – acts as an antioxidant; helps to dissolve clots; lowers cholesterol and blood pressure
- ginger – lowers cholesterol levels; makes the platelets less liable to adhere to arteries
- ginkgo – improves circulation; helps prevent blood clots
- ginseng – lowers cholesterol; normalizes blood pressure

- hawthorn – helps strengthen blood vessels and heart muscle; maintains steady heart rhythms and oxygen to the heart; lowers blood pressure; works as a diuretic and natural chelator
- motherwort – cardiotonic; helps prevent palpitations
- turmeric – lowers cholesterol; stimulates the production of bile

Homeopathic Remedies
The following homeopathic remedies are a few of the many that are effective for angina. You should consult with a qualified homeopathic physician for advice on these and other homeopathic remedies.

- *Arnica montana* – feels as though heart is being held in a vise; heart pains left to right; worse with movement, slightest touch, damp cold; pain in left elbow; cardiac distress at night; heartbeats shake the whole body.
- *Cactus grandiflorus* – Pain in chest or heart "as if grasped by an iron fist"; severe constricting pain worse when lying on the left side, worse with exertion, extends into left arm.
- *Lachesis lanceolatus* – cramp-like pain with fainting; palpitation of heart and choking from the slightest anxiety; feels as if the heart is hanging by a thread and every beat would tear it off; stitching pain in region of heart.
- *Latrodectus mactans* – great pain in the chest that radiates to the axilla or down the left arm, causing numbness and coldness of the hand.
- *Oxalicum acidum* – sharp and stitching pains that may extend to shoulder, arm, or abdomen; better from rest; palpitations worse when lying down.
- *Rhus toxicodendron* – pain worse with exertion, extends to left arm and hand; anxiety in region of heart.

Take one of the following homeopathic remedies for heart attack and immediately seek professional help.

- Aconitum napellus – mental anxiety, fear of death; oppression and palpitations; numbness in left arm and tingling in fingers; heart pains into left shoulder; worse when sitting erect; tachycardia; pulse fast, bounding, shaking, forcible, and tumultuous.
- *Arnica montana* – feels the heart is being held in a vise; heart pains left to right; worse movement, slightest touch, damp cold; cardiac distress at night; heartbeats shake the whole body.
- *Cactus grandiflorus* – feeling of constriction, contraction, and congestion of heart; fluttering palpitations and prostration; severe constricting pain that is worse lying on the left side and extends into the left arm; worse with exertion.
- *Digitalis* – slowness of pulse; tachycardia; sensation that the heart will stop beating; worse from exertion.
- *Lachesis lanceolatus* – cramp-like pain with fainting; palpitation of heart and choking from anxiety; feels as if heart hanging by a thread and every beat will tear it off; stitching pain in heart.
- *Latrodectus mactans* – great pain in the chest that radiates to the axilla or down the left arm, causing numbness and coldness of the hand.

Many people respond well to complex homeopathic remedies. Also take PHP Heart Liquescence, which aids in strengthening and supporting the heart.

Other Therapeutic Measures

Use acupuncture to relieve heart spasms, help heart pain, and help you relax. It can also help people stop smoking. Try receiving shiatsu from a qualified practitioner. (Pressing specific places along the inner forearm may help relieve symptoms of angina.)

Oxygen therapy with hydrogen peroxide may be helpful (see p. 223). Traditional Chinese medicine or Ayurvedic medicine from trained practitioners can be effective.

Chelation Therapy

Chelation therapy is a cleansing method that removes metal irritants and allows leaking and damaged cell walls to heal. Statistics on survival rates and quality of life show that chelation is substantially more effective and less dangerous than bypass surgery in dealing with the effects of atherosclerosis. In chelation therapy, ethylenediaminetetraacetic acid (EDTA) is injected intravenously. It binds to cadmium, lead, calcium, and iron, making them soluble so that the kidneys can excrete them from the body. Chelation therapy removes the calcium content of plaque from the artery walls and improves circulation to all tissues of the body. It also helps prevent the formation of free radicals, which most scientists now believe are a contributing factor in the development of atherosclerosis.

Chelation therapy has been used safely on more than 500,000 patients in the United States for a variety of health conditions over the past 40 years, and has improved the condition of approximately 80 percent of those patients. Nevertheless, EDTA has not yet received FDA approval as a treatment for anything other than lead and heavy metal toxicity—though under current drug safety standards, aspirin is nearly three and one-half times more toxic than EDTA. Consequently, modern medicine considers chelation therapy an unproven treatment. In Canada, physicians who specialize in chelation therapy can treat patients with heart disease as well as heavy metal toxicity, but treatment is not covered by medical plans.

Hundreds of articles on chelation have appeared in the medical literature, almost all favorable to the therapy. For example, Dr. Efrain Olszewer and Dr. James Carter of Tulane University carried out a study in 1988 that followed 2,870 patients suffering from heart disease who had EDTA chelation therapy. Significant improvement was seen in 94 percent of those patients. In the 1980s Dr. Robert Atkins in New York found that 79 percent of the patients in his chelation program improved, 13 percent noted no real change, and 8 percent became worse. (During the course of standard medical treatment, 40 percent of heart disease patients feel worse.)

EDTA can be taken orally, and still provides chelating activity even though only about 5 percent is absorbed when this method is used. Symptoms do not resolve as quickly as when chelation is carried out with intravenous EDTA, but oral chelation therapy is more convenient and costs less. Oral chelation Pack II by AMNI (Advanced Medical Nutrition Inc.—see Sources) contains oral EDTA as well as important heart nutrients. In addition to containing EDTA, Beyond Chelation (Longevity Plus) supplies vitamins and minerals to the cardiovascular system, mind, and body (see Sources).

Patients who are interested in chelation therapy should choose a physician who follows the protocol of the American Board of Chelation Therapy or the American College of Advancement in Medicine (ACAM).

CHAPTER 16

Hypertension

Blood pressure is a measure of the force exerted by the blood against the walls of an artery. It varies according to the strength of the heart's output and the amount of resistance offered by the blood vessels themselves. The blood pressure measured while the heart contracts fully and pumps is called the systolic pressure. The blood pressure measured while the heart relaxes fully between pumps is called the diastolic pressure, and is lower than the systolic pressure. Blood pressure figures are reported as a ratio: systolic pressure over diastolic pressure.

The arteries, too, contract and relax to help keep the blood circulating. If arteries remain contracted and fail to relax sufficiently, high blood pressure results. High blood pressure (hypertension), the most commonly seen cardiovascular disease, is usually said to be present if the systolic blood pressure reading is higher then 140 to 150 and/or the diastolic pressure reading is higher than 90. At one time it was thought that high systolic pressure was not a very significant indicator of risk. However, recent studies sponsored by the National Heart, Lung, and Blood Institute in Bethesda, Maryland show that systolic hypertension may be a greater indicator of cardiovascular risk than diastolic pressure.

Hypertension is a major contributor to the annual incidence of 1.5 million heart attacks, 500,000 strokes, and 400,000 new cases of heart failure in the United States. High blood pressure affects 20 percent of people in their forties, and is the most common chronic disease in people over 40 years of age. Uncontrolled high blood pressure is directly associated with more than 35,000 deaths per year in the United States. In Canada, an estimated 4.1 million people suffer from hypertension, and almost half are unaware of it or of the consequences of letting it go unchecked.

In the earliest stages of hypertension, the patient has no symptoms, and for this reason the disease is called "the silent killer." If high blood pressure is not recognized and treated, blood pressure continues to rise and the patient may eventually have symptoms of headache, lightheadedness, dizziness, ringing in the ears, fatigue, nervousness, vision problems, shortness of breath, abnormal sweating, and a flushing sensation of the head. Nose bleeds may occur, and these usually indicate that the diastolic pressure is persistently above 100. At that point the patient will likely develop enlargement of the heart, heart failure, heart disease, bleeding into the eyes, or a stroke.

ESSENTIAL HYPERTENSION

High blood pressure is of two types: essential (or primary) hypertension and secondary hypertension. Essential hypertension is the most common type of high blood pressure, accounting for 92 to 94 percent of all cases. In almost all essential hypertension patients, the underlying cause of the condition is not known, but risk factors for essential hypertension include genetics, gender, an imbalanced diet, lack of exercise, obesity, and chronic stress. Statistically, the natural history of high blood pressure is likely to be more severe in males, in people whose diastolic blood pressure persistently remains higher than 115, people with African ancestors, older people, those who smoke, people with diabetes or increased blood cholesterol levels, those who are obese, and those with heart failure.

Many researchers believe that hyperinsulinemia is a common cause of essential hypertension (see pp. 232). Others, such as Dr. Robert Atkins, believe that in addition to hyperinsulinemia, prostaglandin problems, mineral imbalances, and magnesium deficiency account for 90 percent of all cases of high blood pressure.

Dr. F. Batmanghelidj, researcher and author of *Your Body's Many Cries for Water*, believes that essential hypertension is an adaptive process that occurs in response to a gross water deficiency in the body. When there is not enough water to serve the body's needs, some cells lose their water to the circulation, as the body attempts to maintain blood volume. The capillary beds and blood vessels close to cope with the loss in blood volume, causing resistance to the passage of blood in the vessels. Increased force (increased blood pressure) is then needed to allow the blood to circulate. The use of diuretics to treat high blood pressure only makes the body more dehydrated.

SECONDARY HYPERTENSION

Only a small number of people have secondary hypertension. Secondary hypertension results from underlying diseases of the kidneys, adrenal glands, blood vessels, or the brain; narrowing of the artery that supplies the kidney; congenital narrowing of the aorta; or the use of birth control pills. High cadmium and lead levels can also cause high blood pressure, and these can be treated with chelation. Certain medications can increase blood pressure—for instance, nonsteroidal anti-inflammatory drugs (Motrin, Aleve, Anaprox, Advil, Naprosyn, Nalfon), steroids, and drugs that affect the sympathetic nervous system (such as phenylpropanolamine, or PPA, which is found in some cold remedies).

OTHER CAUSES OF HIGH BLOOD PRESSURE

High blood pressure has many other causes, including excessive blood volume in the system, constriction of the arteries, or overexertion of the heart. Regardless of the cause, sustained high blood pressure decreases life expectancy, and if untreated can cause congestive heart failure, a stroke, heart attack, or kidney failure. As people age, systolic hypertension becomes more common because the arteries calcify and stiffen from arteriosclerosis. This increases resistance to blood flow, and the heart has to pump harder to force blood through the arteries.

Stress can also cause high blood pressure. Studies show that tense middle-aged men are twice as likely to develop high blood pressure as are calm middle-aged men. In addition, chronic stress is often associated with the use of addictive drugs such as alcohol, tobacco, and caffeine, all of which raise blood pressure. Biofeedback, yoga, and meditation have all been shown to lower blood pressure, although the benefit is often temporary.

Renin is an enzyme secreted by the kidney that has an effect on salt and fluid balance. Some people have high-renin hypertension and others have hypertension with normal renin levels, which is known as low-renin hypertension. Knowing a patient's renin level is important in some drug therapies and for selecting natural treatment.

"White coat hypertension" has recently been described in medical literature. In this syndrome, patients have increased blood pressure while at the doctor's office, but not at home. If you have high blood pressure at the doctor's office, be sure to regularly monitor your blood pressure at home. Consider using a 24-hour ambulatory blood pressure monitoring system. High blood pressure should not be diagnosed on the basis of one high reading, but only after a series of readings over time.

MODERN MEDICAL TREATMENT

Diet

The modern treatment for high blood pressure includes eating a low-salt and/or low-fat diet. Twenty-five percent of all cases of essential hypertension can be reduced to safe levels simply by doing these things. Excess salt seems to affect about 70 percent of patients with high blood pressure; Blacks and older people are more likely to be "salt sensitive." More than 80 percent of sodium in the North American diet comes from processed foods (cereals, cookies, cheeses, crackers, luncheon meats). Foods high in potassium lower blood pressure by balancing the sodium-potassium ratio; potassium supplements are less effective in balancing the ratio than is dietary potassium. Foods high in potassium include bananas, cantaloupes, tomatoes, oranges, potatoes, and leafy green vegetables.

Fiber intake helps to decrease or prevent high blood pressure. Only fruit and vegetable fiber affect systolic pressure, but fruit, vegetable, and cereal fiber all lower diastolic pressure.

Exercise and Lifestyle

Exercise helps to lower blood lipids, decrease body fat, increase blood levels of high-density lipoprotein, and reverse insulin resistance, but more than 25 percent of North Americans get no regular exercise. To help reduce blood pressure, patients should exercise three to four times a week for 20 to 30 minutes, and aim to reach about 50 percent of their maximum pulse. In some cases, walking or other low-intensity exercises may be more beneficial than jogging or running.

Smoking should be eliminated and alcohol intake reduced.

For those who are overweight, weight loss is the most effective nondrug method of lowering blood pressure.

Stress reduction combined with drug therapy may decrease blood pressure more than drugs by themselves.

Drug Therapy

The major categories of anti-hypertensive medications used to treat high blood pressure are diuretics, ACE inhibitors, beta blockers, and calcium channel blockers. Diuretics decrease blood volume, while beta blockers, calcium channel blockers, and ACE inhibitors affect the hormonal and nervous systems, causing the artery walls to increase in diameter or the heart to pump less forcefully. Drugs usually have a long half-life and duration of action, so that when a patient misses a dose, the blood pressure does not rise right away.

Diuretics are usually the first drugs tried in treatment of hypertension. Diuretics stimulate the kidneys to excrete water, sodium, and a large number of minerals (chiefly potassium and magnesium). Deficiencies in those minerals cause weakness and fatigue, and low potassium levels can cause a disturbance of the heart rhythm (especially for a person taking a form of digitalis). There are potassium-sparing diuretics available, but these still cause a loss of magnesium, an important mineral needed for proper heart rhythm.

If high blood pressure is normalized by diuretics, the risk of stroke is decreased, but not the risk of heart attacks, since diuretics often raise cholesterol levels and lower HDL levels. If you take diuretics in the morning, you tend to have to go to the bathroom frequently during the day; if you take diuretics in the evening, you have to get up every hour or so all night long to go to the bathroom.

Beta blockers are the second most commonly used anti-hypertensive medication. These drugs block the ability of the heart to respond to epinephrine (adrenaline), which raises blood pressure and increases the heart rate. Beta blockers are useful temporarily, but used long term can themselves cause heart failure, since they lessen the activity or force of the heart tissue.

Calcium channel blockers are used to treat hypertension as well as angina. Calcium channel blockers decrease blood pressure by preventing calcium from entering the cells, which lets the arterial wall relax and thus decreases blood pressure. Calcium channel blockers can weaken the heart, and individuals on calcium channel blockers experience more heart attacks than those who are on diuretics or beta blockers. Calcium channel blockers should not be used as first-line anti-hypertensives, because they do not cause a decrease in heart disease and often increase it.

ACE (angiotensin-converting enzyme) inhibitors block the renin-angiotensin portion of the hormone system, which constricts blood vessels and increases pressure in the arteries. A patient will respond to an ACE inhibitor only if renin is a factor in causing the high blood pressure. Because excessive renin is produced when the arteries going to the kidneys are narrowed, if you respond to an ACE inhibitor consider having the renal arteries examined. (If an ACE inhibitor does *not* work, that suggests a salt-dependent type of high blood pressure, for which calcium channel blockers or diuretics work more effectively.) The most dangerous side effect of ACE inhibitors is an acute swelling of the face, tongue, lips, vocal cords, and extremities, but 20 percent of patients on ACE inhibitors develop a dry cough after a few weeks on the medication, which goes away when the drug is stopped.

Alpha-agonists reduce sympathetic output from the brain, affecting the "fight or flight" response. They also decrease peripheral resistance (pressure and tone in vessels), renal vascular resistance, heart rate, and blood pressure. These drugs are used to manage hypertension both alone or in combination with other hypertensive agents such as thiazide-type diuretics. Alpha-agonists should not be given with other CNS-depressant drugs or to patients with coronary insufficiency, conduction disturbances, recent heart attack, cerebrovascular disease, or chronic renal failure. These drugs should not be stopped suddenly.

Anti-hypertensive drugs can have the following side effects:

- *Diuretics:* chlorothiazide, hydrochlorothiazide, chlorthalidone, and furosemide can produce fatigue, depression, headaches, diarrhea, impotence, reduced kidney function, potassium deficiency, muscle cramping, elevated levels of uric acid (which can cause gout), and aggravation of any insulin disorders. In the Multiple Risk Factor Intervention Trial (MRFIT, a large, double-blind, placebo controlled, multicenter study done in the United States in the 1970s), diuretics increased the risk of sudden cardiac death for patients with borderline hypertension.
- *Potassium-sparing diuretics:* amiloride, spironolactone, and triamterene can produce fatigue, headache, high potassium levels, nausea, dizziness, muscle cramps, impotence, depression, fainting, and aggravation of insulin disorders.
- *Beta blockers:* nadolol, propranolol, and metoprolol may produce depression, slow heartbeat, nausea, worsening of peripheral vascular circulation, fatigue, dizziness, heart failure, insomnia, elevated blood triglycerides, sexual dysfunction, triggering of asthma (in people with pre-existing asthmatic conditions), and shortness of breath.
- *Calcium channel blockers:* diltiazem, nifedipine, verapamil, and amlodipine may produce headaches, flushing, dizziness, heart attacks, potassium loss, elevated cholesterol, nausea, cramps, swelling of one or both feet and ankles, rash, constipation, interference with

normal carbohydrate metabolism, and may promote cancer.

- *ACE inhibitors:* captopril, enalapril, and saralasin reduce systematic vascular resistance, and may produce anxiety, headaches, dizziness, faintness, exhaustion, nausea, dry cough, rash (which clears up when drug is stopped), and elevated potassium levels.
- *Alpha-agonists:* guanfacine and clonidine can cause headaches, depression, delirium, hallucinations, dry mouth, heart problems, itching, drowsiness, weakness, impotence, constipation, and fatigue.

Because of the side effects of medication, between 16 and 50 percent of patients newly diagnosed with hypertension will stop their anti-hypertension medication within the first year of treatment. Moreover, in one survey, fewer than half the patients being treated pharmacologically had their hypertension under control. The Multiple Risk Factor Intervention Trial showed that increased drug treatment did lower blood pressure, but did not decrease the death rate. In patients with borderline hypertension (whose diastolic readings were between 90 to 94), the death rate actually increased.

Note: If you are on medications for high blood pressure, never stop them suddenly. Work with your physician to gradually reduce the dosages as you change to natural remedies.

ALTERNATIVE TREATMENT

Diet

Drink 12 eight-ounce glasses of water a day, since dehydration can cause high blood pressure. Drink two to three glasses before exercise, and four to six ounces every 15 minutes during exercise.

If you have severe hypertension (systolic pressure 180 or higher, or diastolic pressure of 110 or higher) try the Quick Start Diet for High Blood Pressure. This diet was designed by Dr. Walter Kempner of Duke University. You eat only rice, fruit, and vegetables. You may use spices, but avoid salty condiments such as soy sauce. Follow the diet for one to six weeks.

Make permanent dietary changes, using the following guidelines:

- Eat more whole, unprocessed foods.
- Add 9 to 10 servings a day of high-potassium foods (fruits and vegetables).
- Eat more fish.
- Decrease the amount of red meat in your diet.
- Use only non-fat or low-fat dairy products.
- Eat magnesium-rich foods (broccoli, low-fat dairy products, fish, and green leafy vegetables).
- Decrease consumption of sugar and refined carbohydrates (sugar increases blood pressure in some people, and causes significant excretion of calcium and magnesium).
- Eliminate caffeine and alcohol.
- Avoid potato chips, catsup, pickles, most canned food, and other highly processed foods.
- Eat 1 to 3 Tbsp. a day of oat fiber, guar gum, apple pectin, psyllium seed, and fennel seed powder (helps in some cases by increasing dietary fiber).

If you have migraine headaches or nasal congestion, consider eliminating food allergens.

Try eating a vegetarian diet, which can help lower blood pressure in some people. If you have hyperinsulinemia, eat a low-carbohydrate diet, with 15 to 40 grams of carbohydrates a day. (See chapter 18, Metabolic Disorders.)

Exercise and Lifestyle

Perform aerobic exercise three to four times a week for 20 to 30 minutes at 50 to 60 percent of your maximum pulse (calculated as 220 minus your age).

Do not smoke and avoid all types of tobacco.

Be sure to rest and get sufficient sleep.

Nutrient Therapy

Take the following multivitamin and mineral supplements. Be certain they contain the amounts of nutrients listed:

- vitamin A – 5,000 IU a day. *Caution:* Do not exceed 8,000 IU a day if you are pregnant or think you might be pregnant (destroys free radicals).
- beta carotene – 15,000 IU a day (reduces cardiovascular problems; destroys free radicals)
- B-complex vitamins – 400 mcg of folic acid, 50 to 75 mg of vitamin B_6, 100 mcg of vitamin B_{12} a day (aid circulatory function and lower blood pressure)
- vitamin C – 2,500 to 5,000 mg a day (improves adrenal function; reduces blood-clotting tendencies; lowers blood pressure)
- vitamin E – 800 to 1,200 IU a day (improves heart function)
- calcium aspartate – 1,000 to 1,500 mg a day (works in people with low renin, but not in people with high renin) (deficiency has been linked to high blood pressure)
- copper – 1 to 2 mg a day (to balance long-term zinc use)
- magnesium aspartate, magnesium arginate, or magnesium taurate – 1,500 to 3,000 mg a day (150 to 300 mg elemental magnesium) (helps control the influx of calcium into cells, just as calcium channel blockers do; protects against blood pressure changes; helps prevent cardiovascular disease)
- potassium aspartate – 300 mg three times a day (needed for electrolyte balance; deficiency related to high blood pressure)
- zinc – 30 mg a day with a meal (to help chelate toxic metals; necessary for healing)
- inositol – 1,500 to 2,000 mg a day (for stress; helps prevent hardening of the arteries)

Take the following amino acids in divided doses:

- L-arginine – 4,000 to 6,000 mg a day (participates in the production of nitric oxide, which relaxes blood vessels and lowers blood pressure)
- L-carnitine – 1,000 mg a day (prevents heart disease)
- L-taurine – 2,000 to 3,000 mg a day (helps high blood pressure and heart disease)

Take the following nutrients:

- essential fatty acids and fish oils – 1,600 mg of borage oil, EPO, or flaxseed oil each day (important for circulation; lowers blood pressure)
- coenzyme Q_{10} – 50 mg three times a day, up to 360 mg total if it is affordable (this takes several months to work) (improves heart function; lowers blood pressure)
- DHEA (dehydroepiandrosterone, an adrenal hormone needed for immune system function) – 25 to 1,000 mg a day, enough to return the DHEA to what it was when you were in your 20s (between 200 and 400 mcg/dl in women and between 500 and 700 mcg/dl for men) (helps reduce heart disease and blood pressure; deficiency leaves body vulnerable to high blood pressure)

Herbal Therapy

Take a botanical supplement.

- garlic and onion – effective in lowering blood pressure by affecting autonomic nervous system
- hawthorn berry tincture – increases blood flow to the heart; lowers blood pressure; works as a diuretic; dilates blood vessels
- mistletoe tincture – regulator of blood pressure. *Caution:* Use only under medical supervision.
- sarpaganda – for nervous types of people

with high blood pressure. *Caution:* Use only under medical supervision.

Homeopathic Remedies

Seek the help of a qualified homeopathic practitioner and consider using one of the following remedies that best describes your symptoms.

- *Cratageus* – worse in a warm room, but better with rest, quiet, and fresh air; weak and exhausted; sometimes suddenly weak, with accelerated, irregular pulse.
- *Lachesis* – worse on waking; restless; pulsations in ears; coma and delirium from stroke.
- *Natrum muriaticum* – craving for salt; patient worries a lot and has suppressed anger; headaches and digestive disturbances.

- *Veratrum album* – exhausted vitality; excessive discharges; an intense, unquenchable thirst; cold perspiration on the forehead.

Other Therapeutic Measures

Use stress reduction and management methods such as biofeedback, meditation, progressive relaxation, touch, deep relaxation, deep breathing, listening to music, and drinking soothing teas such as chamomile, peppermint, and lemon balm.

Learn to take your own blood pressure readings in order to monitor your blood pressure regularly. Correct hypothyroidism if it exists (see p. 252). Have acupuncture treatments or bodywork. Consult a Chinese medicine or an Ayurvedic practitioner. Consult a chiropractor.

CHAPTER 17

Cancer

Cancer is a disease in which healthy cells fail to mature properly. They become unresponsive to normal controls and to the organizing influences of adjacent tissues. Cancer cells therefore multiply uncontrollably and develop their own blood supply, eventually forming a tumor. Cancer invades local tissues and spreads by metastasis to distant parts of the body. Cancer is a systemic disease and is almost always fatal if untreated.

TYPES OF CANCER

There are more than 150 different types of cancer, and every part of the body can be affected by one or more of them. Cancers are classified according to the type of tissue and the type of cell in which they originate, because the cell type determines the appearance of a cancer, its rate of growth, and its degree of malignancy. Cell type is a determining factor when choosing the treatment to be used for a given malignancy.

Cancers are usually placed into one of five basic categories:

- Carcinomas are tumors that originate in tissue covering the surface or lining of an internal organ. Carcinomas are the most common type of cancer, and can affect the breasts, intestines, lungs, prostate, and skin.
- Leukemias originate in the tissues of the bone marrow, spleen, or lymph nodes. These cancers do not form solid tumors, but present as an overproduction of white blood cells.
- Lymphomas are cancers of the lymph glands (the filter system for the body). Lymph glands (or nodes) are located in the armpits, the groin, the neck, and the spleen.
- Myelomas are rare tumors that begin in the plasma cells of the bone marrow.
- Sarcomas are the rarest and most deadly malignant tumors. They originate in connective tissues and muscles and attack bones, cartilage, the lymph system, and muscles.

DEVELOPMENT OF CANCER

Cancer seems to develop in two stages, called initiation and promotion. In most cancers, DNA in the cells is transformed by an initiator (a substance that starts the carcinogenic process), resulting in an oncogene (a gene that can transform a cell into a cancer cell). Initiators include tobacco smoke, pesticides, toxic metals, radiation, and hormones. Some viruses (such as the hepatitis B, Epstein-Barr, and papilloma viruses) can be initiators for cancer.

The oncogene often remains "unexpressed" until an added stimulus known as a promoter (such as stress, illness, or toxins) "turns it on." Cancer then develops: there is an increased production of cancer cells, and decreased removal of them from the body because of weakened immunity or clogged lymphatic drainage.

Any cell in the body can become cancerous, and an estimated 300 cells in your body do so every day. The immune system normally destroys these cells, or causes them to function normally again. However, if the immune system is not functioning properly, cancer may develop. Carcinogens (substances that can lead to cancer) do not so much cause cancer, but rather facilitate the development of cancer by weakening the immune system.

For the immune system to be effective, it has to recognize the difference between "self" and "non-self." Cancer cells are in the middle: they are neither normal "self" cells nor foreign protein, so a poorly functioning immune system is tolerant of them. Furthermore, cancer cells seem to produce chemicals that signal the immune system to shut down some of its crucial functions.

One out of every three people will develop cancer within their lifetime. The most common cancer in men is cancer of the prostate, with lung cancer a close second. The most common cancer in women is breast cancer. Cancer of the colon and rectum is seen frequently in men and women. For both genders, lung cancer causes the greatest number of deaths. Cancer is the second leading cause of death in children, with leukemia and cancers of the lymphatic and nervous system the types most often seen.

Cancer is occurring at younger ages in each succeeding generation, and overall cancer *rates* are increasing in the industrialized countries. Dr. Debra Davis, assistant secretary for the Department of Health and Human Services, notes that cancer incidence in North America is increasing in all age groups, while mortality rates for the most common cancers continue to rise, and five-year survival rates have not changed in 25 years.

In 1971, President Richard Nixon declared a war on cancer. Since then, the chances of an American developing cancer have risen from one in six to nearly one in three.

CAUSES

Cancer is triggered by many factors, including tobacco smoke, environmental radiation, asbestos, benzene, vinyl chloride, aflatoxins (found most commonly in peanuts), genetic diseases, overexposure to sunlight, and the body's production of free radicals. Other factors that contribute to cancer include chlorinated water, fluoridated water, hormone therapies, food additives, mercury toxicity, dental factors, chronic stress, toxic emotions, depressed thyroid action, parasites, cellular oxygen deficiency, intestinal toxicity and digestive impairment, and diet and nutritional deficiencies. It is estimated that 10 percent of cancers are related to exposures to chemicals at work.

The National Academy of Science states that 60 percent of all cancers in women and 40 percent of all cancers in men could be caused by dietary and nutritional factors. Consequently, control of diet and nutrition is the principal way to *prevent* cancer. Animal fat intake is a risk factor for cancer; it is believed that a high-fat diet may function as a promoter. Dr. Samuel Epstein, of the University of Illinois School of Public Health, notes that many cancer-causing pesticides and chemicals accumulate in fatty tissue. Smoked, pickled, salt-cured, and barbecued foods contain known carcinogenic substances, and food additives have been linked to an increase in some cancers.

Smoking is a known cause of cancer; the nicotine in tobacco acts as a promoter. Cigarettes also contain many additives, including over 4,000 known toxic poisons. Smoking causes lung, head and neck, bladder, mouth, cervix, pancreas, and kidney cancers, as well as some leukemias. In addition, second-hand smoke causes lung cancer.

In a 1976 study undertaken in Israel by M. Wasserman and others, many chemicals (including DDT and PCBs) were found to be present in cancerous breast tissue. In 1978, Israel banned many of those chemicals, and over the next 10 years the rate of breast cancer mortality among Israeli women decreased by 30 percent. During this same period of time, breast cancer deaths worldwide rose by 4 percent.

Hormones are also implicated in breast cancers. In two large studies carried out in the United States in 1990, the results showed that women who have taken oral contraceptives for more than four years are almost twice as likely as non-users to develop breast cancer by age 50. Also, women who take estrogen after menopause have a higher rate of breast cancer than those who do not use estrogen replacement therapy.

Indoor air pollution can contain cancer-causing chemicals. Radon, a gas that seeps into homes from the ground, can cause cancer. There is some evidence that chlorine in drinking water can cause cancer. Fluoride added to water causes cancer in laboratory animals.

Electromagnetic fields, generated by transmission lines and electric wiring, have been associated with some cancers. Children living near electric power lines face five times the risk of all forms of cancer compared to children who do not have that exposure. Dr. Marjorie Speers, of the University of Texas Medical Branch in Galveston, found that workers exposed to electromagnetic fields showed a 13-fold increase in brain tumors compared to an unexposed group.

Many studies have linked stress to a person's susceptibility to cancer. Loss of a loved one or loss of hope, especially when combined with the repression of emotions, seems to be an antecedent for cancer in some people, as does loneliness and a lack of close friendships. Dr. David Spiegel of Stanford University found that women with breast cancer who met in a weekly support group lived twice as long, on average, as those who did not.

COMMON CANCERS

Cancer can develop at many sites in the body, and there can be more than one type of cancer

cell at a given location. Because space limitations make it impossible to discuss all types of cancer, the following section is limited to some of the more common types of cancer in North America.

BREAST CANCER

Breast cancer occurs in one in every nine women in North America between the ages of 12 and 85. It is the leading cause of death in women who are between 40 and 55 years of age, and the second leading cause of cancer-related death among all women.

The incidence of breast cancer is increasing, but it is not known if this is a true increase, or simply a reflection of better and earlier diagnosis. Some scientists believe that the increase in the number of women with breast cancer is related to estrogenic environmental pollutants.

The death rate from breast cancer has not changed since 1935, which indicates that chemotherapy, radiation, and surgery have not affected the mortality rate for the disease. Many physicians believe that early diagnosis of breast cancer is the best way to save lives. However, this may prove to be an illusory gain. With earlier detection, breast cancer is diagnosed at a smaller size, and there is a longer period between diagnosis and metastasis of the cancer. If the size at diagnosis today is extrapolated to what the size at later diagnosis was a decade or two ago, however, actual life expectancy has not changed.

Populations with the highest intake of dietary fat have the highest mortality rates from breast cancer. An excess of estrogen relative to progesterone appears to be associated with an increased risk of breast cancer. Asian women, who consume a diet that includes many soy-based products, excrete estrogen at a higher rate than do Western women, and they also have a lower rate of breast cancer.

Italian researchers noted in *Lancet* (347, May 1996) that women who eat a lot of pasta, white bread, and other starchy foods increase their risk of breast cancer by as much as 39 percent, while eating olive oil and other unsaturated fats decreases their risk.

Other risk factors include a family history of breast cancer, early menarche (onset of menstruation), and late first pregnancy (or no pregnancies). A gene that is associated with breast cancer and cancer of the ovaries and uterus has recently been discovered. However, fewer than 5 percent of breast cancers are attributable to this gene.

Some health care practitioners feel that the use of commercial underarm deodorants and the wearing of bras contribute to breast cancer. They believe that deodorants put chemicals that are toxic to some women over the breast's lymphatic drainage system, where they are absorbed and over time trigger cancer in the breast. Many brassieres compress the lymph nodes beside the breast, impairing their ability to remove toxins.

Regular breast self-examination is important in the early detection of breast cancer. Breast self-exams should be performed just after the menstrual period, or at one specific time of the month for postmenopausal women.

Examine your breasts to feel for any lumps or other changes in the breast tissue:

- Lie down with your right hand behind your head and a pillow supporting your right shoulder. This helps to flatten the breast against the chest wall.
- Feel the right breast with the flat part of the fingers of your left hand. Palpate superficially—then deeper. Examine the entire breast, including the area around the armpit. Divide the breast into four imaginary quadrants, and examine each quadrant, one at a time; or examine the breast in circular patterns, working from the nipple to the outside or from the outside to the nipple. Breast tissue is densest in the upper, outer, quadrant.
- When you have finished examining your right

breast, put your left hand behind your head, and examine your left breast with your right hand.
- Finally, examine the breasts while sitting or standing, watching for dimpling, changes in the shape of the breasts and changes in the nipples. And remember that most lumps in the breast are benign (non-cancerous).

Mammography

There is much controversy and confusion regarding mammograms. Mammography can detect tumors six months to three years before they can be felt. Women with breast cancers in the early stage (those typically detected by mammography) have an overall five-year survival rate of over 95 percent.

However, almost half of all breast cancers are discovered by self-exam. Only one-third are detected by mammograms. The accuracy of a mammogram is dependent in part on the skill of the radiologist reading it, and on the age of the woman. The U.S. National Cancer Institute notes that in women ages 40 to 49, mammograms have a 40 percent false negative rate (because breast tissue is denser in younger women, making tumors more difficult to detect). Figures regarding the accuracy of mammograms vary from source to source, some sources stating that mammograms can detect 85 to 90 percent of all breast cancers.

Some sources state that the false positive rate (when the mammogram suggests something is abnormal, but in fact nothing is wrong) is about 10 percent. However, other sources state that 70 to 80 percent of positive mammograms do not show any cancer on a biopsy. False positive results are costly, lead to unnecessary tests, and cause great emotional distress. Women taking estrogen replacement therapy are much more likely to have false positive mammograms.

Mammography does save lives in older women (whose breasts are less dense, so that cancers can be better visualized), as they make early treatment possible for those women. However, each mammogram constitutes a radiation exposure. Women who have mammograms yearly beginning at age 50 (and who can expect to live to age 85, statistically) will therefore be exposed to considerable radiation. Such radiation may stimulate tumor growth in high-risk women—the very ones who are urged to have regular mammograms. As well, mammograms require compression of the breasts, and this can rupture some cancers and spread cancer cells into the surrounding tissue.

The question is still debated: Do the benefits of mammograms outweigh their risks? Drs. Wright and Mueller state in *Lancet,* July 1995, that the reported 30 percent reduction in mortality in women over age 50 attributed to mammograms was not confirmed by repeat research groups. They suggest restriction on the use of mammograms because most positive screenings are false positives; screening leads to unnecessary testing and surgery; a negative screening does not mean that there is no breast cancer; and when the breast cancer is diagnosed by screening, the outcome is unchanged.

A better screening test for breast cancer is the anti-malignin antibody screen test (AMAS—see Diagnosis, below). It detects malignant growth only. If it is positive, then a mammogram or ultrasound can be done to locate the tumor. If two AMAS tests are negative, a mammogram is not necessary. The AMAS returns to normal within three months after a breast cancer and its metastases are removed.

COLORECTAL CANCER

Colorectal cancer, affecting the last 10 inches of the colon and the rectum, is the second most common cancer (after lung cancer) in North America. One out of five cancer deaths in the United States is caused by colorectal cancer. About half of those diagnosed with this cancer will die because it is not diagnosed until it is in the later stages. Researchers think that it takes about 20 years for colorectal cancer to develop.

Overweight men are particularly at risk for this type of cancer. Polyps, inflammatory bowel diseases such as ulcerative colitis or Crohn's disease, and family history are the most common risk factors.

In a multi-year study in the United States, reported in 1994, a diet high in red meat, including beef, lamb, or pork, was linked to colon cancer. A diet high in refined sugar and white flour products and low in fruits and vegetables is also a risk factor. People with low folic acid levels develop colon cancer more frequently, as do people with high sodium levels and low potassium levels. Ninety percent of colon cancer is estimated to be avoidable through dietary changes, as a low-fat, high-fiber diet can dramatically reduce the development of benign polyps that can lead to colon cancer.

Dr. Martin Lipkin, of the Irving Weinstein Laboratory for Gastrointestinal Cancer Prevention at Memorial Sloan-Kettering Cancer Center in New York, reports that preliminary findings link higher levels of calcium intake with a lower incidence of colorectal cancer.

Symptoms of colorectal cancer include rectal bleeding; red blood in the stools or black stools; abdominal cramps, pain, and tenderness in the lower abdomen; a change in bowel habits; persistent diarrhea, changing to persistent constipation for no reason; a change in shape of the stool to a thin ribbon-like appearance; weight loss; loss of appetite; weakness; and paleness.

LUNG CANCER

Lung cancer is the leading cause of cancer deaths for both men and women. The prognosis for people diagnosed with lung cancer is usually very poor and has not improved significantly over the past 25 years.

Cigarette smoking and secondhand smoke

exposure is generally attributed as the cause of 85% of all lung cancers. Children and teens who grow up in a smoking household are more likely to develop lung cancer at some time in their adult lives. Asbestos exposure, exposure to chemical pollutants such as coal tars, radiation exposure, chronic bronchitis, and tuberculosis are all risk factors and are responsible for the other 15% of lung cancer. Many physicians who specialize in treatment with nutrients think that deficiencies of beta carotene, vitamin E, and B vitamins may be related to lung cancer.

Lung cancer presents as a cough or a change in a chronic cough, sometimes producing blood-streaked mucus. Other symptoms include fever, chills, sweating, weakness, loss of appetite, weight loss, chest pain, and enlarged neck lymph nodes. At least 10 percent of patients have no symptoms, and the cancer may show up unexpectedly on a chest X-ray. There are several different types of lung cancer.

PROSTATE AND TESTICULAR CANCER

The third most common site for a tumor in males is the prostate gland. Such growths include prostate cancer, which is one of the cancers most often seen in older men. There may be a link between prostate cancer and BPH, and about 20 percent of enlarged prostates are caused by cancer. The incidence of prostate cancer is increasing explosively. One of every five men in the United States will develop prostate cancer, and more than 40,000 men will die from it this year. This type of cancer is uncommon in men under the age of 40; most men who develop prostate cancer are between 60 and 80 years of age. The highest incidence of prostate cancer is found among African-American males.

Prostate cancer is usually a slow-growing cancer. Fewer than 20 percent of prostate cancers spread beyond the prostate gland. The five-year survival rate is 89 percent for white men and 73 percent for African-American men, and approximately one of every eight men diag-nosed with prostate cancer will die from it. For men, prostate cancer is the second-leading cause of death from cancer, behind lung cancer, which is number one. Most cases of prostate cancer are not directly diagnosed, but are found after surgery for BPH. Prostate cancer itself is usually not symptomatic, because it rarely causes enlargement of the entire gland.

Cancer of the prostate is common among workers in the petrochemical, rubber, and textile industries. Cadmium, found in battery factories, has also been implicated as causing prostate cancer. Men who live in urban areas have a higher incidence of cancer of the prostate than men who live in rural areas.

A study done in the 1980s at Johns Hopkins University and Roswell Park Memorial Institute found that the risk of prostate cancer is four times greater in men who have BPH than among men with normal prostates. Studies done in 1979 by Dr. Peter Hill at the American Health Foundation in New York showed that a high-fat diet causes a higher excretion of hormones that are associated with prostate cancer. In countries where people eat a lot of meat and fat, the incidence of prostate cancer is high. Vasectomy, a history of venereal disease, and recurrent prostate infections are also risk factors.

Testicular cancer occurs mainly in younger men and is responsible for 14 percent of the cancer deaths in males between the ages of 15 and 34. Testicular cancer is the most common solid tumor in males. It is always a diagnostic consideration for a male with chronic scrotal symptoms, particularly if there is an undescended testicle. If a testicular mass is discovered that cannot be separated from the testes, it must be considered malignant until proven otherwise. Most young men do not get adequate information from their physicians regarding testicular cancer, their risk for the cancer, and how to perform testicular self-examination. All men, of all ages, should do regular testicular exams (see p. 359).

SKIN CANCER

Skin cancer is the most common cancer (one in three cancers) and the fastest rising cancer in North America. According to the American Cancer Society, there are over 800,000 new cases each year in the United States, and over 10,000 will die from the disease. The average age of people with skin cancer is dropping, and twice as many women under 40 are developing the disease as men in the same age group. Overall, however, 50 percent more men than women develop skin cancer.

Over 90 percent of skin cancers are caused from overexposure to the sun's ultraviolet (UV) rays. There may be a genetic predisposition to react to ultraviolet rays, but exposure to radium, creosote, and coal tar can also be a factor in skin cancer.

Skin cancer is the most treatable of the cancers, and more than 90 percent of all cases of skin cancer are completely cured if treatment is timely.

Caucasians, particularly those with fair skin, are more at risk for skin cancer, as they have less protective pigment in their skin. People who have received a blistering sunburn at any time during their lives are also at higher risk. The ultraviolet rays of the sun disrupt the genetic material of the skin cells, damaging it as well as the normal repair mechanism of the skin. Without the ability to repair the skin, damaged cells can continue to reproduce, and the skin becomes even more vulnerable to subsequent exposure to UV rays.

There are several different types of skin cancer. The two most common are basal cell carcinoma and squamous cell carcinoma, which are quite curable if treated early. The third major type of skin cancer, malignant melanoma, is a serious disease, and can be fatal because of its ability to metastasize (spread to another part of the body).

Basal cell carcinoma is the most common and the least dangerous of the skin cancers and is more prevalent in blond, fair-skinned men. It is more common after the age of 40, and it does not spread until it has become a long-standing lesion. The first sign of basal cell carcinoma is a small, shiny nodule that develops a central ulcer after several weeks. The center will be raw and moist, and will have a hard border that may bleed. Scabs form over the ulcer, but come off without the ulcer healing. Cell damage results from this ulcer-like growth, which destroys tissue as it slowly spreads. Basal cell carcinoma usually occurs on the face by the nose or ears, but can occur on the back or chest as flat sores that grow slowly.

Squamous cell carcinoma develops as a tumor or lump under the skin, usually resulting from damage to the underlying skin cells. This cancer most often appears on the ears, hands, face, or lower lip. Like basal cell carcinoma, the lesion never heals, and may resemble a wart or a small ulcerated spot. Sometimes it appears to be a psoriasis-looking patch or a red papule on sun-exposed areas of skin; with time it becomes hard. Fair-skinned men over 60 are the group that most commonly develops this type of skin cancer, but the risk is higher for people who have outdoor occupations. Squamous cell carcinoma is generally curable with appropriate treatment, but is more invasive when it appears on skin not normally exposed to the sun.

Malignant melanoma is the least common, but the most dangerous skin cancer. The tumor arises from pigmented cells of the deep skin layers. Half of the cases of melanoma may originate in moles. These moles are irregular in shape and color and may be quite large, as much as half an inch in diameter. Early melanomas may resemble a freckle or mole, and warning signs include itching, tenderness, hardening, or a visible change in the size or color of the mole. If not treated early, melanoma can be fatal, spreading through the bloodstream and lymph nodes to internal organs. However, if treated early, the chances of recovery are good.

MODERN MEDICAL PREVENTION

Modern medicine suggests that people act to prevent cancers by not smoking, by cutting down on alcohol consumption, and by eating less fat and more fiber. Minimal warnings are given against industrial carcinogens and exposure to substances such as asbestos. Safety standards for radiation exposure have also been developed.

Early detection is considered by modern medicine to be part of prevention, but this is not true prevention.

The easiest cancer to prevent may be skin cancer, and modern medicine agrees with alternative practitioners on preventative measures. You should do a full-body self-examination every three months. Examine your whole body under good lighting in a full-length mirror, using a hand mirror for hard-to-see areas. Look for changes in moles, or for other marks on your body. Use the ABCD checklist recommended by the Skin Cancer Foundation in New York:

- **A**symmetry: Moles should be symmetrical in shape.
- **B**order: Edges of moles should be smooth.
- **C**olor: Tan, brown, and dark brown are normal colors, not red, white, black, or blue.
- **D**iameter: Watch any mole larger than ¼ inch in diameter, or one whose diameter is increasing.

Watch for any unusual growths or spots, and report any irregularities or changes to a dermatologist. Regular checkups are important to be certain no problems are developing, particularly after recovery from skin cancer.

Take the following protective measures:

- Wear protective clothing and a hat when out in the sun.
- Avoid tanning salons.
- Wear sunscreen, even on cloudy days.
- Stay out of the sun from 10 A.M. until 2 P.M. when the ultraviolet rays are the strongest.

Avoid medications that make the skin more susceptible to sun damage. These include antibiotics, antidepressants, antihistamines, diuretics, estrogen, sedatives, acne medication such as retinoic acid, and any skin care product containing alphahydroxy acid.

ALTERNATIVE PREVENTION

Because alternative medicine sees cancer as an opportunistic disease that can only develop in unhealthy bodies, approaches to prevention emphasize good nutrition. In general, it is recommended that people eat organically grown fresh fruits, vegetables, and whole grains, with little meat and fat (except for people with hyperinsulinemia). Highly processed food should be avoided, and the use of sugar, caffeine, and alcohol should be minimized or eliminated. Dairy products are also a problem for many people. It is important to drink eight 8-ounce glasses of water daily.

Foods rich in the following nutrients should be eaten daily. (The nutrient content of foods varies according to soil quality and mineral content. If you question the quality of your diet, take vitamin E (400 IU a day), selenium (100 to 200 mcg a day), and beta carotene (25,000 to 50,000 units a day) as supplements.)

- beta carotene (found in carrots, sweet potatoes, spinach, and leafy green vegetables)
- vitamin B$_6$ (in bananas, leafy green vegetables, carrots, apples, organ meats, and sweet potatoes)
- vitamin C (in citrus fruits, cantaloupe, broccoli, green peppers, other fruits and vegetables)
- vitamin E (in dark green vegetables, eggs, wheat germ, liver, and unrefined vegetable oils)
- selenium (in fruits and vegetables)
- folic acid (in beets, cabbage, dark green leafy vegetables, eggs, dairy products, citrus fruits, liver, and fish)

- calcium (in dark green vegetables, most nuts and seeds, milk products, sardines, and salmon)
- iodine (in seafood, sea vegetables, and iodized salt)
- magnesium (in most nuts, fish, green vegetables, whole grains, and brown rice)
- zinc (in whole grains, most seafoods, sunflower seeds, soybeans, and onions)
- omega-3 fatty acids (in salmon, mackerel, sardines, haddock, and cod, evening primrose oil, and flaxseed oil)

These cancer-fighting foods should also be part of the regular diet:

- garlic (contains allium compounds that detoxify potential carcinogens and may stimulate cancer-fighting immune cells)
- tomatoes (contain, among other anti-cancer agents, the antioxidant lycopene, thought to be protective for colon and bladder cancer)
- soybeans (contain genistein, an estrogen lookalike that may reduce estrogen exposure both at receptor sites and by lengthening the menstrual cycle slightly)
- grapes (contain ellagic acid, which blocks the production of enzymes cancer cells need in order to grow)
- oranges, lemons, and limes (contain limonene, which boosts enzymes that stimulate cancer-killing immune cells, and glucarase, which inactivates carcinogens)
- licorice root (contains glycyrrhizin, which may be a defense against cancer)
- green tea (laced with polyphenols, which prevent cancer cells from multiplying)
- hot peppers (contain capsaicin, which prevents the formation of nitrosamines)
- cabbage and other cruciferous vegetables, such as broccoli, cauliflower, kale, brussels sprouts (contain brassinin and sulphoraphane, both of which boost enzymes that defuse carcinogens and flush them out)

Avoid food additives, including:

- butylated hydroxyanisole (BHA) and butylated hydroxytoluene (BHT), which are used to prevent fats, oils, and fat-containing foods from becoming rancid;
- citrus red dye #2, used to color orange skins;
- monosodium glutamate (MSG), used as a flavor enhancer;
- nitrites, used as preservatives in cured meats;
- tertiary butylhydroquinone (TBHQ), used to spray the inside of cereal and cheese packages;
- saccharin, used as an artificial sweetener;
- sulfur dioxide, sodium bisulfite, and sulfites—all used to preserve foods such as dried fruits, shrimp, and frozen potatoes; and
- yellow dye #6, used in candy and carbonated beverages.

In addition to these nutritional precautions, do not smoke, and avoid secondhand smoke.

Reduce stresses in your life. If you are overweight, lose weight and exercise regularly. The rate of several types of cancer, including skin cancer and prostate cancer, is lower in people who exercise regularly. Avoid toxins in both the home and workplace, and reduce exposure to electromagnetic fields.

WARNING SIGNS OF CANCER

There are several early warning signs *indicative* of cancer. They are not *definitive*, but are a signal that a physician should be consulted for an evaluation. These early danger signs include:

- Any lump or thickening, especially in the breasts, testicles, lip, or tongue.
- Any irregular or unexplained bleeding, including blood or any bloody discharge from the nipple; unexplained vaginal bleeding or discharge; or vaginal bleeding after menopause.
- Changes in the breast such as a lump; thick, swollen, or dimpled areas; tender, painful,

distorted nipple; irritated or scaly skin; or discharge from the nipple.

- Persistent change in normal bowel or bladder habits. Blood in urine or stools.
- Any sore that does not heal; oozing, scaly patches of skin; bleeding bumps or lumps; itchy or tender areas, particularly around the lips, mouth, or tongue, or anywhere on the skin.
- Changes in the color or size of a birthmark, mole, or wart.
- Loss of appetite, continual indigestion, or heartburn.
- Persistent sore throat, hoarseness, cough, difficulty swallowing, or a constant feeling of a "lump in the throat."
- Persistent cough, blood in sputum, chest pain, unpleasant sweet taste to food, and repeated pneumonia and bronchitis.
- Fatigue, pale skin, repeated infections, unexplained weight loss, easy bruising, and nosebleeds.
- *Pain is not usually present in early cancer; it appears only in the later stages of the disease.*

DIAGNOSIS

Early, accurate diagnosis of cancer is a key factor in evaluating the patient and determining treatment. It takes years or decades for visible tumors to develop, and it is important to detect the cancer before this stage. Even before a tumor is visible, the cancer is adversely affecting the patient's health. Screening tests that detect cancer early allow immediate treatment and increase the chance of survival.

To be of value, screening tests for cancer must be accurate, offering high sensitivity and high specificity. Sensitivity is the probability that a test will show positive results when cancer is present, and specificity is the probability that a test will show negative results when cancer is not present. Many types of tests can be used to help a physician make a diagnosis of cancer and plan treatment for the patient. A few of the more common tests are listed below.

Several blood tests are used by modern medicine to diagnose cancer:

- The PSA (prostate specific antigen) can detect tumors of the prostate too small to be detected on manual exam, but false positive results are common, occurring in approximately 50% of all PSA test results. In addition, men who have cancer may show a normal or low PSA value. However, this test is still of value when used in conjunction with other methods. (See p. 208 for more information on prostate cancer.)
- The AMAS (anti-malignin antibody screen) detects malignin, the inner protein layer of a cancer cell. AMAS is a reliable screen for all types of cancer (95 percent accuracy on a first test, and 99 percent accuracy when repeated) and it can detect cancer up to 19 months before conventional medical tests can find it. It has been shown to be particularly useful in early detection of breast and prostate cancer. The test is available through Oncolab (see Sources).

The PAP smear was developed 50 years ago by Dr. George N. Papanicolaou. This test examines stained cells from the mucus membrane of the cervix for pre-cancerous changes, allowing early detection of cervical cancer. It is generally reported that this test has resulted in 70 percent fewer deaths from cervical cancer. However, false negatives occur in about 30 percent of all cases.

Several imaging techniques are used to detect and diagnose cancers.

- Mammograms are used to detect breast cancer (see p. 49).
- CT scans can detect cancer of the liver, lymph nodes, kidneys, pancreas, and bile ducts (see p. 50).

- MRI scans can detect cancer of the head and neck (see pp. 51–52).
- X-rays can detect cancer of the lung and GI tract (see p. 48).
- Nuclear scanning can detect cancer of the liver, bone, and lymph nodes (see pp. 52–53).
- Ultrasound can detect cancer of the thyroid, ovary, and uterus (see pp. 53–54).

The hemoccult test detects the early signs of colorectal cancer—blood on the surface of, or mixed in, the feces. A positive result with a hemoccult test should be followed up with more extensive testing.

Endoscopy is a procedure using a flexible tube that is inserted in the colon. With this lighted instrument the lower interior portion of the colon can be examined. Two out of every three cases of colorectal cancer are accessible to detection by this method. (For more information on endoscopy see pp. 48, and for more information on colorectal cancer see p. 207.)

Biopsy is a procedure in which a small amount of tissue is taken from the suspected cancer site, prepared on a slide, and examined under a microscope in the laboratory. The amount and location of tissue taken is critical, and the malignant (cancerous) tissue can be missed. As with all surgical procedures, there is a possibility of bleeding and the body is vulnerable to infection. Accurate results depend on the skill of the people preparing and reading the slides.

TREATMENT

Before agreeing to *any* cancer treatment, you should ask your health care provider the following questions:

- What are the expected benefits of the treatment regimen proposed for my specific type and stage of cancer?
- How well does this type of treatment work against my particular tumor type? What can I realistically expect as the results of the treatment?
- Will this treatment (alone or in combination with other treatments) actually cure my cancer, or will it only cause a remission?
- If remission is the intention of the treatment, how long is the remission likely to last?
- If the treatment is not curative, how long will it prolong my life and what is my quality of life likely to be?
- If the treatment is potentially curative, what percentage of patients undergoing this treatment have been cured?
- What factors influence who survives and who does not after undergoing this treatment?
- How long is my survival likely to be if I do *not* undergo treatment?
- What are the side effects of this treatment?

MODERN MEDICAL TREATMENT

Modern medical theory teaches that cancer will spread throughout the body unless it is caught at its early stages. Therefore, surgery, chemotherapy, and radiation therapy are used to prevent metastasis. Once cancer spreads, neither surgery, radiation therapy, nor chemotherapy can bring about a cure, and we have not yet found (and probably never will find) the "magic bullet"—a medication that will cure cancer.

Over half of the cases diagnosed are considered incurable with modern medical therapies, usually because the disease has spread too far for chemotherapy and radiation therapy to be effective. About 50 percent of people with cancer survive for five years after diagnosis and are considered cured; most of these cures are achieved with surgery. Approximately 10 percent of patients are cured by radiation therapy alone, and 5 percent are cured by radiation therapy combined with chemotherapy. Chemotherapy by itself rarely produces a cure, except in childhood cancers (and a few adult cancers, such as lymphomas).

Any one of these techniques may be used alone, or in combination with one or more of the others. The choice of therapy to be used against a particular cancer is based upon protocols developed for each type of cancer. Protocols are changed and improved as studies provide physicians with additional information. However, none of these techniques change the conditions that allowed the tumor to develop initially.

Modern medical cancer treatment has numerous side effects, many of them uncomfortable and severe. You will have to determine if the benefits you may receive from such treatment will be worth the trauma, pain, and discomfort of the treatment itself and its side effects.

Surgery

If the tumor is well defined or well differentiated, with clear margins, and there is no concern for metastasis, then surgery may be indicated in some cases. Surgery can remove the tumor or reduce the size of tumor mass. However, not all tumors are operable, normal tissue is excised with the malignant tissue, and cancerous cells released during surgery can travel to other parts of the body and begin growing there. Surgery does help to reduce the cancer burden, but it does not eliminate the underlying cause of cancer.

Although there can be side effects from surgery (see chapter 5, Surgery), the damage from surgery is generally less than that from chemotherapy and radiation therapy.

BREAST SURGERY

When breast cancer is diagnosed, a lumpectomy (removal of the tumor and a small amount of surrounding tissue) or mastectomy (removal of part of the breast or the entire breast) is performed to remove the tumor. The status of the breast lymph node drainage is checked and any cancerous nodes found are removed. A staining technique allows the surgeons to know which

nodes are cancerous. If lymph nodes are removed, the arm on the surgical side can swell because of accumulation of lymphatic fluid. Arm exercises, manual lymph drainage, and physical therapy help keep the arm from becoming stiff and assist in healing.

After surgery the tumor is tested to determine whether the cancer is estrogen dependent. If it is estrogen dependent, tamoxifen (Nolvadex) may be prescribed as an alternative to chemotherapy. This drug blocks estrogen from binding with receptors on any developing breast cancer cells, starving the cancerous cells and preventing their growth. However, tamoxifen does have side effects, including hot flashes, nausea, and vomiting in one-fourth of the women taking it. Less common side effects include vaginal bleeding and discharge, skin rash, and menstrual irregularities.

COLORECTAL CANCER SURGERY

Surgery is the primary modern medical treatment for colon cancer, involving the removal of the cancerous tumors or the diseased portion of the colon. When the colon has to be shortened considerably, a colostomy (a procedure in which the remaining colon is attached to an opening in the abdominal wall through which the bowels are evacuated) may be necessary.

LUNG CANCER SURGERY

Lung cancer is difficult to treat surgically. Usually, chemotherapy is given first to shrink the size of the tumor. Then, if the cancer is operable, the diseased lobe of the lung is removed. If both lobes are involved, surgery may not be an option.

PROSTATE AND TESTICULAR SURGERY

If prostate cancer is found and it has not spread, surgery may be performed or, in some cases, the cancer may simply be monitored. If the cancer cells do not look aggressive and the patient is elderly or a high surgical risk, monitoring may be the best choice, with re-evaluation every three to four months.

The surgical method for dealing with prostate cancer is removal of the whole prostate gland, known as a radical prostatectomy. After this surgery, 1 to 2 percent of men will develop complete incontinence, 20 to 30 percent will have stress incontinence, and 90 percent of men over age 50 will be impotent. Nerve-sparing surgery, in which nerves to the penis are spared, is somewhat less damaging, causing a 50 percent rate of impotence. Cryosurgery, which involves freezing the cancer cells with liquid nitrogen, causes a 60 percent rate of impotence.

With testicular cancer, the testes may be removed in a relatively easy surgical procedure. Plastic balls are inserted into the scrotum for cosmetic reasons.

After surgery, both for prostate and for testicular cancer, particularly if the cancer has spread, treatment aims to reduce the amount of testosterone produced by the body. Testosterone causes these cancers to grow more rapidly. Patients can take anti-testosterone drugs or female hormones, but all of these cause temporary impotence.

SKIN SURGERY

Surgery is the most common modern medical treatment for skin cancer. Excisional biopsy, where the growth is removed for analysis, is performed in about 95 percent of cases. If treatment is delayed, radical surgery may be necessary to remove the growth, and skin grafts may be needed afterward.

Cryosurgery is sometimes used to treat skin cancer, particularly for people with bleeding disorders or those who cannot tolerate anesthesia. Liquid nitrogen is used to freeze and kill the cancerous tissue, which later peels off.

With electrosurgery, the cancer is scooped out with a circular blade and a border is burned around the excision with an electric current to kill any remaining cancer cells.

Laser surgery cuts away damaged tissue and seals off surrounding blood vessels as it cuts.

A specialized surgical procedure, called Moh's technique, is used for recurrent cancers, large tumors, or when the extent of the cancer is not known. The surgeon shaves off cancerous tissue one thin layer at a time and examines it under a microscope. This procedure is repeated until healthy tissue is reached, guaranteeing removal of the cancer with minimum removal of healthy tissue.

In cases of superficial basal cell carcinoma, if the treatment site is difficult to reach or when there are multiple lesions, fluorouracil (Efudex) solution and cream may be applied topically. It can cause harm to the fetus if given to pregnant women, and exposure to ultraviolet rays should be minimized during and immediately after treatment to avoid exacerbation of the intensity of the reaction. Side effects include localized reactions such as contact dermatitis, rash, irritation, pain, itching, ulceration, and photosensitivity.

Chemotherapy

Chemotherapy is the intravenous administration of a cytotoxic agent (poisonous to cells), and it is given to control tumor mass. Chemotherapy destroys both normal and cancerous cells, and when given full strength, it can destroy the immune system and increase the risk of eventually dying from cancer.

Chemotherapy is used alone or in conjunction with other therapies. As a follow-up treatment, it is given after breast cancer, lung cancer, and colorectal cancer surgery to destroy metastatic cells. Chemotherapy may also be used to shrink lung and colon tumors prior to surgery to make them more operable.

Chemotherapy reverses only 7 to 15 percent of a few types of cancer. It can be effective for acute leukemia in children, Hodgkin's disease, Burkitt's lymphoma, choriocarcinoma, lymphosarcoma, Wilm's tumor, Ewing's sarcoma, rhabdomyosarcoma, and retinoblastoma. Dr. John Cairns of the Harvard University School of Public Health notes that only 2 to 3 percent of people with cancer gain any benefit from chemotherapy.

Radiation Therapy

If tumors are encroaching on a vital part of the body, radiation may be necessary to shrink the tumor. However, extreme care should be exercised and low-dose radiation should be used, as radiation therapy can cripple and even destroy the immune system. It produces free radicals, which can damage DNA.

Radiation therapy can itself cause cancer, shorten life, intensify suffering, and inhibit the action of the body's curative processes. Radiation therapy causes diarrhea, mouth ulcers, painful sores in the throat, and weight loss. Patients who receive radiation therapy are at increased risk for developing leukemia.

Radiation therapy may be given after breast cancer to destroy cancer cells that have spread. After colorectal cancer surgery and lung cancer surgery, radiation is almost always used as follow-up treatment.

Radiation therapy is a treatment option for prostate cancer. At least 85 percent of men who undergo radiation therapy live for 10 or more years, although cancer returns within 10 years in 75 to 80 percent of patients. The side effects of radiation for prostate cancer include chronic diarrhea, rectal pain, fissures, incontinence, infections, and impotence. Another method of delivering radiation therapy is through an implant procedure, in which radioactive palladium capsules are injected into the prostate. The radiation is delivered directly into the prostate for seven days, shrinking the tumor and allowing the dead tissue to be absorbed by the body. This procedure avoids the side effects of standard radiation and the pain of surgery, and surrounding tissue is not damaged. Both forms of radiation therapy, as well as proton beam therapy (an ex-

perimental form of radiation), cause impotence in 10 to 50 percent of men treated.

Radiation therapy is also used for skin cancer. X-rays or electron beams are trained on the diseased area, killing the cancerous tissue.

(For more information on radiation therapy, see chapter 6, Radiology.)

ALTERNATIVE TREATMENT

Cancer is a complex disease and there is no single therapy, technique, or substance that is curative. Alternative medicine approaches cancer as a systemic illness that can develop only in an unhealthy, weakened body. Treatment is therefore centered on strengthening the immune system. Alternative cancer treatment almost always involves the use of a number of different therapies. The combinations used depend on both the patient and the skill and knowledge of the treating physician. Among the alternative therapies used for cancer are nutrition, botanicals, immune stimulators, metabolic factors, new types of less toxic pharmaceuticals, enzyme therapy, glandular therapy, and physical and energy support therapies. The proper combination of therapy modalities can allow people to survive cancer and live productive, healthy lives.

These nontoxic medicines and other treatments are considered unproven and therefore dangerous by the medical establishment. When patients ask about alternative cancer treatments, many physicians try to dissuade them from using alternative approaches. However, most physicians actually know very little about alternative treatments for cancer or the theory behind them. Although information about alternative approaches to cancer treatment does appear in standard medical journals, most physicians ignore it. Alternative treatments represent a new paradigm for most physicians (see chapter 8, Overview) and they are not yet ready to accept it.

Consequently, your physician will probably discourage you from going this route—but it is *your* life, and *your* decision. As you read about and become more familiar with both modern and alternative cancer treatment, careful consideration will help you choose the therapy with which you feel most comfortable, and which you feel offers you the most hope.

The following is a synopsis of some of the alternative therapies that have been used successfully by alternative physicians. Because of space limitations, all the alternative therapies in use cannot be discussed here. The reader is referred to *An Alternative Medicine Definitive Guide to Cancer*, by Drs. W. John Diamond and W. Lee Cowden, with Burton Goldberg, for a more in-depth discussion of these therapies. See Recommended Reading.

Diet

Alternative medicine regards nutrition as foremost in the treatment of cancer. The prevailing nutritional deficiencies in today's world weaken the body and its immune system, leaving it more vulnerable to the onset of cancer. The functions of the body are profoundly affected by the way nutrients work in concert, and providing the correct nutrients can reverse chronic conditions. Although there have been no definitive studies proving their effectiveness, many physicians have used nutritional therapies successfully against cancer, and patient records demonstrate their efficacy.

The importance of the preventative role of diet is becoming increasingly more obvious in the treatment of cancer. Not only can diet and nutritional supplementation reduce the risks of some forms of cancer, but they can help nurture the body and enable healing as well as prevent the recurrence of cancer. The dietary suggestions made above in Alternative Prevention are also helpful in treating cancer.

A macrobiotic diet has been found to be effective for several types of cancer, including prostate cancer and pancreatic cancer, according to Dr. Sherry Rogers in her book, *Wellness Against All Odds*. The medical survival time for prostate cancer patients with modern medical treatment is six years. Three months or more on a macrobiotic diet can improve median survival to over 19 years.

Nutrient Therapy

The following nutrients are among many that are helpful in treating cancer. Consult an alternative physician to plan the best nutritional treatment program for you.

- vitamin A – 50,000 to 100,000 IU a day. *Caution:* Do not exceed 8,000 IU a day if you are pregnant or might be pregnant (powerful antioxidant that destroys free radicals).
- beta carotene – 100,000 IU a day (needed for cellular repair and rebuilding)
- B-complex – 150 mg a day (necessary for normal cell function and division)
- folic acid – 180 mcg a day total, including amount in B-complex (important for cell division and replication)
- vitamin C – 5,000 to 20,000 mg a day in divided doses (boosts immunity and acts as an anti-cancer agent; important for collagen production and connective tissue growth)
- vitamin E – 1,000 IU a day (powerful antioxidant and cancer fighter; promotes healing and tissue repair)
- calcium – 2,000 mg a day (essential for normal cell division and function)
- copper – 2 to 3 mg a day (to balance zinc)
- magnesium – 1,000 mg a day (essential for normal cell division and function)
- selenium – 200 mcg a day (protects against free radicals and some types of tumors)
- zinc – 75 mg a day (important in cell division, growth, and repair; also important for enzyme activity and immune function)
- *Lactobacillus acidophilus* – three times a day with meals (normalizes colon environment)
- coenzyme Q_{10} – 100 mg a day (improves oxygenation at cellular level)

- evening primrose oil – 1,000 mg a day (improves cellular oxygenation)
- flax oil – 1 Tbsp. three times a day (reverses pre-cancerous changes in the bowel)
- L-carnitine – 500 mg a day (protects against damage from free radicals)
- organic germanium – 200 mg a day (immunostimulant; increases cellular oxygenation)
- proteolytic enzymes – three to six tablets two to three times a day, between meals (reduce inflammation; act as free radical scavengers; aid in breakdown and absorption of nutrients from foods when taken with meals)

Herbal Therapy

Herbs or botanicals can be used to treat cancer because they contain biologically active chemicals. They are effective against cancer through several mechanisms, including stimulating DNA-repair mechanisms, inhibiting cancer-activating enzymes, producing antioxidant effects, increasing protective enzymes, and producing oxygenating effects. This section will discuss only a few of the many herbs used in alternative cancer therapies.

Hoxsey herbs are a cancer treatment developed by the Hoxsey family from Illinois and were first used in veterinary medicine. The original formula is in a potassium iodide solution and contains red clover, buckthorn bark, burdock root, stillingia root, barberry bark, chaparral, licorice root, *Cascara amarga,* and prickly ash bark. It is for both internal and external use; the external formula also contains bloodroot. Lymphoma, melanoma, and skin cancer have responded favorably to the Hoxsey formula. The Bio-Medical Center in Tijuana, Mexico, one of the clinics where Hoxsey therapy is practiced, estimates that 80 percent of their patients who use this formula benefit substantially. A five-year multi-center study at three alternative clinics was reported in the *Journal of Naturopathic Medicine* in 1994. It stated that six of sixteen patients

treated with Hoxsey combinations were alive and disease-free after five years, and two of the patients had cancers normally considered incurable, or terminal. All the other patients from the clinics that did not use Hoxsey herbs had died by the end of the five years.

Grape seeds contain several chemicals, including bioflavonoids such as proanthocyanins and anthocyanins. These compounds are effective scavengers of harmful free radicals, and have been shown in numerous studies to be up to 50 times more effective than vitamin E and 20 times more effective than vitamin C in free-radical neutralizing power. Also called pycnogenols, these compounds help decrease cell mutation, which in turn helps to prevent cancer.

A preparation derived from mistletoe, Iscador, increases the activity of several immune cells, including natural killer (NK) cells. In a 1970 article published in *Elemente Naturowissenschaft,* J. Nienhaus reported that Iscador selectively inhibits the growth of different types of tumor cells. In the early 1990s, a German study followed 36 patients with stage 3 ovarian cancer treated with Iscador. Fifteen experienced a halt in tumor growth, eight had partial remission, three had full remission, and ten experienced progression of their cancer. Patients treated with Iscador have increased survival rates over those treated with other therapies alone, including chemotherapy, radiation, and surgery.

Two reviews of clinical research on Iscador have shown that it increases the length and quality of life, causes tumors to shrink, stabilizes cancer, and improves the general condition of the patient.

Amygdalin is a substance that is concentrated in the pits of apricots and other stone fruits. It is also called laetrile or vitamin B_{17}. Amygdalin has a selective toxicity to cancer cells and a relative non-toxicity to normal cells because of its cyanide content. It has strong cancer-fighting potential, especially for secondary cancers, which develop after chemotherapy and radiation therapy. According to Dr. Ralph Moss in *The Cancer Industry: Unraveling the Politics,* it reduces lung metastases by as much as 60 percent. Animal studies, epidemiologic studies, and clinical studies have all demonstrated the efficacy of amygdalin. It may be given orally or intravenously.

In the late 1920s a Canadian nurse named Rene Caisse developed an herbal tea for the treatment of cancer, which she named Essiac tea. Although it has never undergone clinical trials, thousands of case histories have documented its success in treating several different types of cancer. Dr. Charles Brusch and Dr. Charles McClure, of the Brusch Medical Center in Massachusetts, state that in their patients Essiac tea has reduced pain and caused a recession in the growth of the cancer. Patients have also gained weight and shown an improvement in general health. Dr. Brusch attributes his own recovery from colorectal cancer to Essiac tea alone. Other alternative physicians recommend that Essiac tea be combined with other cancer treatments. They think that it may be less effective than it was earlier in the century because of increased pollution in the environment. A review of the anti-cancer activity of substances isolated from the herbs in Essiac may be found in *Cancer Therapy: The Independent Consumer's Guide* by Dr. Ralph Moss.

Some of the other many botanicals that are useful in treating cancer include:

- astragalus – has a regulatory effect on NK cells
- cat's claw – has antioxidant and anti-tumor properties
- Chinese cucumber seeds and peel – inhibits cancer cells
- chlorella – has neutralizing action against free radicals
- echinacea – increases NK cell activity
- garlic – appears to stop the growth of several cancers
- ginkgo – interferes with platelet activating

factor (PAF), which may act as a tumor-promoting agent
- ginseng *(Panax ginseng)* – has anti-tumor and immune enhancement properties
- green tea – has anti-cancer properties
- licorice – retards growth of certain cancerous tumors
- maitake mushroom – inhibits both formation of cancer and metastasis
- red clover – fights cancerous growths
- reishi mushroom tea – helps with interferon production and has anti-tumor properties

Skin cancers may be helped by topical applications of herbs. Those that are helpful include tea tree oil, hot comfrey compresses, and dry mustard plasters.

Homeopathic Remedies

Although there is a misconception that homeopathy cannot be used to treat or cure cancer, the homeopathic oncology repertory is over 100 years old. Late in the last century and early in this century, several homeopathic physicians, including Dr. A. H. Grimmer, Dr. Stuart Close, and Dr. J. G. Gilchrist, reported cancer cures using homeopathy. Their patients remained cancer-free throughout the rest of their lives. Furthermore, those they were unable to save maintained a better quality of life and had more peaceful deaths.

For homeopathic treatment of cancer, consult a skilled homeopath, as a number of issues must be dealt with in order to treat the patient adequately and accurately.

First, there must be proper clinical diagnosis. It is imperative to know which tissue(s) is affected by the cancer so that the remedy that fits the tissue, as well as the nature of the patient, can be used.

The proper layer must be selected for treatment. The cancer layer must be treated first, and then other problems must be treated in reverse hierarchy. As well, proper potency must be used.

Treatment must be continued after the tumor has disappeared. The body—not the tumor—is the guide, and treatment may be necessary for weeks or months after the tumor is gone.

Furthermore, treatment for the next layer of health problems must begin as soon as possible to prevent a return of the cancer.

All obstacles to cure must be removed. These include drugs, alcohol, tobacco, meat (for some people), and stimulants like spicy food and coffee. All allopathic treatments (surgery, radiation, and chemotherapy) must be antidoted with the proper homeopathic remedy.

Finally, other therapies (including oxygen, hydrogen peroxide, diet, and herbs) are frequently helpful as adjuncts to homeopathy.

Note: Patients using homeopathy for *any* condition should avoid coffee, eucalyptus, camphor, menthol, recreational drugs, and electric blankets while taking a homeopathic remedy. Creams containing steroids, antibiotics, and antifungals should also be avoided, and acupuncture should not be used while receiving homeopathic treatment.

Some of the many remedies that the homeopathic practitioner may use to treat cancer are:

- *Arsenicum album* – great fear of death and cancer; marked weakness, rapid loss of weight; extreme burning pains and cancer pain; marked tendency to ulcerations and destruction of tissues; cancerous ulcers; leukemia in children; cancer of the stomach, intestines, ovaries, uterus, skin.
- *Cadmium sulfuratum* – main cancer remedy for the gastrointestinal tract; weakness and tiredness; cachexia; nausea, vomiting of black blood from cancer of the stomach; vomit looks like coffee grounds; marked increase in irritability; sleeps with eyes open; stops breathing on going to sleep; wakes up suffocating; symptoms worse after sleep; insomnia.

- *Carbo animalis* – malignancy of testes; worse with cold; coldness at night in bed; swollen lymph glands; weakness.
- *Carcinosin* – helps relieve pain of cancer; fear of the unknown, dark, death, and of being alone; thyroid cancer; general remedy for people with cancer or history of cancer.
- *Conium maculatum* – cancer of the breast after bruises or injuries; hardness and inflammation of the breasts and nipples; vertigo; mental faculties and memory are profoundly affected; cancer of the bones, skin, glands, tongue, stomach, pancreas, penis, testicles, uterus, ovaries; ulcers on face; lead remedy for cancer of the lips, cervix, and prostate.
- *Cundurango* – cancer of the skin, lips, esophagus, stomach, intestines, anus; painful cracks at the angles of the mouth; cancers with hardened glands, lymphoma; allays pain of cancer of the stomach with constant burning and vomiting; cancer of the breast with retraction of the nipples and sharp pains.
- *Hydrastis canadensis* – probably leading homeopathic cancer treatment; great assistance in pain relief; disturbance in digestion, worse after meals; stomach cancer with progressive debility; wasting emaciation and hypochlorhydria present before and during cancer; breast cancer; mammary gland tumor that is hard and painful; uterine cancer; cancer of the glands, tongue, colon, and pancreas.
- *Phytolacca* – breast cancer and cancer of the tongue, uterus, penis, and rectum; cancer of any gland; Hodgkin's disease; irritable and nervous; cannot endure pain; pains are burning in the ulcerations of cancer.
- *Thuja:* prostate cancer; enlarged prostate; offensive-smelling semen and genitals; bladder feels paralyzed; must wait for urination; sensation of trickling after urination; urge to urinate sudden and cannot be controlled.

Other Therapeutic Measures

BIOCHEMICAL THERAPIES

Chemotherapy is a common modern medical treatment for cancer. However, the chemotherapeutic agents used are cytotoxic (poisonous to cells) and kill both malignant and normal tissue, and in some cases can increase the risk of dying from cancer. Alternative practitioners suggest that using weakened or diluted doses of chemotherapy agents produces cancer cell–killing effects without causing toxicity to the body. In the discussion that follows, a few of these less toxic substances that can be used in chemotherapy are presented. As in the case of nearly all alternative cancer therapies, their use is combined with other treatment modalities.

Carnivora is an extract of the carnivorous plant, Venus flytrap (Dionaea muscipula). It contains one-third pressed Venus flytrap juice, one-third alcohol, and one-third purified water. One of its active ingredients is plumbagin, which has anti-cancer properties. Carnivora stimulates T-helper cells, which allows the body to wage a vigorous defense. Used for several types of cancer, it is given both intravenously and topically, and has led to a total reversal of skin cancer when applied topically. Dr. Helmut Keller, medical director of the Chronic Disease Control and Treatment Center in Bad Steben, Germany, studied the effects of Carnivora on 210 cancer patients. Sixteen percent experienced remission of their tumors and forty percent had a halt in tumor growth. In the other 44 percent, the cancer continued to grow but the patients experienced improved appetite and vitality.

Developed by Canadian biologist Gaston Naessens, 714X is a compound containing nitrogen-rich camphor and organic salts. It seems to neutralize the cocancerogenic K factor (CKF) that paralyzes the immune system. In a paper presented at a 1991 symposium, Dr. Naessens cited hundreds of human case histories in which melanomas, carcinomas, lymphomas, osteosarcomas, and other types of cancer were effectively treated with 714K. It is injected directly into the lymph nodes of the groin and, although it can cause burning sensations around the injection site, has no harmful side effects.

Ukrain is a combination of an extraction from the celandine weed (Chelidonium majus) and thiophosphoric acid (also called thiotepa), which is one of the original chemotherapy agents. This combination appears to neutralize the toxic effect of the alkaloids in the plant, making Ukrain almost non-toxic. It does not harm healthy tissues and appears to fortify anti-cancer defenses. Dr. Robert Atkins of the Atkins Center for Complementary Medicine in New York considers it a non-toxic tumor destroyer, and the most effective anti-cancer agent he has used to date. He reports that Ukrain targets cancer cells, bolsters immunity, and helps to prolong life. It is injected, usually three times a week, depending on the condition of the patient. Unfortunately, it is a very expensive treatment.

Hydrazine sulfate seems to inhibit the loss of weight caused by cancer as well as to exert indirect anti-tumor effects. In a 1990 article in the Journal of Clinical Oncology, R. T. Chiebowski reported that hydrazine sulfate significantly improved the nutritional status and survival rate of lung cancer patients. Another study, by V. A. Filov published in 1990 in the Russian medical journal Vaprosy Onkologii, reports that of 740 cancer patients treated with hydrazine sulfate, 51 percent had tumor stabilization or regression and 46.6 percent reported symptomatic improvements. Even patients with metastatic bone cancer reported decreased pain.

Hydrazine sulfate blocks a liver enzyme and interferes with glucose metabolism, inhibiting the cancer and allowing normal cells to thrive. It also improves appetite and increases the sense of well-being. However, even though the compound is inexpensive and unpatentable, the FDA has made sales of hydrazine sulfate illegal in the United States, because it is not yet a sanctioned cancer treatment.

Angiogenesis, the development of new blood vessels, is essential for tumor growth. Cartilage from either cows or sharks has been shown to stop this process and prevent tumor development. In 1985, Dr. John Prudden used bovine tracheal cartilage (BTC) to treat cancer patients, all of whom had failed to respond to traditional cancer therapy. Ninety percent of the patients had either a partial or complete response to the therapy, as reported in 1985 in the *Journal of Biological Response Modifiers*. BTC seems to also stimulate the activity of macrophages (cells that "eat" foreign material, including cancer cells), as well as to stimulate the immune system and decrease the size and number of malignant cells. Dr. Prudden has not seen any toxic side effects in the more than 25 years he has used BTC, even with very high doses. Bovine tracheal cartilage is not a cancer cure in itself, as patients must take it daily for the rest of their lives to avoid a possible recurrence of their cancer. BTC is taken orally. The standard dosage is 9,000 mg daily, taken in three doses.

Shark cartilage has the same effects as BTC, and has been found very effective against solid tumors, including ovarian cancer, and pancreatic tumors that are not too advanced. The amount for a therapeutic dose is much higher than BTC and it contains 22 percent more calcium, which may be too high for some people. Shark cartilage is administered either orally as a powder or by retention enema. For people with advanced cancer, the dosage is 500 to 1,000 mg per pound of body weight, taken in divided doses.

In the 1960s Dr. Stanislaw Burzynski of Houston, Texas, discovered antineoplastons, peptide molecules that inhibit cancer cell growth at a genetic level. He found that there are five antineoplastons that work against different cancers, including brain tumors, breast cancer, non-Hodgkins lymphoma, leukemia, and lung, colon, bladder, and liver cancers. Many studies have shown the efficacy of antineoplastons against cancer.

IMMUNE STIMULATION

Some alternative cancer therapies use the principle of vaccination with nontoxic substances to provoke strong immune responses to reverse the cancer process. There are a number of these therapies, all of which utilize different substances to stimulate the immune system. Several examples are presented below.

In the 1920s, the late Dr. William B. Coley used a sterilized mixture of heat-killed bacteria and the toxins they produced as a vaccine. He felt that the bacteria would help mobilize anticancer defenses. He reported 41 percent success in reversing cancer in his patients. In the 1960s, the late Dr. Virginia Livingston, at the Livingston-Wheeler Medical Clinic in San Diego, found a form-changing bacteria, *Progenitor cryptocides*, in high concentration in her cancer patients. She administered autogenous vaccines made from the patient's own bacteria. She also included vitamins and minerals in the vaccine to strengthen the immune system. Drs. Vincent Speckhart and Alva Johns of Virginia have conducted a study using Dr. Livingston's vaccine. Of forty patients, three with advanced cancer had complete remission and four experienced dramatic improvement with shrinkage or disappearance of tumors. Greater success was observed when tumors were localized, as in breast and prostate cancer.

Koch vaccine was developed by Robert Koch in 1883 as a medical response to typhoid and tuberculosis. It is based on the bacillus *Mycobacterium tuberculosis* and is used today as a preventative inoculation. This vaccine enhances the immune system and causes it to target cancer cells.

Another vaccine approach is the immunoaugmentative therapy (IAT) developed by Dr. Lawrence Burton, who in the 1960s was a biologist and cancer researcher at St. Vincent's Hospital in New York and the California Institute of Technology. He found that an imbalance among four blood protein components makes it impossible for the body to defend itself against cancer. When the proper amounts of the necessary blood components are injected into the body, a remission of cancer may be achieved, even in cancers that are normally terminal. Dr. Burton claimed tumor reduction and complete remission in 40 to 60 percent of patients who received IAT.

The primary target of cancer vaccines today is malignant melanoma (a type of skin cancer), and about 10 to 20 percent of patients respond to such vaccines. Research continues on perfecting a cancer vaccine, but few clinical trials have as yet been carried out.

METABOLIC THERAPIES

Because cancer growth depends on imbalanced conditions in the body, correcting the imbalance makes it impossible for cancer cells to live and grow. Introducing sufficient oxygen into the cells of the body suffocates cancer cells, as they grow only in the absence of oxygen. With oxygen therapies, normal cells thrive and cancer cells become depleted and die, or become normal again. The body is revitalized, helping to reverse cancer and prevent a recurrence.

Hydrogen peroxide and ozone therapies are two methods used by alternative physicians to introduce oxygen into cells. Hydrogen peroxide is produced by healthy cells in the body to destroy invaders and to regulate metabolism. Research by several North American investigators over the past 15 years indicates that hydrogen peroxide stimulates natural killer cells, which attack cancer cells throughout the body. Intravenously adminstered hydrogen peroxide is reported to regulate tissue repair and improve immune system and hormonal function. Several researchers have stated that hydrogen peroxide improves results with chemotherapy and radiation therapy.

Ozone is administered intravenously or injected directly into the patient. For intravenous administration, blood is removed from the patient, mixed with ozone, and re-injected into the patient. It may also be mixed with water or olive oil and applied topically, or, as a gas, blown in vaginally or rectally. Ozonated water may be taken orally, rectally, or vaginally. Several physicians, including Drs. Joachim Varro and Horst Kief of Germany and Dr. Jonathan Wright, director of the Tahoma Clinic in Kent, Washington, have successfully used several types of ozone treatment to treat patients with lung, breast, or uterine cancer.

ENZYME THERAPY

Enzymes are the substances that keep the body's metabolism running smoothly by speeding up biochemical reactions and causing transformation of organic substances. Disease, including cancer, can result when enzyme levels are too low, dietary elements are lacking, or when minerals or trace elements are missing. The inability of the body to effectively metabolize protein may promote cancer, as can an increase in free radicals caused by enzyme dysfunction.

Proteolytic enzymes, which digest protein, help treat cancer in several ways. They expose foreign antigens on the surface of cancer cells, allowing them to be destroyed by the immune system. They stimulate T-cells and natural killer cells. They reduce the invasive or metastatic potential of cancer cells and can enter them during their reproductive phase, deactivating them.

Enzymes are given in cancer treatment to increase the metabolic enzymes available at the site of a malignancy and to normalize the enzyme chemistry of the body. Enzymes, including bromelain, papain, pancreatin, trypsin, chymotrypsin, lipase, and amylase, are used, and may be administered as an injection, tablet, or suppositories. Enzymes taken between meals have been shown to reduce tumor mass, but the dose is high, up to 40 capsules a day. Organic pork pancreatic enzymes are recommended by Dr. William Donald Kelley, a dentist who successfully treated his own pancreatic cancer. In his book, *One Answer to Cancer: An Ecological Approach to the Successful Treatment of Malignancy,* he calls his program "metabolic ecology," and states that the entire way of life for the cancer patient must be changed. When using enzyme therapy, patients should also use coffee enemas (sometimes several times a day) to help detoxify metabolic waste products.

GLANDULAR THERAPY

Some alternative physicians make use of purified extracts from the endocrine glands of animals to help restore the overall metabolism of cancer patients. These glandular extracts, as well as organ extracts, are known as protomorphogens. They provide both immediate and long-term benefits when an organ is weakened or when the patient is not producing hormones in the correct amounts. These protomorphogens act by providing raw material, active components, nutritional factors, and support for the patient's body. Most of the materials for the glandular products used for this cancer treatment come from lambs raised in New Zealand. This tissue is preferred because most patients tolerate lamb, the animals are raised on pesticide-free ranges, and sheep produce enzymes more similar to human enzymes than either pigs or cows, the source of most glandular extracts used in other types of treatments.

Although it is not known how glandular therapy works in the treatment of cancer, Dr. Jeffrey Bland of HealthComm in Gig Harbor, Washington, has suggested that the glands contain a protein-like substance that has specific messenger activity, which acts on the target tissues.

Another form of glandular therapy is live cell therapy. Live cells, derived from embryonic calf tissue, are injected. Once in the patient, the injected embryonic tissue cells migrate to the organ of origin, where they support and heal. This therapy is used to bolster the endocrine system. One of the hormones replenished by this therapy is DHEA (dehydroepiandrosterone), an adrenal hormone necessary for the proper function of the immune system. According to L. L. Pashki in a 1993 article published in the *Journal of Cell Biochemistry,* DHEA inhibits the proliferation of cancer cells by blocking an enzyme that stops the synthesis of nucleic acids required for cell division. Live cell therapy is available in Europe and at the American Biologics Hospital in Tijuana, Mexico. The FDA has not approved its use in the United States.

PHYSICAL AND ENERGY SUPPORT

Patients who develop cancer generally have an accumulation of toxins in their bodies. One task of alternative cancer therapies is to rid the body of toxins in order to help it heal. Physicians use a number of different techniques to accomplish detoxification, including massage, water therapy, heat therapy, exercise, lymph and circulation detoxification, colon cleansing, environmental cleanup, removal of toxic metals, and biological dentistry.

Disease states, including cancer, are preceded by a change in energy in the organ or part of the body that is affected. Qigong is a hands-on energy technique that helps with cancer prevention and treatment by improving the oxygen supply, the balance of the autonomic nervous system, and lymphatic function. It includes exercises for moving chi (vital life force) throughout the body to direct vital energy to internal organs. A study in China involved 93 cases of advanced cancer that were treated with Qigong and drugs, and a control group treated with drugs alone. Of the Qigong group, 81 percent experienced an increase in strength, 63 percent had improved appetite, and 33 percent became free from diarrhea. The figures for the control group were 10 percent, 10 percent, and 6 percent.

In electrodermal screening, energy and changes in energy are measured based on acupuncture meridians. It is used by many alternative therapists for detection of disease, therapy selection, and proof that therapy is working.

Transcutaneous Electrical Nerve Stimulator, or TENS, units are helpful in treating cancer pain. Cold laser therapy is used to stimulate natural healing processes and control pain (see Light Therapy in chapter 10, Alternative Therapies). Magnetic field therapy, in which the body's normal healthy magnetic fields are restored, is also used to treat cancer and relieve pain.

EMOTIONAL SUPPORT

The diagnosis of cancer is one of the most devastating a person can receive. After receiving such a diagnosis, many people will despair and begin to fail rapidly.

However, if patients acknowledge the depth of its impact, a diagnosis of cancer can provide an opportunity for personal growth in all areas: physical, emotional, and spiritual. Treatment can take care of the physical needs of a cancer patient, but the patient must personally seek help for the mind and spirit. For spiritual needs, many people turn to the church or a spiritual organization of their choice. For those people, prayer—both by patients for themselves and by other people for them—can bring both spiritual comfort and serenity. Faith and trust in a higher being has sustained many people through serious illnesses and led them to recovery. The fellowship offered by churches and other religious organizations is also very important. The laying-on of hands, both spiritual and literal, is healing. The fellowship and positive interaction offered by special support groups has the same effects and benefits.

Meditation in any of its many forms helps the mind, body, and spirit. Meditation can be done alone or with another person, and helps with stress control, controlling the immune system, and managing pain. As a result, most people who meditate feel less anxious and more in control of their situation. Meditation allows people to heal old traumas, finish "old business," confront death anxieties, forgive, and enhance self-esteem and self-acceptance. Many people develop more sensitivity, a more open heart, greater compassion, and less negative judgment of self and others as a result of meditation.

Breathing exercises also relieve anxiety, stress, and emotional upset. The following exercise, adapted from *Natural Health, Natural Medicine* by Dr. Andrew Weil, can be helpful:

- Sit with your back straight. Place the tip of your tongue against the ridge of tissue behind your upper front teeth. Keep your tongue there for the entire exercise.
- Exhale completely through your mouth, making a noise as you do so. Close your mouth and inhale quietly through your nose to a count of four. Hold your breath for a count of seven, then exhale completely through your mouth to a count of eight, making a noise as you do so.
- You have completed one cycle. Repeat the cycle three more times, taking a total of four breaths. Begin by doing this exercise twice a day. Once you become used to it, you cannot do it too frequently. Always keep the ratio 4:7:8, regardless of the speed with which you do the exercise. This exercise can help you through stressful situations and also help you go to sleep.

Imagery is a technique that involves mind, body, and spirit. It is a powerful tool in battling many diseases, including cancer. Several studies suggest imagery can boost immunity. For example, Dr. Carl Simonton of Los Angeles began using imagery in the 1970s to help cancer patients. He tracked 159 patients, all of whom had been told they had incurable cancer and only about a year to live. It turned out that people who used imagery together with medical care lived twice as long as those who used medical care alone. Forty percent were still living four years later; 22 percent went into full remission, and in 19 percent, the tumors shrank.

There are many ways of attending to the mind (and thus the emotions). Physical touching, hugging, and caring by family and friends comforts and heals; there is no substitute for loving parents, spouses, family, and friends. Even hugs from caring medical professionals is healing. Laugh Therapy, originated by Norman Cousins during his illness, has a healing effect on the body and the immune system. It involves watching funny movies; reading funny books; looking at pretty pictures, sunsets, and sunrises; reading joke books; and watching children at play. In fact, any activity that makes you laugh can be part of Laugh Therapy—indeed, any activity that makes you smile is a part of it, because a smile is the beginning of a laugh!

COMBATING SIDE EFFECTS OF CHEMOTHERAPY

During chemotherapy, free radicals develop as a result of damage to cells, both normal and cancerous. These free radicals cause further damage to the body.

Nutrient Therapy
Use the following nutrients before chemotherapy, and for several months afterward, in lower amounts.

- vitamin A – 25,000 IU a day. *Caution:* Do not use more than 8,000 IU a day if you are pregnant or might be pregnant (protects cell membranes from oxidation).
- beta carotene – 25,000 IU a day (converts to vitamin A; prevents damage to cellular components, especially DNA and cell membranes)

- vitamin B_1 – 50 to 100 mg a day (works with other antioxidants, vitamin C, and cysteine to combat free radicals)
- vitamin C – 1,000 mg three to four times a day (a powerful antioxidant)
- vitamin E – 600 to 800 IU a day (an important antioxidant)
- organic germanium – 150 mg one to three times a day (a free-radical scavenger that also aids in oxygen utilization. Cancer cells are anaerobic, and increasing oxygen in the body helps prevent their growth.)
- selenium – 100 to 200 mcg a day (an antioxidant that protects cell membranes; enhances the action of vitamin E)
- coenzyme Q_{10} – 50 to 200 mg a day (antioxidant that protects cell membranes)
- N-acetyl cysteine – 500 mg twice a day (helps to prevent liver and heart toxicity; prevents bleeding and inflammation of the bladder; may increase survival time of the patient if given before some types of chemotherapy)

Homeopathic Remedies
Consult a homeopath for the best remedy to help reduce the side effects of chemotherapy. The following remedies are but a few of the possibilities. Take two doses just before the chemotherapy, and two doses again after the therapy. Continue for two to four days after the treatment is given.

- *Arsenicum album* – for diarrhea, weakness, and some kinds of nausea and vomiting.
- *Cadmium sulphuratum* – main antidote to effects of chemotherapy; relieves nausea.
- *China* – for anemia after chemotherapy, digestive disturbances, diarrhea.
- *Ipecac, Opium* – relieves nausea.
- *Nux vomica* – for nausea not relieved by vomiting, diarrhea.
- *Phosphorus* – for bruises and bleeding after therapy; relieves vomiting.

COMBATING SIDE EFFECTS OF
RADIATION THERAPY

Nutrient Therapy

When tissue is exposed to radiation, free radicals are produced. Nutrients can prevent damage to tissue caused by free radicals. Nutrient supplements should be taken both before and after the radiation procedures. These nutrients include:

- vitamin A – 5,000 to 25,000 IU a day. *Caution:* Do not take more than 8,000 IU a day if you are pregnant or might be pregnant (aids in repair and growth of all body tissues; protects the cell membranes from oxidation).
- vitamin B_1 – 500 to 1,000 mg a day (minimizes injury from gamma radiation)
- vitamin B_2 – 50 mg a day (facilitates the use of oxygen by the tissues of the skin, nails, and hair)
- vitamin B_5 – 100 mg a day (helps protect against radiation injury and is helpful after radiation treatment. It is necessary to cell metabolism and is heavily used in times of stress.)
- vitamin B_6 – 50 mg a day (required by the body to make thymidine, which helps prevent cells from becoming abnormal)
- vitamin B_{15} – 50 to 150 mg a day (provides extra oxygen to the cells; has antioxidant properties)
- vitamin C – 5,000 to 20,000 mg a day (depleted from the cells during stress and acts as an antistress factor; also a free-radical scavenger that can be taken orally or intravenously)
- vitamin E – 400 to 800 IU a day (free-radical scavenger that improves oxygen transportation; decreases radiation damage to the DNA and chromosomes)
- calcium – 1,000 mg a day (protects against radiation)

- magnesium – 500 to 800 mg a day (protects against radiation)
- organic germanium – 150 mg per dose, one to five times a day (increases oxygen utilization by the body and helps to prevent radiation sickness)
- selenium – 100 to 400 mcg a day. *Caution:* Do not take more than 200 mcg a day for long periods of time. (antioxidant that enhances the action of vitamin E; necessary to the production of glutathione peroxidase, which is also an antioxidant).
- cysteine – 500 mg a day (prevents inflammation of the intestinal lining caused by radiation)
- glutathione – 10 to 90 mg a day in divided doses (given before radiation therapy, helps to protect cells)
- lecithin – 1 Tbsp. three times a day before meals (necessary for cellular protection)
- coenzyme Q_{10} – 60 mg a day (acts as an antioxidant and protects cell membranes)
- grape seed extract (proanthocyanadins) – as directed on label (powerful antioxidant that protects against free radicals)
- N-acetyl cysteine (NAC) – 500 mg once or twice a day (helps prevent side effects from radiation therapy; used as an ointment, NAC can help to prevent hair loss, decrease skin burns, and protect the eyes)
- methionine – 500 mg a day (protects against toxic effects of radiation. It is converted by the body to glutathione.)

Herbal Therapy

Take a botanical supplement to help control the side effects of radiation.

- algin – prevents tissue damage from the absorption of radioactive material
- celery seed – an antioxidant
- echinacea – promotes white blood cell formation; enhances the immune system

- garlic – an immunostimulant and protector
- kelp – contains essential minerals, especially iodine; protects against radiation sickness

Homeopathic Remedies

Homeopathic remedies are helpful in controlling the side effects of radiation. Consult a homeopathic physician for the best remedy to take. A few of the possibilities are listed below.

- *Cadmium iodatum* – helps with the nausea after radiation; antidotes radiation poisoning.
- *Cadmium sulphuratum* – antidotes radiation poisoning; helps people "never well since X-rays."
- *Ipecac* – helps with nausea after radiation.
- *Nux vomica* – helps with nausea after radiation.
- *Phosphorus* – helps people weak, emaciated, anemic, and with vertigo since radiation.
- *X-ray* (homeopathic potentized X-ray) – antidotes radiation sickness; helps X-ray burns, weakness after X-rays, bone damage from X-rays, and people who are worse after X-rays.

CHAPTER 18

Metabolic Disorders

Metabolism means the total of the physical and chemical processes and reactions taking place among the ions, atoms, and molecules of the body. Metabolic disorders are caused by body metabolism that is not working properly. Chemical processes are taking place too slowly or too rapidly, they are not taking place properly, or they are not taking place at all. Although there are many processes that could be considered, the discussion here will be limited to four major metabolic problems that affect many North Americans: obesity, hypoglycemia, diabetes, and thyroid disease.

OBESITY

"Fatty, fatty, two by four, can't get through the kitchen door." How many overweight children have been taunted by the cruel childhood chant, and how many adults still feel its sting when the memories of those old experiences surface?

Obesity is the medical term used for the condition of being overweight—the excessive accumulation of fat in the body, which creates an increase in weight beyond that considered desirable for a certain age, height, and bone structure. There are many ways of defining obesity, but generally speaking, a person who is 20 percent or more above ideal weight is considered to be overweight. By that definition, in 1995, 33 percent of North Americans were overweight.

The Canadian Heart Health Survey states that during the last two decades 35 percent of Canadian men and 27 percent of Canadian women were technically obese.

It is disturbing that in the last two decades obesity in 6- to 11-year-old children has increased by 54 percent, and in 12- to 17-year-olds, it has increased by 38 percent. The children who were overweight in those decades are probably now overweight adults, since 40 percent of children who were obese at seven years, and 70 percent of obese adolescents, become obese adults. In spite of all the "healthy" diet suggestions and foods available today, obesity is a growing (almost epidemic) problem, and it is estimated that $30 to $50 billion is spent yearly on diet clubs, special diet foods, and over-the-counter "treatments" for weight loss.

EMOTIONAL AND PSYCHOLOGICAL IMPACT

Obesity has an impact on both physical and mental health. Obese people are subject to many forms of discrimination, as well as to humiliations. Many companies will not hire overweight people because of the health risks involved and the effect those risks might have on the company's health insurance costs; obese people themselves frequently have difficulty getting life insurance.

Many people equate slenderness with intelligence, and assume that overweight people are not as smart as slim people.

Our society equates beauty and thinness with success. When people date and/or choose a mate, very few choose an obese person. Overweight people are frequently lonely, though some develop a cheerful facade to hide their frustration and disappointment. Although the situation has improved immensely in the last 10 years, obese men and women may still have difficulty finding attractive clothes and shoes that fit, and watchbands that are long enough.

Other humiliations occur when obese people try to fit into a world made for people of normal weight. Chairs may not be sturdy enough to hold them, and chairs with arms may not be wide enough. Airplane seats may be an impossible fit for some obese people, and seat belts in cars and planes may not fasten. Driving may be uncomfortable because there is not enough room behind the steering wheel, and eating at a booth in a restaurant may be out of the question. Bending over to pick up an object from the floor or to tie a shoelace may prove impossible. Many of these situations, of course, are endured only by the extremely overweight; however, similar problems exist for all obese people to some degree.

PHYSICAL IMPACT

In addition to the psychological problems that come from being overweight, people who are obese are at high risk of developing high blood pressure, diabetes, and heart disease. The heart of an obese person is overworked, and shortness of breath develops with even slight physical activity. The death rate from circulatory conditions is 45 percent higher in obese men than in those who are closer to normal weight, and obesity shortens life expectancy by 11 percent in men and 7 percent in women, even if they are as little as 10 percent above average body weight.

As well, cancer of the colon and the rectum in men is related to obesity, and endometrial cancer is strongly linked to obesity in women. Women who carry their excess weight around their middle (rather than on their hips and thighs) have a higher-than-normal risk of developing breast cancer after menopause. In fact, both men and women who gain weight around the waist are at greater risk for *all* obesity-related diseases.

Extra weight puts undue stress on the back, legs, and internal organs, and can cause joint pain, foot and ankle pain, and chronic back pain. There is a link between osteoarthritis of the knees and hands and obesity. Obesity is also a primary nonoccupational risk factor for carpal tunnel syndrome.

CAUSES

Overeating

Most people assume that overweight individuals are fat because they eat too much. Some cases of obesity may indeed be caused by compulsive eating, eating too much food, and consuming too many calories. In some individuals, overeating may be induced by stress, and some people eat for comfort and reward themselves with food.

However, many overweight people do *not* eat constantly. They may eat far less than their slender contemporaries and still gain weight. Most overweight people do not lack self-discipline and are not lazy. Other problems are causing their obesity.

Thyroid Disorders

It has been known for many years that a tendency to be overweight can be a symptom of hypothyroidism, because people with sluggish thyroids do not burn calories as efficiently as they should, and their metabolism is slow. For people with hypothyroidism, supplementation with the proper form of thyroid hormone can help. However, sluggish thyroid function is the cause of obesity in only one out of ten overweight people. (For more information on hypothyroidism, see p. 252)

Genetic Problems

Genetics are usually thought to play a role in obesity, and children of obese parents are often also overweight. Some researchers point out that the children of obese parents are usually exposed to the same external risk factors that cause obesity in their parents. However, the issue of hereditary factors in obesity is becoming better understood. A study published in the 1986 *New England Journal of Medicine* shows that adopted children tend to be obese if their biological family is obese, regardless of the weight tendencies of their adoptive families.

Bad Eating Habits

Eating habits, good or bad, often develop in childhood, and most people are unconscious of them. Bad habits, however, can contribute greatly to obesity. Eating habits that can create problems include seasoning food before you taste it, eating when you really are not hungry, eating everything on your plate regardless of hunger, eating while reading or watching television or a movie, eating frequently at fast food restaurants, finishing a full meal in less than 20 minutes, and drinking sodas as thirst quenchers.

Impaired Thermogenesis

The body has two types of adipose (fat) tissue: white fat tissue (which stores fat) and brown fat tissue (which burns fat to produce energy for the body). Impaired thermogenesis (heat production) can lead to obesity if fat from the diet is not burned up by the brown adipose tissue. This dietary fat is stored in the white adipose tissue, resulting in a weight increase.

Chronic Dieting

Chronic dieting is a way of life for many North Americans. At any given time 40 percent of women and 26 percent of men are trying to lose weight by dieting—as well as with exercise, behavior modification, and drugs. While some people do lose weight on the typical low-calorie diet, they tend to regain the weight (and more) when they go off the diet, because chronic dieting can lower thermogenesis. Many people have been through numerous cycles of weight loss/weight gain—and with each cycle their thermogenesis becomes less efficient.

This loss/gain, loss/gain cycle is known as yo-yo dieting, and must be avoided. The reduction in calories taken in by the yo-yo dieter causes the body to decrease its metabolic rate to conserve energy. According to Dr. Majid Ali, author and president of the Capitol University of Integrative Medicine in Washington, D.C., this slows down the metabolic enzymes and leads to emaciation of muscle cells, bloating of fat cells, accumulation of toxic fat in the tissue, and fatigue. Low-calorie diets also fail because their restricted nutritional intake leaves people feeling weak, jittery, irritable, and headachy. The lack of nutrients decreases the brain's production of neurotransmitters—and it is neurotransmitter levels that determine mood (and affect will-power). Low-calorie diets also encourage the setting of unrealistic diet goals or deadlines. Moreover, the desire to binge when going off the diet reflects one of the body's survival mechanisms: feasting after famine. This type of dieting can actually cause obesity, rather than weight loss.

Insulin Imbalance

Insulin imbalance is a major cause of obesity. When we eat food, the body breaks it down into its basic components (macronutrients): protein, carbohydrates, and fat. These macronutrients are absorbed into the bloodstream, causing a rise in blood sugar. Insulin, a pancreatic hormone, is released in response to the rise in blood sugar and attaches to special receptor sites on the cells, enabling the sugar to enter the cells. The sugar is either burned by the cells for energy or stored for later use (as fat in the fat cells, or as glycogen in the muscles).

Some people have a problem with their insulin metabolism; either they have too few insulin receptor sites, or the sites are insulin-resistant and the insulin cannot attach to them. This causes chronically elevated levels of insulin in the bloodstream. Elevated levels of insulin tend to push the system toward storage of fat and sugar, which leads to the development of excess body fat. Years of dieting and excess carbohydrate consumption increase the malfunction of the insulin receptors. Eventually, the sugar metabolism system simply does not work, no matter how much insulin the pancreas makes. High insulin levels and increasing blood sugar levels damage the pancreas and limit its ability to produce insulin. When this happens, blood sugar increases even more and adult-onset diabetes (type II diabetes) results.

Elevated insulin levels (hyperinsulinemia) also lead to increased feelings of hunger. Our feelings of satiety come from serotonin release by the brain, and serotonin release is triggered by the drop in blood levels of insulin when it attaches to the cells. In people with too few or resistant receptor sites, blood insulin levels do not go down appreciably, and very little serotonin is released. Such individuals are therefore hungry most of the time, and so tend to overeat and become obese. This condition is known as hyperinsulinemia.

Most people who have hyperinsulinemia also crave carbohydrates—they are "carbohydrate addicts." Eating a lot of carbohydrates triggers an increase in the amount of insulin released, and the pancreas of carbohydrate addicts always releases more insulin than is needed—compounding and perpetuating the cycle. Because people with hyperinsulinemia are nearly always overweight and always hungry, it is very difficult for them to lose weight. Many are yo-yo dieters, unable to maintain any weight loss they may achieve.

Hyperinsulinemia is probably a major cause of high blood pressure (hypertension). It elevates blood pressure in several ways. It prompts the kidneys to hold on to salt and fluid; it causes the muscular layer of the artery wall to grow, making the arteries thicker and less pliable; and it increases the levels of the neurotransmitter norepinephrine (a compound similar to adrenaline), which raises the heart rate and constricts the blood vessels.

Hyperinsulinemia also plays a role in heart disease. When insulin levels remain high, the pancreas cannot produce glucagon (the pancreatic hormone that signals the liver to stop production of cholesterol). Insulin thus causes an increase in the liver's production of LDL cholesterol, increases the thickness and rigidity of the artery walls, and increases deposits of cholesterol beneath the artery lining where it hardens, creating plaques. These plaques obstruct blood flow through the arteries, eventually leading to a heart attack. The major disease conditions of Western civilization (obesity, high blood pressure, elevated blood fats, and diabetes) are almost always actually symptoms of a single disorder: hyperinsulinemia and insulin resistance.

While most people with hyperinsulinemia show signs of carbohydrate addiction, some people without this symptom are nevertheless hyperinsulinemic. In all, hyperinsulinemia affects 75 percent of all obese people (as well as some individuals of normal weight). Drs. Rachael and Richard Heller of the Mt. Sinai School of Medicine in New York refer to hyperinsulinemia as Profactor-H, which they define as a continuous excess of insulin that can lead to (or contribute to) heart disease and atherosclerosis, stroke, adult-onset diabetes mellitus, polycystic ovary disease, some types of cancer, and vascular disease. It also leads to many health risk factors, such as undesirable levels of fats in the blood, excess weight, and high blood pressure.

Hyperinsulinemia is a genetic tendency, and acanthosis nigricans (a faint mottling of pigment around the neck, more obvious in darker-skinned individuals but also detectable in very fair individuals) is a physical marker for this problem.

Catabolic Maladaption

Obesity can also be caused by catabolic maladaption, which is a profound disturbance of energy enzymes and defective catabolism (breakdown) of nutrients (such as amino acids, sugars, vitamins, and minerals). Fat-processing enzymes in fat cells malfunction, as do the fat-burning enzymes in muscle cells. The muscle fibers become emaciated from disuse, metabolic efficiency of all tissues is impaired, the internal ecology of the bowel is disturbed, and the individual is constantly tired.

This catabolic maladaption (and the resulting obesity) is caused by injured molecules and cells, sluggish enzymes, sore muscles, swollen fat cells, toxic and oxidized fats, denatured and cross-linked protein, heavy metals, and toxins in food. Dieting makes this condition worse, since the injured molecules and cells need more food for healing, but are starved instead.

Other Causes

Excess weight can be caused by eating foods to which we are allergic, as the body floods itself with fluid in an attempt to dilute toxins. This results in allergic edema, and can cause an overnight weight gain of as much as five pounds. Mold allergy can elicit the same response in allergic individuals, and even more problems can develop in some people as a result of exposure to toxic chemicals. Fat-soluble chemicals are deposited in our fat cells, where they are stored until we undergo detoxification. Some overweight people are carrying a high toxic load because of their increased numbers of fat cells.

Several nutritional deficiencies can also play a role in obesity. Chromium is essential for the control of sugar metabolism, and people with a chromium deficiency will have blood sugar

problems together with their obesity. Zinc is needed for normal taste acuity (as well, it enhances the effectiveness of chromium) and some people with a zinc deficiency overeat because their food seems to have no flavor.

Dr. Gus Prosch, an obesity specialist with Biomed Associates in Birmingham, Alabama, says that there are seven facts about obesity that are true for about 99 percent of all patients. These facts are:

1. Obesity is a lifetime disease.
2. In an obese individual, metabolic processes will always tend to be abnormal.
3. Obese people cannot eat what others eat and stay thin.
4. Anyone can lose weight and stay slim if the causes of obesity are identified and treated.
5. Insulin metabolism is the key to losing weight intelligently.
6. There is no physiological requirement for sugar and processed foods.
7. To lose weight and successfully keep it off, you must address all of the factors that contribute to obesity.

MODERN MEDICAL TREATMENT

Diet

Modern medicine counsels obese people to go on a reduced-calorie diet. Many people are able to lose weight on this type of diet, some more easily than others, but most people regain the weight. Their bodies adjust to the lower calorie intake in two to three weeks by lowering metabolic rate. This allows their bodies to use calories more efficiently, preventing them from losing additional weight unless they exercise or lower calories even further. When these people return to their normal diets, they gain back the weight they have lost.

Exercise and Lifestyle

Exercise is advised to help burn off calories and increase metabolic rate. In addition, exercise helps to preserve lean body tissue. Suggested exercises usually involve large muscle groups and include walking, running, cycling, or swimming.

Drug Therapy

At one time many patients were given thyroid supplementation, which can help speed up a sluggish metabolism caused by an underactive thyroid gland and help with weight loss. However, it is now known that not all obese people have hypothyroidism.

Diet pills may also be prescribed. These medications work by either stimulating the nervous system or suppressing appetite. Amphetamines curb the appetite and stimulate calorie-burning. However, they are potentially dangerous in that they promote insomnia, agitation, and excitability, and they are addictive. Other side effects include elevation of blood pressure, blurred vision, dry mouth, headaches, digestive disturbances, and sexual dysfunction. People taking amphetamines without proper supervision risk physical exhaustion and malnutrition because they do not get enough sleep and may not be eating the proper foods.

Appetite suppressants work by several mechanisms. Some stimulate the release of dopamine, a neurotransmitter that makes a person feel less hungry. Others increase serotonin levels and inhibit its reuptake, making a person feel full more rapidly when eating. These drugs have the same side effects as amphetamines. Some of these drugs, the fenfluramines and phentermines, have additional side effects that are serious and life-threatening. Fenfluramine has been removed from the market because it was associated with heart valve damage and increased pressure in the lungs.

Sibutramine hydrochloride (Meridia) is a new diet drug that inhibits the reuptake of norepinephrine, serotonin, and dopamine. Side effects of Meridia include seizures, formation of gallstones, an increase in heart rate and heart problems, and dilation of pupils. It should not be used with MAO inhibitors (see pp. 409–10).

Surgery

Surgical methods can also be used to help people lose weight. Liposuction is a technique that removes fat from the chin, back of the arms, thighs, abdomen, and the waist—areas that do not respond well to exercise and dieting. It is not a substitute for dieting or exercise, and will not work for someone who is seriously overweight, because no more than four to eight pounds of fat can be removed in one operation. Liposuction is performed under local anesthetic; a cannula (a blunt-tipped hollow instrument) is inserted through a small slit and works like a vacuum cleaner, sucking up fat particles.

The procedure normally takes less than an hour, and there is usually little discomfort—though some people have reported significant pain. The American Society of Plastic and Reconstructive Surgeons reports that over 100,000 liposuctions are performed in the U.S. each year, most often on women. It is performed on people of all ages, but those with healthy, elastic skin will have the best results. Some people are very pleased with their results and try to maintain their new look with diet and exercise programs. Other people report failure, continued pain, lumpy flesh in the surgical area, and misshapen areas of their bodies. There have been rare instances of death during the procedure due to shock.

An iliojejunal bypass is another surgical method that can help people lose weight. In this operation most of the small intestine is bypassed, so that the person will absorb fewer nutrients. This procedure is recommended only for people who are 100 percent or more overweight, because it is a major operation and obese people are poor surgical risks. Such bypass surgery can lead to diarrhea, liver disease, arthritis, and kidney stones. Undernutrition frequently results because of the reduced ability to absorb nutrients. This surgery is rarely done now.

In stomach reduction, the stomach is stapled so that it becomes smaller, and its decreased size limits the amount a person can eat. This kind of surgery is not as complicated as bypass surgery, and has fewer side effects. Although people do lose weight after this procedure, many tend to gain it back in a short time.

ALTERNATIVE TREATMENT

Diet

Drink plenty of fluids and do not overeat when tired or stressed, or out of boredom, loneliness, or frustration. Do not skip meals or fast, making sure to eat your meals and snacks (if allowed) at scheduled times. Eat slowly and chew your food well. Find a buddy so that you have someone to talk to when you are tempted to eat improperly. Stay busy, and drink a glass of water if you are hungry at unscheduled times. Sometimes thirst is mistaken for hunger.

Add fiber to your diet, 20 to 40 grams daily in the form of vegetables, fruit, and grains. (But be careful of fruits and grains if you have hyperinsulinemia; see recommended diets below.) Do not use sugar substitutes, as this increases the appetite, as well as increasing cravings for sugar and salt. Check labels on low-fat products as they often contain added sugar to compensate for the taste lost by removing the fat. Also, avoid foods containing fat substitutes because the fat substitute prevents absorption of fat-soluble nutrients, in addition to causing abdominal cramping and loose stools in many people.

Alternative medicine stresses the need to identify the cause of obesity, and to adjust the diet accordingly. If food allergies or sensitivities are contributing to your weight problem, identify and treat these allergies, in addition to using a rotation diet (see pp. 385–86).

If you are hyperinsulinemic, use one of the following insulin-control diets.

Insulin is one of the major hormones. It controls storage of fat; regulates synthesis of cholesterol in the liver; directs amino acids, fatty acids, and carbohydrates to the tissues; is involved in appetite control; functions as a growth hormone; and affects fluid retention by the kidneys. It affects every cell in the body, but too much insulin causes health problems.

Diet is the best method available to treat chronically elevated insulin levels and insulin resistance. The four diets described below are all designed to control insulin metabolism—treating the root cause of health problems, rather than just treating symptoms. Troglitazone (Rezulin), a recently released medication, also treats elevated insulin levels; however, there have been reports of liver injury associated with its use.

While these methods of hormone control are called "diets," they should really be considered a lifetime eating plan rather than a temporary dietary manipulation. Because of the neurotransmitter shift the diets may cause initially, mood swings may occur, but will stabilize after several days to a week.

Carbohydrate Addict's Diet

Drs. Rachael and Richard Heller, in their book *The Carbohydrate Addict's Diet*, present their diet for the control of hyperinsulinemia (a hormonal problem in which too much insulin is produced for the amount of carbohydrate consumed).

Carbohydrate addicts are caught in a vicious cycle of biological origin, in which eating food (particularly carbohydrates) only makes them hungrier. The Hellers' book contains a quiz for identifying carbohydrate addiction.

The Carbohydrate Addict's Diet involves a change of eating habits in which insulin release is controlled. It is not a quick-weight-loss program, as the suggested weekly weight loss is 1 percent of the dieter's current weight. The diet calls for two "complementary" meals daily—

which are high in fiber, and low in fats and carbohydrates. The third meal is a "reward" meal—which is a balanced meal, and contains carbohydrates. All foods are allowed for this meal and quantities are not limited, but the meal must be completed in one hour. No snacking is allowed between meals.

This meal arrangement is the secret of controlling insulin levels. Insulin is released twice during a meal. The first release is at the beginning of a meal, and the amount released is based on the carbohydrate content of the *previous* meal. The second release is 75 to 90 minutes after the meal has begun, and the amount released is based on the carbohydrate content of the *current* meal. The two complementary meals keep the initial release low, and completing the reward meal within one hour keeps the second release low.

This schedule of eating allows a person to eat desired foods once a day while controlling insulin release, thus preventing the health problems that occur when insulin levels are too high. It also controls hunger and cravings, because the proper amounts of serotonin are released by the brain to produce satiety. Because of the genetic involvement most people with hyperinsulinemia must continue to eat at least a modified version of the diet plan in order to control insulin release and maintain their normal weight.

Protein Power Diet

The book, *Protein Power,* by Drs. Michael and Mary Eades, presents a diet plan in which food is used as a tool to reverse or improve a metabolic insulin imbalance.

This plan is structured to minimize the release of insulin (thus preventing insulin resistance) and to maximize the release of glucagon (a pancreatic hormone that counters the action of insulin) creating the correct balance between these hormones.

The diet plan helps achieve metabolic balance by signaling the kidneys to release excess salt and fluid; the liver to slow down production of cholesterol and triglycerides; the fat cells to release stored fat to be burned as energy; and the walls of the arteries to relax and thus drop blood pressure. This plan also causes the action of glucagon to predominate over that of insulin, which allows the metabolic disturbances created by insulin resistance to improve or disappear. Weight loss is gradual, and other medical problems improve as body weight falls and metabolic changes occur and stabilize.

The protein power diet first determines individual protein requirement for preserving lean body mass, and then uses fish, poultry, red meat, low-fat cheese, eggs, and tofu to fulfill those requirements. In addition to the protein, 30 grams of carbohydrate are eaten throughout the day and 25 grams of fiber are to be eaten daily, as are healthy fats (olive oil, nut oils, avocado, and butter). In addition, the protein power diet calls for a high-quality vitamin supplement plus 90 mg of potassium each day, and eight glasses of water a day. Unless insulin excess has triggered the fat storage metabolism, dietary fat will be burned as fuel to meet energy needs.

After obtaining the weight loss goal, the dieter enters a transition period during which carbohydrates are slowly increased. This is continued until the added carbohydrate is sufficient to produce a weight gain. Carbohydrate intake is then reduced to the level at which the weight was stable, and that regimen is maintained.

Although this diet results in size and weight changes (according to the Eades, six pounds of fat represents one gallon in volume), insulin control is its major goal.

The Zone Diet

In his books (*The Zone* and *Mastering the Zone*) Dr. Barry Sears presents a diet that allows people to achieve hormonal equilibrium as well as permanent (and maximum) fat loss. He calls the diet state that allows hormonal equilibrium "the Zone."

Being in the Zone eliminates hunger between meals and the need to count calories or grams of fat. Lack of carbohydrate cravings, good mental focus and clarity, and good physical energy and performance indicate that a person is in the Zone. Being in the Zone should become a lifetime habit, as it will support excellent health, reduce the likelihood of developing chronic disease, and control hormone levels.

As in all insulin-control diets, protein is all-important. However, people on the Zone diet should never consume more low-fat protein in one sitting than they can fit on the palm of their hand. This amount will vary slightly from person to person, but is approximately 5 ounces.

On the Zone diet, people eat no more than five blocks of any macronutrient (protein, carbohydrate, and fat) per meal, with the protein portion eaten first. Three Zone meals and two Zone snacks are eaten each day, with breakfast taken within one hour of rising. No more than five hours should elapse without eating either a meal or a snack. Water is also important. A total of 64 ounces of water is to be drunk each day, including 8 ounces 30 minutes before each meal.

Vitamin and mineral supplementation is neither forbidden nor encouraged, as Dr. Sears feels ample amounts of these nutrients are obtained from the diet.

The Atkins Diet

The Atkins Diet, developed by Dr. Robert Atkins of New York, is a high-protein/low-carbohydrate weight loss diet described in his book, *Dr. Atkins' New Diet Revolution*. This diet controls insulin, by eliminating sugar and refined carbohydrates (such as white flour). It does permit an unlimited variety of meat, fish, salads, and vegetables. Butter, cream, spices, and herbs to taste are also allowed. This is a high-energy, healthy diet that allows people to recover from illnesses as well as lose weight.

The diet has several phases. The Introduction Diet is a 14-day program in which the dieter is carried past most weight-loss barriers: the body is switched from carbohydrate burning to fat burning, blood sugar is stabilized,

cravings are stopped, and addictive patterns are broken. The Introduction Diet puts the body into a state of ketosis/lipolysis, a condition in which stored body fat is burned for energy. The second phase of the diet is Ongoing Weight Loss, during which the dieter must determine his or her Critical Carbohydrate Level for Losing—the maximum level of carbohydrate consumption that will permit weight loss. Utilizing low-carbohydrate vegetables and nuts is very important during this phase, to ensure that ketosis/lipolysis is not disturbed.

Pre-Maintenance is the third phase of the diet. It prepares people for permanent slimness, and is begun when a person is 5 to 10 pounds from the desired weight. By then, weight loss is slowing down, and the pre-maintenance diet phase slows it even more. "Deviations" are added, for instance the addition of a fruit or a starch dish (wild rice or a baked potato).

Maintenance is the final phase of the diet. If it is carefully followed, it allows people to stay slim for the rest of their lives. They must determine their best carbohydrate level—the level at which they feel best without weight gain. People on maintenance should weigh themselves daily. If they gain five or more pounds over their ideal weight, they must immediately go back to the introduction phase of the diet, and should not resume the maintenance diet until the weight is lost.

Exercise and Lifestyle

Engage in regular exercise (preferably aerobic), after first checking with your physician to be certain you are capable of that level of activity.

Nutrient Therapy

Nutrients are essential for weight loss and management. Those listed below are some of the possibilities. Consult a nutritional specialist for advice on the best nutrients for you to take.

- vitamin A – 10,000 IU a day. *Caution:* Do not exceed 8,000 IU a day if you are pregnant or think you might be pregnant (aids in the proper function of the immune system, which is frequently weak in obese people).

- beta carotene – 15,000 IU a day (the body converts beta carotene into vitamin A, which is frequently depleted in dieting)
- vitamin B_2 – 50 mg three times a day (required to burn calories efficiently)
- vitamin B_3 – 50 mg three times a day. *Caution:* Do not take if you have a liver disorder, high blood pressure, or gout (lessens sugar cravings).
- vitamin B_5 – 100 mg a day (essential for the conversion of fat and sugar into energy, and for adrenal gland function)
- vitamin B_6 – 50 mg three times a day (boosts metabolism)
- vitamin B_{12} – 50 mcg three times a day (needed for proper digestion and absorption of nutrients)
- folic acid – 400 to 800 mcg a day (aids in protein metabolism and sugar and amino acid storage)
- biotin – 300 mcg a day (essential for normal metabolism of fat and protein)
- vitamin C – 3,000 to 6,000 mg a day (necessary for normal glandular function; speeds up metabolism, causing the burning of more calories)
- vitamin E – 600 IU a day (an antioxidant that helps the immune system, which can be weak in obese individuals)

In addition, the following supplements are helpful:

- calcium – 1,500 mg a day (involved in the activation of lipase, the enzyme that breaks down fats)
- chromium – 200 to 600 mcg a day (be certain to take a Glucose Tolerance Factor chromium and not other forms) (reduces sugar cravings and stabilizes carbohydrate metabolism)
- copper – 2 to 3 mg a day (to balance zinc)

- iron – 15 mg a day (frequently deficient when calories are reduced)
- magnesium – 500 to 1,000 mg a day (marginal deficiencies occur when dieting and losing weight and can lead to potentially fatal heart abnormalities)
- potassium – 1,000 mg with each meal. *Caution:* This size dose must be taken under the supervision of a physician (helps with sugar metabolism and water balance).
- zinc – 80 mg a day (frequently deficient when calories are reduced)
- alpha-lipoic acid – 50 to 200 mg a day (controls proper functioning of two key enzymes that convert food into energy; helps control sugar metabolism)
- arginine and ornithine – 500 mg of each (elevate levels of human growth hormone; help to burn fat)
- choline – 1,000 mg a day (helps the body burn fat)
- DHEA (dehydroepiandrosterone) – 15 to 25 mg a day (converts calories to heat rather than fat by inhibiting an enzyme involved in fat production; increases sensitivity of the cells to insulin; the body to thyroid hormone)
- inositol – as directed on label (metabolizes fats; aids in redistribution of body fat)
- lecithin – 1 Tbsp. three times a day before meals (makes fat soluble so that it can be transported in the blood)
- L-carnitine – 500 mg a day (reduces cholesterol and triglycerides; speeds up fat burning; controls blood sugar; works as an appetite suppressor)
- L-phenylalanine (LPA) – to be taken on an empty stomach, as directed on the label (suppresses the appetite)
- pancreatin – 250 to 500 mg between meals (supplements digestive enzyme deficiencies; allows better absorption of foods, which results in decreased food intake)

Herbal Therapy

Try the following herbs to help with obesity. If you are extremely overweight, find an herbalist to help you.

- dandelion root and burdock root – enhance liver function
- ephedra tea and green tea – enhance fat burning. *Caution:* Use only under medical supervision and do not use if you have high blood pressure.
- fennel seed – aids digestion
- HCA (hydroxycitric acid extracted from *Garcinia cambogia*) – inhibits conversion of excess carbohydrates to body fat, decreases appetite, and increases ability to burn calories. *Caution:* Do not take if you have high blood pressure.
- kelp and bladderwrack – help sluggish thyroid function
- plantain – for reducing absorption of fats and giving "full feeling"
- spirulina or chlorella – suppresses appetite, keeps blood sugar at a steady level (Some people do not tolerate these substances well)
- yohimbine – blocks fat receptor sites and causes fat burning. *Caution:* Use only under medical supervision.

Homeopathic Remedies

Take the homeopathic remedy that best describes your symptoms. If you are extremely obese, seek the help of a homeopathic physician.

- *Calcarea carbonicum* – constitutional remedy for reducing fat; craving for indigestible things such as dirt, chalk, coal, pencils; milk disagrees; repugnance to hot food; cravings for eggs, ice creams, salt, and sweets; worse after eating smoked meats, milk.
- *Capsicum* – flabby and obese appearance; craves pepper, stimulants such as coffee, spices, and alcohol; heartburn and indigestion; great thirst before chill; takes cold drinks that bring on chill; great thirst after stool.
- *Ferrum metallicum* – obesity with anemia; face puffy with pitting of flesh, rosy flushed face; regurgitation or nausea and vomiting; worse after or even while eating; worse after midnight; ravenous appetite alternates with loss of appetite; diarrhea, often painless, worse during or after eating; craves sweets, bread, butter; aversion to eggs; either craves or has an aversion to tomatoes.
- *Graphites* – tendency to obesity; particularly in females with delayed menstruation; classical obese, thick-skinned, and slow thinking; desires chicken, beer, bland food; aversion to sweets, salt, meat, fish, soup; gastritis or ulcers with pains better by eating or better from drinking milk; thirsty for cold drinks; sensation of trapped gas; appetite lost with nausea; nibbling at food all the time out of boredom; craving for sweets; thirsty most of the time.
- *Phytolacca* – obesity; refuses food in spite of continuous insistence; violent vomiting with retching, desires death to relieve vomiting every few minutes; cannot swallow anything hot; intense thirst; intense hunger, soon after eating.
- *Thyroidinum* – obesity from hypothyroidism; decided craving for sugar; great hunger; easy fatigue; cold hands and feet; sensitive to cold; desire for sweets and thirst for cold water; aversion to greasy foods; insatiable appetite, always wants something more interesting to eat.

Other Therapeutic Measures

Have your thyroid function checked. If you prove to be hypothyroid, take the appropriate form of thyroid supplementation, using a natural supplement rather than a synthetic preparation. (See the section on hypothyroidism and Wilson's syndrome, pp. 252–54.)

Reduce any catabolic maladaption you may have by undergoing testing and treatment for food allergies. Eat only quality foods, including foods that are high in antioxidants, such as vitamins A, C, and E. Correct any enzyme deficiencies you may have by taking digestive enzymes.

Be certain your bowel is healthy, ruling out a Candida overgrowth and parasites. Undergo detoxification procedures to rid your body of any toxins that may be reducing the efficiency of your cells.

Identify and treat any chemical sensitivities that you may have. Have an NAET treatment for your chemical sensitivities. Undergo detoxification procedures to rid your body of any toxins that may be contributing to your obesity. Do any necessary environmental cleanup or alterations to your home.

Consult an Ayurvedic physician.

Learn biofeedback techniques to help with appetite control and weight loss.

HYPOGLYCEMIA

Hypoglycemia (low blood sugar) is a condition in which the blood sugar (glucose) levels are abnormally depleted. Low blood sugar levels may result from decreased secretion of glucose into the blood, or from excessive removal of glucose from the blood. An excess of insulin, either produced by the pancreas or resulting from an overdose of insulin from an external source, can remove sugar from the blood at an accelerated rate, dropping the blood glucose levels.

Hypoglycemia affects over 20 million North Americans. This condition does not develop overnight, but evolves over the years as the pancreas and adrenal glands are stressed by poor diets high in carbohydrates, sugar, coffee, and soda pops. The use of cigarettes and alcohol also plays a role. Some people seldom have symptoms, and others will have them after every meal—but generally, as the pancreas and adrenal glands become weaker, symptoms of hypoglycemia begin, and become worse and worse. Early morning headaches, a wave of fatigue at mid-morning or mid-afternoon, a craving for sweets, or constant hunger are likely to be the first symptoms of this problem.

TYPES OF HYPOGLYCEMIA

Classical hypoglycemia occurs only in people with insulin-dependent diabetes. Their attacks come from an overdose of their insulin medication. This is the only type of hypoglycemia recognized by the majority of modern medicine physicians, who do not accept hypoglycemia as a carbohydrate metabolism dysfunction, and dismiss the phenomenon and its effect on blood sugar levels. These physicians scoff at the idea of hypoglycemia, believing it is a fad that has been popularized by magazines and renegade physicians.

Crying episodes that occur two to four hours after eating indicate reactive hypoglycemia (low blood sugar levels that occur as a reaction to eating). Symptoms commonly occur between 2 and 3 P.M.

Functional hypoglycemia is precipitated by inadequate diet, although heredity can play a role. Around half of all people over 50 who have hypoglycemia also have reduced thyroid function, as people tend to have more than one metabolic problem.

Emotional stress, too, can trigger hypoglycemia. In particular, flat glucose-tolerance curve hypoglycemia is likely to be caused by emotional stress. People with this type of hypoglycemia demonstrate a characteristic flat curve on the graph of their diagnostic test for hypoglycemia. While this type of low blood sugar is not extreme, it has a devastating effect on the life and function of the affected person. The patient has a "flat" life also, and will complain of constant fatigue, apathy, exhaustion, disinterest, boredom, and lack of motivation.

CAUSES

Coffee and cola drinks may be major contributors to the hypoglycemia epidemic, especially when coffee is combined with sugar. Coffee stimulates the adrenal glands, which in turn stimulate the liver to release more sugar into the blood. The sugar in the coffee also enters the bloodstream very quickly. Cola drinks have an even stronger effect than coffee, because they contain huge amounts of sugar in addition to caffeine, and thus stimulate the release of too much insulin, causing blood sugar to plummet.

Alcoholic beverages operate differently, but have an equally serious effect on blood sugar levels. Alcohol reduces the output of glucose by the liver, which precipitates or exaggerates hypoglycemia.

The nicotine in tobacco causes a rapid rise in the blood sugar of smokers, followed by a rapid drop shortly after the cigarette or cigar is finished. The fall in blood sugar leads to the craving for another "pick-me-up" and contributes to chain smoking. Smoking also causes a vitamin C deficiency, which in turn is linked to disorders in the sugar control mechanism.

Salt is another contributor to hypoglycemia, as excessive intake causes a loss of blood potassium, which leads to a drop in blood sugar. Potassium is necessary to treat sugar metabolism abnormalities, and potassium tablets are sometimes useful for those hypoglycemics who tend to experience blackouts. Craving for salt can be a symptom of adrenal exhaustion, and adrenal inefficiency or malfunction is almost always a causative factor in hypoglycemia. Hypoglycemics should use only moderate amounts of sea salt (table salt contains cornstarch and dextrose).

In alternative medicine, hypoglycemia is considered to result from overproduction of insulin by the pancreas. Normally, about two teaspoons of glucose circulate in the blood. To help keep this level constant, extra glucose is stored in the liver and muscles, ready to be released when blood glucose drops below the normal levels. The average American eats 30 teaspoons of sugar a day (plus refined carbohydrates such as white flour and starches, which the body converts to blood sugar). This flood of glucose causes the pancreas to secrete so much extra insulin that not only the excess sugar, but also the sugar that *should* circulate in the bloodstream, is removed, resulting in hypoglycemia.

Both low and high levels of blood sugar can be caused by foods of all types (including fats, carbohydrates, and proteins), and dust or mold allergies can cause the same blood sugar response. A variety of chemicals, including hydrocarbons of all kinds, pesticides, detergents, food additives, and even tobacco, can trigger abnormal sugar levels in susceptible people. These abnormal sugar levels are caused by allergic reactions to specific substances. Both hypoglycemia and hyperglycemia (high blood sugar levels) can be more than just a carbohydrate metabolism dysfunction.

Nutritional deficiencies aggravate hypoglycemia. Deficiencies of chromium, zinc, B vitamins, vitamin C, vitamin E, magnesium, and potassium have all been linked with hypoglycemia. Vitamin B_5 deficiency is a major contributing factor in both hypoglycemia and adrenal exhaustion, as this vitamin is essential to adrenal gland function.

SYMPTOMS

All the body's organs and muscles use glucose, but the brain's demand for glucose as an energy source is much higher than that of any other organ. While the brains of normal people can tolerate hypoglycemia for brief periods without evidencing symptoms, if blood sugar remains low for long periods of time, the brain is unable to function properly. Such a long-term drop in blood sugar will result in the release of hormones (adrenaline, glucagon, cortisol, and growth hormone) that increase blood sugar levels.

When blood sugar drops significantly, a number of symptoms can occur: cold sweats; dizziness; faintness; headaches; nervousness and anxiety; rapid heart rate; extreme hunger; poor or double vision; sensitivity to noise; irritability; depression; pounding head; irrational behavior; digestive problems; muscle aches; suicidal tendencies; confusion; and difficulties with memory, concentration, and learning. A person with hypoglycemia may also have swelling of the feet, weakness in the legs, and a feeling of tightness in the chest. Onset of symptoms and their degree of severity are related to the length of time since the last meal and the type of foods that were consumed at that meal.

DIAGNOSIS

Hypoglycemia can be difficult to diagnose because the symptoms may mimic those of other health problems. A diagnosis can be particularly difficult when hypoglycemia is present concurrently with other problems. Hypoglycemia is usually diagnosed by using a glucose tolerance test, in preparation for which the patient eats nothing after 10 or 11 P.M. on the day preceding the test. The first blood drawn the next morning gives a fasting blood sugar level. The patient then drinks a glucose solution, after which five more blood samples are taken at hourly intervals.

In a healthy person, the blood sugar level will rise following ingestion of the sugar solution, and then gradually fall back down to normal range. It may drop to slightly below the fasting level briefly, but will then return to the fasting level. In diabetics, the blood sugar level rises much higher than in normal people, and then goes down very slowly, returning to normal levels only after five or six hours. In hypoglycemic people, a normal rise in blood sugar levels is followed by a very rapid drop to *below* the normal fasting range. The more severe the hypoglycemia, the faster the blood sugar levels drop, and the lower the level reached.

Dr. Jonathan Wright (a leading scientist and

physician in the therapeutic use of nutrients at the Tahoma Clinic in Kent, Washington) feels that to achieve an accurate diagnosis of hypoglycemia, it is necessary to test both glucose and insulin levels at the time each blood sample is drawn.

Because most allopathic doctors are trained to recognize only one out of five possible hypoglycemic responses to the glucose tolerance test, the test is frequently read incorrectly. There are no set numbers that constitute hypoglycemia; the most important factor in interpreting the glucose tolerance test is not how low the blood sugar level drops, but how rapid the drop is, how long it remains at the low point, and the speed at which it returns to normal. Furthermore, some physicians will mistakenly interpret a rapid drop in blood sugar that remains within normal limits as a normal test. However, the body does not respond to *absolute* levels of glucose, but to *changes* in glucose levels, and the body responds to the blood sugar drop as hypoglycemia. Many physicians also make the mistake of ordering only a three-hour glucose tolerance test. This may be sufficient to diagnose diabetes, but not to identify hypoglycemia, for which a five-hour test is necessary.

Test results should be correlated with symptoms at the lowest point on the test. The glucose tolerance test itself exerts a considerable stress on the person, and full-blown symptoms of low blood sugar often occur around the fourth hour of the test. Both physicians and patients should be aware that taking steroids, salicylates, diuretics, oral contraceptives, and diphenylhydantoin (an anti-epileptic drug) can cause severe repercussions for people during a glucose tolerance test.

MODERN MEDICAL TREATMENT

Except for the classical hypoglycemia that results when diabetics take too much insulin, modern medicine does not recognize or treat this condition.

Diet

Regular meals and snacks are required and the carbohydrate content of meals is kept constant.

Exercise and Lifestyle

Exercise early in the day is recommended. Aerobic exercise that gets the heart rate up to 120 to 140 beats per minute helps oxygenate the body.

Drug Therapy

Blood sugar levels are tested frequently and insulin doses adjusted accordingly. Patients are urged to carry emergency foods and simple sugars to take in case of a sudden drop in blood sugar levels, and an injection of glucagon is given if the patient becomes unconscious.

ALTERNATIVE TREATMENT

Diet

Use the following dietary guidelines for treating hypoglycemia. Avoid all alcohol; sugar; refined, canned, and processed foods; saturated fats; soft drinks and cola drinks; and white flour. Avoid exceptionally sweet fruits such as grapes, pineapple, and prunes. Do not drink coffee or caffeinated beverages, particularly in the morning. Avoid fatty foods, including bacon, fried foods, cold cuts, ham, sausage, red meat, and high-fat dairy products. Do not use products that contain preservatives and artificial colors and flavors.

Eat starchy foods such as brown rice and potatoes in moderation. Eat foods high in fiber and include vegetable protein at each meal. Add fresh fruits and vegetables, seafoods, sea vegetables, soy foods, brown rice, and whole grains to your diet. Include cultured foods such as kefir and yogurt to help balance the bacteria in the intestines. Eat whole fruits instead of juices or sauces. The fiber in the whole fruits will slow the hypoglycemic response.

Use moderate amounts of sea salt, and eat fiber combined with protein for a low blood sugar reaction. Follow a rotation diet if you have food allergies, as they can exacerbate hypoglycemic symptoms. If you have hyperinsulinemia, follow one of the insulin-control diets. Never go without eating for long periods of time. Eat six to eight small meals throughout the day, as well as a snack at bedtime to keep blood sugar levels up. Large meals, particularly at bedtime, can disturb blood sugar levels.

Exercise and Lifestyle

Exercise every day to eliminate unmetabolized acid wastes and to reduce stress. Never eat when you are under stress.

Be certain that any medications you may be taking, such as oral contraceptives, will not cause glucose intolerance and poor sugar metabolism. Avoid smoking and tobacco use in any form.

Because low oxygen levels contribute to hypoglycemia, try to breathe pure, unpolluted air. Get adequate amounts of sun, as well as rest and relaxation.

Nutrient Therapy

Add the following nutrients to your diet:

- vitamin B-complex – 50 to 100 mg a day and up (important in carbohydrate and protein metabolism)
- extra vitamin B_1 and vitamin B_3 – 100 mg of each a day (aids proper digestion)
- extra vitamin B_5 – 1,000 mg a day in divided doses (important in adrenal gland function and in converting glucose to energy)
- extra vitamin B_{12} – 300 mcg twice a day on an empty stomach (prevents nutrient deficiency that contributes to hypoglycemia. A new form of vitamin B_{12} can be administered as a nasal spray for better absorption.)
- vitamin C – 3,000 to 8,000 mg a day in divided doses (for adrenal insufficiency, which is common in hypoglycemics)
- vitamin E – 400 IU and up a day (improves energy and circulation)

- calcium – 1,500 mg a day in divided doses (works with magnesium)
- chromium picolinate – 300 to 600 mcg a day (vital in glucose metabolism)
- copper – 1 to 2 mg a day (to balance zinc)
- magnesium – 750 mg a day in divided doses (important in carbohydrate metabolism)
- zinc – 50 mg a day (needed for proper release of insulin)
- L-carnitine, L-cysteine, and L-glutathione – as directed on label (convert stored fat into energy; block the action of insulin in lowering blood sugar; reduce craving for sugar)
- pancreatin – with meals, as directed on the label (for high protein digestion)
- proteolytic enzymes – after meals, as directed on label (for high protein digestion). *Caution:* Do not give to a child.

Herbal Therapy

Take the following herbs. If you do not obtain relief of your symptoms, consult an herbalist.

- bilberry and wild yam – aid in controlling insulin levels
- dandelion root – supports the pancreas and liver; an excellent source of calcium
- goldenseal – normalizes blood sugar levels
- licorice – nourishes the adrenal glands. *Caution:* Do not use on a daily basis for more than a week.
- milk thistle – rejuvenates the liver

Homeopathic Remedies

Consult a homeopathic practitioner to determine which remedy best fits your symptoms.

- *Iodium* – emaciation despite a voracious, insatiable appetite; worse from fasting and better from eating; great thirst; nervous agitation; amelioration by moving or exerting; anxious or worried if not eating; drinking cold milk relieves constipation; headache from fasting; trembling of limbs and whole body.

- *Kali carbonicum* – fear impending disease; anxiety and worry; desires sweets, acids; gastritis, stomach pains from cold drinks while overheated; difficulty swallowing; milk and warm food disagree; disgust for food; when hungry feels anxious, nauseated, nervous, tingling, palpitations; wants to eat frequently but the least amount of food oppresses.
- *Lycopodium* – worse from missing a meal or from fasting; craves sweets, alcohol, warm drinks; aversion to oysters, cold drinks, food; disordered by oysters, onions, cabbage; loud rumbling in the abdomen; bloated and distended abdomen, ameliorated by burps and gas; worse eating even small amounts of food; huge appetite, ravenous, appetite increases while eating; wakes at night to eat; stomach pains better by rubbing the abdomen; heartburn, sour burps.
- *Phosphorus* – worse from fasting; amelioration from eating and cold drinks; worse from spicy foods, warm foods, and salt; ravenous appetite, gets up at night to eat; appetite increased with headache; craves chocolate, ice cream or cold foods, salty and spicy foods, rice, milk, fish, fat, hamburger, chicken, cheese; craves alcoholic drinks, especially wine, carbonated drinks; aversion to sweets, warm foods, eggs, oysters, meat (except hamburger), fruit, tea; indigestion, burping, regurgitation.
- *Silicea* – craves sweets, eggs, rarely milk; aversion to fat, meat, salt, milk, warm food; cramps and diarrhea from milk; infants unable to tolerate mother's milk and will frequently vomit it; intolerance of alcoholic stimulants; pain in head better eating; migraines.
- *Sulphur* – anxiety; craves sweets, chocolate, ice cream, fats, spicy foods, alcohol, especially beer or whisky, meat, pungent things, apples; craves sweets and chocolate before menses; aversion to eggs, especially soft egg yolk, fish, sour foods, olives, squash, liver, rarely sweets; big appetite, loves eating; great

thirst for ice-cold drinks; heartburn from dietary indiscretions; indigestion during menses; headache or tired unless eating often.

Many patients respond to complex homeopathic remedies. You may want to try PHP Hypoglycemia Drops for temporary relief of symptoms (see Sources).

Other Therapeutic Measures
Have reflexology treatments, which are beneficial for the pancreas, all glands, and the liver. Practice Qigong daily to balance energy.

Have food, inhalant, and chemical allergies or sensitivities tested and treated by an alternative physician.

Biofeedback training can be effective in dealing with hypoglycemia by helping to relieve stress and promote relaxation. In biofeedback training, a monitor helps patients gain control over body functions such as blood pressure, circulation, digestion, heart rate, and perspiration. This allows the patient to become aware of problem areas and to learn voluntary control of physiological responses. Once the control is learned, the monitor is no longer necessary.

DIABETES

According to the American Diabetic Association, 15.7 million people in the United States have diabetes. This represents 5.9 percent of the population. Of these people, 5.4 million are unaware that they have it. In Canada, the Canadian Diabetes Association estimates that 2.5 million people have diabetes, including 1 million who do not realize they have it. Diabetes is the seventh leading cause of death in the United States and was responsible for 300,000 to 350,000 deaths each year during the early 1990s. Half of those suffering from coronary artery disease and three-quarters of stroke victims developed their circulatory problems prematurely because of diabetes. A person with diabetes is at risk for eye disease and blindness, kidney failure, nerve damage, infections of the skin, foot ulcers, high blood pressure, and heart damage.

Diabetes is a metabolic disease in which carbohydrate metabolism is reduced and disordered because of abnormal insulin function. Insulin is a hormone that is secreted by the pancreas, and it regulates the blood sugar, glucose. It keeps the level of blood sugar normal by allowing glucose molecules to pass through cell membranes into the cells and lowering the concentration of glucose in the blood. All organs, including the brain, depend on glucose for energy. If glucose levels are low, hypoglycemia results; if glucose levels are high, the result is hyperglycemia, or diabetes (see earlier in this chapter for more information).

TYPE I DIABETES

In Type I diabetes, the cells of the pancreas are unable to produce insulin, causing the hormone to be absent or low. The body is unable to utilize its glucose to produce energy, and excretes excess glucose in the urine. As a result, these diabetic patients must take insulin, sometimes several times a day. The majority of children who have diabetes have Type I diabetes.

Symptoms of Type I diabetes include excessive thirst, hunger, urination, and dehydration. Many patients also have weight loss.

TYPE II DIABETES

Type II diabetes accounts for 85 percent of diabetes cases and usually occurs in middle age. However, some cases are now being diagnosed in adolescents. In Type II diabetes, the pancreas is able to produce insulin, but the cells of the body are resistant to it. Glucose cannot pass through cell membranes into the cells. Symptoms of Type II diabetes are the same as those for Type I diabetes, but there is no weight loss.

Poor diet, obesity, food allergies, viral infections, genetics, and stress contribute to or aggravate Type II diabetes. A major factor is a poor diet, composed of high-calorie, low-fiber, high-sugar and carbohydrate, and nutrient-deficient food. Food sensitivity causes inflammation and contributes to autoimmune damage to the insulin-producing cells. Stress increases adrenalin levels, which also increases blood sugar and interferes with the control of diabetes. Type II diabetes runs in families, and is more common in American Indians and Hispanic populations.

Many patients with Type II diabetes are able to control their disorder with a non-insulin oral medication, diet, exercise, and weight control. However, they may need to take insulin if their diabetes is not well controlled.

GESTATIONAL DIABETES

A third type of diabetes, gestational diabetes, occurs in pregnant women and is a temporary condition. Symptoms include excessive hunger, thirst, and the need to urinate. It is a mild condition, but must be treated to prevent damage to the fetus.

Most women can control this type of diabetes with diet and exercise, but some may require insulin. Women who have gestational diabetes are more likely to develop Type II diabetes as they get older.

WARNING SIGNS

Regardless of the type of diabetes, there are two major concerns: control of the blood glucose levels and prevention of the complications of diabetes. Everyone should be aware of the warning signs of diabetes and immediately seek professional help should they occur:

- any change in vision
- slow healing of cuts and bruises
- thirst accompanied by frequent urination
- obesity (more than 20 percent over ideal weight)
- anxiety, sweating, and hunger three to four hours after a large meal
- easy tiring, weakness, irritability, and nausea
- dry, itching skin and frequent skin infections
- vaginal irritation, vaginal yeast infections

- tingling of the hands, feet, and legs
- unexplained weight loss
- frequent bladder, gum, and yeast infections

MODERN MEDICAL TREATMENT

Diet
Proper diet, with regular spacing of meals, is an important factor in treating Type I diabetics. Even though they are permanently insulin dependent, the amount of insulin required can be reduced with diet. The risk of complications is also reduced when diabetes is controlled.

A healthy diet and weight reduction are essential for control of Type II diabetes.

Exercise and Lifestyle
Moderate exercise is an important factor in controlling Type I diabetes and can help reduce the amount of insulin needed.

For Type II diabetics, exercise is essential for control of weight and sugar metabolism.

Drug Therapy
Modern medicine treats Type I diabetes with daily insulin injections. At one time insulin was prepared from pork, beef, and pork-beef combinations, in intermediate-acting, long-acting, and rapid-acting forms. Recently human insulin made from a recombinant DNA technique has come on the market. Humulin, Humalog, and Novolin are DNA-recombinant insulin preparations. Velosulin is a pork insulin preparation that has been enzymatically converted to human configuration. Side effects from these injectable insulins include local allergic reactions that cause redness, swelling, and itching at the injection site. Systemic allergic reactions are characterized by rash, shortness of breath, wheezing, low blood pressure, fast pulse, and sweating. These reactions may progress to severe, life-threatening symptoms.

Insulin dose requirements change and have to be monitored frequently. Illness, pregnancy, puberty, interactions with other medications, exercise, and travel, particularly across time zones, can necessitate a change in insulin dose. Insulin reactions, or severe hypoglycemia, result from taking too much insulin; missing or delaying a meal; exercising or working more than usual; an infection or illness, especially with diarrhea; diseases of the adrenal, pituitary, or thyroid gland; interaction with other drugs; and alcohol consumption.

There are several oral diabetic preparations that lower blood sugar. One type are sulfa drugs that have been altered so they no longer have antibacterial properties. They stimulate the release of insulin from the pancreas. Even after there is a decline of the insulin secretory response to the drug, blood sugar remains lowered. These preparations include glimepiride (Amaryl), chlorpropamide (Diabinese), glipizide (Glucotrol), and glyburide (DiaBeta Tab, Glynase Pres Tab, Micronase). They are ineffective against Type I diabetes, but can be taken orally for Type II diabetes. However, because the major problem in Type II diabetics is insulin resistance and hyperinsulinemia, they can aggravate the course of diabetes for some people. Side effects from these drugs include gastrointestinal disturbances, severe itching, allergic skin reactions, increased cardiovascular mortality, hypoglycemia, liver function abnormalities, and blurred vision.

Two other drugs are helpful for noninsulin-dependent diabetics. Acarbose (Precose) delays digestion of carbohydrates so that there is a smaller rise in glucose following meals. It does not enhance insulin production. Side effects include gastrointestinal symptoms such as pain, diarrhea, and flatulence. Metformin hydrochloride (Glucophage) decreases liver production of glucose and intestinal absorption of glucose, and improves insulin sensitivity. Diarrhea, nausea, vomiting, abdominal bloating, flatulence, rashes, and anorexia are side effects of Glucophage. Neither of these drugs causes hypoglycemia.

Diabetes, particularly Type I diabetes, must be carefully monitored by regularly determining blood sugar levels. Problems with diabetes treatment arise when insulin levels are too high, resulting in hypoglycemia, or when blood sugar levels are too high, resulting in hyperglycemia. Both conditions require an emergency response. When insulin levels are too high, caused by taking too much insulin, modern medicine advises eating sugar, which will cause insulin levels to fall. Some physicians advise carrying glucagon as a prescription injection, to block insulin and pump glucose into the bloodstream. If blood sugar is not restored to normal levels, coma can result.

When blood sugar is too high, modern medical treatment is an immediate injection of insulin. If blood sugar levels are not lowered, diabetic ketoacidosis results, causing mental confusion, nausea and vomiting, and severe thirst.

ALTERNATIVE TREATMENT

Diet

Because Type I diabetics are insulin dependent, alternative medicine does not attempt to eliminate the insulin injections, but to reduce the amount needed by careful attention to diet. Many times Type II diabetes can be totally controlled by diet. Observe the following dietary guidelines, whether you have Type I or Type II diabetes:

Eliminate refined sugar and sugar products with no exceptions. Avoid saturated fats and "junk foods." Eliminate alcohol, which can cause a drop in blood sugar and interact with medication. Avoid caffeine, particularly coffee, as it triggers the release of glucose from the liver.

Eat complex carbohydrates that release their natural sugars slowly and steadily into the bloodstream (whole grains, fresh fruits, and vegetables). Eat berries, brewer's yeast, dairy products (particularly cheese), egg yolks, fish, garlic, kelp, sauerkraut, soy, and vegetables which help normalize blood sugar. Eat protein for snacks, including nut butters.

Be tested and treated for any food sensitivity and intolerances that you may have. For a hypoglycemic attack during which blood sugar plummets, eat fiber and protein along with sugar to moderate and restore blood sugar levels.

If you are Type II diabetic, take off excess weight by following an insulin control diet (see p. 247 for more information).

Exercise and Lifestyle
Perform aerobic exercise daily or make walking part of your daily routine. Use relaxation and stress reduction techniques such as meditation, guided imagery, massage, and yoga.

Do not use tobacco in any form, as it constricts the blood vessels and impairs circulation. Because adult diabetics can develop foot ulcers caused by poor circulation, pay close attention to foot hygiene. Do not ignore injuries, wear well-fitted shoes, and keep your feet clean and dry.

Nutrient Therapy
Take the following nutrients:

- vitamin A – 15,000 IU a day. *Caution:* Do not exceed 8,000 IU a day if you are or might be pregnant (needed to maintain eye health).
- B-complex – 50 mg three times a day (needed for B vitamin balance with B_{12})
- vitamin B_6 – 50 to 100 mg a day (needed for proper absorption of B_{12})
- vitamin B_{12} – as directed on your product (needed to prevent diabetic neuropathy)
- biotin – 50 mg a day (needed for metabolism of carbohydrates)
- vitamin C – 3,000 to 6,000 mg a day (deficiency can lead to vascular problems in diabetics)
- vitamin E – 400 IU and up a day (improves circulation)
- calcium – 1,500 mg a day (important for pH balance)
- chromium picolinate – 400 to 600 mcg a day (improves the efficiency of insulin)

- copper – 2 mg a day (to balance zinc)
- magnesium – 750 mg a day (important for enzyme systems and pH balance)
- manganese – 5 to 10 mg a day (needed for repair of the pancreas; a cofactor in enzymes for glucose metabolism)
- potassium – 99 mg a day (deficiency associated with glucose intolerance; necessary for insulin formation)
- selenium – 200 mcg a day (needed for pancreatic function)
- vanadium (vanadyl sulfate) – 100 to 150 mg a day (works with chromium in regulating blood sugar)
- zinc – 50 to 80 mg a day (deficiency has been associated with diabetes)
- alpha-lipoic acid – 300 to 600 mg a day (stabilizes blood sugar)
- coenzyme Q_{10} – 80 mg a day (stabilizes blood sugar; improves circulation)
- L-carnitine – 500 mg twice a day (mobilizes fat; with glutamine reduces the craving for sugar)
- L-glutamine – 500 mg twice a day on an empty stomach (with L-carnitine reduces craving for sugar)
- taurine – 500 mg twice a day on an empty stomach (aids in insulin release)
- digestive enzymes – as directed on your product (aids in proper digestion, which is essential in diabetes)

Herbal Therapy
Consult a trained herbalist to determine which botanical supplements might help you. The following are but a few of the many possibilities.

- bilberry – helps prevent eye damage; improves sugar tolerance
- bitter melon – lowers blood sugar
- blueberry leaves – lowers blood sugar; helps treat eye problems
- fenugreek – reduces blood sugar and harmful fats

- garlic and onion – both have blood sugar lowering action
- goat's rue – lowers blood sugar levels
- milk thistle – drops and stabilizes glucose; helps with insulin utilization

Homeopathic Remedies

Consult a homeopathic physician to determine the remedy that best fits your symptoms.

- *Bovista lycoperdon* – diabetes with frequent desire to urinate, even immediately after urination.
- *Lycopodium* – addicted to sugar; craves sweets, starches, and alcohol; huge appetite, ravenous, appetite increases while eating; wakes at night to eat.
- *Phosphoric acid* – craving for fruit, fruit juices, and refreshing things; urine is increased, milky color, and contains sugar; great debility and bruised feeling in muscles.
- *Phosphorus* – restlessness and dryness of mouth; thirst for cold water; quantity of urine passed is about 4 to 5 pints in 24 hours; craves chocolate ice cream, cold drinks; "spacey."
- *Plumbum* – diabetes with constipation; albumin and clumps of white blood cells in urine.
- *Uranium nitricum* – diabetes with indigestion and debility; sugar in the urine; great thirst, excess urination, and dry tongue; big appetite even when the stomach is full.

Other Therapeutic Measures

Consider using Chinese medicine, both herbal and acupuncture treatments. Seek the help of an Ayurvedic practitioner. Take chelation therapy to prevent circulation complications.

To help improve circulation, get biofeedback training or reflexology treatments. Dry brushing is another technique to improve circulation. Brush the skin with a soft brush, then compress each joint by gently but firmly pushing from each end toward the center of the joint.

THYROID PROBLEMS

The thyroid is a butterfly-shaped gland found at the front of the neck, lying on either side of the trachea (windpipe). The thyroid gland releases hormones that regulate every cell in the body, so a deficiency or excess of a thyroid hormone can affect all body systems. Thyroid hormones increase the total body consumption of oxygen and regulate the uptake of oxygen by individual organs. They increase enzyme activity in many biochemical systems, and help form protein RNA (ribonucleic acid) for every cell. In addition, thyroid hormones help release fatty acids from fat tissue to act as fuel for muscles, and they help in the incorporation of amino acids into protein.

The thyroid synthesizes L-thyroxine (T_4) and L-triiodothyronine (T_3) from elemental iodine and the amino acid tyrosine. The daily requirement for iodine is estimated to be between 100 and 200 mcg a day. (Potassium iodide–enriched salt contains 1 mg of iodine per 10 grams of salt.) Not only iodine is necessary for the proper function of the thyroid gland: zinc, vitamin E, vitamin A, vitamin C, riboflavin (B_2), niacin (B_3), and pyridoxine (B_6) must also be available in order for active thyroid hormone to be produced.

Dysfunction of the thyroid glands affects 5 to 15 percent of older people, but symptoms of thyroid disease are subtle in people over 50, and are difficult to recognize. The incidence of thyroid deficiency (hypothyroidism) is higher in women: it affects 20 percent of all women over 60. Some physicians recommend that all women have their thyroid levels checked beginning at age 35.

People who have a family or personal history of autoimmune disease (diabetes, rheumatoid arthritis, vitiligo) are at high risk for thyroid disease, as are people with prematurely gray hair (appearing before age 30). People who have had past treatment with radioactive iodine or radiation to the head or neck are also at risk of thyroid disease. Two medications (lithium and amiodorone) can increase the incidence of thyroid disease. People who have high cholesterol levels (over 200 mg/dl or LDL 130 mg/dl) should have their thyroid glands checked because hypothyroidism can cause elevated cholesterol.

Pregnancy is a common cause of temporary thyroid dysfunction. About 5 percent of new mothers develop thyroid dysfunction; typically the woman becomes first hyperthyroid, and then hypothyroid. Postpartum thyroiditis lasts for three to six months, and up to half of these mothers develop persistent thyroid problems.

Babies can be born with no thyroid function. This is the most common metabolic defect among newborns, occurring in 1 of every 3,700 live births in North America. Because thyroid hormone is essential for both brain and body growth, mental development will be affected if a baby does not promptly receive proper thyroid hormone replacement.

Diffuse enlargement of the thyroid gland is known as a goiter, which is caused by a deficiency of iodine. Goiters are common in areas of the world where the soil lacks iodine, but are now rare in industrialized countries because of the addition of iodine to salt. Some foods contain substances that block the utilization of iodine, including turnips, cabbage, mustard, soybeans, peanuts, and millet, but cooking usually inactivates those substances.

If the thyroid is enlarged and smooth, there is probably a goiter. If the thyroid has a single nodule (lump) it could be cancer. Multiple nodules are less likely to be cancer. Pain in the thyroid with swallowing, and pain radiating up the neck to the ear are suggestive of thyroiditis, an inflammation of the thyroid gland.

HYPERTHYROIDISM

Hyperthyroidism occurs when the thyroid hormones manufactured from tyrosine and iodine are produced in excess. It is much rarer than hypothyroidism. It can be caused by a toxic nodular goiter (a nodule that secretes too much thyroid hormone), but Graves' disease (an autoimmune disease) is the most common hyperthyroid problem. Its most obvious symptom is exophthalmos, or bulging eyes. A substance known as "long-acting thyroid stimulator" (LATS) is present in most patients with Graves' disease. Stress may contribute to some types of hyperthyroidism.

Patients with hyperthyroidism experience weight loss despite an increase in appetite, heart palpitations, jitteriness, loss of muscle mass and strength, excessive sweating, heat intolerance, and fast heart rate. The difference between the upper and lower numbers of the blood pressure reading is widened, and the patient may have chest pain. The heartbeat can become irregular to a life-threatening degree, and osteoporosis occurs. Patients should not drink alcohol because it worsens their symptoms.

Patients may also have fatigue, shortness of breath, and lowered tolerance to exercise. Their eyes are more prominent, they have widened eye openings, and they blink less often than is normal. Protrusion of the eyes may affect only one eye, or may affect the eyes unequally.

The patient has an inability to concentrate, rapid speech, and tremors, and can be more irritable and nervous than usual. Some patients experience restlessness, apprehension, and insomnia, which can progress to severe agitation and even frank psychosis. It can be difficult to distinguish the symptoms of hyperthyroidism from those of anxiety. In anxiety states, however, the hands and feet are wet but cool to touch, and the tremor is usually slower and more noticeable with large movements. In hyperthyroidism, the hands and feet are warm and moist, and the nails may be concave and separated from the nail bed. The hair is often fine, silky, and thinned out. The skin in the area about two inches above the ankle becomes raised, hard, and reddish-brown.

In older patients, hyperthyroidism can be "masked"—that is, they may have very few symptoms, which are not classical hyperthyroid symptoms. Cramps and severe diarrhea may signal the onset of hyperthyroidism. Patients may also present with heart failure, angina, or heart arrhythmias. Older people can become so weak they cannot rise from a chair.

MODERN MEDICAL TREATMENT

Drug Therapy

Modern medicine treats hyperthyroidism by prescribing pharmaceuticals such as propylthiouracil (PTU) and methimazole (Tapazole). These preparations inhibit the synthesis of thyroid hormone. Side effects include inflammation of the liver, hair loss, low white blood cell count, rash, anemia, and bleeding.

If the thyroid gland needs to be suppressed rapidly, large doses of iodine, which immediately inhibit thyroid hormone production, may be given.

Radiation Therapy

For cases in which there is no response to drug therapy, for patients who do not want to take the medications, and for teenagers, radioactive iodine is given to destroy some of the overactive cells. If too many cells are damaged during radiation therapy, patients will become hypothyroid and must take thyroid supplementation for the rest of their lives.

Surgery

Another alternative is to surgically remove part or all of the thyroid gland. If all of the thyroid gland is removed, lifetime supplementation with thyroid hormones is necessary.

ALTERNATIVE TREATMENT

Alternative treatment may not completely control hyperthyroidism, and some medication may still have to be used.

Diet

Increase your caloric intake to compensate for the increased metabolism. Eat a whole-food diet, and include goitrogens, foods that help to suppress thyroid hormone production. These foods should be eaten raw as cooking usually inactivates most of the thyroid-lowering activity. They include broccoli, brussels sprouts, cabbage, cauliflower, kale, mustard, rutabagas, spinach, turnips, peaches, pears, soybeans, peanuts, and millet. Avoid high-iodine foods such as dairy products, seafood, processed foods, and iodized salt. Significantly reduce or avoid consumption of stimulants such as coffee, tea, and caffeinated soft drinks. Also reduce consumption of spicy and highly seasoned foods.

Reduce or avoid alcohol consumption. People with hyperthyroidism tend to deplete their glucose stores, and alcohol prevents the liver from making glucose.

Because hyperthyroidism causes you to excrete more fluid each time you urinate, increase fluids so that you are drinking more than eight 8-ounce glasses of water each day (unless you have heart or kidney problems).

Exercise and Lifestyle

Stop smoking and avoid all sources of nicotine, as it is a stimulant.

Exercise daily to the point that you are breathless and sweaty. If possible, swim in the ocean to absorb the naturally occurring minerals. Expose the skin to early morning sun as often as possible.

Nutrient Therapy

Take nutritional supplements under a physician's supervision. Requirements for nutrients are increased because excess thyroid hormone speeds up the metabolic rate.

- vitamin A – 25,000 to 50,000 IU a day. *Caution:* Do not take more than 8,000 IU a day if you are or might be pregnant (needed for thyroid function).
- vitamin B-complex with 50 mg of most Bs (needed for thyroid function; for stress)
- vitamin B_1 – 50 mg over that in the B-complex (used up by overactive thyroid; needed for energy levels)

- vitamin C – 1,000 mg three times a day (needed for stress)
- multivitamin/mineral complex – one capsule a day (needed because of increased metabolism)
- calcium – 800 to 1,000 mg a day (needed for the stress imposed on the body)
- choline – 100 mg three times a day (aids in hormone production)
- magnesium – 400 to 800 mg a day (balances calcium)
- iodine and kelp – 1 mg of iodine a day (suppresses thyroid function)
- amino acid – one capsule three times a day (needed because of increased metabolism)
- coenzyme Q$_{10}$ – 60 mg three times a day (immune enhancer)

Herbal Therapy

Consult a trained herbalist to select the best herbal therapy for you. The herbs listed below are a few that can be helpful.

- astragalus – balances thyroid function
- bugleweed – inhibits iodine metabolism and production of thyroid hormone
- ginkgo – balances thyroid function
- hawthorn – balances thyroid function
- lemon balm – blocks attachment of antibodies to thyroid gland

Homeopathic Remedies

Consult a homeopathic physician to help you select the best remedy for your symptoms. Hyperthyroidism is more easily managed before the patient is on pharmaceuticals, but as improvement results from homeopathic treatment the drugs can be tapered. A few of the possible remedies are listed below.

- *Arsenicum iodum* – hyperthyroidism; exophthalmus; feeling of constriction in the heart; may have goiter, indurated thyroid gland; marked emaciation despite eating ravenously.
- *Iodium purum* – goiter, hyperthyroidism; worse heat, rapid metabolism, emaciation, weight loss; trembling of limbs or body; always feels too hot, better cold air.
- *Kali iodatum* – hyperthyroid; goiter; thyroid enlarged and very sensitive to touch, exophthalmus.
- *Lachesis* – hyperthyroid; thyroiditis; left-sided goiter; tightness in throat, difficulty swallowing; hyperthyroidism after disappointed love, jealousy, or suppression of intense emotions.
- *Thyroidinum* – metabolic disorders, goiter, myxedema, hyperthyroidism; better during and after menses; better in evening, with rest, lying on abdomen or reclining; worse during and after menses, worse least exertion or stooping, with cold.

Other Therapeutic Measures

See an alternatively oriented family practitioner or internal medicine physician. Do not take over-the-counter medications, as the ingredients in some of them can aggravate or bring on a thyroid problem.

Use ice packs on the thyroid gland to slow its activity. Use biofeedback to slow the activity of the thyroid gland. Press on acupressure points on both sides of the spinal column at the base of the neck three times, for 10 seconds each time.

HYPOTHYROIDISM

Some people in the medical field suggest that 25 percent of the population may have hypothyroidism. The onset of hypothyroidism is usually gradual and subtle, but it can present prominently with obvious symptoms, as in myxedema. With myxedema there is dry, waxy swelling of the skin. Facial changes include swollen eyes and a thickened nose.

Hypothyroidism can be associated with a goiter. It can occur because of pituitary failure or because of primary thyroid failure. Primary thyroid failure usually occurs because of an autoimmune condition, Hashimoto's thyroiditis (see below).

Hypothyroidism causes an accumulation of connective tissue in the skin, skeletal muscles, and heart muscle, and probably in the nervous system. There is a slowing of metabolic processes, the heart rate slows, nervous function is depressed, and motility of the gastrointestinal system is decreased. Body temperature and skin temperature may fall. The person is cold intolerant, and sometimes heat intolerant. The patient gains weight (but only an average of 5 to 10 pounds), is exhausted, and may complain of dizziness and vertigo. Numbness of the hands and feet may occur. The patient's limbs may feel heavy as he or she drops off to sleep, and the muscles and joints may ache. Nocturnal cramps are common.

There is water retention and the patient appears puffy, especially around the lips and eyelids, and in the skin of the face. The skin is pale, cool, and dry, and flakes when it is rubbed. The palms may be yellow from an accumulation of carotene. The outside of the eyebrows thin, and the scalp hair becomes scarce, coarse, brittle, and dry. The nails become brittle and dry, and may develop transverse grooves. Wounds heal poorly.

Patients with hypothyroidism are hypersensitive to small doses of sedatives and narcotics. They are prone to infections, but do not produce a fever. The patient may be constipated, but in some cases diarrhea develops, which is related to colonic obstruction with dried feces. Some patients may develop anemia. Cholesterol and triglyceride levels increase, and this may lead to accelerated atherosclerosis. The patient may develop high blood pressure and become short of breath.

Some patients have mood swings and others may become depressed or psychotic. Patients may also have difficulty with concentration and can be extremely forgetful. In women, there may be profuse menstrual bleeding. There is loss of libido, and decreased fertility. Impaired kidney function can also occur. Patients may have an increase in allergic reactions, and in older patients, hypothyroidism can mimic alcoholism, depression, or dementia.

There is controversy over the diagnosis of hypothyroidism. Many patients have all the symptoms of hypothyroidism and may feel better taking thyroid hormone, but have normal hormone levels. Because the laboratory test for thyroid hormones is now very sensitive, most physicians believe that a patient cannot be hypothyroid with normal laboratory levels of these hormones. Many alternative physicians, however, feel that patients with mild hypothyroidism are underdiagnosed.

In the late 1930s and early 1940s, Dr. Broda Barnes, author of *Hypothyroidism: The Unsuspected Illness,* found that basal body temperature was an easy way to diagnose hypothyroidism. Body temperature reflects the body's metabolic rate and may be a more accurate indication of thyroid function than the laboratory tests that show circulating hormone rather than hormone utilization. Dr. Barnes suggested measuring the axillary temperature before a person gets out of bed in the morning. The thermometer is held under the arm for 15 minutes. The basal body temperature should be between 97.6° and 98.2°F. A temperature below 97.4° to 97.5°F may indicate a problem with the thyroid gland. The temperature is taken and averaged for at least three mornings, although some physicians feel temperatures should be taken for two weeks to be accurate. For menstruating women, the temperature record should start the second day of menstruation and continue for 14 days.

HASHIMOTO'S THYROIDITIS

Hashimoto's thyroiditis (chronic thyroiditis, lymphadenoid goiter) is a disease of unknown etiology that can be associated with other autoimmune diseases. In Hashimoto's disease the thyroid gland is infiltrated with white cells, and there are autoantibodies to thyroid tissue antigens.

Early in the course of Hashimoto's, the patient may be hyperthyroid, and thyroid hormone is released by injured thyroid cells. Most patients then develop some degree of hypothyroidism.

The thyroid gland may be painful and tender, and it is firm and diffusely enlarged. The diagnosis of Hashimoto's thyroiditis is suggested by a goiter and hypothyroidism. Hashimoto's is more common in women, especially those between the ages of 40 and 70.

WILSON'S SYNDROME

In 1990, Dr. Denis Wilson (of the Wilson's Syndrome Foundation in Florida—see Sources) described Wilson's syndrome (not to be confused with Wilson's disease, an inherited disease with abnormal copper metabolism). Patients with Irish, Native American, Scottish, Welsh, or Russian backgrounds (or those of any nationality whose ancestors survived famine) are more prone to develop Wilson's syndrome. Eighty percent of patients with Wilson's syndrome are women.

Wilson's syndrome occurs in response to stress, when the thyroid gland reduces the amount of active thyroid T_3, converted from thyroxine (T_4) in an attempt to conserve energy. Normally, when the stress is over, the body resumes production of normal levels of T_3. In Wilson's syndrome patients, the thyroid does not resume normal function because the stress forces hormone production into alternative pathways. The enzyme needed to convert T_4 to T_3 is used in the production of inactive hormones. Because this enzyme is not available to convert T_4 to T_3, the amount of T_3 available to the body is reduced.

Wilson's syndrome has four major characteristics:

- The symptoms are typical for low thyroid function: fatigue, headaches, irritability, depression, decreased memory and concentration, hair loss, decreased sex drive, constipation, dry skin, dry hair, cold and/or heat intolerance, irregular menstrual periods, fluid retention, easy weight gain, and anxiety and panic attacks.
- Symptoms often develop or worsen after a major stress such as childbirth, divorce, death of a loved one, surgery, accidents, or excessive dieting.
- Patients with Wilson's syndrome have low body temperature. Temperatures are usually below 98°F, and in some cases are as low as 93°F. A small percentage of patients have temperatures in the 98.0° to 98.4°F range. Low body temperature is essential for a diagnosis of Wilson's syndrome.
- Laboratory tests for patients with Wilson's syndrome are typically normal. Because of this, most physicians do not accept this syndrome as a valid condition. Patients are told by these physicians that their TSH is normal and that they do not have a thyroid problem.

The diagnosis of Wilson's syndrome is made by body temperature. The temperature should be checked by mouth (using a mercury thermometer) every three hours, three times a day, beginning three hours after you wake up. Hold the thermometer in your mouth for five minutes (but wait for 20 minutes if you have drunk hot or cold liquids). Women should start keeping temperature records on the second day of the menstrual period. Despite the low body temperature, some patients with this syndrome feel hot all the time.

MODERN MEDICAL TREATMENT
Drug Therapy
Patients are usually given levothyroxine (Synthroid or Levothroid), which is a synthetic thyroid preparation. Side effects include bone loss,

heart palpitations, insomnia, nervousness, diarrhea, and hyperthyroidism if the dose is too large. Thyroid supplementation should not be taken with iron or antacids as it is bound up by these substances.

ALTERNATIVE TREATMENT

Alternative treatment may not completely control hypothyroidism, and some medication may still have to be used.

Diet

Avoid eating goitrogens (foods that suppress thyroid hormone production), such as broccoli, brussels sprouts, cabbage, kale, spinach, turnips, peaches, pears, soybeans, peanuts, pine nuts, and millet. If you do eat them, cook them to inactivate the goitrogens. Eat foods that are naturally high in iodine such as fish, kelp, mushrooms, garlic, onions, watercress, vegetables, and root vegetables such as potatoes.

Increase fiber in the diet to compensate for the slowed metabolism that can result in constipation. Eat vitamin A–rich foods such as yellow and dark green vegetables, eggs, carrots, and raw dairy products. Also eat foods high in vitamin B-complex, including raw nuts, seeds, and whole grains. Avoid sugars, white flour, refined foods, saturated fats, and red meats.

Exercise and Lifestyle

Exercise aerobically 15 to 20 minutes a day. This stimulates thyroid gland secretion and increases tissue sensitivity to thyroid hormones. A brisk walk for 30 minutes a day increases metabolism and stimulates circulation. Sun- and sea bathe whenever possible.

Avoid sulfa drugs or antihistamines (which can act as goitrogens) unless your physician prescribes them. Avoid fluorides, commonly found in toothpaste, and chlorine, found in tap water. These substances block the iodine receptors in the thyroid gland, resulting in reduced hormone production.

Nutrient Therapy

Take the following nutritional supplements:

- vitamin A – 25,000 IU a day. *Caution:* Do not take more than 8,000 IU a day if you are or might be pregnant (helps manufacture thyroid hormone; some patients cannot convert carotenes to the active form of vitamin A).
- B_2 – 15 mg a day (for normal manufacture of thyroid hormone; to reactivate the thyroid gland)
- B_3 – 25 to 50 mg a day (for normal manufacture of thyroid hormone)
- B_6 – 25 to 50 mg a day (for normal manufacture of thyroid hormone)
- vitamin C – 1,000 mg a day (for normal manufacture of thyroid hormone)
- vitamin E – 400 IU a day (helps manufacture thyroid hormone)
- calcium/magnesium supplement – 800 to 1,000 mg a day/400 to 800 mg a day (to help prevent bone loss that thyroid supplementation can cause if the dose is very high)
- iodine – 300 mcg a day (needed to produce thyroid hormone)
- manganese – 10 mg a day (essential for the formation of thyroid hormone)
- selenium – 200 mcg a day (essential for the enzyme that activates T_4)
- tyrosine – 250 mg a day (precursor to thyroid hormone)
- zinc picolinate – 30 mg a day (helps manufacture thyroid hormone)
- essential fatty acids – 1 Tbsp. three times a day (for proper functioning of thyroid gland)
- DHEA – 10 to 25 mg a day (increases cell sensitivity to the natural thyroid hormone of the body)

Herbal Therapy

Take the following herbs for hypothyroidism. If you have multiple symptoms of hypothyroidism, the help of a trained herbalist may be necessary.

- bayberry – has a stimulating effect
- cascara – for constipation
- gentian – normalizes thyroid function
- kelp – has high iodine content; normalizes thyroid function
- mustard – high in iodine and tyrosine
- sarsaparilla tea – stimulates metabolic processes

Homeopathic Remedies

Consult a homeopathic physician to help in selecting the best remedy for you. Thyroid hormone supplements do not interfere with homeopathic treatment, but it is important to continue to monitor thyroid hormone levels. If the thyroid gland regenerates with homeopathic therapy, the supplementation can cause you to become hyperthyroid.

- *Calcarea carbonicum* – chilly, better warmth; tendency to be overweight; pale skin with chalky look; thyroid dysfunction; leg cramps, worse cold, wet weather, exertion; worse puberty, menopause.
- *Calcarea iodata* – hypothyroidism; thyroid tumors, enlarged glands; indifference and indolence; obesity.
- *Graphites* – hypothyroidism and hyperthyroidism; thyroid nodules; chilly, intolerant of heat and cold, indoors and out; delayed menstrual history; obesity, fatigue, and constipation with full feeling in rectum; skin thick and hard, cracked skin; hair coarse.
- *Iodium purum* – thyroid swollen and hard, great debility, slightest effort induces perspiration; out of breath going upstairs.
- *Kali carbonicum* – hypothyroidism; diffuse enlargement of thyroid gland; chilly and sensitive to drafts; constipation without urge.
- *Natrum muriaticum* – thyroiditis, hyperthyroidism, hypothyroidism; diffuse goiter; intolerance to heat or sun; thyroiditis after grief or disappointed love.
- *Sepia* – hypothyroidism; goiter more on right side; cold hands and feet; sallow, yellow complexion with thickened skin; constipation without urging.

If no homeopathic therapists are available to help you, take Th'ro by Vibrant Health—a complex remedy for thyroid gland regulation and support (see Sources).

Another complex remedy that gives temporary relief of hypothyroidism and related endocrine problems is Thyroid Liquescence by PHP (see Sources).

Other Therapeutic Measures

Use contrast hydrotherapy daily, alternating hot and cold compresses over the thyroid, to stimulate glandular function.

Have reflexology treatments or press on the acupressure point in the hollow at the base of the throat to stimulate the thyroid. Press three times for 30 seconds each time.

See an acupuncturist for treatments to stimulate thyroid function, and use traditional Chinese medicine treatments.

Take natural thyroid hormones, such as Armour thyroid or Westhroid.

Undertake treatment for Wilson's syndrome. Liothyronine, a long-acting hormone medication, is used to reset the thyroid gland. It must be taken every 12 hours—not even minutes late. The hormone level in the blood must be kept steady and the medication should never be stopped abruptly.

The dose is determined by body temperature. If the body temperature is low, the dose is increased until the temperature rises to and stays at a normal, steady level.

Dr. Wilson has a complex protocol to begin and continue the medication, and it must be followed closely with your physician's help. Patients with Wilson's syndrome do not need to take lifelong thyroid medication, because once the metabolism is normalized, it stays that way unless the patient is subjected to another serious stress.

CHAPTER 19

Gastrointestinal Problems

The gastrointestinal (GI) tract begins in the mouth and includes the esophagus, stomach, small intestine, large intestine, and the anus. The liver, gallbladder, and pancreas are also part of the GI system. The role of the GI tract is to break food down so that it can be used as energy for the body.

One-third to one-half of all North Americans suffer from some type of digestive disorder, and complain of chronic abdominal pain. The National Center for Health Statistics notes that five million Americans have ulcers, six million have frequent indigestion, and eight million are constipated.

Zantac, a medication that blocks acid secretion from the stomach, was the best-selling prescription drug in the late 1980s. It is now sold as an over-the-counter drug. Prescription and over-the-counter drugs do not address the cause of digestive problems, and relieve symptoms only temporarily. Gastrointestinal complaints are rarely life-threatening, and most patients are simply told to live with their symptoms.

CAUSES OF GASTROINTESTINAL PROBLEMS

There are many causes of gastrointestinal problems, but they basically fall into four categories: diet, medications, organisms, and structural problems. One of the major causes is diet, with the Standard American Diet (SAD) being the culprit. (See Diet section in chapter 10, Alternative Therapies.) In general, North Americans eat a very poor diet, low in fiber and high in sugar and processed foods. They consume many food additives, preservatives, and artificial sweeteners, colors, and flavors.

Several major national surveys have shown that the number-one favorite food of Americans was white bread—followed by doughnuts, cookies, cake, hot dogs, and hamburgers. Soft drinks were the favorite beverage, followed by coffee, tea, and whole milk. Alcoholic beverages also rank high on the list of desired beverages for many North Americans.

Caffeine, which is in coffee, tea, many soft drinks, and chocolate, speeds up intestinal peristalsis (the contractions that move food through the intestines). Coffee has a laxative effect, and can cause intestinal spasms. It also reduces the flow of chemicals that help protect the stomach against its own acid secretion, and may worsen heartburn. Sugar, which is a major component of many prepared foods, is devoid of nutrients, causes gas and bloating, and contributes to the development of ulcers. Excess consumption of alcohol causes malnutrition, liver problems, diarrhea, loss of appetite, and inflammation of the stomach. Alcohol also depresses the number of friendly bacteria in the intestines and contributes to leaky gut syndrome—in which the intestines absorb large molecules of food intact into the bloodstream, leading to food sensitivities. (There is now a laboratory test available for leaky gut syndrome, Intestinal Permeability—see Sources.)

Medications can contribute to or cause gastrointestinal problems. Medications for gastrointestinal complaints can cause constipation themselves, as well as malabsorption of nutrients, gas, and diarrhea. Medications used for other problems can also cause gastrointestinal symptoms. For example, antibiotics kill friendly bacteria in the intestine and can impair the production of vitamin K. Non-steroidal anti-inflammatory agents can cause loss of appetite, vomiting, nausea, diarrhea, ulcers, a leaky gut, bleeding from the gastrointestinal tract, and loss of iron, vitamin C, and folic acid. Medications to lower cholesterol can cause constipation, malabsorption of fat (and fat-soluble vitamins A, D, E, and K), and deficiencies in iron, carotene, and vitamin B_{12}. Antihypertensive medications can cause constipation, diarrhea, and loss of potassium, zinc, and magnesium.

Organisms, including bacteria, viruses, parasites, and fungi (yeast) can cause gastrointestinal symptoms (see chapter 20, Parasites). Constipation, diarrhea, gas, intestinal cramping, and abdominal pain and bloating are common symptoms caused by organisms. In severe cases, intestinal ulceration and bleeding may occur.

Among the structural causes of gastrointestinal problems are a weak esophageal sphincter that allows gastric juice reflux into the esophagus, a hiatal hernia caused by an enlarged opening in the diaphragm, allowing the stomach to protrude, and weaknesses in the wall of the large intestine, which allow food-trapping pouches to form, causing diverticulosis.

PEPTIC ULCER DISEASE, STOMACH ACHES, AND ABDOMINAL PAIN

The stomach secretes digestive juices, pepsin, and hydrochloric acid to digest food. Special cells secrete a slightly alkaline mucus that coats the stomach surface, forming a chemical barrier between the stomach contents and the cell surface to protect cells from the acid and pepsin. In addition, the stomach repairs and replaces lining cells rapidly. If this protective coating is damaged, some of the outer mucosa is literally eaten away by the stomach acid, causing the pain of an ulcer or gastritis. Three-quarters of all ulcers, though, are actually found in the duodenum (the first part of the small intestine). Duodenal ulcers are four to five times more common in men than in women. Smoking increases the chance of developing both types of ulcers, and also slows down their healing process.

Many people react to stress by producing high levels of acid secretion, which leads to damage of the gastric or duodenal mucosa. However, half the people with ulcer disease do not have excess acid secretion. Alcohol, use of non-steroidal drugs such as aspirin and ibuprofen, and use of steroid drugs can all cause ulcers.

It is now known that most ulcers are primarily caused by a bacteria known as *Helicobacter pylori* (previously known as *Campylobacter pylori*). Ulcers tend to run in families because this bacteria is contagious. Such ulcers are typically chronic, unless the bacteria are eradicated.

Ulcer pain presents as pain between the end of the breastbone and the navel. The pain is often described as gnawing, burning, and aching. It is sharp and constant and occurs especially between meals, during the night, and 45 to 60 minutes after meals. Eating, or taking antacids, usually gives pain relief. Caffeine, alcohol, milk, and smoking can stimulate acid secretion from the stomach, which increases the pain. Fried foods, citrus fruits, and decaffeinated coffee can also stimulate acid production.

Peptic ulcers occur in the stomach or duodenum. They can bleed, perforate, or cause obstruction, in addition to causing pain. All of these conditions are life-threatening, and when they occur, patients must be hospitalized. The diagnosis of peptic ulcer disease is verified by a barium swallow or endoscopic examination. Endoscopic studies can also obtain gastric juice samples to test for the presence of *H. pylori*. As well, there are now blood tests that indicate the presence of antibodies against *H. pylori*.

Most stomach pain is not caused by ulcer disease. Stress or a reaction to a specific food are more common causes. Lactose intolerance (an inability to digest milk sugar) is a common cause of stomach pain, and the digestion of other sugars can also be a problem. According to Dr. Ronald Hoffman, founder and director of the Hoffman Center for Holistic Medicine in New York, 71 percent of adults cannot completely absorb fructose (the sugar found in fruits). Fructose intolerance can cause cramps and diarrhea, and may also cause irritable bowel syndrome (see below). Beans and other legumes contain oligosaccharides, which are long chains of sugars that the small intestine cannot break down; they are broken down into carbon dioxide, hydrogen, and methane by bacteria in the large intestine. Consequently, some people whose diet is high in legumes can develop stomach pain, gas, and diarrhea.

Dyspepsia is discomfort in the upper abdomen that is felt after eating, and is sometimes accompanied by nausea or vomiting. Dyspepsia can be a symptom of an ulcer or hiatal hernia, and can be related to stress or worry. However, a simple lack of sufficient stomach acid is one of the most common causes of dyspepsia. In addition, Dr. Hoffman has found that symptoms of food intolerance include heartburn and dyspepsia, about half an hour after eating (see Food Allergy in chapter 25, Allergy).

When people complain of abdominal pain, most physicians consider the possibility that the stomach is overproducing acid, but it has been estimated that from 10 to 15 percent of the general population does not produce *enough* stomach acid. Patients who do not produce adequate stomach acid develop indigestion, bloating, belching or burning immediately after meals, bad breath, a feeling that food stays in the stomach without being digested, and a full feeling after eating a small amount of food. These people are aware of the taste of food for many hours after eating, and many (but not all) are also constipated, or have diarrhea.

Because of poor absorption of minerals caused by low stomach acid, these patients have weak fingernails, hair loss, gas in the upper abdomen, and dilation of the capillaries in the cheeks and on the nose. Low stomach acid is associated with diabetes mellitus, asthma in childhood, acne rosacea, chronic hepatitis, rheumatoid arthritis, eczema, and osteoporosis. Taking an antacid or acid-blocker is the worst thing to do if a person produces too little stomach acid.

Modern medical diagnosis is usually made by means of a gastric lavage, in which a patient swallows a tube, and a sample of gastric juice is taken and analyzed. The best way to diagnose low stomach acid (hypochlorhydria) is to have a Heidelberg test. In this test the patient swallows a capsule that contains a radiotransmitter, which signals the pH of the stomach and small intestine to a recording device. This test also gives information regarding transit time through the GI tract (see Sources). Hair analysis can also indicate hypochlorhydria, but only if there are low levels of essential minerals such as zinc, manganese, copper, and chromium. Dr. Jonathan Wright of Tahoma Clinic in Kent, Washington, and Dr. Alan Gaby of Bastyr College in Seattle, Washington, suggest that when hair analysis shows low readings for five or six minerals, a Heidelberg test is the next logical step.

Finally, a deficiency of bile (a dark pigment produced by the liver and stored in the gallbladder) can cause poor digestion and its accompanying symptoms, because bile helps digest fat and increases peristalsis in the intestines. People who do not produce adequate bile have light yellow or tan stools.

MODERN MEDICAL TREATMENT

Diet
Patients are advised to eat a bland diet.

Drug Therapy
The standard medical recommendations for dealing with abdominal pain are largely based on treatment with medications. People are told to take an antacid or an acid-blocker such as Tagamet, Axid, Zantac, or Pepcid.

Antacids can cause constipation or diarrhea, and malabsorption of nutrients (in particular iron, vitamin B_{12}, folic acid, and calcium). It has been demonstrated that antacids for chronic upset stomachs perform no better than placebos—simply because most upset stomachs are not caused by ulcers. Antacids also cause "acid rebound," in which the stomach produces more acid when the antacids wear off, and they cause the intestines to become alkaline, which allows pathogenic bacteria to overgrow. In addition, the kidneys have to excrete the extra alkaline in order to maintain the proper acid-base balance; otherwise, an acid-base imbalance can lead to kidney stones and urinary tract infections.

Antacids typically contain the following ingredients.

- Calcium carbonate (the main ingredient in Tums) comes from chalk. Calcium carbonate combined with a large amount of milk can cause an excess of calcium in the body, lead-

ing to kidney stones and calcification of the kidneys.
- Sodium bicarbonate can make the gastrointestinal tract too alkaline and affect the kidneys. The sodium content can also lead to hypertension (see chapter 16).
- Magnesium hydroxide is a potent laxative, and can cause diarrhea. This includes Milk of Magnesia.
- Aluminum hydroxide depletes phosphorus, and can thin bones and waste muscles. Aluminum also can cause constipation and delays the stomach from emptying into the small intestines. Gelusil, Maalox, and Mylanta all contain aluminum, which has been implicated in Alzheimer's disease, pulmonary disease, and bone disease.

The most common medications used for any type of stomach pain (regardless of the cause) are acid blockers, called histamine H_2-receptor antagonists: rantidine (Zantac), cimetidine (Tagamet), nizatidine (Axid), and famotidine (Pepcid). They are sold either as prescription drugs or over-the-counter medications, depending on the dosage. These medications prevent the release of hydrochloric acid from the stomach, and change the structure and function of the cells that line the digestive tract. There is a high relapse rate when these drugs are discontinued.

Patients taking acid blockers have less pain, and need to take less antacids, than do people taking placebos. The side effects of these medications can include malaise, dizziness, sleepiness, insomnia, changes in heart beat, headaches, constipation, diarrhea, nausea, vomiting, abdominal pain, dry mouth, taste disorder, liver problems, joint pain, enlarged breasts in males, impotence, loss of libido, hives, and anaphylaxis. The manufacturers suggest consulting a physician if the need for the over-the-counter versions of these medications persists daily for two continuous weeks.

Omeprazole (Prilosec) and lansoprazole (Prevacid) are known as gastric acid–pump or proton pump inhibitors. They reduce gastric acidity by blocking the final step in acid production. The medication effects occur within one hour of ingestion, and last for 72 hours. In animal studies, these medications caused a significant increase in gastric tumors and hyperplasia of some of the cells, and may affect other cells in the gastrointestinal tract. Side effects of proton pump inhibitors can include diarrhea, abdominal pain, muscle weakness, joint pain, nausea, vomiting, rashes, fatigue, constipation, gas, hypoglycemia, weight gain, depression, hepatitis (including hepatic failure), enlarged breasts in males, testicular pain, and taste perversion.

The least recognized side effect of both the histamine H2-blockers and the proton pump inhibitors results directly from their ability to suppress gastric acid secretion. As noted earlier, gastric acid is necessary for proper digestion, and lack of adequate amounts of stomach acid can cause anemia related to iron deficiency; anemia, nerve damage, and neurological disease related to vitamin B_{12} deficiency; and osteoporosis related to calcium malabsorption. People with low stomach acid are more likely to get bacterial intestinal infections, intestinal yeast infections, and parasitic infections. Low stomach acid is also associated with cancer of the stomach.

Patients are also given sucralfate (Carafate), which accelerates healing of duodenal ulcers. Because it is poorly absorbed from the gastrointestinal tract, it covers the ulcer site and protects it against further attack by acid and pepsin. Side effects of this medication can include constipation, diarrhea, nausea, vomiting, indigestion, gas, dry mouth, sleepiness, hives, and runny nose.

Because *Helicobacter pylori* infections are a cause of ulcers, patients may be treated with antibiotics. Treatments typically include clarithromycin plus omeprazole (Prilosec), a gastric acid suppressor; clarithromycin plus rantidine-bismuth-citrate (RBC), a gastric acid suppressor; or clarithromycin plus a second antibiotic and omeprazole or RBC.

Antibiotics of the erythromycin class (such as clarithromycin) can cause nausea, vomiting, abdominal pain, diarrhea, and loss of appetite; elevation of liver enzymes; confusion and hallucinations; cardiac rhythm disturbances; and hives and rashes. Antibiotics can also cause an overgrowth of yeast in the intestines (see Irritable Bowel Syndrome, p. 269) and vaginal yeast infections in women.

Pepto-Bismol, an over-the-counter medication, contains bismuth subsalicylate as its active ingredient. It is used for indigestion, to help eradicate *H. pylori* in the stomach, for diarrhea, and as a preventative against traveler's diarrhea. It also contains salicylates, and can cause ringing in the ears, inflammation of the stomach, thinning of the blood, and dizziness. Patients should not take Pepto-Bismol while they are taking aspirin products. Pepto-Bismol can also cause a blackened tongue and/or black stools.

Other Therapeutic Measures
Some physicians still advise patients to drink milk. Patients are also advised to stop smoking.

ALTERNATIVE TREATMENT FOR ULCERS
Antibiotics may be necessary if *H. pylori* cannot be eradicated with alternative methods. Treatment will be less stressful for the body and more successful if alternative measures are used with the antibiotics.

Diet
To reduce the recurrence rate of ulcers, eat a high-fiber diet, including barley, oats, brown rice, and kudzu. Cut back on meat and eat more fish.

Eat dark green leafy vegetables, which contain vitamin K, needed for healing. Avoid tea and coffee (even decaffeinated), chocolate, strong spices, fried foods, animal fats of any kind, alcoholic beverages, and carbonated drinks. Do not drink cow's milk, as it can stimulate the production of more acid; use almond milk instead. Because hot beverages can cause gastric discomfort, be sure to allow them to cool before drinking.

Eat frequent, small meals, eat slowly, and chew your food well. Avoid late night snacks. If your symptoms are severe, eat soft foods or purée your food in the blender. For bleeding ulcers, eat organic baby food and use psyllium seed or guar gum for fiber.

Drink six to eight glasses of water a day. For relief of acute ulcer pain, drink two glasses of water. Drink a glass of water half an hour before eating and two and a half hours after a meal.

Exercise and Lifestyle
Perform aerobic exercise for 20 minutes each day.

Stop smoking as it can delay or prevent healing.

Avoid taking salicylates such as aspirin, and other anti-inflammatories. Read labels carefully, as salicylates are in many over-the-counter preparations. Also avoid ibuprofen (Advil, Nuprin, and other preparations).

Nutrient Therapy
Take the following nutritional supplements:

- vitamin A – 20,000 IU a day. *Caution:* Do not take more than 8,000 IU a day if you are pregnant or might be pregnant (heals stomach lining; protects mucus membranes).
- vitamin B$_6$ – 50 to 150 mg a day (heals stomach lining)
- folic acid – 2 to 5 mg a day (to heal an ulcer)
- vitamin E – 400 to 800 IU a day (reduces stomach acid; relieves pain)
- zinc picolinate – 30 mg a day (promotes healing)
- fish oil Max EPA – two capsules three times a day (protects stomach and intestines from ulcers)

- pectin – as directed on label (creates protective coating in intestines)

Herbal Therapy
Use the following botanical treatments.

- cabbage juice – 1 quart a day, using spring and summer cabbages, which contain more healing factors (helps heal ulcers)
- unripe plantain banana powder – 1 tsp. in a glass of water three times a day (heals ulcers)
- DGL (deglycyrrhizinated licorice) – two to four 380 mg tablets between meals, or 20 minutes before meals (continue for 8 to 16 weeks) (stimulates normal defense mechanisms that prevent ulcer formation; promotes healing of gastric and duodenal ulcers)
- aloe vera gel – 3 ounces, 20 minutes before meals (aids in pain relief; speeds healing)
- slippery elm – drink as a tea (soothes irritated mucus membranes)
- chamomile – take 1 tsp. of an infusion made of one part chamomile and two parts marshmallow root, three times a day (soothes mucus membranes; helps decrease spasms and inflammation)
- cayenne pepper – ½ tsp. in a glass of water two to three times a day (stops bleeding of ulcers)
- Robert's formula – ¼ to ½ tsp. (or one to two capsules) three times a day, between meals (see Diarrhea, below, for formula) (helps heal ulcers)

Homeopathic Remedies
Take the homeopathic remedy that best describes your symptoms. If you do not obtain relief, seek the help of a homeopathic practitioner.

- *Anacardium* – dull pain radiating to the back two hours after eating; tasteless or sour belches; eating gives relief; sensation of a band around a single part of the body; sensation of a blunt plug stuck in a location in the body (stomach, joints).

- *Arsenicum album* – burning in the esophagus or stomach with desire to sip on water; liquids are poorly tolerated and often immediately vomited; desires fat, sour foods, especially lemon and alcohol; inability to digest food, loss of appetite, pains immediately after eating, nausea and vomiting; stomach pains ameliorated by drinking milk.

- *Lycopodium* – vigorous appetite that increases while eating; full, bloated feeling after a few mouthfuls of food, ameliorated by burping and flatus (gas); worse eating even small amounts of food; sleepy feeling after eating; excessive flatulence (gas) may press upwards and cause difficulty with breathing; loud rumbling in the abdomen; heartburn; sour burps.

- *Nux vomica* – pain about an hour after eating; pain after mental overwork; nausea, empty retching, and sour belching; bad-tempered and worse in the morning; peptic ulcers in the workaholic patients; gastritis from alcohol abuse; stomach pains; worse with anger; worse tight clothes; better with warmth, warm applications, or warm drinks.

- *Pulsatilla* – dry mouth, putrid taste in the morning; sensation of food stuck under the breastbone; tongue is thick, rough, and white; nasty taste of food eaten previously; pain one or two hours after eating; flatulence seems to move around; worse in the evening; craves butter, cheese, ice cream, cold food; thirstless; bloating and abdominal distension.

Other Therapeutic Measures

Take bismuth (Pepto-Bismol) for a limited time, which acts as an antibiotic against *H. pylori*.

Get acupuncture, or see an Ayurvedic physician.

Press on the following acupressure points:

- halfway between the lower end of the breastbone and navel, in the midline
- between the tendons of the big toe and the first toe, two thumbs' width towards the top of the foot from the web
- three thumbs' width below the joint under the kneecap lying on the outer side of the knee, one finger's width back from the sharp edge of the shin bone
- one hand's width (four fingers) up from the inner ankle joint, just behind the tibia.

Be tested and treated for food allergies, either with NAET treatment (see Chiropractic section in chapter 9, Alternative Medical Disciplines), or by an environmental medicine physician using food extracts. Follow a rotation diet to help control allergies and prevent new allergies from developing (see chapter 25, Allergy).

ALTERNATIVE TREATMENT FOR STOMACH AND ABDOMINAL PAIN

Diet

Avoid sugar, processed food, coffee, alcohol, and artificial colors and sweeteners. As well, avoid foods to which you are sensitive. If you do not know which foods are a problem, have food allergy testing performed or go on an elimination diet.

Drink six to eight glasses of water a day.

Exercise and Lifestyle

Perform aerobic exercise for 20 minutes a day.

Stop smoking and do not use tobacco in any form.

Nutrient Therapy

Take the following nutrients for stomach and abdominal pain.

- betaine hydrochloride or glutamic acid capsules with pepsin – start with one capsule or tablet before each meal, and increase the dose gradually to six capsules or two to five tablets, depending on the quantity and type of food ingested (to treat inadequate levels of hydrochloric acid as demonstrated by Heidelberg test—see Other Therapeutic Measures—or symptomatology. Also see Sources.)

- minerals – as directed on the label of your multimineral, or individual replacement minerals (inadequate levels of any mineral as demonstrated by hair analysis) (provides essential nutrients)
- bile salts – as directed on the label of your product (insufficient bile or removal of gall bladder)
- taurine – 500 to 1,500 mg a day (for light stools)

Herbal Therapy
Take an herbal remedy for general pain.

- bitters in water – soothes stomach upsets
- meadowsweet tea – protects and soothes the stomach
- Stomach Tonic, made of bitter herbs (from Herbs Etc.) – soothes stomach upsets (see Sources)
- chamomile, peppermint, or raspberry leaf tea – for cramps
- ginger root as a tea (using a few slivers), taken 10 to 15 minutes before meals – helps stimulate gastric juices
- garlic – one to three odorless garlic capsules a day – serves as a digestive aid and relieves gas
- cumin, coriander, turmeric, anise, or fenugreek tea – soothes stomach
- chlorophyll tablets, as directed – prevents inflammation, combats toxins
- half a lemon squeezed into ½ cup water, taken 10 to 15 minutes before meals – helps stimulate gastric juices
- Trikatu (a mixture of Indian long pepper, black pepper, and ginger) – ½ tsp. before meals – stimulates gastric juices

Mix a few drops of soy sauce, a pinch of ginger, and kudzu powder. Mix. Bring to a boil, and stir into a smooth cream. Then add uemboshi plum paste and eat the mixture (soothes stomach upsets).

Homeopathic Remedies
Take the following homeopathic remedy that best fits your symptoms. If you do not obtain relief, consult a homeopathic practitioner.

- *Anacardium orientale* – nervous indigestion relieved by food; sensation of a plug in the intestines; flatulent colic with rumbling, pinching, and griping.
- *Arsenicum album* – stomach pains from fruit, acid foods, and ice cream or cold drinks.
- *Causticum* – acid indigestion; desire for water but makes sick; loss of appetite; craving for sour.
- *Hydrastis* – poor digestion, bitter taste, feeling of weakness.
- *Lycopodium* – food tastes sour; distension and indigestion from eating carbohydrates; great hunger but the stomach feels full after eating only a very small amount.
- *Nux vomica* – a liking for highly seasoned foods and coffee, all of which disagree; preceded by a ravenous appetite.
- *Pulsatilla* – distension after eating; aversion to fat, warm food, and drink.

Other Therapeutic Measures
If there are clinical symptoms that suggest low stomach acid, have a Heidelberg test done.

See a chiropractor or an Ayurvedic physician.

Practice biofeedback or have hypnotherapy or acupuncture.

Press on the following acupressure points:

- halfway between the lower end of the breastbone and the navel, in the midline
- at the tip of the ninth rib on the front of the

body, halfway along the lower end of the ribcage from the midline to the side

- one hand's width (four fingers) up from the inner ankle joint, just behind the tibia bone
- below the inside of the kneecap and below the top of the tibia (this point is usually tender when pressed with a finger tip)
- on the back of the wrist, three thumbs' width towards the elbow from the wrist crease.

HEARTBURN

The lower esophageal sphincter (which acts as a valve) separates the stomach from the esophagus. If the valve is weak, it allows gastric juices, including acid, to feed back into the esophagus. This is gastroesophageal reflux, also known as heartburn. The acid causes a burning pain in the chest, which can be mistaken for a heart attack. It can cause a bad taste in the mouth, bad breath, and can make food (with an acidic or bitter taste) come back toward the mouth. Heartburn symptoms typically occur right after a meal, or when a person lies down in bed. At least 10 percent of Americans have heartburn every day.

Many people with gastroesophageal reflux have a hiatal hernia, in which the stomach protrudes above the opening for it in the diaphragm. This causes pressure on the lower esophageal sphincter, and can contribute to heartburn, but there is no direct relationship between a hiatal hernia and reflux. More than half of all people over age 50 have a hiatal hernia.

Smoking can weaken the lower esophageal sphincter by causing bile (a digestive juice produced by the liver) to back up into the stomach and then into the esophagus—and bile may be carcinogenic when it is in contact with cells that it normally does not touch. Other causes of heartburn are pregnancy; obesity; alcohol; aging; and eating certain foods (fatty foods, tomatoes, citric fruits, coffee, and chocolate).

Some people develop chest and stomach pain simply because their pants are too tight. Wearing pants that are as much as three inches too small in the waist can cause "tight pants syndrome," in which pain is caused by increased pressure on the abdomen. Over time tight pants syndrome can result in the development of a hiatal hernia.

MODERN MEDICAL TREATMENT

Diet
People with heartburn and hiatal hernia are told to avoid eating citrus fruits, chocolate, caffeine, and spicy foods, or drinking peppermint tea, which aggravates reflux.

Drug Therapy
Many of the medications used to treat ulcers and stomach pain are also used for heartburn. Antacids are used, but it has been demonstrated that antacids for chronic upset stomachs or heartburn are no more effective than placebos, and can cause constipation or diarrhea (see Modern Medical Treatment for Peptic Ulcer Disease, Stomach Aches, and Abdominal Pain, above, for more information on antacids).

Perhaps the medications most commonly used to treat any type of stomach pain are the histamine H2-receptor antagonists: rantidine (Zantac), cimetidine (Tagamet), nizatidine (Axid), and famotidine (Pepcid). These medications are sold either as prescription drugs or over-the-counter medications, depending on the dosage.

Gastric acid–pump or proton pump inhibitors (Prilosec and Prevacid) that block the final step of acid production are sometimes used for heartburn (see Modern Medical Treatment for Peptic Ulcer Disease, Stomach Aches, and Abdominal Pain, above, for further details on these medications).

Pepto-Bismol is also used for heartburn (see Modern Medical Treatment for Peptic Ulcer Disease, Stomach Aches, and Abdominal Pain, above, for information on this medication).

Other Therapeutic Measures
People with heartburn and hiatal hernia are advised to elevate the head of their bed 6 inches.

ALTERNATIVE TREATMENT

Diet
Avoid eating large meals, and eat several smaller meals instead. Eat meals slowly and chew food thoroughly. Avoid citrus fruits, chocolate, and spicy foods as well as peppermint, peppermint tea, and spearmint, all of which aggravate reflux. Also avoid alcohol, coffee, teas, colas, and any foods or drinks containing caffeine. Include extra fiber in your diet.

For hiatal hernia and heartburn, do not eat within three hours of bedtime.

With the first symptom of heartburn, drink a large glass of water to reduce the acid levels in the esophagus. In addition, drink water every three hours during the daytime, even if you do not feel thirsty.

Exercise and Lifestyle
If running causes heartburn, wait for an hour or more after eating before you begin. Or try swimming or another form of exercise instead. Do not smoke.

If you have a hiatal hernia, avoid becoming constipated and straining during bowel movements.

Take medications and supplements with plenty of water, and stand or sit up while taking them to be sure they reach the stomach.

Practice Tai Chi or Qigong daily to relieve stress.

Nutrient Therapy
Take the following nutrients for heartburn and hiatal hernia.

- vitamin A – 20,000 IU a day. *Caution:* Do not take more than 8,000 IU a day if you are or might be pregnant (aids in combating excess acid; enhances immune function).
- beta carotene – 25,000 IU a day (antioxidant; precursor to vitamin A)
- vitamin B-complex – 100 mg twice a day with meals (needed for all enzyme systems in the body and for proper absorption of nutrients)
- vitamin C – 1,500 mg a day (needed for healing of tissues and proper immune function)
- vitamin E – 400 IU a day (antioxidant; protects cell membranes)
- copper – 2 to 3 mg a day (balances zinc)
- zinc – 50 mg a day (necessary for healing and repair of tissues)

Herbal Therapy
Take the following botanical supplements.

- aloe vera gel – soothes stomach; helps prevent reflux
- comfrey – helps wound healing; helps to produce mucus. *Caution:* Do not take in excess, as comfrey can lead to liver disease.
- licorice root – stimulates normal defense mechanisms. *Caution:* Do not take in excess, as licorice root can cause hypertension.
- meadowsweet – protects and soothes stomach

Homeopathic Remedies
Take the homeopathic remedy that best fits your symptoms. If you do not obtain relief, consult a homeopathic practitioner.

- *Ammonium carbonicum* – pain in the pit of the stomach; nausea; chilliness.
- *Conium maculatum* – nausea, acrid heartburn and acid belches; worse after going to bed and lying down; eating gives temporary relief.
- *Kali carbonicum* – indigestion in the elderly; burning acidity; bloating of the abdomen.
- *Lobelia* – acidity; flatulence and shortage of breath after eating; profuse flow of saliva.

- *Natrum phosphoricum* – sour belches and taste; a yellow-creamy coating on the tongue.
- *Sulphur* – great acidity; complete loss of or excessive appetite; milk disagrees; the patient feels weak and faint at about 11 A.M., so must eat.

Other Therapeutic Measures

Elevate the head of your bed 6 inches by using blocks.

If you have a hiatal hernia, get chiropractic care for it. Also consider bodywork such as massage or reflexology.

Press on the following acupuncture points:

- one and a half thumbs' width below the navel
- halfway between the lower end of the breastbone and navel, exactly in the midline
- between the tendons of the big toe and the first toe, a thumb's width towards the top of the foot from the web
- two thumbs' width to each side of the navel.

Keep the pressure off your waist by giving the stomach two hours to empty before lifting, bending, or other physical exertion. Also, do not wear clothing that is tight in the waist.

NAUSEA

Nausea occurs when you have an upset stomach and begin to feel that you are going to vomit. Anxiety, stress, food poisoning, food sensitivities, stomach flu, morning sickness, certain smells and odors, seeing blood, giving blood, motion sickness, and other people vomiting can all be causes of nausea. In addition, there are at least 25 different diseases that can cause chronic nausea.

MODERN MEDICAL TREATMENT

Diet

Patients are told to drink small amounts of fluid, such as Pedialyte, for vomiting. After an attack of nausea, patients are advised to eat light car-bohydrates, such as toast or crackers, in small amounts, then graduating to light protein.

Drug Therapy

When it is necessary in cases of food poisoning, syrup of ipecac (available from drugstores) is used to induce vomiting. This syrup should be used only under the direction of a physician or a poison control center.

Patients are told to take an anti-nausea medication or suppository.

Prescription anti-emetics (anti-vomiting medications) include antihistamines, phenothiazines (strong tranquilizers), metoclopramide (Reglan), and ondansetron (Zofran). In addition to prescription antihistamines, Bonine is used. It is an over-the-counter chewable antihistamine that helps settle the stomach. Antihistamines can cause dry mouth, drowsiness, and tremor, or rarely, convulsions.

Phenothiazines can cause sedation, sleepiness, blurred vision, dry mouth, rash, low white blood cell and platelet counts, vomiting, a lowered seizure threshold resulting in seizures in some patients, blood pressure problems, jaundice, disorientation, motor restlessness, altered libido, enlarged breasts in males, urinary incontinence, and neuromuscular symptoms such as rigidity of the jaw and neck or tongue protrusion. Phenothiazines used over the long term can cause neuroleptic malignant syndrome, a potentially fatal syndrome with high temperature, altered consciousness, muscular rigidity, and dysfunction of the autonomic nervous system.

Metoclopramide increases peristalsis of the upper small intestine, causing the stomach to empty more rapidly. It can cause fatigue, headaches, confusion, neuromuscular symptoms (rigidity of the jaw and neck, or tongue protrusion), motor restlessness, impotence, diarrhea, urinary frequency, and visual disturbances. Metoclopramide can also cause neuroleptic malignant syndrome.

Ondansetron (Zofran) blocks one of the serotonin receptors; it is used for nausea and vomiting caused by chemotherapy. It can cause constipation, rash, seizure, spasms of the bronchial tubes, elevated liver enzymes, neuromuscular symptoms, and blurred vision.

Exercise and Lifestyle
Patients who are nauseated are advised to rest, and not to exercise.

Other Therapeutic Measures
Patients are advised to allow themselves to vomit, and to drink clear liquids, an electrolyte solution, or flat carbonated drinks. Coke syrup, Emetrol (a phosphorated carbohydrate solution), or the sugar-containing syrup from canned fruit (not the fruit packed in its own juice) are also recommended.

ALTERNATIVE TREATMENT

Diet
Develop eating habits to minimize the potential for nausea. Avoid overeating, and avoid food allergens. Nausea is a common symptom of food allergy as well as of food poisoning. Do not eat foods that have molded, and do not use cracked eggs.

When eating out, be careful of salad bars that do not look fresh or do not have protective glass covering them. Be wary of food containing mayonnaise, creamed foods, and chicken or fish. Refuse any food served you that is not at the proper temperature or that looks "shop-worn," as though it has been sitting around and not maintained at the proper temperature.

Exercise and Lifestyle
Rest when you have nausea, regardless of the cause. Do not exercise until you have fully recovered and no longer feel nauseated.

Learn proper food-handling methods to prevent the nausea that accompanies food poisoning. Keep food at the appropriate temperature, either hot or cold, and refrigerate perishable leftovers as soon as possible. Never leave foods at room temperature, or in the sun at outdoor events. Cook meats thoroughly and thaw all frozen foods, particularly meats, in the refrigerator. Store foods properly and immediately after completing grocery shopping. Throw away any bulging cans or cracked jars. Before using them again, thoroughly wash or disinfect any utensils that have come in contact with raw foods or meats.

Nutrient Therapy
Take the following nutrients to help with nausea.

- charcoal tablets – five tablets at first sign of nausea and again at six hours (removes toxic substances from the colon and bloodstream)
- garlic – two capsules three times a day (detoxifier that kills bacteria in the colon)
- potassium – 99 mg a day (restores electrolyte balance)
- vitamin C – 8,000 mg a day in divided doses (detoxifies the body; helps remove bacteria and toxins)
- vitamin E – 600 IU a day (enhances immune function, reducing symptoms)
- *Lactobacillus acidophilus* – up to 3 tsp. of powder a day (repopulates "good" intestinal bacteria)
- Aerobic 07 – 20 drops in a glass of water every three hours (destroys harmful bacteria) (see Sources)

Herbal Therapy
Take a botanical supplement.

- cinnamon – relieves upset stomach
- clove oil – stops vomiting
- colombo – stops nausea and vomiting
- ginger root tea – helps relieve nausea so severe the person feels that death is near
- peppermint tea – stops stomach cramps and nausea

Homeopathic Remedies

Take the homeopathic remedy that best fits your symptoms. Those listed below are but a few of the many possibilities. If you do not obtain relief and the nausea and vomiting continue for more than a day, consult a homeopathic physician.

- *Antimonium crudum* – nausea and/or vomiting immediately after eating; tongue coated white; nausea and loss of appetite; distension from overeating; nausea worse during headache, worse from drinking, worse from dietary indiscretions.
- *Arsenicum album* – burning pain soon after eating; sensation of a stone in the stomach; better after a warm drink or after vomiting; loss of appetite; nausea comes on after midnight; vomiting and extremely violent nausea; food poisoning; thirsty for small sips frequently; loss of appetite.
- *Ipecac* – constant nausea that is incapacitating; stomach seems to hang loose inside; nausea unrelieved by vomiting; loathing food or even the smell of food; abdominal cramping or colic; tongue remarkably clean despite constant nausea.
- *Nux vomica* – discomfort about an hour after eating, makes the patient bad-tempered; nausea with empty retching; excessive hunger; symptoms from too rich a diet; symptoms are worse in the morning.

Many patients respond to complex homeopathic remedies. You may want to try Food Poisoning Detox by PHP, which aids in the relief of acute food poisoning and removal of toxin residue.

Other Therapeutic Measures

Take Magic Brew. (See Other Therapeutic Measures for Pollen Allergy in chapter 25, Allergy for the recipe and instructions.)

Sip all fluids carefully, ½ to 1 ounce every 30 minutes. Drink a balanced electrolyte solution, such as Recharge.

Use the following acupressure points:

- two thumbs' width up from the palm wrist crease toward the elbow, directly in the center between the two tendons
- three thumbs' width below the joint under the kneecap, lying on the outer side of the knee
- one finger's width back from the sharp edge of the shin bone.

Take a plain water enema or a coffee enema (see p. 119) to remove toxins from the colon.

IRRITABLE BOWEL SYNDROME

Irritable bowel syndrome (IBS) is the second most common American medical complaint. It is estimated that 15 percent of the population has irritable bowel syndrome, with almost two times as many women as men experiencing symptoms of the condition. It is the most common gastrointestinal complaint seen by physicians, and the reason for a large proportion of all referrals to gastroenterologists.

Irritable bowel syndrome is also known as spastic colon or mucus colitis, and it can cause significant discomfort. The most common symptoms of IBS are abdominal pain, bloating, alternating constipation and diarrhea, and mucus in the stools. Other symptoms include gas, more frequent bowel movements with pain, relief of pain with bowel movements, nausea, loss of appetite, and anxiety or depression. Studies demonstrate that patients with IBS show symptoms from overdistention of the colon sooner than people who do not have IBS. People with irritable bowel syndrome are also prone to have asthma and mitral valve prolapse (a floppy heart valve).

CAUSES OF IBS

Food intolerance is a common cause of IBS. Many studies document that patients with IBS who go on an elimination diet will improve, and when foods are added back to their diet, their symptoms recur. Common food triggers are wheat, corn, dairy products, coffee, tea, and citrus fruits. According to Dr. Alun Jones at

Cambridge University in England, at least two-thirds of patients with IBS have at least one food intolerance. Studies indicating that food allergies do not play a role in IBS have been flawed: most of those studies failed to eliminate wheat from the diet, which is one of the most common causes of food sensitivities and malabsorption. In addition, food challenges were performed using food capsules, which provide only small quantities of food, much less than the amount that a person would actually eat. Dr. Ronald Hoffman, founder and director of the Hoffman Center for Holistic Medicine in New York, has found that 40 percent of his patients with food allergies and intolerances and IBS improve significantly after one week on a common food allergy elimination diet.

In patients with IBS, barium enemas, colonoscopy, and upper GI test results are all normal, so the diagnosis of IBS is made by a process of elimination. Conditions that can mimic IBS are inflammatory bowel disease (Crohn's disease and ulcerative colitis); laxative abuse; overgrowth of candida; malabsorption diseases such as celiac disease; metabolic diseases such as adrenal insufficiency, diabetes, and hyperthyroidism; diverticulosis; cancer; or a chronic parasitic infection (amebiasis or giardiasis). For many people, stress is a major trigger of IBS.

Overgrowth of *Candida* (a yeast) can also cause symptoms of IBS. Everyone has yeast in the intestines, which is normally kept under control by digestive secretions and beneficial bacteria. If the number of helpful bacteria are decreased (usually through the ingestion of antibiotics, but also due to a high-sugar diet, impaired immunity, nutrient deficiency, use of drugs, and impaired liver function), candida increase in number in the intestines. An overgrowth of candida increases the risk of food allergies by increasing the permeability of the intestines, permitting large food molecules to cross the intestinal barrier, get into the bloodstream, and cause food sensitivities. Candida

overgrowth is a controversial diagnosis. While physicians admit that antibiotics, diabetes, and birth control pills favor the overgrowth of yeast, and recognize that babies with thrush (yeast infection of the mouth) typically have yeast in their intestines, many are reluctant to make or accept a diagnosis of candida overgrowth.

Gluten intolerance may mimic IBS and can present in different degrees. Gluten is a protein found in wheat, rye, barley, oats, spelt, kamut, and other closely related grains; buckwheat (which is not a grain) also contains some gluten. Corn, millet, teff, and rice do not contain gluten. In glucose-intolerant people, gluten damages the lining or villi of the small intestines, and prevents the absorption of nutrients. Gluten intolerance can cause only mild symptoms (occasional gas and bloating) or can produce celiac disease or celiac sprue, with malabsorption so severe that children with the condition do not grow properly, and adults lose weight. Patients who are gluten-intolerant are commonly also milk-intolerant. New tests are available to help in the diagnosis of gluten intolerance.

There are several other forms of malabsorption that can mimic irritable bowel syndrome. Lactose intolerance is caused by the absence of the enzyme lactase, and causes gas, bloating, pain, and chronic diarrhea. Fructose intolerance is the result of the inability of many people to properly digest fructose (the sugar found in fruits), and causes cramps and diarrhea.

Defective carbohydrate metabolism is an inability to completely break down the complex carbohydrates of beans in the small intestines. When these carbohydrates are eventually broken down by bacteria in the large intestine, carbon dioxide, hydrogen, and methane are formed, causing stomach pain, gas, and diarrhea.

Fat malabsorption creates a strong stimulus to intestinal contractions, causing people to have to defecate after eating.

Dr. Leo Galland of New York, and author of

The Four Pillars of Healing, has found that half the patients he has seen for IBS have chronic infections with *Giardia lamblia,* a common intestinal parasite. He believes that 25 percent of IBS patients in the United States may have giardiasis (see chapter 20, Parasites). Other parasitic infections, such as *Blastocystis hominis,* can also mimic IBS (see chapter 20, Parasites).

MODERN MEDICAL TREATMENT

Diet
Patients with IBS are told to increase the amount of fiber in their diets. They are also told to increase the bulk by taking a supplement such as Metamucil.

Drug Therapy
Simethecone, which is in such over-the-counter preparations as Maalox, Mylanta, and Gelusil, is suggested for the gas symptoms of IBS. Simethecone has a defoaming action that relieves gas by dispersing and preventing the formation of mucus-surrounded gas pockets in gastrointestinal disease. This drug can cause belching or the passage of large quantities of gas.

Depending on the symptoms, an antidiarrheal or antispasmodic medication may be necessary.

Diphenoxylate hydrochloride with atropine sulfate (Lomotil) is an antidiarrheal and is sometimes given for the diarrhea of IBS. Diphenoxylate hydrochloride is chemically related to the narcotic meperidine (Demerol). It is not an innocuous drug, and dosage has to be strictly watched, especially for children. In children under two years of age, overdosage can result in severe respiratory depression and coma. Because this is an addictive medication, a subtherapeutic dose of atropine is added to discourage deliberate overdosage. This can cause numbness of the extremities, itching, vomiting, abdominal discomfort, high temperature, urinary retention, flushing, dryness of the skin and mucus membranes, hives, restlessness, headaches, and cessation of normal peristalsis of the intestines.

Difenoxin hydrochloride (Motofen) is also similar to meperidine (Demerol). Motofen slows intestinal motility. Again, atropine is added to discourage deliberate overdosage. There must be strict adherence to dosage recommendations for Motofen. It is not recommended for children under two years of age, as overdosage may result in severe respiratory depression and coma. Its side effects can include dizziness, constipation, nausea, dry mouth, drowsiness, headaches, insomnia, and blurred vision.

Dicyclomine hydrochloride (Bentyl) is an antispasmodic and anticholinergic; it blocks the effect of acetylcholine on nerves, and relieves smooth muscle spasms of the gastrointestinal tract. Bentyl can cause a dry mouth, dizziness, blurred vision, nausea, nervousness, and heat stroke and fever with high environmental temperature. The drug is contraindicated for patients with obstruction of the bladder neck related to enlargement of the prostate, glaucoma, obstructive disease of the gastrointestinal tract, myasthenia gravis (a neurological disease), and hiatal hernia with inflammation of the esophagus.

Hyoscyamine sulfate (Levsin) inhibits gastrointestinal motility and decreases gastric acid secretion. It is an anticholinergic and is used for IBS, diverticulitis, and mild diarrhea. Side effects include dryness of the mouth, urinary hesitancy and retention, blurred vision, increased pressure in the eyes, weakness, nausea, vomiting, impotence, constipation, a bloated feeling, mental confusion, decreased sweating, and heat stroke and fever with high environmental temperature. Contraindications for Levsin are the same as those for Bentyl.

Donnatal is a medication that combines phenobarbital, hyoscyamine sulfate, atropine sulfate, and scopolamine hydrobromide. Side effects include dry mouth, urinary hesitancy and retention, blurred vision, fast heart rate, increased ocular pressure, headaches, insomnia, nausea, vomiting, impotence, constipation, muscle pain, and decreased sweating. Phenobarbital may produce excitement in some patients. Older patients, especially, may react with symptoms of excitement, agitation, and drowsiness, even when given small doses. Donnatol is contraindicated in patients with obstruction of the bladder neck related to an enlarged prostate, obstructive disease of the gastrointestinal tract, myasthenia gravis (a neurological disease), and hiatal hernia with inflammation of the esophagus.

Other Therapeutic Measures
Because of the emotional component of IBS, counseling is advised.

ALTERNATIVE TREATMENT

Diet
Eat small frequent meals. Avoid processed foods, preserved or prepared meats, and gum and candy sweetened with sorbitol, a sugar that is not absorbed and which causes loose stools. Avoid acid foods such as oranges, grapefruits, tomatoes, and vinegar for several weeks to see if symptoms improve. Also avoid spices to see if this helps. Many people who are food sensitive are sensitive to the aromatic chemicals in spices. Avoid alcohol, especially beer and red wine, and drink six to eight glasses of pure water a day.

Be tested for food allergies by an environmental medicine physician, or use an elimination and rechallenge diet. If food allergies are present, have appropriate treatment for them.

Add vegetables, beans, and whole grains to the diet for fiber. Use oat bran, crushed psyllium seeds (the main component of Metamucil), pectin, or 5,000 mg of guar a day.

Reduce fat in the diet by avoiding heavy sauces, fried foods, and salad oils. Fat stimulates contractions of the colon.

If you eat meat, eat organic free-range meat and poultry if possible. Animals raised in confined spaces are given massive doses of antibiotics.

Avoid foods to which you are allergic. Consider avoiding wheat fiber, because many people with IBS are sensitive to it. Eliminate sugar, fruit juices, and white flour from your diet. To reduce bowel irritability, eliminate caffeine.

Consider eliminating all forms of milk (lactose intolerance is very common, especially in Black, Hispanic, Native, Mediterranean, and Asian populations) as well as fruit, because some people are fructose intolerant.

Also avoid foods such as beans, cabbage, brussels sprouts, broccoli, cauliflower, and onions, if they cause gas for you. There are several ways to improve your tolerance for gas-producing foods. Try using an enzyme such as Beano. When preparing beans, soak them in water for four or five hours and then discard the water. Cook the beans for half an hour, and discard the water again. If you need to cook the beans longer, discard the next cooking water also. Add kombu (a sea vegetable) while cooking beans, and discard it after they are cooked. Try eating legumes sprouted, rather than cooking them.

Eat rejuvelac, miso, or sauerkraut, which are fermented and rich in enzymes that help you digest food.

Exercise and Lifestyle
Exercise, but not to the point of causing diarrhea.

Avoid running if it causes cramps. Change to another form of exercise, such as biking, swimming, or walking.

Do not smoke, and avoid tobacco in any form, including secondhand smoke.

Practice Tai Chi and Qigong daily to relieve stress.

Nutrient Therapy
Take the following nutritional supplements.

- vitamin A – 20,000 IU a day. *Caution:* Do not take more than 8,000 IU a day if you are pregnant or might be pregnant (protects mucus membranes; helps heal mucosa).

- vitamin B-complex – 50 to 100 mg three times a day (needed for proper muscle tone of gastrointestinal tract)
- calcium – 2,000 mg a day (helps "nervous stomach" and the central nervous system)
- magnesium – 1,000 mg a day (balances calcium; helps prevent colon cancer)
- zinc picolinate – 30 mg a day (helps heal inflammation)
- lipase – as directed on your product (helps digest fat)
- quercetin – 500 mg twice a day between meals (for food sensitivities; strengthens capillary walls)
- evening primrose oil – two capsules three times a day (anti-inflammatory)
- digestive enzymes – take as directed with each meal (to help digest food)
- *Lactobacillus acidophilus* – ½ to 1 tsp. three times a day. Make your own yogurt, which is high in live acidophilus (for *Candida* overgrowth; soothes the intestines; helps repopulate normal flora).
- caprylic acid – 100 to 300 mg with meals (for *Candida* overgrowth)

Herbal Therapy
Take a botanical supplement. Seek the help of a trained herbalist if you do not obtain relief.

- barberry – promotes the secretion of bile
- chamomile, passion flower, valerian, rosemary, or lemon balm teas – all are antispasmodic (but chamomile tea can be constipating)
- ginger – calms an upset stomach
- goldenseal – helps stomach ailments and is a laxative. *Caution:* Do not use if you are pregnant.
- peppermint oil – aids in healing and digestion; relieves gastrointestinal contractions and gas
- Formula SF-722 (Mycocidin) from Thorne Research – for *Candida* overgrowth (see Sources)

- ParaMicrocidin from Nutricology – for *Candida* overgrowth (see Sources)
- Pau d'arco tea – for *Candida* overgrowth

Homeopathic Remedies
Consult a homeopathic physician to help select the best remedy for your treatment. The remedies listed below are a few of the many possibilities.

- *Antimonium tartaricum* – diarrhea alternates with constipation; stool is slimy with much mucus, but also contains hard lumps; tongue coated, thick, and white; craving for acids and pickles.
- *Argentum nitricum* – great distension of the stomach with much gas; diarrhea immediately after eating or drinking; loose stools made much worse by anxiety or fear; anticipation of an ordeal, such as an exam or interview, may produce the symptoms; burping, loud and frequent enough to earn a "reputation" with friends and family; burping after eating sweets; desires sweets; forceful vomiting in morning with anxiety about the coming day.
- *Colocynthis* – painful area just below the navel; stool is loose and like jelly; severe colic pains in the abdomen are eased by bending double and pressing on the abdomen, or from local warmth, such as a hot water bottle; abdominal pains worse from anger, indignation, or excitement; abdominal pains worse before diarrhea, worse from drinking, worse from eating, worse from fruits, better from coffee.
- *Natrum sulphuricum* – loose stools, more frequent during the morning; are yellow and watery, the amount passed is huge; tight clothing around the waist causes burning sensation in the colon and abdominal pain as if bruised; diarrhea in the morning after rising; sudden urging to stool; diarrhea with gas mixed causes a sputtering stool; diarrhea from vegetables or acid foods; loud rumbling in the abdomen.

- *Nux vomica* – stomach pains, worse with anger, worse with tight clothes, better with warmth, warm applications, or warm drinks; cramping or sharp pains in abdomen; worse after eating, worse with cold; better following stool; diarrhea alternating with constipation; constant urging for stool but passes small amounts; urging for stool during urination.

Other Therapeutic Measures

Take two tablets of activated charcoal before a meal rich in gas-producing food, and two tablets afterward. Be careful, though, because activated charcoal can bind medications so they are not absorbed.

For abdominal pain, place a hot water bottle over the painful area or soak in a tub of warm water.

Practice progressive relaxation, biofeedback, self-hypnosis, or meditation to relieve stress (see Anxiety section in chapter 27, Mood Disorders). Keep a stress diary, and work on the issues that cause you to be stressed.

See a chiropractor, or have acupuncture.

Press on the following acupressure points:

- one and a half thumbs' width to each side of the second lumbar vertebra
- one and a half thumbs' width below the navel
- halfway between the lower end of the breastbone and the navel, exactly in the midline
- two thumbs' width to each side of the navel
- three thumbs' width below the joint under the kneecap lying on the outer side of the knee
- one finger's width back from the sharp edge of the shin bone
- below the inside of the kneecap and below the top of the tibia. This point is usually tender when pressed with a finger tip.

Take one of the following substances:

- buffered vitamin C – 1,000 mg every 15 to 30 minutes (for acute abdominal pain)

- "Magic Brew" (1 tsp. baking soda and 1 tsp. sea salt in 1 quart of water) – drink 1 cup chilled, to be sipped gradually (soothes abdominal pain and nausea)
- Alka-Seltzer Gold – one tablet in water (for abdominal pain)
- Bi-Carb Formula from Klaire Laboratories – one to three capsules, as needed (for abdominal pain) (see Sources)

DIARRHEA

Diarrhea is the passage of unformed, loose, or watery stools. Stools that are frequent but solid are not considered to be diarrhea. Diarrhea can be acute or chronic, and can be a mild or severe condition. Diarrhea usually lasts from one to ten days. If it is accompanied by fever and severe abdominal cramps, blood or pus in the stools, or jaundice, contact your physician.

Diarrhea is often a way for the body to get rid of some type of toxin. If the course of diarrhea is halted, the illness can be prolonged, so it is often better to let the diarrhea run its course. Especially in children and infants, the main worry with diarrhea is the risk of dehydration, which is what makes diarrhea the leading cause of death of children in developing countries. Signs of dehydration include dry-looking sunken eyes, skin that stays tented when pulled up, dry mouth, decreased urination (no urination for 10 to 12 hours), and lack of tears when crying.

CAUSES OF DIARRHEA

Acute diarrhea is usually caused by bacterial or viral infections of the gastrointestinal tract; by eating a food to which you are sensitive; by food poisoning; or by overeating some kinds of food, such as fruit. Acute or chronic diarrhea can be caused by excessive vitamin C intake, excessive magnesium intake, excessive laxative intake or laxative abuse, fat or carbohydrate malabsorption, inflammatory bowel disease (Crohn's disease or ulcerative colitis), antibiotics, tumors of the bowel, surgical removal of a large part of the intestine, excess fiber, alcoholism, menstrual periods (because of hormones the body secretes), AIDS, cystic fibrosis, diabetes, irritable bowel syndrome, radiation treatment for a cancer in the lower abdomen, chronic stress, subclinical thiamine deficiency, various medications, antacids, quinidine, or toxins secreted by bacteria. The excessive intake of non-absorbable sugars can also cause diarrhea. Those that most commonly cause malabsorption are milk sugars, fructose, beans, mannitol, and sorbitol.

"Traveler's diarrhea" is thought to be caused by the ingestion of unfamiliar intestinal bacterial flora in the food and water supply of foreign countries. If you travel in Latin America, South America, Asia, or Africa, do not drink the water or eat the food unless you peel it, boil it, or otherwise cook it. Make sure that you eat food just after it has been prepared. Do not drink bottled water or soda pop with ice cubes made from local water. Do not brush your teeth with the local water. If you have diarrhea for more than seven days, see a physician. You may have a parasitic infection (*Entamoeba histolytica* or *Giardia lamblia*).

Some children have painful, hard bowel movements. This sets up a vicious cycle. They hold their bowel movements to avoid pain, and become more constipated as the stools become larger and more painful to pass. These children then develop impacted stools, and have loose stools that leak around the impaction. Parents think the children have diarrhea and are not aware that these children are in fact constipated (see treatment for constipation, below).

Lactose intolerance, caused by a lack of the enzyme lactase, is one of the most common causes of chronic diarrhea. Lactose intolerance causes gas, bloating, pain, and diarrhea. People with this condition often react to even a small amount of lactose. Approximately 70 to 90 percent of Asian, Black, Native American, His-

panic, and Mediterranean adults lack this enzyme, compared to 10 to 15 percent of western Europeans. Yogurt and aged cheeses contain the enzyme lactase, which helps break down lactose.

Chronic diarrhea in children is often related to drinking too much fruit juice. Fruit juice contains sugars that are often poorly absorbed by children, and hence cause diarrhea. Pear juice (which contains sorbitol) seems to be the worst offender, but apple juice (which has fructose) can cause a problem too. In some children, as little as one teaspoon of juice in a day can trigger diarrhea. Drinking any cold fluids can often cause diarrhea too.

MODERN MEDICAL TREATMENT

Diet
Patients are told to avoid eating poorly absorbed carbohydrates (bread, pasta, other wheat products, pears, prunes, corn, beans, cabbage, Brussels sprouts, and oats). They are also told to avoid coffee, which is an irritant to the bowel.

Drug Therapy
Lomotil (diphenoxylate hydrochloride with atropine sulfate) is an antidiarrheal that is frequently prescribed for recurring diarrhea as well as for the diarrhea of IBS. Difenoxin hydrochloride is also used for diarrhea, and it slows intestinal motility. Motofen is difenoxin hydrochloride with atropine sulfate (see Irritable Bowel Syndrome, above, for the side effects of these drugs).

Codeine is a narcotic that also slows intestinal motility. It can cause lightheadedness, dizziness, sedation, shortness of breath, nausea and vomiting, allergic reactions, euphoria, constipation, abdominal pain, and itching. Drug dependence can occur with any narcotic.

Antacids that contain aluminum hydroxide (Amphogel or Alternagel) are sometimes taken for diarrhea as they can cause constipation—but they can also cause diarrhea. They can cause malabsorption of nutrients (in particular iron, vitamin B_{12}, folic acid, and calcium). Antacids cause the intestines to become alkaline, and allow pathogenic bacteria to overgrow. The kidneys have to excrete extra alkaline to maintain the acid/base balance of the body. Antacids can lead to kidney stones and urinary tract infections because of the acid/base imbalance.

Pepto-Bismol is used for indigestion, for diarrhea, and as a preventative against traveler's diarrhea. When traveling, patients are advised to take two chewable tablets of Pepto-Bismol four times a day to prevent traveler's diarrhea (see Peptic Ulcer Disease, Stomach Aches, and Abdominal Pain for side effects). If you develop traveler's diarrhea, you will be told to take one tablet every hour, or take a prescription antidiarrheal medication (Lomotil, Motofen, or codeine), or an antibiotic such as a sulfa drug.

Kaopectate is commonly used to control diarrhea. It contains Kaolin (a type of clay) and pectin (a type of fiber). It can cause nausea and constipation. Imodium (loperamide hydrochloride) slows intestinal motility and affects water and electrolyte movement through the intestines. Side effects include constipation, nervous system depression, and nausea.

Other Therapeutic Measures

To avoid dehydration patients are told to drink an electrolyte fluid, such as Pedialyte, Lytren, or ReSol. After drinking clear fluids, they are told to progress to bananas, rice, applesauce, and yogurt as the diarrhea clears.

They are cautioned to wash their hands thoroughly if they are taking care of someone who has diarrhea, or if they have diarrhea themselves.

ALTERNATIVE TREATMENT

Diet

Drink plenty of liquids, mainly pure water. Also drink rice or barley water, made by boiling 1 cup of rice or barley in 4½ cups of water. Boil for 45 minutes and strain off the water. Add a little sugar and drink.

Drink Recharge, a balanced electrolyte solution. Also drink sauerkraut and tomato juice, mixed in equal parts. Cabbage juice helps heal intestinal lesions.

Eat a high-fiber diet, and include oat bran and rice bran. Increase your intake of fluid when you increase fiber.

Avoid milk and ice cream as well as alcohol, caffeine, and spicy foods. Do not consume any dairy products, as the enzyme needed to digest them is temporarily lost during diarrhea. Restrict intake of fats and gluten grains such as barley, oats, rye, and wheat. Be careful to avoid any foods to which you are sensitive.

For children with chronic diarrhea, remove fruit juices from the child's diet.

Observe modern medical dietary suggestions as well.

Exercise and Lifestyle

Do not exercise when you have acute diarrhea. Wait until you have recovered to resume your regular exercise program.

Nutrient Therapy

Take the following nutritional supplements.

- *Lactobacillus acidophilus* – ½ to 1 tsp. a day. Eat yogurt with live cultures. Take acidophilus before you travel and while traveling (replaces normal bacteria).
- pectin – 1 Tbsp. three times a day (helps bind stools together)
- whey – as directed on the label of your product (helps heal intestines)
- B-complex – 50 mg of each B vitamin. Some people have an extra need for vitamin B_1, especially if the diet is high in refined carbohydrates (helps heal intestines; necessary for digestion and absorption of nutrients).

Herbal Therapy
Take a botanical supplement.

- aloe vera gel – soothes inflamed intestines
- blackberry root – long-standing remedy for diarrhea
- goldenseal – has a significant antibiotic effect against the bacteria and parasites that cause diarrhea. It can also be used prophylactically for a week before and after a trip to prevent traveler's diarrhea. *Caution:* Do not take if you are pregnant.

Use Robert's formula, a complex herbal preparation: ¼ to ½ tsp. (or one to two "oo" capsules) between meals, three times a day. This preparation contains the following herbs:

- althea – for soothing mucus membranes
- comfrey – an anti-inflammatory; promotes wound healing
- echinacea – an antibacterial and immune stimulant
- goldenseal – inhibits the growth of bacteria and parasites. *Caution:* Do not take if you are pregnant.
- pokeweed – heals ulcerations of the intestinal mucosa
- slippery elm – a demulcent that soothes irritated mucus membranes
- spotted cranesbill – stops bleeding in the intestinal tract
- wild indigo – for gastrointestinal infections

Homeopathic Remedies
Take the homeopathic remedy that best fits your symptoms. If your diarrhea does not stop, consult a homeopathic practitioner. The remedies listed below are but a few of the many possibilities.

- *Arsenicum album* – for food poisoning with vomiting; worse during the night (midnight to 3 A.M.); rectum feels burned by watery diarrhea; thirst for small, warm drinks; restlessness and anxiety; diarrhea with acrid, offensive, watery stool; diarrhea worse from cold drinks, worse from ice cream, worse from fruit.
- *Chamomilla* – worse in the evening; stool is frothy, offensive, and greenish like cut grass or spinach; patient is restless and irritable; diarrhea during teething; stool with "rotten egg" odor, thirsty for cold drinks.
- *China officinalis* – painless, watery, offensive, yellow stools; extreme weakness; diarrhea after eating excessive fruit; diarrhea worse from fish, milk; anorexia.
- *Mercurius solubilis* – acute gastroenteritis with strong urging for diarrhea and the "never get done" sensation; stool offensive; craving bread and butter.
- *Podophyllum* – profuse, spluttery, watery, pasty, yellowish, diarrhea; worse in the early morning; painless stool is extremely offensive; followed by a weakness of the rectum; explosive diarrhea, soils the whole toilet bowl; gurgling in the abdomen before stool.
- *Veratrum album* – diarrhea with vomiting; patient is icy cold with cold sweat; asks for large amounts of cold drinks; desire to be in the cold, fresh air; patient may faint after defecation; profuse, watery stools preceded by abdominal pain.

Many patients respond to complex homeopathic remedies. You may want to try BHI Diarrhea to relieve your symptoms (see Sources section at back of book).

Other Therapeutic Measures
Evaluate medications and artificial sweeteners that you are using to see if they may have caused your diarrhea. Medications such as antacids (Maalox and Mylanta) as well as quinidine, lactulose, and colchicine can often cause diarrhea.

Press on the following acupressure points:

- one and a half thumbs' width below the navel
- two thumbs' width to each side of the navel
- three thumbs' width below the joint under the kneecap, on the outer side of the knee, and one finger's width back from the sharp edge of the bone
- one hand's width (four fingers) up from the inner ankle joint, just behind the tibia bone.

Have acupuncture treatments, or get NAET treatments for allergies contributing to your diarrhea (see Chiropractic section in chapter 9, Alternative Medical Disciplines).

Make your own rehydration solution by adding 1 tsp. of sugar and a pinch of salt to 1 quart of water.

CONSTIPATION

Constipation is the passage of dry, hard stools. Difficulty passing stools is also known as constipation, although it is more correctly designated as obstipation. Constipation is the leading disorder of the digestive tract; people over 65 are five times more likely to have problems with constipation than are younger people. If you suddenly develop constipation, have abdominal cramps, and cannot pass stool or gas, see a doctor immediately. This could be caused by a tumor blocking the intestine, or by a stool impaction.

The most common cause of constipation is the Standard American Diet (see Diet section in chapter 10, Alternative Therapies). Some other causes of constipation include drinking insufficient fluid, eating too little fiber, lack of exercise, laxative/enema abuse, taking medications that can slow down bowel transit time (narcotics, cholesterol-lowering medications, antidepressants, beta blockers, iron pills, diuretics, muscle relaxants), toxic metal poisoning (lead, arsenic, mercury), irritable bowel syndrome, hypothyroidism, diverticulosis, nerve disorders of the bowel, neurological disorders (Parkinsonism,

strokes), organophosphate pesticide exposure, aging, voluntary stool withholding because of painful defecation, or bowel tumors.

Naturopathic physicians feel that diabetes mellitus, meningitis, myasthenia gravis, thyroid disease, ulcerative colitis, and rheumatoid arthritis are associated with antigens and toxins absorbed from intestinal bacteria, made more likely by slow transit time of the stool through the intestine. It is difficult to define the "normal" number of stools a person should pass. Most alternative physicians feel that two to three stools a day is normal, but many modern physicians feel that daily stools are neither normal nor necessary.

MODERN MEDICAL TREATMENT

Diet

Patients are told to eat foods high in fiber, especially fruits and vegetables, six to eight servings a day. They are told to drink prune juice daily as well as eight glasses of fluid (preferably water) every day.

Exercise and Lifestyle

Patients are advised to exercise for 20 minutes, three times a week.

They are also told to set aside a time to have a stool daily.

Drug Therapy

Over 40 million Americans take laxatives, and 1 percent of doctor's prescriptions are for laxatives. Laxatives can cause gas, diarrhea, and rebound constipation. They can decrease transit time and cause malabsorption of nutrients, especially minerals and vitamin D. All laxatives (except the bulking agents) are habit-forming. If people use them frequently, their bowels can become sluggish, and they can become dependent upon these preparations.

Different kinds of laxatives have different mechanisms of action.

- Bulk-forming laxatives, such as Metamucil, work by absorbing water into the bowel, making the stool larger, softer, and easier to evacuate. Metamucil contains colors and additives, and some people can become sensitized to it. If Metamucil is added to water and not drunk soon afterward, it will form a big clump, which can block the esophagus. If not taken with sufficient water, bulk-forming laxatives can make constipation worse.

- Hydrophilic and osmotic laxatives, such as Milk of Magnesia, cause water to be secreted into the large intestine, and decrease water reabsorption into the body. They are typically salts containing phosphates, citrates, magnesium, and sulfates. *Caution:* Do not use this kind of laxative if you have kidney disease, high blood pressure, or heart failure.

- Lubricant laxatives soften the stool and allow it to be passed more readily. Mineral oil is a common lubricant and laxative, but it interferes with the absorption of fat-soluble vitamins; it also leaks between bowel movements, and is very messy. If a person has difficulty swallowing (for instance, a child who is neurologically damaged or an older adult), mineral oil can be accidentally inhaled into the lungs and can cause pneumonia.

- Stool softeners, such as docusate sodium, moisten the stool and prevent it from becoming too hard and dry. They are useful for people who have painful hemorrhoids or cracks in the anus, and after childbirth. Stool softeners coat the lining of the bowel and prevent absorption of vitamins and minerals. Some ingredients in stool softeners are absorbed from the bowel, and no one knows what the long-term effects may be.

- Contact stimulants or irritant laxatives cause rhythmic contractions in the small or large intestines. Castor oil is the most common ingredient in irritant laxatives, and it can damage the lining of the intestinal tract. Other stimulants include Ex-Lax, in which the main ingredient is phenolphthalein, and Dulcolax. If chewed, Dulcolax can damage the lining of the mouth and the upper intestinal tract on contact. The suppository form of Dulcolax can cause rectal irritation and cramps. Other stimulants may contain senna, aloe, and cascara, which can color urine brown or violet.

- Suppositories are also used as laxatives. They are inserted into the rectum where they melt or are softened at body temperature. Glycerin suppositories work by irritating the lining of the rectum, causing the reflex that results in a stool. They take about half an hour to work. They can cause burning and pain in the rectum.

Patients are told to take a laxative, but for no longer than two weeks. Metamucil, antacids, Ex-Lax, Dulcolax, and Neoloid (castor oil) are common medications used. Stool softeners, such as docusate (Colace), are also used. Mineral oil is sometimes given, but not at the same time as a stool softener, because it will cause absorption of the mineral oil. A glycerin suppository, or a plain tap water enema, may be suggested.

ALTERNATIVE TREATMENT

Diet

Eat foods that are high in fiber, especially fruits and vegetables: six to eight servings a day. Eat corn bran, wheat bran, or oat bran (¼ to ½ cup a day), if you are not sensitive to any of those foods. Eat fresh rhubarb and drink prune juice or eat figs daily.

Drink at least 10 glasses of fluid (preferably water) every day. For acute constipation drink a large glass of water every 10 minutes for half an hour. This can flush out toxins and relieve constipation.

Avoid dairy foods, salt, coffee, sugar, processed foods, soft drinks, alcohol, meat, and white flour. In addition to having little fiber, these foods are difficult to digest. Do not eat fried foods, fats, and spicy foods.

Eat foods that are high in pectin, including apples, carrots, beets, bananas, cabbage, citrus fruits, dried peas, and okra.

Exercise and Lifestyle

Set aside a time each day to have a stool, preferably after breakfast or after exercise. Retrain the intestine; do not repress an urge to have a bowel movement.

Exercise regularly for 20 minutes, three times a week, as physical activity encourages the movement of waste through the intestines.

Nutrient Therapy

Take a nutritional supplement to help correct constipation.

- folic acid – 2 to 5 mg a day (deficiency results in constipation)
- vitamin C – 1,000 mg every hour up to the point of loose stools (bowel tolerance) (will encourage regular bowel movements)
- calcium – 1,000 mg a day (needed for proper muscular contraction)
- magnesium – 400 to 800 mg a day; an extra 500 mg capsule at bedtime will encourage a morning bowel movement (balances calcium)
- *Lactobacillus acidophilus* – 1 tsp. twice a day (helps survival and rapid passage of "good" bacteria into the small intestine)
- pectin – 500 mg a day (source of fiber that helps relieve constipation)

Herbal Therapy

Take one of the following botanical supplements, all of which have a laxative effect.

- dandelion or senna tea in small doses
- goldenseal, buckthorn bark, flax or linseed oil, or psyllium – 1 Tbsp. in a large glass of water daily. *Caution:* Buckthorn should not

be used for long periods of time. Do not take goldenseal if you are pregnant.
- rhubarb, in pills or as a tea (unless you are prone to calcium kidney stones)
- psyllium in the form of Konsyl, which does not contain either sugar or aspartame – 1 to 2 rounded tsp., after meals in a full glass of water

Homeopathic Remedies

Take the following homepathic remedy that best fits your symptoms. If you do not obtain relief from your constipation, seek the help of a homepathic physician. The remedies listed below are but a few of the many possibilities.

- *Alumina* – severe constipation, usually without urge for stool; constipation so stubborn that the patient must assist the evacuation with fingers; constipation during pregnancy with great dryness of the rectum; constipation with soft stool; constipation of newborns.
- *Calcarea carbonica* – constipation without an urge for stool; patient feels no ill effects from constipation; clay-like stool.
- *Causticum* – constipation better from standing; stool covered with mucus; rectal fissure.
- *Graphites* – constipation with large, hard stool; stool stays in rectum with no urge to expel it; sensation of trapped gas; rectal itching; hemorrhoids.
- *Nux vomica* – constipation with constant, ineffectual urging for stool; small amounts are passed which temporarily relieves the urging only to return moments later; constipation in children with hard, painful stool; the child fears going for stool; hemorrhoids; pains better with warmth, better after stool.
- *Ruta graveolens* – constipation alternating with mucus, frothy stools, discharge of blood with stool; difficult feces, evacuated only with straining; rectal prolapse.

Many patients respond to complex homeopathic remedies. You may want to try BHI Constipation, which helps relieve constipation (see Sources).

Other Therapeutic Measures
Do a colon cleanse every six months by using the following procedure.

Add 1 Tbsp. of psyllium seed husks to 8 ounces of water; shake well in a jar and drink immediately. Then drink 8 ounces of water followed by 4 ounces of bentonite solution (Somes #7 from NEEDS—see Sources). Repeat three times a day, between meals, a total of 15 times.

Avoid calcium carbonate (Tums), as it is constipating.

Press the following acupressure points:

- on the side of the bone which runs from the forefinger knuckle down toward the wrist
- one finger's width up from the web between the big toe and the second toe tendons
- two thumbs' width to each side of the navel.

Have acupuncture or NAET treatments for allergies that may be contributing to your constipation (see Chiropractic section in chapter 9, Alternative Medical Disciplines). Consult an Ayurvedic physician, or Chinese medicine physician.

Take a cleansing enema, but only if constipation is persistent. Use laxatives if necessary, but take acidophilus to replace "friendly" bacteria.

If constipation becomes constant, have a proctoscopic exam or barium enema radiology procedure to rule out bowel cancer and obstruction of the lower bowel.

DIVERTICULOSIS

Diverticulosis is a condition in which the walls of the large intestine weaken and balloon out, forming pouches called diverticula, which are most often located in the lowest part of the large intestine, the sigmoid colon. Diverticulosis is related to constipation; the stool is unusually dry and difficult to move. The diverticula may become inflamed and infected when food particles and bacteria are trapped in them. This can cause an attack of diverticulitis, which is the most severe form of diverticulosis. Complications from diverticulitis can be fatal.

Many people develop diverticula without being aware of it. By age 60, more than half of all Americans have diverticulosis, although it was very rare in the early 1900s and is rare today in Africa and Asia. The main cause is a diet high in meat and refined foods, and low in fiber.

Symptoms of diverticulosis include bloating and constipation alternating with diarrhea, nausea, and pain in the lower left quadrant. Because of this pain, diverticulosis is sometimes referred to as "left-sided appendicitis." The pain worsens with stress, after meals, and when passing gas. With diverticulitis there may be vomiting, fever, chills, and rectal bleeding.

MODERN MEDICAL TREATMENT
Diet
Increasing dietary fiber is very helpful in preventing and treating diverticulosis. However, do not suddenly switch from a low-fiber diet to a high-fiber diet, as this can cause gas and bloating. Dietary fiber consists of soluble fiber and insoluble fiber. Soluble fiber dissolves in water and is found in fruit; beans, peas, and other legumes; psyllium; rice; and oats. Soluble fiber decreases the cholesterol levels in the blood. Wheat cereal contains insoluble fiber, which pulls water into the intestines, causes the stools to be softer and heavier, and increases transit time.

Patients are advised to change to a high-fiber diet that is low in sugar and fat, and to avoid whole nuts, seeds, and fruits and vegetables with tiny pits or seeds.

Exercise and Lifestyle
Patients with diverticulosis are advised to exercise regularly.

Drug Therapy

Patients who develop diverticulitis are given antibiotics. (See Strep Throat in chapter 13, Respiratory System Problems, for a discussion of antibiotics.)

ALTERNATIVE TREATMENT

If you develop diverticulitis, you will likely need to take antibiotics. The following alternative measures should be followed whether or not you take medication.

Diet

Control your diverticulosis with adequate fiber and lots of pure water. Change to a high-fiber diet that is low in sugar and fat. Avoid foods with small seeds or pits, and foods that are difficult to digest. Also do not eat nuts or grains except for well-cooked brown rice. Do not eat sugar, fried foods, dairy products, red meats, spices, or processed foods.

Eat a low-carbohydrate diet with high levels of protein from fish and fiber from vegetables. Also eat green leafy vegetables that contain vitamin K, which is important for intestinal disorders.

After an attack of diverticulitis, do a vegetable juice fast for one to three days. Then eat a soft-fiber diet for a week, eating steamed root vegetables, or vegetable soups mixed in the blender. After this, eat beans, cooked leafy green vegetables, oats, miso, and agar.

Exercise and Lifestyle

Perform aerobic exercise for 20 minutes three times a week, or take a brisk walk outdoors daily. Activity reduces diverticulosis and walking outdoors boosts vitamin D.

Nutrient Therapy

Take the following nutrients.

- vitamin A – 25,000 IU a day. *Caution:* Do not exceed 8,000 IU a day if you are pregnant or might be pregnant (heals and protects the lining of the colon).
- B-complex vitamins – 100 mg three times a day (needed for proper digestion)
- vitamin C – 3,000 to 8,000 mg a day in divided doses (reduces inflammation; boosts immune system)
- vitamin E – 800 IU a day (protects mucus membranes; antioxidant)
- vitamin K – 100 mcg a day (deficiency linked to intestinal disorders)
- proteolytic enzymes – as directed on label, between meals (helps digestion; reduces inflammation)
- *Lactobacillus acidophilus* – up to 3 tsp. a day in divided doses (recolonizes intestines with "good" bacteria)
- flaxseed oil – as directed on the label three times a day or ground flaxseed, 1 to 3 tsp. three times a day (anti-inflammatory; helps protect cells lining the walls of the colon)

Herbal Therapy

Take the following botanical supplements.

- aloe vera gel – 2 to 4 Tbsp. of the gel a day in divided doses (soothes inflamed intestines)
- chlorophyll capsules or liquid – as directed on the label of your product (prevents inflammation; heals colon)
- DGL (deglycyrrhizined licorice) – two to four 380 mg tablets between meals, or 20 minutes before meals (stimulates normal defense mechanisms that prevent inflammation)
- garlic – one capsule of odorless garlic, three times a day (a natural antibiotic)
- Robert's formula – see Diarrhea, above (heals intestines)
- slippery elm bark, comfrey, or mullein as a tea, 1 to 3 cups a day (soothes inflamed mucus membranes of intestines). *Caution:* Do not drink comfrey tea for long periods of time.

Homeopathic Remedies

Take the homeopathic remedy that best matches your symptoms. The remedies listed below are a few of the possibilities. If you do not obtain relief, seek the help of a homeopathic physician.

- *Belladonna* – pain and cramping along the transverse colon; pains aggravated by touch, better from general, firm pressure.
- *Bryonia* – pain worse from motion, worse after eating, worse after vomiting, worse from dietary indiscretions, better with heat.
- *Colocynthis* – abdominal pain helped by pressure, by lying face down, by bending double; pains worse from anger, indignation, or excitement; severe cutting, cramping pains in the abdomen; cramps radiating to the pubic region; cramping around the umbilicus.

Other Therapeutic Measures

Get massage therapy. Apply wet, hot compresses to abdomen and lower back to stimulate intestinal action.

Because food allergies or sensitivities, especially milk allergy, can cause constipation, be tested and treated for food sensitivity by an environmental physician. Have NAET or EPD treatments for food allergy (see Chiropractic section in chapter 9, Alternative Medical Disciplines).

Use the following mixture: soak 1 Tbsp. of a mixture of psyllium, bentonite, and myrrh in a cup of water with raisins and prunes. The next morning, combine the mixture with grated, peeled apples and pears to taste, and eat.

Press on the following acupressure points:

- one and a half thumbs' width to each side of the second lumbar vertebrae
- on the side of the bone which runs from the forefinger knuckle down toward the wrist
- halfway between the lower end of the breastbone and the navel, exactly in the midline
- two thumbs' width to each side of the navel

- just below the inside of the kneecap and below the top of the tibia. This point is usually tender when pressed with a finger tip.

HEMORRHOIDS

Hemorrhoids (also known as piles) are enlarged veins or varicose veins around the anus. Hemorrhoids can be caused by weakness of the veins, straining to produce a stool, standing or sitting for long periods of time, and heavy lifting. The veins swell under pressure, and straining to expel the stool leads to internal hemorrhoids (inside the rectum) or external hemorrhoids (under the skin around the anus). Either kind causes bright red, painless bleeding during defecation, and external hemorrhoids may itch.

Hemorrhoids are common during pregnancy, and they affect half of all Americans by age 50. They are rarely seen in parts of the world where people eat a high-fiber, whole food diet.

MODERN MEDICAL TREATMENT

Diet

Patients with hemorrhoids are advised to add fiber to their diet.

Drug Therapy

Hemorrhoids are usually treated with external steroids.

Surgery

If hemorrhoids remain a problem, laser surgery, cryosurgery, or ligation (tying off hemorrhoids) is performed.

Other Therapeutic Measures

Patients are advised to cleanse the rectum after defecation and to take warm sitz baths, alternating with ice packs.

ALTERNATIVE TREATMENT

Diet

Include plenty of fiber in your diet, eating vegetables, fruits, beans, and grains. Eat blackberries, cherries, and blueberries to strengthen the veins. Include psyllium and guar gum in your diet, as they have a laxative effect.

Avoid fats and minimize animal products, which are hard on the intestines. If your hemorrhoids bleed, eat dark green leafy vegetables, alfalfa, and blackstrap molasses. These foods are high in vitamin K.

Drink six to eight glasses of pure water a day. Water is a natural stool softener and helps prevent constipation that can aggravate hemorrhoids.

Exercise and Lifestyle

Do Kegel exercises. Practice by stopping your urination in midstream, tightening and then relaxing the muscles. Do the exercises 30 times, two to three times a day.

Do exercise that is vigorous enough to raise your pulse to 220 minus your age × 60 percent. (For example, a 40-year-old should attain a pulse rate of 108: 220–40 = 180 × 60% = 108.)

Nutrient Therapy

- vitamin A – 10,000 IU a day. *Caution:* Do not exceed 8,000 IU a day if you are or might be pregnant (aids in healing mucus membranes and tissues; heals hemorrhoids).
- vitamin B-complex – 50 to 100 mg three times a day (vital for good digestion, which takes stress off rectum; helps heal hemorrhoids)
- vitamin C – 3,000 to 5,000 mg a day (aids in healing and blood clotting)
- vitamin D – 400 IU a day (aids in healing mucus membranes; needed for calcium)
- vitamin E – 600 IU a day (promotes healing and blood clotting)
- calcium – 1,500 mg a day (necessary for blood clotting)
- magnesium – 750 to 800 mg a day (needed to balance calcium)
- potassium – 99 mg a day (constipation common in deficiency; causes hemorrhoids)

- zinc – 15 mg a day (heals inflamed tissue)
- bioflavonoids – 100 mg a day (aids in healing and normal blood clotting)
- coenzyme Q_{10} – 100 mg a day (increases cellular oxygenation; improves healing)
- flaxseed oil – 1 to 2 Tbsp. a day (softens stools)

Herbal Therapy

Use the following botanical supplements.

- stoneroot – as a cream, externally or internally; or stoneroot and witch hazel in a solution, applied externally – eases itching and irritation
- witch hazel, goldenseal, plantain, Solomon's seal, white oak bark, bayberry, yellow dock, yarrow, spearmint, comfrey, chickweed, wheatgrass, horse chestnut, or mullein – as a tea eases itching and irritation
- butcher's broom – eases itching and irritation
- equal parts of stoneroot, cranesbill, and ginkgo – for internal relief
- salves of calendula, aloe, or plantain, applied externally – helps heal hemorrhoids

Homeopathic Remedies

Take the homeopathic remedy that best fits your symptoms. If you do not obtain relief, consult a homeopathic practitioner. The remedies listed below are but a few of the possibilities.

- *Aesculus* – sensation of splinters in the rectum; aching in the lower part of the back; purple hemorrhoids; burning, itching, dryness of the anus.
- *Arsenicum album* – bluish-colored hemorrhoids; burning pain.
- *Capsicum* – bleeding hemorrhoids; anal burning, itching, smarting, and stinging during defecation.
- *Collinsonia* – sensation of sticks in the rectum; constipation from bowel inertia; itching around the anus; hemorrhoids during pregnancy.

- *Graphites* – hemorrhoids protrude, burn, and sting; worse when sitting.
- *Hamamelis* – hemorrhoids with copious bleeding; excessive soreness, the anus feels raw.
- *Nux vomica* – large hemorrhoids; burning, stinging, constricted sensation in the rectum; bruised pain in the small of the back; itching that prevents sleep; cold-water applications relieve the itch; with bleeding and a constant desire to defecate.

Many patients respond to complex homeopathic remedies. You may want to try PHP Hemorrhoid Drops, which provides support for the itching, pain, and bleeding of hemorrhoids.

Other Therapeutic Measures
Take warm sitz baths, at a temperature of 100° to 105°F.

Do not read while you sit on the toilet. The longer you sit, the more the veins will swell.

Crouch on the toilet (with both feet on the porcelain rim) and keep your head forward while having a bowel movement.

To avoid putting pressure on the rectum, and developing hard stools, which aggravate the condition, do not delay elimination.

Avoid hemorrhoid-reducing over-the-counter remedies. Most do not work, and the FDA has recently banned the key ingredient in the most popular hemorrhoid-reducing ointment. Instead, use zinc oxide cream or vitamin E capsules on hemorrhoids.

Take a plain water enema to relieve discomfort.

Press on the following acupuncture points:

- directly behind the knee joint in the center of the crease
- right at the base of the spine below the tip of the coccyx, midway toward the anus
- right at the top of the head where two imaginary lines cross, one drawn from the top of one ear to the top of the other ear, the other line drawn from the top of the nose right over the top of the skull to the back of the skull.

CHAPTER 20

Parasites

Parasites are organisms that take up residence, either temporarily or permanently, on or within another organism for the purpose of obtaining food. The parasite obtains the benefit from the association, receiving food and shelter from its host. At times the relationship between a parasite and a host may be mutual, where both organisms benefit, or it may be commensal, where one partner benefits and the other is unaffected. In some cases, the parasite will cause disease in the host.

Many modern medicine practitioners consider parasites to be a thing of the past, a problem that exists only in developing countries, or at worst, a very minor problem in North America. Unfortunately this is not true, and parasitic infections are a type of "silent epidemic." Over 500 million people worldwide are infected with parasites, and three out of five North Americans will be infected by parasites at some time in their lives. Dr. Leo Galland of New York, and author of *Four Pillars of Healing*, estimates that at least 10 percent of all Americans have parasites.

SPREAD OF PARASITES

Parasitic diseases have no geographical boundaries, and make no distinctions of class or gender. They have been carried all over the world by travelers, immigrants, and armed forces members returning from overseas. The increase in daycare centers contributes to the spread of parasites, and many sources of water (municipal, rural, and natural) are now contaminated. Many people have pets, some of them from other countries, and these animals, too, can be a reservoir for parasites, as can wild animals. Consumption of foods prepared by people carrying parasites, and the sexual revolution are other major factors in the spread of parasitic disease. The wide range of exposure complicates diagnosis of parasitic disease, and parasitic symptoms can also mimic those of other diseases. Unfortunately, most physicians do not consider parasites as a possibility when they are diagnosing their patients' problems.

Although parasites are distributed worldwide, the humidity and moisture of the tropics assures their abundance in those areas. Moisture is essential for parasites with free living stages; short summers and low temperatures arrest the development of larvae and eggs. Economic and social conditions that include low standards of living, lack of information, and inadequate personal and community sanitation encourage the prevalence and spread of parasites.

The spread of parasites requires:

• a source of infection. Sources of infection are many and varied; contaminated air, water, food, dirt, and dust are primary sources of infection. Household pets and wild animals can transmit many of their parasites to humans.

- a mode of transmission. Transmission takes place through direct contact; indirect contact; contaminated air, food, or water; soil; and vertebrate and invertebrate (insect) vectors, a living carrier that transports the parasite to its new host. In rare cases, parasites may be transmitted from mother to child.
- the presence of a suitable host. Humans may be the only host, the main host, or an incidental host, with animals as the principal host.

SYMPTOMS OF PARASITIC INFECTIONS

People can have parasites for years without being aware of them and experiencing few or no symptoms. These people become carriers. When symptoms do occur, they can easily be attributed to another cause. Many parasites have incredible longevity, some worms being capable of persisting in the intestine for 20 to 30 years.

In other cases, the infection is acute, and people may have serious symptoms. People who have the following symptoms should be tested for parasites:

- bloating and excessive gas
- diarrhea, colitis, dysentery, and chronic bowel symptoms
- alternating diarrhea and constipation
- chronic constipation
- abnormal stool formation and appearance (floating, frothy, blood-tinged, mucus-laden, or crumbling)
- chronic or unexplained fatigue
- nutrient malabsorption and metabolism disruption
- increased food intolerance
- allergic responses
- night sweats, fever
- asthma
- teeth grinding
- sleep disturbances
- skin problems

- rheumatologic symptoms (which may be an immunologic response in the joints to intestinal parasites)
- eosinophilia (an increase in specific white blood cells)

Major health problems can be caused by even mild parasitic infections. Although digestive symptoms are frequently present, it is important to remember that digestive symptoms may not be the predominant feature in parasitic infections. These infections may present as aching joints and muscles, fatigue, and chronic asthma. Parasitic infections may contribute to a variety of major diseases, including arthritis, Crohn's disease, rheumatoid symptoms, chronic fatigue syndrome, ulcerative colitis, and AIDS.

A number of digestive complaints, not formerly attributed to parasites, are now being linked both to past and present parasitic infections. Dr. Galland found that nearly half of his patients with irritable bowel syndrome were relieved of their symptoms when they were treated for parasites. In a 1990 study by Dr. Galland and his colleagues, 46 percent of 96 patients with chronic fatigue syndrome (CFS) were shown to be infected with *Giardia lamblia*. Dr. P. H. Levine in the *Archives of Internal Medicine* in 1992, reported the results of studies in four clusters of chronic fatigue syndrome. In one cluster in a California town, a CFS epidemic occurred at the same time as a *Giardia* epidemic.

COMMON PARASITES

Parasites of medical importance include protozoa (usually one-celled, microscopic animals), and helminths (worms). The severity of illness depends on the number of parasites, their tissue specificity, and the mechanisms and type of tissue damage they produce. Damage to the host is caused by:

- the sheer numbers of parasites as they multiply

- mechanical damage as vessels are obstructed
- destruction of host cells by parasitic invasion
- inflammatory reaction to the parasite and its metabolic products, affecting many systems of the body and producing varying symptoms
- depletion of the host body through competition for nutrients
- the immune system being overwhelmed

PROTOZOA

The most common parasitic infections are those caused by protozoa, which are usually one-celled, microscopic organisms. There are four major classes of protozoa:

- *Rhizopods* – include *Entamoeba histolytica, Entamoeba coli, Entamoeba gingivalis, Entamoeba hartmani, Dientamoeba fragilis, Endolimax nana, Iodamoeba buetschlii,* and *Blastocystis hominis.* All of these amebas live in the intestine, except for *Entamoeba gingivalis,* which is found in the mouth. Transmission of these organisms is through ingesting the cysts in food, in drink, from the fingers, and from other objects. Flies can transport the cysts, and poor personal hygiene plays a large role in transmission of amebas.
- *Flagellates* – *Giardia lamblia* is the most common flagellate and the most widespread protozoan infection in North America. This organism has flagella (whip-like appendages) that aid in propulsion, and a concave sucking disk that allows it to attach to the small intestine. Transmission of *Giardia* is through food and water contaminated by feces; food handlers; flies; and (in cases of poor hygiene) from hand to mouth. Sometimes even chlorine treatment of water does not kill this parasite. Campers and travelers should exercise care, because many water sources are contaminated by animal feces—thus the disease's common name in North America, beaver fever. *Trichomonas vaginalis,* a sexually transmitted parasite that causes vaginitis

in females and urethritis and prostatitis in males, is also a member of this class.

- *Ciliates* have thread-like cilia that cover the body and aid in locomotion. *Balantidium coli,* which lives in both the large and small intestine, is the only pathogen in this class. It causes liquid stools containing blood and pus. This parasite is transmitted through hogs and their contaminated feces, and by poor personal hygiene.
- *Sporozoa* – This class of parasites has no method of locomotion. *Cryptosporidium* infects the stomach and small bowel and causes diarrhea. It is spread hand-to-mouth and has been found in male homosexuals and among children in daycare. *Pneumocystis carinii* infects the lungs and can cause death by respiratory failure. Its transmission is through respiratory exposure, but affects only people with suppressed immune function. The *Plasmodium* species cause malaria, a disease characterized by recurring high fever, shaking, chills, and other flu-like symptoms. It is spread by the bite of the *Anopheles* mosquito, and although it is commonly found in Africa, South America, and Southeast Asia, cases are now being reported in the United States.

HELMINTHS

Helminths are any of the many species of worms. Most are free living, but some can be parasites of humans. Over one billion people worldwide are host to many different intestinal worms, and it is estimated that 25 million Americans, many of them children, have worms.

Parasitic worms usually have some type of device that allows them to attach to, penetrate, or abrade the tissues of the host. Most worms have a life cycle that includes the passage of eggs (or larvae hatched from the eggs) out of one host into an external environment, where they wait for another host. Many eggs and larvae perish before they can reach another host, and some species have several hosts.

Malnutrition plays a major role in worm infestation. It interferes with antibody production and can increase inflammatory reactions, both of which lower host resistance.

There are several classes of worms:

- Annelids – segmented worms. These include the leeches, which are external parasites that occur mainly in Asia.
- Nematodes – round worms. Hookworms, pinworms, roundworms *(Ascaris),* and the worms that cause trichinosis and filariasis make up this class of worms. Hookworms enter through the skin (usually through a bare foot) and live in the small intestine. *Ascaris* enter the body as eggs from contaminated soil or vegetables and subsequently live in the small intestine after they hatch. The worms causing trichinosis live in the small intestine as adults, and the larvae form cysts in the muscles. The filarial worms reside in the lymph system. This class of worms causes a variety of symptoms including anemia, GI symptoms, growth retardation, failure to thrive, muscle pain, eosinophilia, anal itching, bloody stools, and inflammation of lymph glands.
- Flatworms. This class of worms has two important subclasses: tapeworms and flukes.

  Tapeworms normally live in animals. Humans become infected with these worms when they ingest inadequately cooked animal flesh (beef, pork, or fish) containing the cysts, or feces containing the eggs. Pets may also carry and transmit tapeworms.

  Tapeworms live in the small intestine and can become quite long; their segments sometimes appear in the stool when they break off from the worm. Tapeworms usually do not cause symptoms, other than an increased appetite as the worm depletes the host of nutrients. A few species (the dwarf tapeworms and fish tapeworms) can cause digestive disturbances or abdominal discomfort. Pork tapeworms can cause brain infections in humans.

Flukes are internal parasites and are parasitic during nearly all of their life cycle. Most of the flukes that cause disease are from Asia, although the sheep liver fluke has been reported in Central and South America and Africa as well. Flukes burrow into the skin and are carried through the bloodstream to the liver, intestines, or bladder. Liver flukes include *Clonorchis sinensis, Fasciola hepatica,* and several species of *Schistosoma.* One type of fluke *(Paragonimus westermani)* is found in the lung, and *Fasciolopsis buski* is found in the small intestine.

Fluke infections used to be rare in North America, but with the increase in world travel and the increase in immigrants and refugees they are becoming more common. Symptoms of a fluke infection may include intestinal symptoms, urinary bladder symptoms, lung symptoms, and liver symptoms, depending on the infecting organ.

DIAGNOSIS OF PARASITIC DISEASE

The difficulty in diagnosing parasitic diseases is compounded by the fact that many parasitology laboratories fail to find the majority of the intestinal parasites in the stool samples submitted for their examination. Some laboratories, particularly hospital laboratories, do not have the trained staff or sufficient time for careful analysis of stool samples, or for the multiple procedures (that may take several days) that are needed for accurate testing.

Another complicating factor in diagnosing intestinal parasites is that they usually live buried in the mucosa of the intestines. Unless they happen to break off into the stool the day the sample is taken, they may simply not be present in the sample. The life cycles of the parasites and the different forms taken in these life cycles (eggs, cysts, larvae, trophozoites, etc.) can make a definitive sample difficult to obtain. The cyst and egg excretion rate varies from day to day, as does segment excretion in the case of worms. The larvae do not produce eggs that can be found in the stool. The age of the specimen can lessen the possibility of finding the parasites, and the amount of stool submitted can also be a problem, since both too much and too little material can lower the possibility of finding parasites.

The test most commonly used to diagnose intestinal parasites is the purged stool specimen, in which stools are chemically induced. A purged stool is a better sample than the normal random stool, and is useful in identifying giardia, amoeba, roundworm, hookworm, tapeworm, threadworm, cryptosporidium, and liver and blood flukes. However, the purged stool cannot be used if the patient is pregnant, or has an intestinal obstruction, appendicitis, or debilitation. Individuals with high blood pressure will have to exercise caution if a saline laxative is used.

New techniques involving smears taken from the rectal mucosa are also used to diagnose parasites. These specimens are stained with immunofluorescent stains for examination under special microscopes. In some cases these techniques will give a positive diagnosis when the purged stool sample is negative; however, insufficient swabbing can miss parasites. The best results are obtained by using both a purged stool examination and a rectal smear.

In the string test, another method of diagnosis, a gelatin capsule containing a string is swallowed, with one end of the string tethered to the patient's cheek. The string is withdrawn through the mouth after three or four hours and a microscopic examination of the string will often demonstrate organisms that reside in the duodenum of the small intestine.

Parasites that are found in the tissues and blood can sometimes be diagnosed by a blood test, since many worm infestations will cause a pronounced increase in the eosinophil (a type of white blood cell) count—as much as 25 percent or more. Many physicians attribute this increase to an allergy, not realizing that the allergic reaction is to parasitic worms. Microscopic examination of blood and blood smears will identify parasites such as malaria and filarial worms.

Abnormally low levels of vitamins and minerals can also indicate the presence of some parasites, as can abnormal levels of liver enzymes. Antibody tests performed on blood serum can measure antibodies produced by the immune system in an attempt to eliminate the parasite. However, with immuno-compromised patients these tests may not be reliable.

Other diagnostic tests for parasites utilize other body fluids and materials.

- Sputum tests can diagnose several species of worms and protozoa.
- Urine tests can detect blood fluke eggs, microfilariae, and trichomonas.
- Tissue scrapings (perianal scrapings) will show amoeba, eggs from several worms, and blood flukes.
- Radiologic tests (CAT scan and MRI scan) can detect the lesions of several parasites.
- Aspiration (removal of fluid from body cavities) can demonstrate the presence of several protozoa.
- A biopsy (removal of tissue that is examined microscopically) can demonstrate parasites in various tissues, depending on the life cycle.
- Several parasites can be cultured in an appropriate growth medium from vaginal, stool, and blood samples.

MODERN MEDICAL PREVENTION

Parasites can be very difficult to treat and to eliminate, and the relapse rate is high. It is far better to prevent a parasitic infection than to have to treat it. Because the sources of parasitic infections are many and varied, care must be exercised in many areas to prevent infection by these organisms.

Food Handling

Patients are told to drink only safe water that is either filtered, treated with chlorine or iodine, or has been boiled for 20 minutes.

Meat, poultry, and fish should be rinsed in cold water before cooking. In addition, patients are to cook the meat well, because tapeworms and other parasites may be transmitted by improperly cooked (or raw) meat, poultry, and fish.

Patients are warned to choose carefully when eating at salad bars. Improperly cleaned salad ingredients, or ingredients prepared by employees with poor personal hygiene, can be a source of parasites.

A Clorox solution should be used to clean cooking utensils, cutting boards, and all surfaces that come in contact with uncooked and raw foods. Hands must be washed before each meal and before preparing food. Food should be protected from exposure to insects such as houseflies and cockroaches, which can be carriers of parasites.

Animal Care

Because wild animals and household pets are often infected with parasites and can transmit them to humans, patients are told to take the following precautions. Cat litter should be changed regularly and the person doing this chore should wear gloves and a mask. Pregnant women and immuno-compromised people should not be exposed to or change cat litter. Pets should be wormed regularly and they should be brushed and groomed outdoors.

Food preparation and eating areas should be totally off limits to all pets, and they should not eat off the family dishes. Children should not eat dirt, or play in dirt and sand where cats and dogs relieve themselves. Neither adults nor children should kiss pets, and pets should not be allowed to lick their faces. Both children and adults should wash their hands after handling pets, and pets should not play with children's toys.

Personal Hygiene

Patients should thoroughly wash their hands with soap before each meal, and after using the toilet, changing a diaper, or handling pets. Both adults and children should keep their nails short and scrub under them with a nailbrush. They should not put their hands in their mouths unless they have just washed them.

Sterilized lens cleaning preparations or safe water (never tap water) should be used to clean and sterilize contact lenses, and patients should not wear contact lenses while swimming.

Patients should also be aware of sexual risk factors. Oral sex, anal sex, and multiple sex partners play a role in the spread of parasites.

If using a strange bathroom, patients should protect toilet seats or wipe them with toilet paper. Squatting is preferable to sitting when cleanliness is questionable. Toilet seats at home should be cleaned with Clorox, both the top as well as underneath.

Traveling Precautions

The following general precautions will help prevent parasite infestation, both at home and when traveling. Patients are warned to be careful of food when traveling in developing countries. They should avoid dishes containing pickled, dried, raw, or smoked fish, crabs, and crayfish. Patients should drink only bottled water and avoid ice cubes, as they are usually made from tap water. They should never drink from streams or rivers unless they sterilize the water by boiling it, using iodine, or filtering it.

Patients should always wash their hands after handling soil of any kind, and should not walk barefoot on moist, warm, sandy soil. Insect control must be exercised over flies, cockroaches, mosquitoes, and ticks, which can all carry parasites. Patients should wear long sleeves and pants to avoid insect bites, and sleep under netting.

People who eat out regularly or travel frequently should be tested for parasites twice a year.

ALTERNATIVE PREVENTION

Food Handling

To prevent parasitic infections, observe the following food-handling guidelines in addition to those under Modern Medical Prevention. Drink only bottled water or safe water. If there is any doubt regarding the purity of the water, add a stabilized oxygen product like Aerobic 07 (see Sources section at back of book). Have your tap water tested or use a water treatment system that helps block parasites.

Soak all vegetables, both organic and nonorganic, for 30 minutes in a saltwater solution made of 1 Tbsp. salt to every 5 cups of water before cooking them. Wash all fruit and vegetables in water to which Clorox has been added. Use Clorox brand bleach only; its safety record is well known, and other brands of bleach may have undesired additives in them. Use ½ tsp. Clorox in each gallon of water, and soak the food for 15 to 30 minutes. Chlorine-sensitive people will have to substitute hydrogen peroxide or NeoLife Green soap (see Sources) for Clorox, or use ozonated water. (These substances may not work as well as Clorox for some people.) Rinse the food thoroughly in plain water, then store or cook. Peel fruits and vegetables whenever possible.

Thaw meat (except ground meat) in a Clorox bath (½ tsp. Clorox to 1 gallon water) and then rinse in cold water to help lower the risk of getting parasites. This does not adversely affect the taste. Freezing meat will also kill larvae. Beef and pork require 24 hours at −4°F, while fish must remain at 0°F for 48 hours. Never sample meat dishes before they are fully cooked.

Animal Care

Observe the modern medical precautions for animal care. If you have a pet, wash your children's toys regularly in soapy water. If you bathe your pet in the bathtub, clean the tub with a Clorox solution afterward.

Personal Hygiene

In addition to the modern medical guidelines, do the following: Bathe or shower daily. Wear close-fitting underpants even under sleepwear. Wash bed clothing and bed linens frequently. Clean the bedroom and bathroom frequently and be certain there is adequate circulation.

Traveling Precautions

Use the modern medical traveling precautions in addition to the following. Carry Aerobic 07 or other stabilized oxygen product to treat water. If possible, carry a water filter.

Take 1 Tbsp. of Bentonite liquid (a clay solution available in health food stores) morning and evening as a natural parasite preventative. It absorbs toxins in the intestinal tract and helps to flush them out of the system. Do not take with meals.

MODERN MEDICAL TREATMENT

Drug Therapy

There are many pharmaceuticals available for the treatment of parasites. Following are a few of the drugs used: for protozoans—Yodoxin, Humatin, Flagyl, Aralen, Atabrin, Furoxone; for tapeworm—Niclocide and Biltricide; for hookworm, pinworm, and ascaris—Vermox, Antiminth, or Zental; for flukes—Biltricide, Bitin, or Niclocide; for malaria—Chloroquine or quinine.

Drugs for treating parasites have many unpleasant side effects. Among the more common are:

- Yodoxin – occasional rash, acne, slight enlargement of the thyroid gland, nausea, diarrhea, cramps, anal itching, and eye problems (if used for long periods of time).
- Humatin – GI disturbances
- Flagyl – nausea, headache, dry mouth, metallic taste
- Aralen, Chloroquine, or quinine – itching, vomiting, headache, confusion, depigmenta-

tion of hair, skin eruptions, corneal opacity, weight loss, partial hair loss, extra-ocular muscle palsies, exacerbation of psoriasis, eczema and other exfoliative dermatoses, myalgias, photophobia

- Atabrin – dizziness, headache, vomiting, diarrhea, jaundice
- Furoxone – nausea, vomiting
- Niclocide – nausea, abdominal pain
- Biltricide – malaise, headache, dizziness
- Vermox – diarrhea, abdominal pain, migration of *Ascaris* through mouth and nose
- Antiminth – GI disturbances, headache, dizziness, rash, fever
- Zental – diarrhea, abdominal pain, migration of *Ascaris* through mouth and nose
- Bitin – photosensitivity reactions, vomiting, diarrhea, abdominal pain, hives

Because there is a very high relapse rate in parasitic infections, treatment must be continued long enough to ensure that the infection is gone. Parasites can also develop resistance to drug therapy, and this possibility should be considered if therapy first appears to be effective and then the patient begins to relapse. In these cases, the drug will have to be changed, perhaps several times, until treatment is effective and complete.

Other Therapeutic Measures
Because of the difficulty in eradicating parasites, repeat tests should be performed at the discretion of the physician to confirm that treatment is complete. If any of the repeat tests are positive, treatment must be continued and/or changed. Further repeat tests must be done until several consecutive tests are negative.

ALTERNATIVE TREATMENT
Diet
Avoid sugar, honey, malts, and fruit juice sweeteners, as sugars encourage the growth of some parasites. Eat small amounts of properly washed whole fruit, but do not drink fruit juice.

Avoid pasteurized milk and dairy products, as they are mucus producers, which makes parasites more difficult to eradicate. Avoid alcoholic beverages, including beer and wine, which can decrease immunity. Do not eat junk food or food low in nutrients.

Eat a high vegetable-protein diet and cultured foods, such as yogurt. Include garlic and onion in your diet regularly. Drink extra water daily to help flush out dead parasites. Be certain to consume cold-pressed or expeller-pressed safflower, flax, sesame, or sunflower oils that strengthen the immune system by fortifying the cell membrane walls.

Adding specific foods to your diet can help rid your body of parasites. Eat one ounce of pumpkin seeds each day to aid in the expulsion of intestinal worms. Eat nothing but pineapple for three days to clear up tapeworms. Drink a strong clove tea for intestinal worms and other parasites, or add powdered cloves to pineapple or papaya juice. Eat curry dishes that contain turmeric, which is effective for nematodes. Mix the juice from three cloves of garlic with carrot juice and take every two hours to help rid the body of roundworms, pinworms, and protozoans. To help with amebic dysentery, use cubeb, a relative of black pepper, on your food. While these dietary additions are helpful, they may not be adequate for some parasites, and additional treatment will be necessary.

Exercise and Lifestyle
Exercise daily for 30 minutes to aid bowel elimination, and be certain you have a bowel movement daily.

Keep the immune system strong and the intestines healthy, both to prevent parasites and to make parasite treatment more effective. Do not smoke, so that your body and immune system will be stronger.

Use condoms and avoid oral and anal sex to reduce the spread of parasites.

Nutrient Therapy
Take the following nutritional supplements.

- vitamin A – 10,000 IU a day. *Caution:* Do not use more than 8,000 IU a day if you are pregnant or might be pregnant (strengthens immune system; helps support mucus membranes).
- beta carotene – 50,000 IU a day (an anti-infective)
- vitamin B_{12} – 300 mcg a day (needed for proper assimilation of foods; helps with fatigue)
- vitamin C – 2,000 to 8,000 mg a day (strengthens immune system; anti-inflammatory)
- calcium – 1,000 mg a day (helps maintain proper cell membrane permeability)
- magnesium – 500 to 1,000 mg a day (balances calcium; helps reduce spasms of all muscles)
- coenzyme Q_{10} – 30 mg twice a day (enhances effectiveness of and produces energy for immune system)
- organic germanium – 150 mg one to three times a day (oxygenates tissues)
- *Lactobacillus acidophilus* – ½ tsp. three to four times a day (recolonizes the gut with "good" bacteria)
- probiotic culture – as directed for your product (must contain *Lactobacillus acidophilus*, *Bifidobacteria*, and *Lactobacillus bulgaricus*) (recolonizes the gut with "good" bacteria)
- proteolytic enzymes – take the dosage recommended on your product between meals (helps expel dislodged worms)
- betaine hydrochloride – follow the directions on your product (increases stomach acid, which is a good defense from parasites)
- borage oil, black currant oil, flaxseed oil, or evening primrose oil – as directed on your product (strengthens the immune system by fortifying cell membrane walls)

Herbal Therapy
Take a botanical supplement.

- barberry – for amebic dysentery
- barberry, bayberry, echinacea, garlic, elecampane, turmeric, and goldenseal – for giardia
- chinchona bark tea – for malaria and ameba
- elecampane – for amebiasis
- goldenseal – for intestinal parasites. *Caution:* Do not use if you are pregnant.
- ipecac – for amebiasis (a one-dose, one-time treatment only)
- Qing hao – for amebiasis
- sweet Annie – for amebas, malaria
- wormseed – for worms

Take one of the following complex herbal preparations by UniKey (see Sources).

- Paratox 11 – four capsules of 400 mg each, three times a day. Contains black walnut, senna blend, pink root, slippery elm, and garlic. It is effective against worms, but must be taken in four cycles to be certain all the parasites are gone. *Begin treatment with Paratox 11 and follow up with Paratox 22.*
- Paratox 22 – four capsules of 400 mg each, three times a day. Contains grapefruit seed extract, garlic, slippery elm, and cranberry concentrate. It is effective against protozoa, and must also be taken in four cycles.
- Verma-Key – two capsules 20 minutes before meals, three times a day, for worms. Take for two weeks, followed by a five-day rest period. Do two to three repetitions.
- Verma-Plus – 15 to 20 drops between meals, twice a day and before bedtime, for worms. Take for two weeks, followed by a five-day rest period. Do two to three repetitions.
- Para-Key – two capsules 20 minutes before

meals, three times a day, for protozoa. Take for two weeks with a five-day rest period. Do two to three repetitions.

- Para-Plus – 15 to 20 drops between meals, two times a day and before bed, for protozoa. Take for two weeks, followed by a five-day rest period. Do two to three repetitions.

Use a botanical supplement by Nutricology (see Sources section at back of book).

- ParaMicrocidin – a grapefruit seed extract; take two capsules three times a day (for protozoan infections)
- ParQing – contains *Artemesia annua;* work up to three capsules three times a day, then increase by one capsule every two to three days (for protozoan infections)

Homeopathic Remedies

Take a homeopathic remedy that is specific for your type of parasite. Because of the difficulty in eradicating parasites, the help of a homeopathic practitioner may be necessary. The remedies listed below are but a few of the many possibilities.

- *Chenopodium* – for hookworm disease; also treats roundworm; disagreeable belching, nausea; regurgitation of yellow frothy material smelling of worm-seed.
- *China officinalis* – for giardiasis, watery diarrhea; stools undigested, frothy, yellow, dark, foul, bloody, painless.
- *Cina* – remedy for roundworms, threadworms, and tapeworms; grinding of teeth; restless, constant rubbing of the nose; loss or increase of appetite; itching rectum.
- *Ipecac* – for amebic dysentery; dysentery with hot head and cold legs; pain so great it nauseates; stool brown, green, or yellow-green; stool molasses-like or bloody, slimy.
- *Mercurius sulphuricus* – for ameba; watery stools; burning in anus; intense evacuation like rice water.
- *Natrum phosphoricum* – intestinal longworms, roundworms, or threadworms; picking of nose; tendency to rheumatism; recurrent worms; greenish diarrhea; itching of anus.
- *Phosphorus* – amebic dysentery; little or no abdominal pain; no rectal spasm; person is able to walk despite abdominal pain.
- *Ratanhia* – pinworms, ascaris; dry itching anus; fetid, thin diarrhea; discharge of blood with or without stools.
- *Sinapis nigra* – remedy for pinworms.
- *Spigelia* – abdominal pain around the navel caused by worms; faint nauseated feeling, blue rings around the eyes.
- *Sulphur* – remedy for tapeworms; must be taken for a long time; chronic amebic dysentery; worse hot weather, hot rooms; urge to pass diarrhea drives from bed in morning; resistant giardiasis.
- *Terebinth* – burning and crawling in anus as though worms are creeping out, discharges roundworms and tapeworms.

Complex homeopathic remedies are helpful for many people. Take any one of the following complex remedies that describes your symptoms.

- Bowel Pathogen Nosodes from PHP – aids in enhancement of response to typical bowel pathogens.
- Vermex from PHP – assists in eradication of intestinal parasites.
- Amebex from PHP – assists in eradication of amebic infections.
- P'sites from Vibrant Health – a comprehensive parasite remedy covering all aspects of a parasitic infection.
- Am'bas from Vibrant Health – amoeba and protozoan infections.

Other Therapeutic Measures

Follow the prevention methods carefully. If any family member tests positive for parasites, treat all family members. Person-to-person contact is the most important factor in the spread of parasites, and even symptom-free family members should be treated.

Be treated for any parasite that you may have. Be aware that when you begin parasite treatment you may experience die-off symptoms (Herxheimer reaction) as the body reabsorbs protein from the dead parasitic cells. You may experience fever, chills, sweating, diarrhea or constipation, headaches, irritation, muscle aches, memory loss or poor concentration, hormonal imbalances, or depression. Die-off may also include a worsening of symptoms already present, but they will subside as treatment progresses.

Have parasite tests at appropriate intervals to be certain you do not have a parasitic infection, particularly if you travel or have pets. Repeat tests are particularly important after treatment to be certain that the parasites are indeed gone.

Breastfeed your baby because the milk provides antibodies that help fight against ameba and *Giardia.*

Consult an Ayurvedic or Chinese practitioner. Have NAET treatments (see the Chiropractic section in chapter 9, Alternative Medical Disciplines) for the parasite that you have. Be tested and treated by an environmental medicine physician for parasites. Allergy extracts for the parasite will reduce allergy symptoms to the body or eggs of the parasite and help to expel fragments of the parasite.

To reduce parasite numbers, use the following colon cleanse between meals three times a day for five days. After completing the 15 doses, take an acidophilus preparation (see Nutrient Therapy, above) to replenish bowel flora.

- Thoroughly mix 1 Tbsp. of psyllium seed husks in 8 ounces of water and drink immediately.
- Follow with 8 ounces of pure water.
- Then drink 4 ounces of a commercial bentonite solution or one prepared from 2 ounces of bentonite powder to 1 quart of water. Bentonite is a clay that absorbs toxins and is available at health food stores.

Urinary Tract Problems

The urinary tract consists of the kidneys, ureters, urinary bladder, and the urethra. The kidneys are paired, bean-shaped organs that lie on the back wall of the body below the ribcage. The primary function of the kidneys is to eliminate waste products from the blood in the form of urine. Two tubes (the ureters) drain urine from the kidneys into the urinary bladder, where the urine accumulates. The urethra leads from the bladder and carries the urine out of the body. In men, it passes through the penis; in women, the urethra exits above the vagina. Tiny valve-like muscles, called sphincters, open and close to control the flow of urine out of the body.

URINARY TRACT INFECTIONS

Bladder infections, known medically as cystitis, are more common in women than in men because of the shorter length of the urethra in women and the proximity of the urethral opening to the rectum and vagina. Bladder infections are the most common reason for women visiting a physician's office. Ten to twenty percent of adult women will have at least one acute bladder infection during their lifetime.

Almost 85 percent of bladder infections are caused by *Escherichia coli,* a bacterium found in the intestines. In women, a tendency to get bladder infections results from either an anatomic irregularity (these are usually discovered in childhood) or a failure of the bladder to function properly. In men, bladder infections are almost always caused by an anatomical problem (such as an enlarged prostate).

The symptoms of a bladder infection are an urgent desire to urinate, burning pain on urination, and pressure. Urination is frequent and painful; soon after the bladder has been emptied, there is an urgent need to urinate again. The urine may have a strong odor, and it may be bloody. Sometimes the infection occurs in the kidney, and in this case is known as pyelonephritis. Symptoms of pyelonephritis include back pain (just below the rib cage in the back), fever, and often nausea and vomiting. People who have kidney infections are usually much more ill than those who have a simple bladder infection. A urinary tract infection (UTI) refers to either pyelonephritis or cystitis.

The male and female urinary tracts serve different purposes. When women urinate, the urine, which is normally sterile, cleans off bacteria from the labia, the vagina, the tissue between the vagina and anus, and the anus. Bacteria can enter the bladder either during intercourse or because of an anatomical problem. However, bladder infections are not related to bacteria getting *into* the bladder, but are caused by bacteria not being able to get *out* of the bladder. There may be an obstruction to urine getting out of the bladder, or there may be a neurological problem that prevents the bladder from emptying completely. To keep the bladder healthy, a woman must be able to empty her bladder completely, she must have a forceful stream of urine, and she must void often.

If a woman has repeated bladder infections, rather than continuing to treat them with antibiotics, she needs to discover the cause of the infections. Antibiotic treatment causes a loss of the normal bacteria in the genital area and their replacement by antibiotic-resistant bacteria. In order to determine the cause of repeated infections, it is important to know when the first bladder infection occurred. If bladder infections started in childhood, there is an increased chance that an anatomical abnormality exists. Occasionally, a woman will have an acquired anatomic problem.

CAUSES OF BLADDER INFECTIONS

Holding urine for long periods of time predisposes people to urinary tract infections. Women must practice good hygiene after urinating and always wipe from front to back.

Women should also always empty the bladder before and after intercourse. Hygiene sprays, douches, scented and/or colored toilet paper, and bubble baths cause irritation and can lead to bladder infections. Some women are sensitive to soap, and should use only water to clean their genital area. Wearing cotton underwear or underwear with a cotton crotch helps prevent bladder and vaginal infections. Some studies show a link between the onset of a bladder infection and a recent pelvic exam.

The use of a diaphragm can cause bladder infections in some women. Diaphragms disturb the flow of urine from the bladder, causing some residual urine to be left in the bladder along with bacteria that enters during sexual intercourse. The size of the diaphragm used is important. Most women are fitted with diaphragms that are too large—if she can feel the diaphragm in place, it is too big. In addition, the spermicide used with the diaphragm alters the vaginal environment and promotes the growth of bacteria that cause infection. Some spermicides can cause bladder or vaginal irritation, but they will cause less irritation if used with an applicator.

Sexual position can be a factor in inducing bladder infections, particularly the angle at which the penis enters the vagina. If the man enters from a high position, the up and down motion of the penis in the vagina causes the woman's urethra to become abraded and sore. If he enters from a lower position, he will not injure the urethra, and can also stimulate the woman's erogenous tissue more easily, because at that angle the penis compresses the clitoris and massages the top wall of the vagina. A woman whose vagina lacks sufficient lubrication can have tissue abrasion from friction during intercourse, and may then develop a urinary tract infection.

Frequent vaginal infections are a risk factor for bladder infections because they increase the number of bacteria in the area. Using a diaphragm can cause a vaginal infection, while wearing tight pants and/or tight underwear can cause irritation of the vagina and urethra. Some women are allergic to the materials used in pads and/or tampons, and will develop a bladder infection by the third or fourth day of their period. Some women also develop an obstruction of their bladder from the tampon. They need to remove their tampon every time they urinate in order to empty the bladder completely.

Women who do not have a strong urine stream are often prone to recurrent infections. These women frequently have a history of a back injury, sometimes caused by wearing heels that are too high. Being overweight also puts extra stress on the back. Bladder dysfunction often is the first sign of back problems, appearing before other nerve abnormalities develop. A uroflow exam, which measures the rate of urine flow, can diagnose this problem. A back radiograph (X-ray) may show narrowing between the disc spaces.

Recent studies at Northwestern University Medical School in Chicago, Illinois demonstrate that some women have a biological defect in the cells lining the urinary tract that may make them more vulnerable to urinary tract infections. As well, women who have blood type B or AB are at higher risk for UTIs, and a high percentage of women who have recurrent UTIs have P_1 negative blood (a specific marker on red blood cells). Women with recurrent UTIs also have urine that is less acidic than normal.

If you have symptoms of a bladder infection, it is important to have your urine cultured. Vaginal infections can cause the same symptoms as a bladder infection. Consider buying urine test sticks from a pharmacist if you get frequent infections. Also keep in mind that antibiotics taken when not necessary may damage the bladder, cause an upset stomach or diarrhea, and lead to vaginal yeast infections.

MODERN MEDICAL PREVENTION

The conventional medical approach to prevention of repeated urinary tract infections is to have patients drink plenty of liquids before and after a pelvic exam, and before (and within 30 minutes after) intercourse. Patients are also encouraged to urinate with a good strong stream.

It is particularly important for women to practice good vaginal hygiene, and to empty the bladder before and after sexual intercourse.

ALTERNATIVE PREVENTION

Take two garlic-parsley tablets three times a day to prevent bladder infections. Garlic has antibiotic action, and parsley is a diuretic. Drink at least 64 ounces of liquids a day, half of which is pure, tolerated water. Avoid citrus fruits and drinks, caffeine, carbonated beverages, tomato sauce, curry, cayenne pepper, chili powder, concentrated fruit juices, chocolate, and alcohol, all of which are bladder irritants.

If you relapse after treatment, or have recurrent infections, have your partner checked for a urinary tract infection also. Consider trying a different size diaphragm, or using a different method of birth control altogether. Learn how to place your diaphragm properly, to prevent the introduction of bacteria into the urethra.

Do not have a urethral dilation unless there is evidence of a stricture. Instead, have your bladder function and back status evaluated.

MODERN MEDICAL TREATMENT

Drug Therapy
Modern medicine prescribes 7 to 10 days of oral antibiotic for urinary tract infections. Azo Standard or Uristat (an over-the-counter pyridium dye that numbs the urinary tract) is also given to reduce sensations of pain and urgency. If there is an anatomic abnormality that predisposes the person to urinary tract infections, suppressive antibiotics may be given daily for three to six months.

Bethanechol chloride (Urecholine), which is a synthetic form of the neurotransmitter acetylcholine, is given when a narrowing between disc spaces in the back causes bladder dysfunction. Often physical therapy is also used to treat this problem.

Urethral Dilation
Modern medicine practitioners frequently suggest urethral dilation to treat repeated urinary tract infections.

ALTERNATIVE TREATMENT

Diet
Avoid the foods listed under alternative prevention. Also avoid simple sugars, and refined and processed foods. Eat natural diuretics such as celery, parsley, and watermelon, which act as cleansers.

Exercise and Lifestyle
Do not delay emptying the bladder, and wear white cotton underwear. Keep the genital area clean and dry, wiping from front to back after

emptying the bladder or bowels. Never sit around in a wet bathing suit. Do not use scented products such as soaps, bubble bath, toilet paper, tampons, sanitary pads, douches, or feminine hygiene sprays.

Nutrient Therapy

- vitamin A – 25,000 IU a day. *Caution:* Do not take more than 8,000 IU a day if you are or might be pregnant (protects against bladder infections; needed for immune response and tissue repair).
- beta carotene – 200,000 IU a day (precursor for vitamin A)
- bioflavonoids – 1,000 mg a day (important in immune function; improves tissue integrity)
- vitamin B$_6$ – 50 mg a day (decreases bladder pain; reduces fluid retention)
- vitamin C – 500 mg every two hours—some people may need to take the buffered form (produces an antibiotic effect through acidification of urine; strengthens immune system; improves tissue integrity)
- vitamin E – 600 IU a day (combats infecting bacteria)
- calcium – 800 to 1,000 mg a day (decreases bladder pain)
- magnesium – 400 to 800 mg a day (decreases spasms of the bladder; works with calcium)
- potassium – 100 mg a day (to replace potassium lost with frequent urination)
- zinc picolinate – 30 mg a day (important in tissue repair and immunity)

Herbal Therapy

Take a botanical supplement three times a day.

- bearberry – urinary antiseptic and diuretic. This works best if the urine is alkaline, so avoid acidic foods, citrus fruits, cranberry, vinegar, and ascorbic acid (unbuffered vitamin C) while taking it. It often turns urine dark green.
- garlic – antibacterial. Can be taken in combination with parlsey.
- goldenseal – enhances the immune system. *Caution:* Do not use during pregnancy.
- hibiscus – for painful urination
- parsley – diuretic. *Caution:* Do not use during pregnancy.
- sandalwood oil – diuretic and urinary tract antiseptic

Homeopathic Remedies

Take a dose of a homeopathic remedy every two hours during intense symptoms and every four hours for less intense symptoms. The correct remedy may need to be taken for up to three days. If the remedy does not work, seek the help of a homeopathic practitioner.

- *Aconite* – sudden onset of symptoms after exposure to dry cold.
- *Apis* – burning, stinging pain or heat; worsened by heat.
- *Belladonna* – acute pain aggravated by any motion or jarring; sensation of something moving inside the bladder; night-time restlessness.
- *Cantharis* – strong burning pains before, during, and after urination; each drop passes as if it were scalding water; despite a constant desire to urinate, the bladder never feels empty.
- *Pulsatilla* – pain during and after urination as well as when lying down; dry mouth but no thirst.
- *Sarsaparilla* – pain felt only after urinating.
- *Staphysagria* – cramping and burning; urination frequent and sometimes involuntary; often follows a sense of assault physically or emotionally.

Many patients respond to complex homeopathic remedies. You may want to try BHI

Bladder, a prescription remedy specifically for bladder infections (see Sources).

Other Therapeutic Measures

Take two capsules of NK 9-1-1, an antibiotic substitute containing echinacea and dairy whey, every four hours. Most patients, including those who are milk sensitive, tolerate this product, distributed by Super Life, quite well (see Sources).

Drink 1 tsp. of baking soda in a glass of water every three to four hours to help decrease symptoms.

Use colloidal silver, a natural broad-spectrum antibiotic that fights infection, reduces inflammation, and promotes healing. Colloidal silver is available at health food stores and can be applied topically or used orally.

Take only three pills of a prescribed antibiotic for an infection; if your bladder can function normally and empty properly, it will repair itself quickly. If your bladder does not empty well or you are pregnant, you will need to take antibiotics for five to seven days.

Take sitz baths (baths in shallow bath water) twice a day for 20 minutes at a time. You may add 1 cup of vinegar to a sitz bath, which increases acidity, helping to kill bacteria. Position yourself so that the water can enter the vagina. Alternate vinegar in the bath water with two cloves of crushed garlic, or with garlic juice, a natural antibiotic.

Drink plenty of liquids, including cranberry or blueberry juice, which help prevent bacteria from sticking to the bladder and urethra. Use pure unsweetened juice, which is very tart, from a natural food store, and sweeten it with apple or grape juice. If you find that cranberry juice increases irritation, take cranactin tablets as an alternative, in an amount equivalent to 16 ounces of cranberry juice daily.

Increase the alkalinity of the urine with citrate salts, such as potassium citrate and sodium citrate. (Both goldenseal and bearberry work most effectively in an alkaline environment.)

Take Azo-Standard or Uristat to reduce pain and urgency.

Try using acupressure at the following points:

- Apply pressure the width of one hand below, and in line with, the navel.
- Apply pressure the width of one hand above the crown (the bump) of the inner ankle, just behind the shin bone (tibia) on the front of the leg.

INTERSTITIAL CYSTITIS

Interstitial cystitis is a disease of the bladder characterized by frequency of urination, spasms, and burning pain in the bladder, which is worse after urinating. Some women have only the burning pain, without the frequency. Pain is relieved only during urination.

Common cystitis is caused by a bacterial infection of the bladder. Interstitial cystitis, however, is an inflammation of the protective mucus-like layer between the bladder lining and the bladder muscle. Although its symptoms appear to be the same as those of a bladder infection, a urine culture will fail to grow any bacteria. Foods such as coffee, tea, and orange juice make the pain worse, as do antibiotics, in particular nitrofurantoin, tetracycline, and erythromycin. Intercourse may also make symptoms worse.

Interstitial cystitis is a progressive disease. At first, there is no visible damage—cystoscopy (an examination of the inside of the bladder through a small scope) often shows nothing abnormal—but as it progresses it can lead to ulceration and scarring of the bladder. Both women and men can develop interstitial cystitis, and men are often incorrectly diagnosed as having bacterial prostatitis or non-specific urethritis. Factors causing this painful bladder syndrome include taking antibiotics when no infection is present; Epstein-Barr virus; scarlet fever; chemical exposure; and certain drugs.

MODERN MEDICAL TREATMENT

Drug Therapy

Antibiotics are the main treatment offered by traditional medicine for interstitial cystitis. They do not cure the problem. Patients are instructed to drink lots of fluids and to take painkillers or Elavil for pain. Elavil is an antidepressant that can reduce pain if it is given in low doses. For more information on Elavil, see Drug Therapy for Depression in chapter 27, Mood Disorders. Dimethylsulfoxide or DMSO, a solvent, is injected into the bladder to ease the pain.

ALTERNATIVE TREATMENT

If you have recurrent pain and continued negative urine cultures, you could have interstitial cystitis. Find a physician who can give you the correct diagnosis. In some cases a cystoscopy may be helpful.

Diet

Eat a diet that emphasizes low-acid foods, and avoid the following:

Alcoholic beverages	Grapes
Apples and apple juice	Guava
Cantaloupes	Peaches
Carbonated drinks	Pineapple
Chilies/spicy food	Plums
Citrus fruits and juices	Strawberries
Coffee	Tea
Cranberries	Tomatoes

Avoid the following foods, which are high in tyrosine, tyramine, tryptophan, and aspartate:

Avocados	NutraSweet
Bananas	Nuts
Beer, champagne	Onions
Brewer's yeast	Pickled herring
Canned figs	Prunes
Cheeses (hard and soft)	Raisins
Chicken livers	Rye bread
Chocolate	Saccharine
Corned beef	Sour cream
Fava beans	Soy sauce
Mayonnaise	Vitamins buffered with aspartate

Exercise and Lifestyle

Do not use tampons if you have interstitial cystitis. Choose birth control with care, as some spermicidal creams and foams can increase the risk of all types of cystitis.

Nutrient Therapy

Take nutritional supplements as follows:

- vitamin A – 25,000 IU a day. *Caution:* Do not take more than 8,000 IU of vitamin A a day if you are or might be pregnant (for immune response; resistance to infection; helps reduce scarring)
- beta carotene – 200,000 IU a. day (precursor for vitamin A; needed for immune response and resistance to infection)
- bioflavonoids – 1,000 mg a day (improves tissue integrity)
- vitamin B$_6$ – 50 mg a day (decreases bladder pain)
- buffered vitamin C – 500 mg every two hours (neutralizes acidity; strengthens immune system; improves tissue integrity)
- vitamin E – 600 IU a day (helps reduce scarring)
- calcium – 800 to 1,000 mg a day (decreases bladder pain)
- magnesium – 400 to 800 mg a day (decreases bladder spasms)
- zinc picolinate – 30 mg a day (for immune response)

Herbal Therapy

The following herbs may help interstitial cystitis. Because of the difficulty in treating this condition, consult a trained herbalist.

- astragalus – promotes healing; protects the immune system
- bearberry – mild diuretic and antiseptic
- bilberry – anti-inflammatory
- echinacea – anti-inflammatory; strengthens immune system; stimulates white blood cells
- goldenseal – anti-inflammatory; strengthens the immune system. *Caution:* Do not take if you are pregnant.

Take Bladder Irritation, a complex herbal remedy from Natra-Bio of Ferndale, Washington (see Sources).

Homeopathic Remedies

Consult a physician trained in homeopathy. The remedies listed on p. 302 can also be helpful for interstitial cystitis.

Take a dose every two hours during intense symptoms and every four hours for less intense symptoms. The correct remedy may need to be taken for up to three days.

Other Therapeutic Measures

Take 1 tsp. baking soda in water for pain, and take four Tums (or another form of calcium carbonate) a few hours later. Repeat the Tums in 12 hours. This will give a slow release of bicarbonate over several hours.

Drink lots of clear fluids. Try ice packs or heating pads for pain, and use the treatment that feels better.

Try using acupressure at the following points.

- Apply pressure the width of one hand below, and in line with, the navel.
- Apply pressure the width of one hand above the crown (bump) of the inner ankle, just behind the shin bone (tibia) on the front of the leg.

Take a sitz bath (see instructions on p. 301).

KIDNEY STONES

Kidney stones develop in the kidney and are excreted through the ureters. The frequency of kidney stones has been increasing. In the United States, one hospitalization out of every 1,000 is for kidney stone removal, and more than 10 percent of men and 5 percent of women will develop a kidney stone in their lifetime.

Kidney stones are usually very painful, and the patient often requires narcotics for pain relief. (However, it is possible to have "silent" kidney stones that produce no pain.) The pain radiates from the lower back area to the abdomen, pelvic area, groin, or thighs. Patients will often have nausea, vomiting, chills, fever, pain with urination, and blood in the urine. The patient will change positions, trying to lessen the pain, and cannot lie still.

The tendency to have kidney stones runs in families. Two-thirds or more of all kidney stones are composed of calcium oxalate, and 5 percent are composed of uric acid (these appear in patients with gout). Patients who develop kidney stones are more likely to excrete large amounts of calcium, and may have a parathyroid gland abnormality. Stones can also be caused by too much vitamin D and (rarely) by leukemia.

Kidney stones typically develop during the early and middle years, and one or more stones may be present. Stones too large to pass out, or stones that have many protuberances, get stuck and must be removed by surgery or broken up with the use of sound waves. Ninety percent of kidney stones can now be removed by means of extracorporeal shock wave lithotripsy, a procedure in which ultrasound is used to break up kidney stones so they can be passed in the urine. Contraindications to lithotripsy include pregnancy, an aneurysm of the aorta, a blood clotting problem, or obesity.

The best way to deal with kidney stones is to prevent them—and most stones are preventable. If you have had one stone, chances are

greater than 50 percent that you will have another one within 5 to 10 years. If you have a kidney stone, it is important to have it analyzed so
that you can carry out the proper preventative
actions.

The high rate of calcium stones in the United
States is caused by diets low in fiber and high in
refined carbohydrates, fat, calcium-containing
food, salt, and vitamin-D enriched food and animal protein. High levels of alcohol are also implicated. Recent studies show that 1,000 mg of
calcium a day (for women) reduces the body's
absorption of oxalate, and decreases the risk of
calcium oxalate stones. On the other hand, taking a calcium supplement slightly increases the
risk of kidney stones—depending on the ratio of
calcium to phosphate, citrate, and oxalate. That
risk may be decreased by taking the calcium
with food.

MODERN MEDICAL PREVENTION

Modern medical prevention for kidney stones
includes drinking at least 3 quarts of fluid a day.
Calcium intake in the diet is decreased, and it is
suggested that calcium-rich antacids and calcium supplements be avoided. Vitamin C is also
avoided.

To help prevent the formation of calcium oxalate stones, a citric acid supplement (potassium
citrate) is suggested. The usual dosage is 60 to
80 mg a day, which will form complexes with
calcium and help prevent the formation of calcium oxalate stones.

ALTERNATIVE PREVENTION

Diet
Avoid or cut back on asparagus, black tea, co-
coa, parsley, cranberry, beets, spinach, Swiss
chard, rhubarb, and other vegetables that contain or produce oxalate.

Eat foods high in magnesium and vitamin B_6
such as liver, fish, nuts, seeds, whole grains,
wheat germ, brown rice, avocado, banana, lima
beans, potato, and soybeans.

Reduce salt consumption to less than 2,000
or 3,000 mg a day.

Increase the amount of fiber, leafy green vegetables, and complex carbohydrates you eat,
and decrease the proportion of protein.

Limit dairy products, especially those for-
tified with vitamin D, and reduce your consumption of sugar and caffeine.

Correct carbohydrate metabolism (see p. 235–
36).

Avoid refined sugar, which stimulates the
pancreas to release insulin, which in turn causes
extra calcium to be excreted in the urine.

Drink 2 quarts of lemonade a day, made from
reconstituted lemon juice, water, and a sweetener (this supplies citrate).

Exercise and Lifestyle
Drink more fluids—at least 3 quarts of liquids a
day. Replace additional lost fluids when you exercise and sweat a lot.

Nutrient Therapy
Take the following nutritional supplements:

- vitamin B_6 – 50 mg a day (decreases the
  amount of oxalate the body produces)
- vitamin K – 200 mcg a day (coenzyme for
  production of a protein that inhibits growth
  of calcium oxalate crystals)
- copper – 2 to 3 mg a day (to balance zinc)
- magnesium citrate – 450 mg a day (increases
  solubility of calcium oxalate)
- potassium citrate – 150 mg a day (inhibits
  crystallization)
- zinc – 50 to 80 mg a day (important inhibitor
  of crystallization)
- glutamate – 300 mg a day (reduces calcium
  oxalate precipitation)

Herbal Therapy
Take aloe vera juice at levels below those that
cause a laxative effect, to help prevent stone formation.

Other Therapeutic Measures

If you produce stones found in acidic urine, keep the urine alkaline by taking sodium ascorbate or vitamin C with baking soda. If you produce stones found in alkaline urine, keep the urine acidic by taking vitamin C (ascorbic acid).

Some physicians think that vitamin C can cause kidney stones. However, a 1981 study by Ringsdorf and Cheraskin published in the *Southern Medical Journal* showed that people can take up to 4,000 mg of vitamin C a day without producing a statistically significant increase in calcium oxalate.

Look for evidence of heavy metal poisoning (have a hair analysis performed). Avoid aluminum compounds and alkalis (antacids). A toxic heavy metal load can contribute to the formation of kidney stones.

MODERN MEDICAL TREATMENT

Diet

If the patient's kidney stones contain oxalate, green vegetables, meat, chocolate, and iced tea are to be avoided. If they are made of uric acid, grapes, instant coffee, berries, citrus fruits, juices, vegetables, and caviar are the foods to avoid.

Drug Therapy

Allopurinol (Zyloprim) is given to lower uric acid if the patient has gout. People who experience gout frequently also have kidney stones. Skin rashes that can be fatal are the most serious side effect of allopurinol, but chills, joint pain, and diarrhea are other side effects. Antibiotics are used to combat any infection that may be associated with the kidney stones.

For the intense pain of kidney stones, an NSAID plus hydrocodone bitartrate (Vicodin) is given. If this combination is not effective, oxycodone (Percodan) plus an NSAID is prescribed. Side effects of these drugs include lightheadedness, dizziness, nausea and vomiting, and sedation.

Surgery

If the stones do not pass spontaneously in three to four days, surgery is usually suggested. Shock wave therapy can be used to dissolve them rather than surgery, unless ultrasound treatment is contraindicated.

ALTERNATIVE TREATMENT

Diet

Follow the dietary suggestions in Alternative Prevention.

Exercise and Lifestyle

Be active and exercise regularly to help pull calcium from the blood into the bones and to keep kidney function optimal. Sedentary people tend to accumulate high levels of calcium in the bloodstream.

Avoid antacids and NSAIDs during treatment.

Nutrient Therapy

In addition to the nutrients listed in Alternative Prevention, take the following preparations:

- vitamin A – 25,000 IU a day. *Caution:* Do not take more than 8,000 IU a day if you are or might be pregnant (promotes healing of the urinary tract).
- vitamin B-complex – 50 mg of each B vitamin a day (B vitamins work best when taken together)
- vitamin E – 600 IU a day (a powerful antioxidant)
- proteolytic enzymes – two to three capsules three times a day, one hour before or two hours after a meal (reduces inflammation; helps with pain)

Herbal Therapy

Take botanical supplements.

- aloe vera juice at levels below those that cause a laxative effect – this may reduce the size of a stone during an acute attack

- cleavers, combined with bearberry and buchu – to eliminate kidney stones
- gingko biloba – normalizes body functions
- goldenseal – soothes irritated mucus membranes. *Caution:* Do not take if you are pregnant.
- marshmallow – drink quart of tea a day to help expel stones

Homeopathic Remedies
Consult a homeopathic physician for the appropriate remedy.

- *Berberis* – sharp pain that radiates around the abdomen into the hip and groin.
- *Lycopodium* – right-sided kidney stones; reddish sediment to urine.
- *Magnesia phosphorica* – kidney pain that makes the person double over and is relieved by heat.

Other Therapeutic Measures
Use acupressure at the following points.

- Apply pressure between the crown (bump) of the inner ankle and the tip of the heel (this may be a larger area than most acupressure points).
- Stimulate the point in the center of the crease at the rear of the knee, between the two ligaments (but do not use this point if you have varicose veins).

Have reflexology treatments.

Place a hot water bottle or ice pack on the area of pain.

URINARY INCONTINENCE

Millions of adults suffer from some degree of urinary incontinence (involuntary leaking of urine from the bladder). Incontinence is particularly troublesome in older people. American nursing homes spend up to $1.5 billion a year dealing with incontinence. Almost half of all women who exercise regularly experience some degree of urinary stress incontinence.

There are three basic types of incontinence: stress incontinence, urge incontinence, and overflow incontinence.

STRESS INCONTINENCE
In urinary stress incontinence, urine leaks when a person laughs, coughs, or sneezes. This is the most common type of incontinence, accounting for 40 percent of incontinence cases.

Stress incontinence frequently occurs after childbirth, usually developing gradually beginning about 10 years after a woman's last baby. It occurs more frequently in women who have had three or more babies. During delivery, the baby's head rests on the neck of the bladder, and stresses the ligaments that support the bladder. As women age, the resulting poor muscle tone causes the bladder neck to descend into the vaginal canal, bringing with it a small part of the bladder, which forms an outpouching known as a cystocele.

The cystocele holds urine, and when a woman urinates, the cystocele does not empty. When there is urine in a cystocele, the weight tends to prevent the bladder neck from closing. When a person with stress incontinence suddenly sneezes or coughs, the weakened bladder neck opens up, letting out some urine.

Some men who have had their prostates removed may develop stress incontinence because their sphincters were damaged by the surgery.

MODERN MEDICAL TREATMENT
Exercise and Lifestyle
Kegel exercises (tightening the muscles used to stop the flow of urine) are done 20 to 30 times a day, in at least two or three sessions, to strengthen the muscles of the bladder neck. If the muscles remain weak, electrical stimulation may be considered. Vaginal cones, which are

available without a prescription, may also be used. They come in graduated sizes, and train the vaginal muscles, which have to tighten in order to retain the cones.

Patients are given training to learn how to contract the sphincters or the muscles of the pelvis, or both. They are also taught to urinate on schedule.

Drug Therapy

Imipramine hydrochloride (Norfranil, Tofranil) is prescribed, 25 to 50 mg, twice a day for one month to a year. This prescription will decrease bladder tone, making it more difficult to urinate. Side effects include nausea, headache, fatigue, dizziness, increased appetite, and dry mouth.

Phenylpropanolamine hydrochloride (Prolamine, Propagest) taken twice a day will stimulate the muscles of the bladder outlet. Constipation, dizziness, blurred vision, and dryness of the mouth, nose, or throat can result from taking this substance.

Women with stress incontinence can also try using a topical estrogen vaginal cream (15 mg twice a day to 60 mg four times a day), either alone or combined with phenylpropanolamine. They may need to use it for several months to a year.

Other Therapeutic Measures

A diaphragm is sometimes used to help support the bladder. It is removed at night to allow the tissues to breathe. The Reliance insert, a new product with a tiny balloon at the tip, can be placed in the urethra to block urine leakage. Vaginal pessaries (Milex incontinence rings, Cook rings, contraceptive diaphragms, or moistened tampons) can be used for stress incontinence associated with exercise. Be aware, however, that these may make incontinence worse for a woman with a cystocele.

For a small cystocele and mild stress inconti-

nence, Teflon or collagen can be injected into the bladder neck to thicken it. Men with stress incontinence can have an inflatable cuff implanted around the urethra.

URGE INCONTINENCE

Urge incontinence occurs in people who have strong involuntary contractions of the bladder, which make the bladder empty on its own. The nerves that normally inhibit bladder contractions do not get their signal through. The most common cause is damage to nerves in the upper back, above the fourth and fifth lumbar vertebrae. Strokes and multiple sclerosis are other causes of urge incontinence.

Be sure this type of incontinence is properly diagnosed, because surgery will usually not help it. Try other treatments before deciding to have surgery performed.

MODERN MEDICAL TREATMENT

Drug Therapy

Patients with urge incontinence are treated with propantheline (Pro-Banthine) or oxybutynin chloride (Ditropan), which both block the transmission of acetylcholine and act as an antispasmodic. Side effects of these drugs include dizziness, constipation, blurred vision, and dryness of the nose, mouth, or throat.

Surgery

If the back has been injured, surgical intervention may be advised. Surgery to enlarge the bladder is another treatment option.

OVERFLOW INCONTINENCE

Overflow incontinence (the rarest type of incontinence) occurs when the bladder muscle is not functioning properly, and allows leakage of urine without any warning. People with diabetes or severe low back problems are prone to develop this type of incontinence.

Be sure your incontinence is properly diagnosed, as surgery will usually not help this type of incontinence. Try other treatments before having surgery performed.

MODERN MEDICAL TREATMENT
Exercise and Lifestyle
Patients are encouraged to void on a schedule. They are also taught exercises to strengthen the bladder muscles.

Drug Therapy
Bethanechol chloride (Urecholine), a copy of the neurotransmitter acetylcholine, is prescribed for these patients. Malaise, abdominal cramps, and flushing are side effects of this drug.

Surgery
If the above measures do not work, surgery may be performed to reposition and strengthen the bladder muscles. In a few cases, this may help.

ALTERNATIVE TREATMENT FOR ALL FORMS OF INCONTINENCE
Diet
Avoid beverages that irritate the bladder, such as alcohol, caffeinated drinks, carbonated drinks, and milk. Citrus, other fruits, tomatoes, and tomato-based products may also have to be avoided. Avoid extremely spicy foods, such as chili, hot mustards, and hot peppers. Sugar, honey, corn syrup, chocolate, and artificial sweeteners can also irritate the bladder. Eat enough fiber to avoid constipation, which can affect bladder control.

Drink enough fluid to keep the urine light yellow. Do not reduce the amount of liquid consumed, as the urine will become more concentrated and irritating to your bladder.

Avoid eating asparagus, as it can cause foul-smelling urine. Cranberry and cherry juices help to deodorize urine, reducing any embarrassing odor.

Exercise and Lifestyle
Do the Kegel exercises described under Modern Medical Treatment, above. Also do daily exercises, such as bicycle riding, to encourage good circulation. Yoga exercises can also help incontinence.

For women, wearing a tampon during exercise may stop leakage.

Stop smoking as tobacco smoke adversely affects the bladder and urethra. Schedule regular bathroom breaks so that your bladder is never overfull.

Nutrient Therapy
The nutrients listed for Urinary Tract Infections and Interstitial Cystitis, particularly those that improve bladder tone, will help incontinence.

If the skin is burned by urine, use a cream containing vitamin A and D to treat it topically.

Herbal Therapy
Take a botanical supplement.

- aloe vera – aids in healing; soothes irritation
- parsley root – improves bladder function

Homeopathic Remedies
Consult a homeopathic physician for advice on the best remedy for your condition.

- *Belladonna* – involuntary urination in daytime and/or nighttime, especially if urine is emitted when the person is cold or chilled; burning pains the length of the urethra during normal, voluntary urination; wild dreams at night, often of urinating.
- *Causticum* – involuntary urination during the first part of sleep; people who wet their pants when they cough, sneeze, blow their nose or laugh; loss of urine without realizing it until they feel wet.

- *Ferrum phosphoricum* – daytime wetting in the pants, especially when the person feels the strongest urges while standing; urge to urinate lessens while lying down.
- *Gelsium* – people who accidentally dribble when they are excited or anxious about an upcoming event.
- *Kreosotum* – a sudden urge to urinate without enough time to get out of bed to go to the bathroom; wet during the first part of the night.
- *Lycopodium* – people who are so anxious they constantly worry about what others think of them; fears of trying anything new; more apt to wet the bed if they sleep in a warm or stuffy room; prefer to sleep with an open window; person concurrently has flatulence.
- *Secale* – men with an enlarged prostate, or elderly women, who feel better in general when exposed to coldness and feel worse when exposed to heat.
- *Staphysagria* – for a person who develops involuntary urination after an embarrassing or abusive experience; this person feels a lot of anger, and these feelings are usually held in for a period of time until they finally explode in a rage.

Other Therapeutic Measures

Consult a chiropractor, osteopath, or massage therapist to determine if a compressed nerve or other type of obstruction can be contributing to the incontinence.

Use biofeedback training to help lessen or conquer incontinence. Reflexology treatments can also help incontinence.

CHAPTER 22

Socially Transmitted Diseases

Socially transmitted diseases, as discussed in this book, are diseases that are transmitted from person to person. Almost all are transmitted through sexual contact. Others can be transmitted through close but more casual contact. For example, most viruses can be passed in airborne droplets and from shared objects.

SEXUALLY TRANSMITTED DISEASES

Sexually transmitted diseases (STDs) were known as venereal diseases in the past. There are over 20 organisms that are sexually transmitted, usually through intimate sexual contact. Some, such as hepatitis B and AIDS, can also be spread by contact with infected blood. People who contract an STD may have severe symptoms, while others may have no symptoms or only mild symptoms. Some diseases, such as syphilis, become dormant, giving the false hope that they are cured.

For this reason, if you are sexually active, regular examinations by a physician are extremely important, whether or not you have symptoms of an STD. If you do experience any symptoms, you should have them checked immediately.

The incidence of STDs is increasing each year, with teenagers and young adults experiencing the highest rate. More than 3 million new cases of STDs occur among American teenagers each year, according to the U.S. Division of STD Pre-

vention. Half of the top 10 reportable infectious diseases in the United States are STDs.

A small population group engaging in high-risk sexual practices with a large number of partners can maintain the spread of an STD. Changing partners dramatically increases the risk of becoming infected. Although condoms can prevent some STDs, among the general population only 5 to 17 percent report that they use condoms consistently, according to a 1995 article in the *American Journal of Public Health*. Even among adult couples with one HIV-positive individual, the reported rate of consistent condom usage is only about 50 percent.

Condoms do not offer reliable protection against genital herpes, chlamydia, or human papilloma virus, which causes genital warts. Abstinence is the only way to be certain of avoiding sexually transmitted disease.

Untreated STDs can cause infertility in men and women, or impotence in men. STDs can be passed to unborn children, causing lung disease, eye disease, and central nervous system infections.

PREVENTION OF STDS

The following measures will help prevent sexually transmitted diseases.

- Remain abstinent, unless you are involved in a monogamous relationship with a partner who is monogamous.

- Find out about your partner's health and sexual history.
- If you are not monogamous, limit the number of your sexual partners.
- Practice "safer" sex by using latex condoms, male or female.
- Have a checkup for STDs yearly if you have more than one partner.
- Do not have sex with anyone who cannot produce recent laboratory tests that show they tested negative for STDs.
- See your doctor if you think you have been exposed. Do not have sex again until you and your partner have been tested.

AIDS (ACQUIRED IMMUNE DEFICIENCY SYNDROME)

Although AIDS is not a common health problem, it is included in this book because it is a contagious STD and its rate of spread is increasing among all population groups. As there is no cure yet, prevention remains the most important factor in slowing the spread of this disease.

AIDS was first recognized as a distinct clinical syndrome in 1981. In 1983, it was shown to be caused by the human immunodeficiency virus (HIV). The main types of transmission are sexual contact, sharing contaminated needles, and reception of contaminated blood or certain blood products. AIDS can also be passed to babies if their mothers are HIV positive.

The U.S. Centers for Disease Control's case definition of AIDS includes being HIV positive and having one of 28 symptoms. The HIV virus attacks a type of lymphocyte (a white blood cell called a T helper cell) in the immune system, and patients develop recurrent, unusual, and severe infections or lymphomas (cancer of the lymph nodes). The infections seen in AIDS are often caused by pathogens that do not cause disease in people with normal immune systems.

AIDS can present as the sudden onset of fevers, sweats, fatigue, muscle pain, joint pain, headaches, sore throat, diarrhea, generalized swelling of the lymph glands, and skin rashes. It may also have a gradual onset, with unexplained fatigue, weight loss, fever, diarrhea, and generalized swelling of the lymph nodes. In some cases, HIV can directly infect the brain and cause dementia. People can be HIV positive for years before they develop any symptoms.

MODERN MEDICAL TREATMENT
Drug Therapy
The first treatment specifically for AIDS was azidothymidine (AZT), now known as zidovudine (Retrovir). Zidovudine interferes with the virus's replication, although HIV readily develops a resistance to the drug. Side effects of zidovudine can include muscle wasting, extreme nausea, anemia (low red blood cell count), diarrhea, rashes, fatigue, dementia, seizures, and the development of lymphoma.

Protease inhibitors, such as indinavir sulfate (Crixivan), are the newest treatment for AIDS. They block an enzyme of the virus that is needed for the virus cells to mature and become infectious. Although they have only been in use for a few years, protease inhibitors have reversed the course of AIDS in patients who were emaciated, had recurrent infections, and had been diagnosed as terminal. These patients have gained weight, regained energy, and are now able to work. The side effects of protease inhibitors can include nausea, vomiting, headache, abdominal pain, and fatigue.

Not all patients tolerate these new drugs, but may be able to if they use alternative methods to strengthen their immune system. Even patients who do tolerate the medications will benefit from alternative therapies.

ALTERNATIVE TREATMENT
Diet
Eat a quality diet that includes a wide variety of foods. Be very careful of your nutrition in order

to minimize weight loss and malabsorption problems. Malnutrition, with inadequate calories and insufficient protein, is a common reason for immune system deficiency.

Eliminate refined carbohydrates such as sugar and white flour. Reduce polyunsaturated and saturated fats and oils and use monounsaturated oils. Eliminate chocolate, caffeine, and alcohol from your diet. Do not eat processed foods or foods with additives such as colorings, flavors, and preservatives. Avoid diet drinks and all artificial sweeteners.

Eat fresh, organic vegetables, fruits, and proteins. Carefully clean all fruits and vegetables so they are free of parasites and pesticides. Always peel non-organic produce.

Drink at least eight 8-ounce glasses of pure water each day. Water is necessary to flush toxins out of the body. You must drink water even if you are not thirsty.

Exercise and Lifestyle

Exercise regularly. Stop smoking, and do not use tobacco in any form, as it reduces immune defenses. Avoid exposure to all tobacco smoke.

Do not take recreational drugs under any circumstances, and select any medicinal drugs you must take with care.

Practice safe sex either by abstaining or by using a latex condom. Avoid sexual excesses and non-monogamous relationships. Be aware that a condom does not guarantee protection against HIV.

Rest as much as possible and get fresh air and sunshine. Develop a habit of daily meditation.

Nutrient Therapy

Take nutritional supplements.

- vitamin A – 25,000 to 50,000 IU a day. *Caution:* Do not take more than 8,000 IU a day if you are pregnant or may be pregnant (strengthens mucus membranes; antioxidant).
- beta carotene – 200,000 IU a day (antioxidant)
- B-complex with 50 mg of each B (necessary for the functioning of all cells)
- vitamin B_6 – 50 to 100 mg a day (anti-cancer; helps immune system)
- vitamin B_{12} – 1,000 mcg a day (needed for cell division; combats fatigue; helps jittery nerves)
- folic acid – 2 to 5 mg a day. This is a large dose of folic acid and is available only by prescription at compounding pharmacies. (needed for cell division)
- vitamin C – 1,000 to 2,000 mg three times a day (boosts immune function and is an antiviral agent)
- vitamin E – 400 to 800 IU a day (antioxidant)
- copper – 2 to 3 mg a day (to balance zinc)
- iron – 50 to 100 mg a day, only if you are shown to be deficient (for anemia)
- selenium – 100 to 200 mcg a day (antioxidant; strengthens immune system)
- zinc – 25 to 50 mg a day (promotes wound healing; boosts immune function to fight a broad range of microbes)
- amino acids – as instructed on the label if malnutrition is a problem (needed for tissue repair)
- bioflavonoids – 1,000 mg a day (strengthens immune system)
- coenzyme Q_{10} – 100 mg a day (antioxidant; immune system stimulant)
- egg lecithin – 20,000 mg a day in divided doses (for cellular protection)
- organic germanium – 200 mg a day (improves tissue oxygenation and interferon production)
- Protozymes by Marco Pharma – three to four tablets two to three times a day between meals (destroy free radicals; reduce inflammation; aid in absorption) (see Sources)
- pycnogenol or grape seed extract – as directed on the label of your product (antioxidant; immune system stimulant)
- raw thymus glandular – as directed on the label of your product (enhances T-cell production)

Herbal Therapy
Take a botanical supplement.

- astragalus – protects the immune system; promotes healing
- echinacea – immune system stimulant
- garlic – natural antibiotic and immune system stimulant
- goldenseal – immune system stimulant. *Caution:* Do not take if you are pregnant.
- licorice root – stimulates the production of interferon
- osha root – strengthens the immune system
- St. John's wort – helps to inhibit viral infections, including HIV
- Siberian ginseng *(Eleutherococcus senticosus)* – enhances immune function

Homeopathic Remedies
Take a homeopathic remedy under the supervision of a homeopathic physician.

- *Arsenicum iodatum* – AIDS; recurring fever; drenching night sweats, swollen glands, emaciated patient; tendency to diarrhea; profound prostration; rapid, weak, irregular pulse.
- *Baptisia tinctoria* – AIDS; high toxic fevers; toxic and drugged; tongue yellow with brown streaks; heaviness of muscles and muscular soreness all over the body; sore throat; indescribable sick feeling all over; prostration; foul odor of the body, breath, and excretions.
- *Ferrum phosphoricum* – AIDS; periodic high fevers; fainting from weakness; fatigue; earaches; sore throat; anemia; inflammatory disorders; vomiting of undigested food; sour belching.
- *Medorrhinum* – AIDS; chronic recurrent infections; unstable vitality; arthritic pains; state of collapse; night sweats; trembling all over; profuse acrid discharges; lymph glands enlarged.
- *Mercurius solubilis* – AIDS; swollen glands;

profuse night sweats; recurring fever; fatigue; sore throat; narrow temperature range for comfort; sweats with fever.
- *Thuja* – AIDS, green mucus in sinus, may have warts and gonorrhea; tearing pain in muscles and joints; rapid exhaustion and emaciation; edema about the joints; better from warmth.

Other Therapeutic Measures
Be tested and treated for food, chemical, and inhalant allergies. Your allergies must be treated and controlled because they can damage the immune system.

If you are taking an antibiotic, take a *Lactobacillus acidophilus* supplement. Also take food-grade aloe vera, which appears to inhibit the growth and spread of HIV. Take 2 cups a day; reduce dose if diarrhea occurs.

Consult an acupuncturist. Take hyperthermia treatments or massage therapy from a trained therapist.

Consider hyperbaric oxygen treatments (oxygen administered in a special chamber under increased pressure) to increase total body tissue and blood oxygenation. This helps combat the opportunistic infections that accompany AIDS.

Take coffee enemas to help eliminate toxins.

Consult a qualified health care practitioner who has experience treating AIDS and educate yourself about your condition. Treatment protocols constantly change, and being as informed as possible is both necessary and helpful.

CANDIDA

Candida albicans is an opportunistic body yeast that lives in small amounts in all people. It normally occurs on the skin, in the vagina, and on the mucus membranes of the gastrointestinal and upper respiratory tracts. If the immune system becomes depressed, inefficient, or overwhelmed, candida can multiply and cause problems.

Because of their complex hormone systems,

women typically have more problems with and severe effects from candida. Increased use of antibiotics has caused increased incidence of candida vaginitis. Symptoms include vaginal and vulvar itching, with a thick cottage cheese–like discharge that does not have an odor. Risk factors for developing candida vaginitis include a diet high in refined sugar, antibiotic use, allergies, diabetes mellitus, oral contraceptives, pregnancy, use of steroids, and wearing nylon tights. Babies can be infected with candida as they pass through the birth canal if their mother has yeast vaginitis, usually resulting in thrush.

Sexual partners may cause re-infections of candida, as men and women can pass it back and forth, causing problems for both. Men can get jock itch, which is a fungal infection of the male genitalia, typically caused by candida. It can be sexually transmitted by a woman who has a yeast vaginal infection. In women there is complete correlation between genital and gastrointestinal candida cultures, but no studies on this correlation in men have yet been carried out. In addition to the rash, men may experience itching in the genital area, and some may have pain when urinating.

Risk factors for jock itch include diabetes, a partner with yeast vaginitis, antibiotic use, and a diet high in refined sugar. Moisture in the groin area also promotes the growth of yeast.

MODERN MEDICAL TREATMENT
Drug Therapy
Modern medicine treats candida vaginitis with monistat cream, nystatin cream, or clotrimazole (Gyne-Lotrimin) vaginal tablets. Monistat and Gyne-Lotrimin are now available over-the-counter. Nystatin cream is still a prescription drug. For jock itch, an antifungal cream such as monistat or nystatin is used. Side effects include irritation, burning, and allergic contact dermatitis.

Fluconazole (Diflucan) or itraconazole (Sporonox) may also be prescribed short term.

Side effects of Diflucan include headache, nausea, and abdominal pain. Adverse reactions to Sporonox include constipation, nausea, stomach ache, headache, and rash.

ALTERNATIVE TREATMENT
Diet
Avoid sugar and simple carbohydrates, such as fruit and white breads. Avoid dairy products; smoked, dried, fermented, or pickled foods; and any food containing yeast. There may be a sensitivity to yeast. Do not eat fruit, fruit juices, dried fruits, or candied fruits. Avoid coffee, caffeine, carbonated drinks, alcohol, and vinegar. Some people may have to limit grains.

Eat fresh and steamed vegetables, poultry, seafood, meats, and eggs. Include garlic and onions, as well as sea vegetables.

Drink eight 8-ounce glasses of pure water each day.

Exercise and Lifestyle
Avoid birth control pills, antibiotics, and steroids unless they are absolutely necessary. Do not smoke, and avoid all forms of tobacco, as it reduces immune defenses.

Perform aerobic exercise for 20 minutes each day or take regular walks. Be sure to get enough sleep.

Avoid fabrics that trap moisture next to your skin and do not wear synthetic fibers, pantyhose, or tight-fitting clothes every day. Wear loose, absorbent clothing. Bathe after any activity that causes sweating, and rinse and dry the groin area thoroughly after bathing.

Avoid sexual activity unless a latex condom is used. Both partners must be treated to stop transferring the infection back and forth.

Nutrient Therapy
Take the following nutritional supplements.

- vitamin A – 25,000 IU a day. *Caution:* Do not take more than 8,000 IU a day if you are or might be pregnant (strengthens mucus membranes).

- beta carotene – 200,000 IU a day (antioxidant; strengthens immune system)
- B-complex with 50 mg of each B – as directed on the product. Be certain it is a yeast-free preparation (helps regulate hormones necessary for functioning of all cells, often deficient in vaginitis).
- biotin – as directed on your product (inhibits yeast)
- vitamin C – 2,000 mg three times a day (boosts the immune system)
- vitamin E – 200 IU two times a day (strengthens immune system)
- zinc picolinate – 15 mg a day (important for the health of the reproductive organs)
- coenzyme Q$_{10}$ – 100 mg a day (stimulates the immune system; increases tissue oxygenation)
- fructo-oligosaccharides – as directed on the label of your product (encourages growth of beneficial bacteria in the intestines)
- *Lactobacillus* species (*L. acidophilus* and *L. bulgaricus*) – ½ tsp. three times a day (a source of beneficial bacteria)
- organic germanium – 150 mg a day (for tissue oxygenation
- thymus glandular – one tablet three times a day (strengthens immune system)

Herbal Therapy

Take the following botanical supplements. If you do not obtain relief, seek the help of a trained herbalist.

- black walnut hulls – antifungal
- caprylic acid – antifungal; inhibits yeast
- echinacea – stimulates the immune system
- garlic – natural antibiotic
- goldenseal – stimulates the immune system. *Caution:* Do not use during pregnancy.
- grapefruit seed extract – antifungal; inhibits yeast
- Pau d'arco tea – antifungal; inhibits yeast

- ParaMicrocidin – two capsules three times a day (antifungal) (Nutricology—see Sources)
- St. John's wort – strengthens the immune system and the mucosa
- undecylic acid – antifungal

Homeopathic Remedies

Below are listed several homeopathic remedies that may be helpful. If your symptoms are not relieved, seek the help of a trained homeopathic practitioner.

- *Borax* – oral thrush, candidiasis; candida rash of anus; vaginal discharge like egg white; white fungus-like growth on mouth; cracked nipples; heat in vagina; discharges hot, thick, biting.
- *China officinalis* – gas, bloating, and diarrhea; night sweats; belching and burping; fermentation in bowel; total exhaustion; liver and colon irritable and sensitive; bloating; sensitive to touch and pressure, particularly on abdomen; stools smell sour and acidic; major remedy for candida.
- *Lycopodium* – craves sweets and starches; depression; problems of self-esteem and low confidence; weakness of digestion; full of gas and bloating; acidity, sour, tasteless belching; fermentation in intestines; excessive hunger; hard, difficult, small stools.
- *Medorrhinum* – craves sweets, oranges, sour things, green fruits, refreshing things; ravenous appetite; itching skin; belching of "rotten egg"; intense itching of anus; vaginal discharge thick, acrid, excoriating, fishy odor; intense itching, vagina better rubbing and by bathing with tepid water; sad; weak memory; feels life unreal, everything seems unreal.
- *Natrum carbonicum* – candida; weak digestion and digestive problems; gas, bloating, belching, heartburn, depressed and melancholy; worse with wine and milk; oversensitive to dietetic errors; puffiness; worse from

vegetable diet, starchy food; worse damp weather; abdomen enlarged and distended; diarrhea from starches and milk; always nibbling.

- *Thuja* – candida; discharges foul, acrid, musty, rancid, or of sweetish odor; flatulence and abdominal distention; vagina itches and is very sensitive, preventing sex; profuse vaginal discharge thick, greenish; sweetish-smelling sweat on scrotum; offensive-smelling genitals; chronic diarrhea with painless, watery, grass-green stools; skin sensitive to touch; persistent insomnia; worse damp, humid atmosphere.

Other Therapeutic Measures

Treat candida vaginitis with a retention douche of a 1:1,000 dilution of betadine, an iodine solution, once or twice a day during the acute phase.

Use one of the following nutritional and herbal douches for several days, or use a tampon saturated in the supplement. The tampon must be removed after four hours. Remember that it is not healthy to douche frequently, as it disturbs the normal bacterial flora of the vagina. Recurrent douching has also been associated with ectopic pregnancy.

- apple cider vinegar – 2 Tbsp. to 1 quart of water (re-acidifies the vagina)
- boric acid capsule – 600 mg per capsule a day, vaginally, for no more than 14 days (re-acidifies the vagina)
- boric acid (powdered) mixed with equal amounts of berberis, hydrastis, and calendula – use vaginally in capsule form (reacidifies the vagina; strengthens the immune system)
- chopped garlic – add to a douche solution or use a clove, peeled, wrapped in gauze to be inserted as a vaginal suppository (antimicrobial). *Caution:* This may cause irritation in some women.
- *Lactobacillus acidophilus* – ½ tsp. in a cup of warm water daily, or use plain yogurt with live cultures (reinoculates the vagina with beneficial bacteria)
- St. John's wort, goldenseal, echinacea, fresh plantain, garlic, and calendula – use in equal parts to make a douche – alternate this douche with acidophilus douches (strengthens immune system). *Caution:* Do not take goldenseal if you are pregnant.
- tea tree oil – soak a tampon with 3 drops of tea tree oil in 1 Tbsp. of yogurt (antifungal)

Treat jock itch topically with tea tree oil on the rash, or a wet Pau d'arco tea bag applied to the area for 10 minutes.

Be sure your sexual partner is also treated.

Be tested and treated for candida allergy with both a *Candida* extract and a T.O.E. extract for common skin fungi.

Have NAET treatments for candida (see the Chiropractic section in chapter 9, Alternative Medical Disciplines).

Have reflexology treatments.

CHLAMYDIA

Chlamydia are bacteria-like organisms that can cause infection of the genitourinary system, eyes, and lungs. Chlamydia is now the most common STD in North America, and at least 4 million people are infected with it each year. It is also known as non-gonococcal urethritis (NGU). Five to ten percent of all women have chlamydia, which often causes a silent infection that can be identified only with special tests. Up to 85 percent of women infected may not have any symptoms, and 50 percent of men have no symptoms.

In women, chlamydia most commonly affects the fallopian tubes, lining of the uterus, and lining of the pelvis. When it infects the lining of the pelvis, it causes a serious condition known as pelvic inflammatory disease (PID). Pelvic inflammatory disease can cause scarring of the fallopian tubes, infertility, chronic pain, and a tenfold risk of ectopic pregnancy. Symptoms include vaginal discharge, pelvic pain, pain with intercourse, and fever. Chlamydia is not a common cause of vaginitis, but it can cause vaginal irritation and a yellowish-green discharge.

If a mother is infected with chlamydia during pregnancy, her baby may develop an eye infection or pneumonia in the first six months of life, and asthma and permanent lung damage later on.

In men, chlamydia causes infection of the urethra (urethritis) and the epididymis. Men with urethritis have discharge from the penis, urethral itching, or changes in urination. An infection of the epididymis causes pain in one side of the scrotum, swelling, and redness. Men should seek medical attention, since epididymitis is difficult to distinguish from torsion of the testicle, which is a surgical emergency (see chapter 24, Male Problems).

MODERN MEDICAL TREATMENT

Drug Therapy

Chlamydia is treated with erythromycin, or azithromycin (Zithromax) or tetracycline (Achromycin), and doxycycline (Doryx, Vibramyacin), all of which are antibiotics. Tetracycline and doxycycline are known as a broad-spectrum antibiotic, which can affect a wide range of organisms. They cannot be used by pregnant women, because they can permanently discolor the teeth of the baby. They can also cause permanent yellow-gray or brown discoloration of the teeth in children less than eight years of age. Side effects include anorexia, nausea, vomiting, diarrhea, pain with swallowing, and inflammation of the intestines. Expired tetracycline and doxycycline can cause kidney damage.

Erythromycin can cause nausea, vomiting, abdominal pain, diarrhea, and anorexia. Since erythromycin is metabolized by a certain enzyme in the liver, it can interfere with the metabolism of such drugs as theophylline (see Asthma in chapter 13, Respiratory System Problems) and phenytoin (Dilantin, used for seizures). Erythro-

mycin has been associated with heart rhythm abnormalities when taken with Hismanal and Seldane (prescription antihistamines).

Both tetracycline and erythromycin can cause overgrowth of yeast and a yeast infection.

Clindamycin (Cleocin) or metronidazole (Metrogel) vaginal creams are used for chlamydia vaginitis. Cleocin can cause vaginal candidiasis, vaginitis, dizziness, headache, heartburn, nausea, vomiting, diarrhea, abdominal pain, and hives. Metrogel can cause vaginal burning and discharge, vaginal candidiasis, pelvic discomfort, abdominal cramps, diarrhea, and nausea.

Other Therapeutic Measures

Abstinence or the use of condoms is suggested until the infection has cleared.

ALTERNATIVE TREATMENT

Consult a physician to determine if antibiotics are necessary, in addition to natural remedies. Pelvic inflammatory disease usually requires treatment with antibiotics.

Diet

Avoid fatty foods, sugar, white flour, coffee, alcohol, and simple carbohydrates such as white breads. Also avoid red meats, pasteurized dairy products,and caffeine during healing. Eat fresh fruits and vegetables.

Increase fluids, including pure water and fruit and vegetable juices. Use juicing therapy, including juices from apples, carrots, celery, cranberry, cucumber, grapes, green vegetables, nectarines, pomegranate, parsley, and watermelon.

Exercise and Lifestyle

Stop smoking and avoid tobacco in any form, as it reduces immune defenses.

Use latex condoms to prevent the spread of chlamydia.

Avoid sexual activity during the infection's acute stage to reduce trauma to inflamed tissue.

Nutrient Therapy

Take the nutrients listed below, as well as taking nutrients that help strengthen the immune system (see the nutrients listed for AIDS earlier in this chapter).

- vitamin A – 25,000 IU a day. *Caution:* Do not take more than 8,000 IU a day if you are pregnant or might be pregnant (necessary for the integrity of vaginal mucosa).
- vitamin C – 750 to 2,500 mg four times a day (boosts immune function)
- vitamin E – 400 IU twice a day (increases tissue resistance to chlamydia)
- copper – 2 to 3 mg a day (balances zinc)
- zinc – 50 mg a day (important for the health of the reproductive organs; promotes wound healing; boosts the immune system)
- coenzyme Q_{10} – 60 mg four times a day (stimulates the immune system; increases tissue oxygenation)
- organic germanium – 150 mg a day (increases tissue oxygenation)

Herbal Therapy

Take a botanical supplement.

- cranberry extract – prevents the spread of bacterial urinary infections
- echinacea – supports the immune system
- goldenseal – strengthens immune system to combat infection. *Caution:* Do not take if you are pregnant.
- horsetail – accelerates healing
- pulsatilla and podophyllum (given by a professional knowledgeable in the use of herbs) – antibacterial activity
- saw palmetto – soothing to sexual organs

Homeopathic Remedies

Consult a homeopathic physician to help you choose the remedy that best fits your symptoms.

- *Arsenicum album* – right ovarian pains; acrid, yellow, thick and offensive vaginal discharge; urinary incontinence; burning in ovarian region; edematous scrotum.
- *Belladonna* – right-sided ovarian pains or cysts; cystitis; sex drive generally low to low-normal; uterine hemorrhage feels hot; violent bearing down towards genitals, as if everything would fall out; orchitis and epididymitis; cutting pains from hip to hip.
- *Cantharis* – urethritis; great burning before, after, but especially during urination, each drop passes as if scalding water; urethritis and purulent or bloody discharge; inflammation of ovaries; worse after suppressed discharges; burning and itching of labia, worse from urination; excessive sexual appetite; vaginal discharge with sexual excitement causing severe itching; swelling of male genitals, bloody semen.
- *Lac caninum* – high sex drive, but worse from sex; pain in ovaries alternating sides; pain in the uterus extending upwards; flatus from vagina; epididymis sore to touch; penis swollen, pain in urethra.
- *Lycopodium* – stomach pains, better rubbing abdomen; abdomen sensitive to the weight of clothing; painful urging for urination; discharge of blood from genitals during stools; vagina dry, burning, worse during and after sex; sex painful; vaginal discharge acrid; sexual exhaustion in male; enlarged prostate; hematuria, urine burning hot.

Other Therapeutic Measures

Wear cotton underwear. Avoid bubble baths. Take warm sitz baths with herbs, plain water, or Epsom salts.

Women should avoid douching with commercial vaginal chemicals. Use retention douches with a 1:100 dilution of betadine, an iodine solution, once or twice a day during the acute phases.

Use one of the following nutritional douches for several days, or use a tampon saturated in the supplement, but it must be removed after four hours. Remember that it is not healthy to douche frequently, as it disturbs the normal bacterial flora of the vagina. Recurrent douching has also been associated with ectopic pregnancy.

- *Lactobacillus acidophilus* – ½ tsp. in a cup of warm water daily, or use plain yogurt with live cultures (reinoculates the vagina with beneficial bacteria)
- zinc sulfate – 1 Tbsp. of a 2 percent solution in 1 pint of water (helps with wound healing; boosts the immune system)

Be treated by an environmental medicine physician with a *Chlamydia* extract.

Have NAET treatments for chlamydia (see the Chiropractic section in chapter 9, Alternative Medical Disciplines).

GARDNERELLA

The bacteria *Gardnerella vaginalis* (previously known as *Haemophilus vaginalis*) is the second most common cause of infectious vaginitis. *Gardnerella vaginalis* causes what is termed non-specific vaginitis, because it is not caused by trichomonas, gonorrhea, or candida. The discharge is a non-irritating, gray, frothy, sometimes thick discharge. It is very foul smelling, described by some women as fishy. The vaginal pH is lowered to 5.0 to 5.5. Some physicians think that gardnerella is a secondary infection that develops after anaerobic bacteria colonize the vagina.

MODERN MEDICAL TREATMENT
Drug Therapy
Oral antibiotics are not normally prescribed for gardnerella vaginitis. Clindamycin (Cleocin) or metronidazole (Metrogel) vaginal creams are used instead. Cleocin can cause vaginal candidi-asis, vaginitis, dizziness, headache, heartburn, nausea, vomiting, diarrhea, abdominal pain, and hives. Metrogel can cause vaginal burning and discharge, vaginal candidiasis, pelvic discomfort, abdominal cramps, diarrhea, and nausea.

ALTERNATIVE TREATMENT
Diet
Follow the dietary recommendations for chlamydia, above. In addition, drink cranberry juice.

Exercise and Lifestyle
Stop smoking and avoid tobacco in any form, as it reduces immune defenses.

Use latex condoms to prevent the spread of gardnerella.

Nutrient Therapy
Take the following nutrients to help with a gardnerella infection.

- vitamin A – 25,000 IU a day. *Caution:* Do not take more than 8,000 IU a day if you are or might be pregnant (necessary for the integrity of vaginal mucosa).
- beta carotene – 150,000 IU a day (helps protect mucus membranes from infection; helps repair damaged cells)
- vitamin B-complex – 100 mg of each B vitamin twice a day (regulates metabolism; usually deficient in vaginitis)
- vitamin C – 750 to 2,500 mg four times a day (boosts immune system; aids tissue healing)
- vitamin E – 400 IU twice a day (powerful antioxidant that aids in healing)
- copper – 2 to 3 mg a day (to balance zinc)
- zinc picolinate – 50 mg a day (important for health of reproductive organs; promotes wound healing; boosts immune system)

Herbal Therapy
Take a botanical supplement.

- garlic – enhances immune function to combat infection
- goldenseal – enhances immune function to combat infection. *Caution:* Do not use if you are pregnant.
- Pau d'arco – antibacterial agent
- tea tree oil suppositories – good for vaginitis and infections

Homeopathic Remedies

Consult a homeopathic physician to help you choose the remedy that best fits your symptoms.

- *Medorrhinum* – vaginal discharge thick, acrid, excoriating, fishy odor; sensitive spot near uterus; intense itching, vagina better rubbing and by bathing with tepid water; pain in ovaries better with pressure; ovarian pain; infertility.
- *Natrum phosphoricum* – infertility with acid secretions from vagina; sour-smelling discharges from uterus; vaginal discharge sour, creamy, honey-colored, or acid and watery.
- *Pulsatilla* – vaginal discharge acrid, milky, thick like cream with pain in the back.
- *Sepia* – vaginal discharge yellow, greenish, foul smelling; itching; pain high in vagina from uterus to navel.
- *Thuja* – profuse, thick, greenish vaginal discharge; vaginal itching; vagina very sensitive.

Other Therapeutic Measures

Alternate saltwater and vinegar douches for a week. For the saline douche, use 1 tsp salt. in 1 quart of water, and for the vinegar douche, use 2 Tbsp. vinegar in 1 quart of water.

Use vaginal packs and suppositories to rebalance vaginal pH. Apply plain yogurt, acidophilus powder, boric acid, diluted tea tree oil, or diluted calendula oil on a tampon. (Note: The tampon should not be left in for more than four hours.)

Use lavender oil in sitz baths, douches, creams, lotions, and tampons.

Have NAET treatments for gardnerella or be treated by an environmental medicine physician with a *Gardnerella* extract.

Be sure your sexual partner is also treated.

GENITAL WARTS

Genital warts are caused by human papilloma virus (HPV). Approximately 40 to 80 percent of the North American population is infected. HPV is the most common STD in adolescents, and as many as 38 percent of sexually active females ages 13 to 21 are infected. There are three times more office visits for genital warts than for genital herpes. Genital warts are difficult to detect and can be spread sexually, but can also be spread by objects that have not been cleaned properly, such as underwear, and sexual aids or devices. The source of a wart infection can be difficult to trace because the warts may not develop for 2 to 18 months after exposure.

Warts may show up as soft, cauliflower-like growths appearing singly or in clusters in and around the vagina, anus, penis, groin, and/or scrotal area. However, only 2 to 3 percent of those infected have visible warts. Some people have only burning, itching redness, and irritation. White vinegar applied to the area can make the warts visible, or a special test to look for the DNA of the virus can be used. HPV has been linked to 90 percent of the cases of cancer of the cervix.

MODERN MEDICAL TREATMENT

The warts are removed with electrocautery, liquid nitrogen, and application of acid or podophyllin. However, they can recur many times, and all of these treatments can be very painful.

ALTERNATIVE TREATMENT

Diet

Eliminate processed foods from your diet. Eliminate dairy products, sugar, and junk foods. Reduce meats, dietary fat, caffeine, and alcohol. Eat fresh fruits and vegetables. Use fresh vegetable juices and "green" drinks such as barley green for immune support.

Exercise and Lifestyle

Stop smoking and avoid tobacco in any form, as it reduces immune defenses.

Alternative treatment for genital warts requires a strong commitment and significant lifestyle changes. Avoid multiple sexual partners, unprotected sex, and oral sex. Use latex condoms to prevent the spread of the virus. However, there is evidence that HPV is small enough to penetrate a condom.

Nutrient Therapy

Take nutrients to support the immune system. In addition to the supplements listed below, see the nutrients listed for immune supported under AIDS, earlier in this chapter.

- vitamin A – 25,000 IU a day. *Caution:* Do not take more than 8,000 IU a day if you are pregnant or might be pregnant (necessary for integrity of vaginal mucosa).
- beta carotene – 150,000 IU a day (helps protect mucus membranes from infection; helps repair damaged cells)
- vitamin B-complex – as directed on your product (combats virus; helps keep it from spreading; works with L-lysine)
- folic acid – 800 mcg a day (needed for cell division)
- vitamin C – 2,000 mg a day (boosts immune function; reduces spread of infection)
- vitamin E – 400 IU a day (antioxidant; prevents cell damage)
- copper – 2 to 3 mg a day (to balance zinc)
- organic germanium – 150 mg a day (increases tissue oxygenation)
- selenium – 200 mg a day (powerful antioxidant)
- zinc picolinate – 50 mg a day (important for reproductive organs; promotes wound healing; boosts the immune system)

- L-lysine – 1,500 to 3,000 mg a day during an outbreak (prevents viral replication)

Herbal Therapy

Take a botanical supplement.

- burdock – stimulates the immune system
- echinacea – stimulates and supports the immune system
- lomatium – antiviral; stimulates the immune system; decreases inflammation
- thuja – helps control warts

Homeopathic Remedies

Consult a homeopathic physician to help you choose the remedy that best fits your symptoms.

- *Aurum metallicum* – venereal warts about the anus and genitals.
- *Medorrhinum* – venereal warts; especially genital warts over penis, glans, and scrotum; warts inside the vagina or on the labia; may also be on the hands or thighs; moist warts, often fleshy, stubby warts; may also be pointed.
- *Nitric acid* – widespread, sensitive warts with splinter-like pains; sometimes soft or cauliflower-shaped warts; may be on genitals, anus.
- *Sabina* – oozing or itching warts on or near the genitalia or perineum; large, impressive, and hard warts; butternut-shaped wart on dorsum of penis; offensive fish-brine odor from wart; on both male and female genitalia.
- *Thuja* – most common remedy for warts; often large and impressive warts; may be rapidly growing; may occur on genitals, inside urethra or vagina, or on penis; may also be on cervix or uterus.

Other Therapeutic Measures

Apply an ointment of vitamin A, thuja, and lomatium (herbs) for antiviral properties and strengthening of mucus membranes.

Use castor oil compresses on genital warts. Use only cold-pressed castor oil on clean white cotton cloth and apply to the area with heat for 30 minutes. Change the cloth each time and discard the used cloths.

Use alternating hot and cold sitz baths to promote immune activity in the pelvic area.

Be sure your partner is also checked for genital warts.

GONORRHEA

Gonorrhea is caused by the bacteria *Neisseria gonorrhoeae*. It can infect the genital mucus membranes, eyes, joints, and throat. There are approximately 2.5 million new cases in North America each year. In major cities in the United States, one out of every three cases of gonorrhea is now resistant to penicillin, and in almost half of the cases, chlamydia is also found.

In women, gonorrhea can infect the vagina, urethra, rectum, uterus, cervix, ovaries, or fallopian tubes. It can also cause pelvic inflammatory disease (PID), which tends to recur (see Chlamydia, above). About half to three quarters of women have symptoms, including pain with urination, urgency, and frequency, and a pus-like vaginal discharge, The remaining women are asymptomatic, although the infection can cause infertility in the future. Gonorrhea may cause vaginitis, but is seen in fewer than 4 percent of vaginitis cases. Vaginitis caused by gonorrhea is more common in prepubertal girls, and is the result of sexual abuse. After puberty, gonorrhea tends to infect the cervix and can spread to the fallopian tubes.

Ninety-five percent of men with gonorrhea have symptoms. They have frequent painful urination, with an urgency to urinate and a pus-like discharge from the penis. A scarring and narrowing of the urethra can occur in men with untreated gonorrhea. It can also cause infection of the rectum, prostate gland, and epididymis. Untreated gonorrhea can lead to sterility.

Gonorrhea can cause a severe eye infection in the newborn and even blindness, so most babies are routinely treated with antibiotic eye drops shortly after delivery. A rare complication of gonorrhea is gonococcal arthritis, which presents a fever, chills, and body aches. If untreated, it can become full-blown arthritis in which there is rapid destruction of cartilage and bone.

MODERN MEDICAL TREATMENT
Drug Therapy
Gonorrhea is treated with antibiotics, such as rocephin (Ceftriaxone), tetracycline (Doxycycline), or quinolones (Ofloxacin). Rocephin has to be given by injection or intravenously. It can cause diarrhea, anemia, pain at the site of injection, high white blood cell count, headache, flushing, and elevation of liver enzymes. Tetracycline cannot be used by pregnant women, because it can permanently discolor the teeth of the baby. Side effects include anorexia, nausea, vomiting, diarrhea, pain with swallowing, and inflammation of the intestines. Expired tetracycline can cause kidney damage. Ofloxacin can cause nausea, diarrhea, vomiting, abdominal pain and discomfort, headache, restlessness, and rash. It should not be used by pregnant women or adolescents, because it may cause damage to the cartilage. All of these antibiotics can cause an overgrowth of yeast (candida).

Exercise and Lifestyle
The use of a latex condom is advised, or remaining abstinent until the infection has cleared.

ALTERNATIVE TREATMENT
Gonorrhea is difficult to cure with alternative measures, and because it is so virulent, antibiotics are nearly always necessary. However, treatment is more successful and less stressful for the body if alternative measures are used along with antibiotics.

Diet
Follow the dietary recommendations for chlamydia, above.

Exercise and Lifestyle
Stop smoking, and avoid all forms of tobacco, as it reduces immune defenses.

Use latex condoms and diaphragms to help reduce the spread of gonorrhea.

Nutrient Therapy
Take nutrients to strengthen your body and help eliminate infection. In addition to the supplements listed below, see the nutrients listed for immune support under AIDS, earlier in this chapter.

- vitamin A – 25,000 IU a day. *Caution:* Do not take more than 8,000 IU a day if you are or might be pregnant (strengthens mucus membranes).
- beta carotene – 150,000 IU a day (helps protect mucus membranes from infection; helps repair damaged cells)
- vitamin C – 2,000 mg every hour during the acute phase; reduce to 5,000 mg a day for a month after the infection (essential to immune function; reduces spread of infection)
- vitamin E – 400 IU two times a day (antioxidant; prevents cell damage)
- copper – 2 to 3 mg a day (balances zinc)
- zinc – 50 mg a day (important for the health of the reproductive organs; promotes wound healing; boosts the immune system)
- coenzyme Q_{10} – 60 mg four times a day (stimulates the immune system; increases tissue oxygenation)
- organic germanium – 150 mg a day (increases tissue oxygenation)

Herbal Therapy

- bayberry – strengthens immune system; antibacterial properties

- echinacea – stimulates immune system
- garlic – a natural antibiotic
- goldenseal – broad-spectrum herbal antibiotic for disorders of vagina and prostate. *Caution:* Do not use if you are pregnant.
- nettle – helps cure vaginal infections

Homeopathic Remedies
Consult a homeopathic physician to help you choose the remedy that best fits your symptoms.

- *Medorrhinum* – chronic vaginitis, urethritis, or cystitis, especially if this occurs after beginning a new sexual relationship; extreme sex drive; arthritis with history of gonorrhea; history of gonorrhea in the patient or parents.
- *Natrum sulphuricum* – gonorrhea, suppressed gonorrhea; greenish urethral discharge.
- *Nitric acid* – gonorrhea; chronic urethral discharge, may be bloody, non-specific urethritis; ulcers of genitals, ulcers or stricture in urethra with stitching pains; vaginitis, itching before or after menses, worse with sex; acrid vaginal discharge; sex drive excessive.
- *Pulsatilla* – acrid, burning, creamy vaginal discharge with back pain; gonorrhea; high sexual energy; gonorrheal orchitis; thick yellow discharge from urethra in late stage of gonorrhea.
- *Thuja* – gonorrhea; sensation of something alive in the abdomen; profuse greenish vaginal discharge; discharges are foul, acrid, musty and on occasion may have a sweetish odor; sex drive generally high; vagina very sensitive, preventing sex; rheumatism from suppressed gonorrhea.

Other Therapeutic Measures
Be treated by an environmental physician with a *Neisseria gonorrhoeae* extract.

Have NAET treatments for gonorrhea (see

the Chiropractic section in chapter 9, Alternative Medical Disciplines).

Be sure your sexual partner is also treated.

HEPATITIS

Hepatitis is an inflammation of the liver that may be chronic and continuous, or acute and will eventually heal. Hepatitis is associated with damage or death of liver cells, causing the liver to function poorly. Hepatitis may be caused by drugs or by a viral infection. Parasites and rickettsia (a form of bacteria) can also cause hepatitis. In the early stages of hepatitis there is fever, nausea, vomiting, and loss of appetite. Rashes and joint pain may occur, as well as extreme fatigue with rapid weight loss. Dark urine and light stools appear, followed by jaundice that may take one to two weeks to reach its peak and two to four weeks to fade. During this time the liver may be enlarged and tender to the touch. Symptoms may be as mild as flu-like symptoms or as serious as liver failure and coma.

According to the American Liver Foundation in Cedar Grove, New Jersey, there are several types of viral hepatitis, including types A, B, C, D, E, F, and G. All hepatitis types can cause acute infection, and B, C, and D can result in chronic infection.

Hepatitis A, also called infectious hepatitis, is spread through fecal-oral contact, oral-anal sex, and through contact with infected items such as food, clothing, bed linens, and other items. It is contagious two to three weeks before the jaundice appears, and for one week afterward, but rarely has any long-term consequences.

Hepatitis E is transmitted through fecal contamination. Both water and food-borne transmission have been documented. Type E hepatitis is rarely seen in North America.

Hepatitis B, also called serum hepatitis, is the most lethal of the group. There are 200,000 new cases annually in North America, and over 6,000 North Americans die from it each year. It accounts for about 50 percent of reported hepatitis cases and is spread through infected blood products and needles as well as sexual contact. Six to ten percent of infected adults will become carriers; there are 300 million carriers of hepatitis B worldwide.

Groups at high risk for hepatitis B infection include healthcare professionals, inmates and staff of institutions, dialysis patients, household contacts and sexual partners of hepatitis B carriers, international travelers, intravenous drug abusers, sexually active adults with more than one sexual partner, and sexually active bisexual and homosexual men. Estimates place hepatitis B infections among all North Americans at 5 percent and among homosexual men at 85 percent. Hepatitis B is not very contagious except among those involved in high-risk behavior. About 10 percent of acute hepatitis B cases progress to the chronic state, damaging the liver.

There are 3.9 million North Americans chronically infected with hepatitis C virus. Acute hepatitis C causes a mild illness, but 80 percent of acute hepatitis C infections become chronic and lead to liver disease. Hepatitis C constitutes 90 to 95 percent of all hepatitis contracted from blood transfusions, even though blood is screened for both hepatitis B and C. It takes six months for antibodies to hepatitis C to develop, making it impossible to identify all infected blood. Hepatitis C can also be contracted through sexual contact, intravenous drug abuse, and broken skin or mucus membranes, but in about 40 percent of hepatitis C cases, no risk factor can be identified.

Hepatitis D is sometimes called a "defective" virus because it can cause infection only in the presence of hepatitis B virus. It can cause both acute and chronic hepatitis and has been responsible for epidemics among high-risk populations such as IV drug abusers, hemophiliacs, and patients with multiple transfusions.

The importance of hepatitis F has not yet been established in human disease. Like hepatitis A and hepatitis E, it is transmitted through fecal contamination, and recovery from the illness confers specific immunity.

Hepatitis G is transmitted by blood and is the cause of some post-transfusion hepatitis. Hepatitis G is found in around 2 percent of blood donors in North America. Healthcare professionals are at risk through occupational exposure to blood or body fluids.

Excessive alcohol consumption; drug abuse, including prescription drugs; overexposure to chemicals; and rare drug reactions can cause toxic hepatitis. The extent of the liver damage is directly related to the amount and length of exposure to the toxin.

MODERN MEDICAL TREATMENT

Diet
In recent years the only dietary recommendation for acute hepatitis has been the avoidance of alcohol, both during the infection, and for three to four months afterward, until the liver enzymes return to normal. Some people may not be able to consume alcohol again after having hepatitis, and people with chronic hepatitis cannot consume alcohol. Many patients find they cannot eat fat or fried foods while they are ill.

Drug Therapy
There is no treatment for acute hepatitis other than rest, good nutrition, and avoidance of alcohol.

Gamma globulin injections will temporarily enhance immunity to hepatitis A, but is of no value for hepatitis B and C. When food-caused outbreaks of hepatitis occur, people who have eaten at the implicated restaurant may be given gamma globulin. Hepatitis B immune globulin injections a month apart will help prevent hepatitis B in those who have been exposed. Side effects of these globulin injections are uncommon but may include pain at the site of injection, hives, and anaphylactic shock.

Interferon (a protein with antiviral and im-

munogenic properties) injections help about 50 percent of patients with acute hepatitis B and C. Interferon is also used with chronic hepatitis C. It is thought to work by stimulating resistance in the non-infected cells in the liver. Intron A, a genetically engineered alpha interferon, reduces liver damage caused by chronic hepatitis C. The fatigue and malaise are also lessened and liver function tests often improve.

Vaccination
A vaccine for hepatitis A has been developed, but there is controversy over its use because infection with hepatitis A confers lifetime immunity. The vaccine could be helpful in preventing an outbreak, however, and would be more helpful for adults than for children. The disease is more severe in adults, and the incidence of hepatitis A is decreasing in children. The vaccine for hepatitis A is useful for travelers who will be staying in an area where hepatitis A is endemic.

Health workers, anyone in contact with hepatitis B patients, and teenagers are advised to be vaccinated against hepatitis B. Babies are now being routinely vaccinated for hepatitis B even though they are not at risk. The vaccine is said to protect for years by stimulating the formation of antibodies to the virus. However, some people do not develop antibodies, even after repeated vaccinations. Side effects from the vaccination include pain at the injection site, fever, hives, and chronic fatigue syndrome. The vaccine for hepatitis B can also protect against hepatitis D. At present there is no vaccine for hepatitis C. (See Hepatitis B section in chapter 7, Childhood Vaccinations for more information.)

Liver Transplant
In cases of chronic hepatitis B and C, where the liver is severely damaged, cirrhosis or cancer of the liver can eventually develop. A liver transplant can be life-saving in some of these cases. However, with hepatitis B, the new liver usually soon becomes infected, and the hepatitis can be

severe and is usually chronic. Re-infection with hepatitis C is almost universal, but the disease is less severe than that of the hepatitis B re-infection.

Exercise and Lifestyle

Patients are advised not to exercise while they are ill.

They are told to avoid intimate contact during the incubation period of hepatitis A if they think they have been exposed. Because it is spread by the oral-fecal route, patients are told to wash their hands thoroughly after each bowel movement; wash their bed linens and underwear alone, not with the family laundry; and avoid sharing toothbrushes or towels with anyone else. Bleach or disinfectants and hot water are advised when washing the patient's linens and underwear.

For hepatitis B and C, razors and toothbrushes should not be shared.

ALTERNATIVE TREATMENT

Diet

Eat only fresh foods and a diet low in protein to minimize stress on the liver. Avoid animal protein, including raw fish and shellfish. Eat small meals throughout the day and avoid processed foods, refined sugar, heavy spices, and caffeine. Eat the grains and seeds that are more easily digested, such as millet, quinoa, and buckwheat. Include at least one salad and one meal of steamed vegetables a day. Also eat artichokes, which help protect the liver.

Avoid alcohol, as it is a liver toxin. Be cautious of contaminated food and water when you travel.

Drink ample distilled or filtered water daily. In addition, drink fresh lemon juice mixed in water followed by vegetable juice both morning and evening as this is very healing for the liver.

Use juice therapy containing the following blends. The concentrated nutrients will help speed recovery from hepatitis.

- beet, carrot, and wheat grass
- garlic, burdock, flax, and black currant

Exercise and Lifestyle

Do not exercise while you are ill. After the jaundice fades, slowly resume your exercise program.

Get plenty of bed rest during the acute stages of the illness. Avoid intimate physical contact until well after you are no longer contagious.

Do not smoke, and avoid tobacco in any form, including secondhand smoke.

Nutrient Therapy

Take the following supplements.

- vitamin A – 15,000 IU a day. *Caution:* Do not exceed 8,000 IU a day if you are or might be pregnant (aids in healing mucus membranes and tissues).
- vitamin B-complex – 50 to 100 mg three times a day, but do not exceed 100 mg of vitamin B_3 in any one day (all B vitamins are essential for normal liver function)
- vitamin C – 5,000 to 10,000 mg a day (powerful antiviral agent)
- vitamin E – 400 to 800 IU a day (a potent antioxidant)
- calcium – 1,500 mg a day (essential for clotting, which is a problem in liver disease)
- magnesium – 1,000 mg a day (essential for clotting; balances calcium)
- coenzyme Q_{10} – 60 mg a day (enhances tissue oxygenation; stimulates immune system; increases cellular energy)
- essential fatty acids – as directed on the label (combats inflammation of the liver)
- free-form amino acids – as directed on the label (supplies necessary protein and takes strain off the liver)
- glutathione – 500 mg a day (protects the liver)
- L-cysteine – 500 mg a day (helps detoxify liver)
- L-methionine – 500 mg a day (helps detoxify liver)

- lecithin – 1 Tbsp. three times a day (protects liver cells; prevents fatty liver)

Herbal Therapy
Take a botanical supplement.

- burdock – cleanses the liver
- dandelion – important in cleansing the liver
- goldenseal – promotes function of the liver. *Caution:* Do not use if you are pregnant.
- licorice – inhibits liver cell injury
- milk thistle – heals and rebuilds liver
- red clover – for liver disease
- yellow dock – improves liver function

Homeopathic Remedies
If you have hepatitis, do not attempt to self-treat. You need professional help. Consult a homeopathic practitioner to determine which remedy is best for you. Below are a few of the possibilities.

- *Chelidonium* – liver disease with marked pain; constricting or cramping pain in right upper quadrant; jaundice frequently marked; tongue yellow and imprinted by teeth; liver enlarged, hard, painful; cirrhosis.
- *Lycopodium* – liver disease with indigestion, bloating, and flatus; soreness as if a blow to the right upper quadrant; pain often extends through to the back; jaundice combined with marked gas; bloating after eating even one or two bites; hard stool followed by soft or liquid stool; enlarged liver.
- *Magnesia muriatica* – liver weakness; hepatitis with fatigue and depression; chronic or acute hepatitis; long smoldering liver diseases; hepatitis of children; pressing pains or heaviness in the liver extending to the back; enlarged, hard, liver.
- *Natrum sulphuricum* – acute and chronic hepatitis with severe nausea and headache; stitching pain, bursting, or soreness in the liver region; jaundice accompanied by diar-

rhea; tongue coated greenish or has a dirty color; asthma and hepatitis as concomitants; liver enlarged or swollen.
- *Nux vomica* – liver disease with fatigue, indigestion, and mental strain; worse with alcohol, fats, spices, overindulgence in food; indigestion, cramps, or reflux symptoms with liver disease; diarrhea alternating with constipation; jaundice; fullness in liver; chronic hepatitis.
- *Phosphorus* – acute hepatitis with much vomiting; gray, pale stool, but can be yellow; hepatitis after exposure to toxins and solvents; liver disease; soreness over whole liver; vomits liquid once it becomes warm in the stomach; atrophy of liver; fatty liver; chronic hepatitis; worse with alcohol.
- *Sulphur* – chronic hepatitis with jaundice, diarrhea, and congested veins; stitching pain or soreness in the liver, worse 11 A.M.; appetite impressive despite the illness; constipation from liver congestion.

Other Therapeutic Measures
Isolate hepatitis A patients and observe the modern medical cautions for clothing and bed linens. Because the feces are infectious, disinfect the bathroom frequently.

Use castor oil packs on the liver (see Alternative Treatment for Genital Warts, above). Keep the pack in place for up to two hours as needed. Use frequently during the first few weeks of infection. Continue for one to three months after the acute phase of the infection, but reduce the frequency.

Use hydrotherapy for acute hepatitis by alternating hot and cold compresses over the liver for one hour, applying the hot compress for one minute and the cold compress for five minutes. Repeat this sequence three times a day. For chronic hepatitis use a cold compress on the liver every night for a few weeks, reducing the frequency to every night for one week a month, for six months.

Take a chlorophyll enema three times a week. Use 1 pint as a retention enema to help cleanse and heal the liver.

Be treated by an Ayurvedic practitioner.

Be tested for hepatitis, and treated with a hepatitis virus extract by an environmental medicine physician.

Have NAET treatments for hepatitis (see Chiropractic section in chapter 9, Alternative Medical Disciplines).

HERPES

Herpes is caused by the virus *Herpes simplex,* which is differentiated into type I and type II herpes. It is a very contagious infection, and is the most common cause of genital ulcers in North America. Herpes can be transmitted sexually, or by contact with infected saliva and skin discharge.

GENITAL HERPES

Genital herpes is typically caused by *Herpes simplex* type II. Symptoms can occur four to seven days after sexual contact with an infected partner. Herpes can appear as a systemic illness, accompanied by fever, swollen glands, severe genital pain, and sometimes in an inability to urinate, secondary to pain in the bladder or urethra. There may be tingling, burning, or itching before the rash breaks out, first as small red pimple-like bumps, which then turn into blisters. The blisters heal in 7 to 14 days. Some people, however, can contract herpes without having any noticeable symptoms. Herpes can also be a dormant virus, so a person may have the first herpes outbreak 20 or more years after infection.

The virus remains in the nerves for the peron's lifetime and most people will experience subsequent outbreaks, which are usually much less severe than the initial one. Recurrences may be triggered by stress, anxiety, menstruation, food allergy, sexual activity, drugs, and minor infections.

In women, the blisters occur on the buttocks, the external genitals, cervix, and around the rectum. In men, the blisters occur on the glans penis, the foreskin, the shaft of the penis, and around the rectum.

ORAL HERPES

Oral herpes, or cold sores (fever blisters), is usually caused by *Herpes simplex* type I. This virus usually blisters the lips, but can also affect the mouth, nostrils, eyelids, and the fingers. The lesions consist of clusters of small fluid-filled blisters surrounded by an area of inflammation, and are often quite painful. The blisters burst after a few days to several weeks, then dry, crust over, and disappear.

The first time cold sores develop, they may be accompanied by fever, neck ache, enlargement of the neck lymph nodes, and fatigue. For many people, however, the initial event may go unnoticed. The infection is usually a lifelong problem, because the virus remains dormant in nerve cells. Some people develop antibodies, which prevent or minimize recurrent attacks, but 40 percent of people who harbor the virus will have recurrences.

People with depressed immune systems may have prolonged, recurrent bouts of cold sores, as may healthy people when they are under high levels of stress. Other trigger factors include fever, trauma, hot or cold weather, nutritional deficiencies, and exposure to sunlight. Cold sores often appear with other illnesses, such as a cold or the flu.

Cold sores are very contagious, and both kissing and oral sex can spread the infection. Children can develop fever blisters from being close to or being kissed by adults who have a herpes infection.

Unless a woman develops her first herpes outbreak during pregnancy (and therefore does not have adequate antibody levels), herpes does not cause problems in pregnancy prior to delivery. But if a woman has a history of herpes, and the virus is active close to the time of delivery, the baby will be delivered by Cesarean section to avoid infecting the newborn.

Oral herpes can be transmitted to the genital area through oral sex. Sexual partners who have inactive herpes can also transmit the disease.

MODERN MEDICAL TREATMENT

Drug Therapy

For genital herpes, acyclovir (Zovirax), famciclovir (Famvir), or valacyclovir (Valtrex) are given for suppressive therapy, either at the time of an outbreak, or daily for prophylaxis. They can cause nausea, vomiting, headache, diarrhea, dizziness, loss of appetite, fatigue, skin rash, and sore throat.

For cold sores, acyclovir (Zovirax) is given, and penciclovir (Denavir), a topical antiviral cream, is prescribed for application to the lesions. Headaches can be a side effect of these preparations.

ALTERNATIVE TREATMENT

People with severe outbreaks may need to use the modern medical drug therapy as well as alternative measures, while others will be able to stop or reduce outbreaks by following alternative treatments alone.

Diet

To minimize outbreaks, avoid foods high in arginine such as chocolate, peas, cereals, nuts, peanuts, beer, gelatin, raisins, and seeds. Arginine "feeds" the herpes virus. Also avoid sugar, simple carbohydrates, alcohol, processed foods, refined carbohydrates, and coffee. Avoid citrus and pineapple during an outbreak. To increase the alkalinity of your diet, eat fewer meats, fish, eggs, milk products, breads, and baked goods. Routinely avoid food allergens or be treated for your food allergies in order not to weaken the immune system.

Eat potatoes, brewer's yeast, chicken, and beans. These foods are high in lysine, which prevents viral replication. Use juice therapy with beet, carrot, and celery juice, which contain nutrients that help strengthen the immune system.

Exercise and Lifestyle

Unless you are having an acute herpes attack, perform aerobic exercise for 20 minutes a day.

Wear white cotton underwear to bed during an outbreak. Launder it after each wearing. Keep the genital area clean and dry. Wash your hands before and after touching your body.

Use latex condoms routinely to prevent transmitting the infection. Herpes can be spread even when it appears to be dormant. Avoid sexual activity during an outbreak to avoid reinfection and to reduce trauma to inflamed tissue.

Do not kiss anyone if you have oral herpes. Do not share towels, razors, drinking glasses, eating utensils, or finish the food of anyone who has oral herpes. Wash your hands thoroughly after touching the blisters, and replace your toothbrush after a cold sore has healed.

Stop smoking and avoid tobacco in all forms, as it reduces immune defenses.

Nutrient Therapy

At the first sign of discomfort, take the following nutritional supplements.

- vitamin A – 50,000 IU a day. *Caution:* Do not take more than 8,000 IU a day if you are or might be pregnant (strengthens immune response).
- beta carotene – 100,000 IU a day (helps protect mucus membranes from infection; helps repair damaged cells)
- vitamin B-complex – one capsule three times a day, or according to directions on product label (combats virus and helps keep it from spreading; works with L-lysine)
- vitamin C – 1,000 mg every two hours as soon as the tingling begins, then 1,000 mg four times a day for several days. 2,000 mg a day routinely, between outbreaks (strengthens

the immune system; prevents sores; inhibits virus)
- bioflavonoids – 1,000 mg as soon as tingling begins, then 500 mg three times a day for the next day or two. Routinely take 1,000 mg a day between attacks (suppresses virus; works with vitamin C).
- vitamin E – 400 IU a day (decreases pain; shortens healing time)
- selenium – 200 to 400 mcg a day (antiviral; suppresses herpes)
- zinc picolinate – 15 mg a day for genital herpes (boosts immune function)
- zinc gluconate – 180 mg lozenge containing 23 mg of elemental zinc every two hours during waking hours for a week for oral herpes. *Caution:* Do not use longer than a week (reduces symptoms; inhibits recurrences).
- L-lysine – 4,000 mg a day for the first four days, then 500 mg three times a day for two weeks or routinely as a suppressive measure. May take 2,000 mg a day in divided doses, for suppression, but be aware that lysine may stimulate the liver to manufacture cholesterol. (prevents viral replication)
- Monolaurin – one to six capsules a day during the acute phase. Drop to one to three capsules a day for two weeks. May be taken regularly as a suppressive measure (prevents viral attachment to cells). (Cardiovascular Research—see Sources)
- thymus extract – two tablets three times a day (enhances immune function)

Herbal Therapy
Take botanical supplements as follows.

- echinacea – strengthens the immune system; antiviral properties
- garlic (deodorized) – has antiviral properties
- goldenseal – a natural antibiotic. *Caution:* Do not take if you are pregnant.
- licorice – inhibits viral growth and cell damage

- St. John's wort – inhibits viral infections, including herpes

Apply an herbal preparation to the affected areas.

- black walnut extract – antiviral activity
- glycyrrhizinc acid ointment three times a day – inhibits herpes growth and cell damage
- goldenseal extract – strengthens the immune system; powerful antimicrobial. *Caution:* Do not take if you are pregnant.
- lemon balm – antiviral
- tea tree oil (Melaleuca oil) to the tingling area before an actual outbreak – antiviral activity

Homeopathic Remedies
Consult a homeopathic physician to help you find the remedy that best fits your symptoms.

- *Arsenicum album* – burning pains in the lesions and the skin affected in the prodrome; initial attack severe with large vesicles followed by superficial ulcers that may fester or blacken; lesions on prepuce, foreskin, penis, labia; pain may extend down back of thigh; frequent mild recurrences without apparent cause; may be more intense or limited to the right side; better warm applications.
- *Natrum muriaticum* – recurring herpes sores of the face; painful lesions about the lips, margin of hair, chin, wings of the nose, and in the beard area; also bends of the knees and elbows; often affects the area where the thigh rubs against the genitals, vesicles on labia or inside vagina; herpes with soreness and stitching pain, preventing intercourse; worse emotional stress, any acute illness or fever, exposure to the sun; lesions with definite periodicity; associated with a generalized malaise and fever.
- *Nitric acid* – very painful herpes outbreaks with small ulcers; crusts may develop;

painful, sensitive ulcers directly on genitals with stitching or splinter-like sensation; ulcers on all parts of penis, labia, or clitoris.

- *Petroleum* – recurring outbreaks of isolated vesicles, which cause yellow, thick crusts that crack; marked itching during the outbreak, coldness in spot after itching; lesions on inner thigh, perineum, scrotum, labia, and anus; worse during menses, winter; combination of herpes with eczema or cracks on hands or fingers.
- *Rhus toxicodendron* – swollen, red, itchy, and angry herpes lesions on the lips, nose, and face; may be behind ears, back of head, fingers, and the cornea; small, burning, intensely itchy vesicles; worse in cold or cold, damp weather, and during fever; eruptions may alternate with respiratory or intestinal symptoms.
- *Sepia* – periodic herpes lesions with chapped, raw, or cracking skin on lower lip; vesicles crust and crack; herpes in women with marked itching and vaginal discharge; commonly associated and worse with the menstrual cycle; periodic outbreaks monthly, yearly in the spring; severe burning or pain preventing intercourse; lesions on genitals, vulva, perineal region, hips, thighs; marked pain during urination.

Many people respond to complex homeopathic remedies. You may want to try HRPZ by PHP or Herps by Vibrant Health for relief of symptoms (see Sources section at the back of the book).

Other Therapeutic Measures

Practice stress reduction techniques such as biofeedback, imagery, and meditation to prevent outbreaks.

Use the following topical ointments on herpes lesions. If you have a cold sore on or around the eyes, see a physician before applying topical treatment.

- aloe vera – apply aloe directly to the blister (aids healing)
- lithium succinate or lithium sulfate ointment – 8 percent solution applied within 48 hours of the outbreak of a sore, with continued applications four times a day until the sore disappears (interferes with replication of herpes)
- lysine cream – apply directly to the blisters (prevents viral replication)
- vitamin E – open a vitamin E capsule and apply the oil directly to the blister (shortens healing time; soothes blisters)
- zinc sulfate solutions – 0.025 percent applied to the lesions three times a day, or zinc oxide ointment – apply the ointment directly to the sore (reduces healing time 30 to 40 percent; strengthens immune system)

Place ice on the lesion during early stages: 10 minutes on, 5 minutes off. This will relieve pain and shorten an attack. Repeat as often as needed. Wrap the ice in a cloth to minimize dripping, and launder the cloth in hot water before using for anything else.

Take hot baths frequently. The heat may temporarily exacerbate symptoms, but will hasten healing.

Get intravenous hydrogen peroxide therapy or ozone therapy from an alternative physician. Have acupuncture treatments.

Be allergy tested by an environmental medicine physician and take a *Herpes* or fluogen allergy extract.

Have NAET treatments for herpes (see the Chiropractic section in chapter 9, Alternative Medical Disciplines).

If your partner has been exposed during a herpes outbreak, a medical examination is important.

MONONUCLEOSIS

Mononucleosis, sometimes called the "kissing disease" and more frequently called "mono," is caused by the Epstein-Barr virus (EBV). It may also rarely be caused by the cytomegalovirus (CMV). Once these viruses are in the body they remain for life, but the acute illness will usually run its course and the individual will recover. Mononucleosis is very contagious and may be transmitted by kissing or sexual contact. Sharing food or utensils can also spread this virus, as can droplets spread through the air, similarly to colds or influenza.

The incubation period is about 30 to 50 days in adults and 10 days in children. Mononucleosis is more common in young adults and children, and by adulthood, 90 to 95 percent of people have demonstrable antibodies to EBV.

Mononucleosis is often mistaken for the flu because the symptoms can be similar. Major symptoms of "mono" are severe fatigue, sore throat, and swollen glands. Sore throat will predominate in 80 percent of patients. Other symptoms include depression, chills, fever, generalized aching, and headache. In some cases the spleen can become enlarged, and liver function may be adversely affected. Some people develop a mild jaundice, and 10 percent of patients may develop rashes.

Acute symptoms can last from two to four weeks and the fatigue can persist for three to eight weeks. Diagnosis is made by a blood test called the heterophil antibody test, which detects the presence of specific antibodies against EBV. Liver function tests may also be valuable.

MODERN MEDICAL TREATMENT

Drug Therapy

Nearly all cases of mononucleosis improve without drugs in four to six weeks. Because mono is a viral infection, antibiotics are not helpful unless there is a secondary bacterial infection. If given during mononucleosis, the antibiotic ampicillin can cause a rash. Aspirin can create complications in some cases. If a medication is needed for pain, acetaminophen is given to lower fever and reduce aches and pain. For a few individuals, the antiviral medication acyclovir may be used.

Steroids are frequently given to shorten the course and lessen the severity of mono, particularly when tonsils are so swollen that the patient is having difficulty swallowing. Almost every university health service treats mononucleosis patients with steroids. However, according to Dr. Samuel L. Katz, Wilburt C. Davison Professor and chairman of the department of pediatrics at the Duke University School of Medicine in Durham, North Carolina, steroids should not be given to teenagers and young adults with acute infectious mononucleosis. Steroids sabotage the normal immunologic suppression of EBV and the immune system of the patient will not learn to "live with" EBV, which remains in the body for life. Steroid use should be limited to patients with extremely severe symptoms.

Exercise and Lifestyle

Strenuous exercise and contact sports must be avoided if the liver and spleen are enlarged. Rest may have to be continued until these organs return to their normal size.

Other Therapeutic Measures

Bed rest is essential when there is fever and fatigue.

ALTERNATIVE TREATMENT

Diet

Avoid excess animal protein. Instead take amino acid blends or vegetable protein drinks as a snack between meals to help build up the organs involved. Eat smaller meals more frequently to avoid overeating at any one meal. Eat raw foods, and be certain to include sprouts, seeds, and nuts.

If your sore throat makes it difficult to swallow, eat organic baby food or purée your food in the blender. Vegetable soups are nourishing and easily swallowed.

Avoid processed foods, sugar, caffeine, white flour, fats, alcohol, soft drinks, and fried foods. Drink at least eight 8-ounce glasses of pure water throughout the day in addition to juices.

Use juice therapy containing the following blends between meals. The concentrated nutrients will help speed recovery and blood sugar balance.

- carrot, beet, tomato, and green pepper seasoned with garlic and onion
- lemon, orange, and pineapple
- wheat grass juice and other fresh green juices

Exercise and Lifestyle
Do not exercise while you are acutely ill. If your liver or spleen is enlarged, you must not participate in strenuous exercise or a contact sport of any kind until the organs return to their normal size.

During the rebuilding stages after mononucleosis, do regular mild exercise. Perform Qigong or Tai Chi.

Do not smoke, and avoid all forms of tobacco, including secondhand smoke.

Avoid close physical contact with others and dispose of your tissues by flushing them. Do not share food, eating utensils, or towels. Wash your hands frequently.

Nutrient Therapy
Take the following nutritional supplements.

- vitamin A – 50,000 IU a day for two weeks, then gradually reduce dose to 15,000 IU a day. *Caution:* Do not take more than 8,000 IU a day if you are or might be pregnant (essential for the immune system).
- vitamin B-complex – 100 mg three times a day (increase energy; essential for digestion and normal liver function)
- vitamin C – 10,000 mg a day in divided doses or up to bowel tolerance (destroys viruses; boosts the immune system)
- vitamin E – 400 to 800 IU a day for a month, then gradually reduce dose to 400 IU a day (essential for the immune system)
- calcium – 1,000 mg a day (necessary for normal cellular function and repair)

- magnesium – 75 to 1,000 mg a day (necessary for normal cellular function and repair)
- potassium – 99 mg a day (necessary for normal cellular function and repair)
- coenzyme Q_{10} – 30 to 90 mg a day (stimulates immune system; increases cellular energy)
- free-form amino acid – as directed on the label, in small divided doses (supply necessary protein for healing and rebuilding tissues)
- proteolytic enzymes – as directed on the label, three to four times a day between meals (reduce inflammation; aid in absorption of nutrients)
- raw thymus glandular – as directed on the label (enhances immune response)

Herbal Therapy
Take a botanical supplement.

- astragalus – boosts immune system
- dandelion – protects the liver
- echinacea – boosts the immune system
- goldenseal – fights infection. *Caution:* Do not use if you are pregnant.
- hawthorn – helps reestablish strength
- milk thistle – protects the liver
- Siberian ginseng *(Eleutherococcus senticosus)* – enhances the immune system

Homeopathic Remedies
Consult a homeopathic practitioner, and take the homeopathic remedy that best describes your symptoms. The remedies listed below are but a few of the many possibilities.

- *Belladonna* – throat red, worse on right side, tonsils enlarged; throat feels constricted, hot, and dry; swallowing difficult, worse with liquids; muscles of swallowing very sensitive; must take drink to swallow solid food; when swallowing bends head forward and lifts up knees; sensation of a lump in the throat; swelling of glands of neck; high fever, delirium; no thirst with fever; hot head with cold limbs.

- *Calcarea carbonica* – swelling of the tonsils and submaxillary glands with stitching pain on swallowing; difficulty swallowing; uvula swollen, edematous; glandular swelling below the jaw and in the neck; chill with thirst, fever with sweat, night sweats, especially on head, neck, and chest; liver region painful when stooping.
- *Carcinosum* – lump in throat; worse at night, on waking, with heat; enlargement of tonsils; lump, plug, sensation on empty swallowing; better with cold drinks; weakness and excessive fatigue; glands enlarged; high fevers; acute or chronic mononucleosis; weariness and fatigue; never well since mononucleosis.
- *Gelsemium* – throat feels rough, burning; tonsils swollen, shooting pains into ears; feeling of a lump in throat that cannot be swallowed; aching, tiredness, heaviness, weakness, and soreness; fever with a stupor, dizziness, faintness; thirstless, prostrated.
- *Mercurius iodum ruber* – swallowing painful; sore throat, left to right; tonsils and the glands greatly swollen, worse on left tonsil; phlegm in nose and throat; disposition to "hawk" with sensation of lump in throat; stiffness of muscles of throat and neck; brings up much mucus from posterior sinuses; tongue wrinkled and stiff at base, pains when moving; much glandular swelling; spleen enlarged; intense shivering followed by fever; night sweats.
- *Phytolacca* – Marked pain in throat; dark red discoloration and inflammation of tonsils, pharynx, or root of the tongue, worse on the right side; throat pain better with cold drinks and worse with warm drinks; throat pain extends to the ears on swallowing; pain in throat as from a "burning hot ball"; hard, painful swelling of the cervical glands; neck pain and stiffness; pains in both ears, worse when swallowing; high fever, alternating with chilliness and great prostration.

Other Therapeutic Measures

Get complete bed rest during the acute stages when you have fever. After you no longer have fever, continue with a reduced schedule and rest periods until your fatigue clears. Be aware that intermittent fatigue can occur for up to a year.

Try acupuncture, Ayurvedic medicine, and Chinese medicine, which have been helpful to some people with mononucleosis. Do biofeedback training to help relieve symptoms.

Be tested and treated with an EBV extract by an environmental medicine physician (see Allergies to Microorganisms section in chapter 25, Allergy). Receive NAET treatments for EBV (see Chiropractic section in chapter 9, Alternative Medical Disciplines).

SYPHILIS

Syphilis is caused by a bacteria *(Treponema pallidum)* that originated in the Americas and was transmitted to Europe. The initial manifestation of syphilis, or the first stage, typically involves a sore on the genital mucus membranes. This disappears without treatment, but surfaces later with symptoms in internal organs. Symptoms of the second stage include rash, patches of flaking tissue, fever, sore throat, and sores in the mouth or anus. In the third stage, syphilis can infect the brain, kidneys, bones, and heart, causing brain damage, hearing loss, heart disease, and/or blindness. This stage is rare in North America, as most people seek treatment earlier.

Syphilis can cause disease in the unborn child, and may cause death of the fetus.

MODERN MEDICAL TREATMENT

Drug Therapy

The antibiotic penicillin is the treatment of choice for syphilis. Its side effects can include skin rashes, chills, fever, joint pain, anemia, and allergic reactions. When syphilis is being treated, many people develop the Jarish-Herxheimer reaction, with fever, myalgias, and malaise. This is an allergic response to the syphilis organisms that are being killed. Penicillin can also cause overgrowth of yeast. However, the full course of antibiotics must be taken even if symptoms abate.

ALTERNATIVE TREATMENT

Dr. Tori Hudson, a naturopath who is the academic dean at the National College of Naturopathic Medicine in Portland, Oregon, notes that syphilis requires treatment with antibiotics. However, natural remedies can be used in addition to antibiotics.

Diet

Avoid refined, starchy, fried, and saturated fat foods. Minimize red meats, pasteurized dairy products, and sugars. Avoid caffeine and alcohol.

Exercise and Lifestyle

Stop smoking and avoid tobacco in any form, as it reduces immune defenses.

Abstain from sex or use a latex condom with each sexual encounter.

Nutrient Therapy

- vitamin A – 25,000 IU a day. *Caution:* Do not take more than 8,000 IU a day if you are or might be pregnant (strengthens mucus membranes).
- vitamin B-complex with 50 mg of each B – follow directions on the label of your product (necessary for functioning of all cells)
- vitamin C – 2,000 mg three times a day (boosts the immune system)
- vitamin E – 200 IU a day (strengthens immune system
- zinc – 15 mg a day (essential for immune system function)
- bioflavonoids – 1,000 mg a day (strengthens immune system)
- coenzyme Q_{10} – 60 mg four times a day (stimulates the immune system; increases tissue oxygenation)
- organic germanium – 150 mg a day (increases tissue oxygenation)

Herbal Therapy

Take a botanical supplement.

- Add 2 Tbsp. of sarsaparilla and 2 Tbsp. of yellow dock root in 1 quart of boiling water. Simmer five minutes and add 3½ tsp. dried thyme. Steep covered for one hour. Drink 1 to 3 cups a day. Women can use as a douche.
- Use calendula ointment on lesions to hasten healing and prevent infection.

Homeopathic Remedies

Take a homeopathic remedy under the supervision of a homeopathic physician.

- *Aurum metallicum* – ulcers that attack the bones, nightly bone pains, especially cranial and nasal; glands swollen; indicated in secondary syphilis with attack of the blood, glands, and bone.
- *Kali iodatum* – deep ulceration on gums, edema in larynx, lungs, or on tongue from syphilis; syphilitic rheumatism, especially of fingers and toes; excoriating discharge blistering the nostrils and lips; throbbing and burning in nasal and frontal bones; gnawing, burning bone pains; papular eruption on the scalp and back; burning pains.
- *Mercurious corrosivus* – chancres with extensive ulceration in mouth, gums, and throat; fetid breath, profuse salivation, enlarged tonsils; syphilitic ulceration on tongue, larynx, or lungs.
- *Mercurious solubilis* – main remedy for all stages of non-congenital and acquired syphilis; chancres red and spread inward with yellowish fetid discharge, tendency to bleed; syphilitic ulceration on tongue, larynx, or lungs; syphilitic rheumatism.
- *Phytolacca* – syphilitic bone pains, chronic rheumatism; glandular swellings with heat and inflammation; sore throats with enlarged and painful cervical glands; aching, soreness, restlessness, prostration, aching all over body; hard and painful nodes.

- *Syphilinum* – syphilitic disorders that affect the nerves, mucus membranes and bones; prostration and debility in the morning; ulceration of mouth, nose, genitals, skin; succession of abscesses; pains worse at night; neuralgia and headache; syphilis in family; brain affected; never well since syphilis; ulcers and bone pain.

Other Therapeutic Measures

Take alternating hot and cold sitz baths daily to stimulate immune activity in the pelvic area.

Be treated by an environmental medicine physician with an extract for *Treponema pallidum*.

Have NAET treatments for syphilis (see the Chiropractic section in chapter 9, Alternative Medical Disciplines).

Be sure your sexual partner is also treated.

TRICHOMONAS

Trichomonas is caused by a protozoan, *Trichomonas vaginalis,* which is a type of parasite. It affects the genital tract of both men and women. It is a sexually transmitted disease that does not have serious side effects. The third most common cause of vaginitis, it causes greenish-yellow, frothy, foul-smelling discharge with itching and burning. It grows best in a vaginal pH of 5.5 to 5.8. In men it causes urethritis, prostatitis, epididymitis, and may cause infertility.

MODERN MEDICAL TREATMENT

Drug Therapy

Metronidazole (Flagyl) is used to treat trichomonas. Flagyl can cause an adverse reaction to any alcohol ingested during treatment. Other side effects can include seizures, numbness of the arms or legs, nausea, loss of appetite, abdominal cramping, and constipation. It can also cause an overgrowth of yeast.

Other Therapeutic Measures

The use of a latex condom is recommended to prevent the spread of trichomonas, or abstinence until the infection has cleared.

ALTERNATIVE TREATMENT

Trichomonas is difficult to treat with natural medicine alone, and is best treated with a combination of modern medicine and alternative medicine.

Diet

Eat fresh vegetables, fruits, and whole grains (unless you are hyperinsulinemic). Avoid refined foods, junk foods, and processed foods. Keep fat and salt intake to a minimum and eat a moderate amount of protein. Avoid sugar, as it encourages parasite growth, as well as coffee, alcohol, and any food allergens.

Exercise and Lifestyle

Use a latex condom to prevent the spread of the parasite.

Stop smoking and avoid tobacco in all forms, as it reduces immune defenses.

Nutrient Therapy

Take the following nutrients.

- vitamin A – 25,000 IU a day. *Caution:* Do not take more than 8,000 IU a day if you are or might be pregnant (antioxidant; strengthens immune system; necessary for integrity of vaginal mucosa).
- beta carotene – 150,000 IU a day (antioxidant; strengthens immune system)
- vitamin C – 2,000 mg every hour to bowel tolerance during acute phase; 5,000 mg a day for a month after the infection is cleared (boosts the immune system)
- vitamin E – 400 IU a day (antioxidant; prevents cell damage)

- copper – 1 to 2 mg a day (to balance zinc)
- zinc – 25 mg two times a day and apply topically (essential for immune function and healing of tissue)

Herbal Therapy
Take the following botanical supplements.

- bayberry – supports the immune system; antibiotic for protozoan infections
- echinacea – stimulates the immune system; antibiotic for protozoan infections
- elecampane – antibiotic for protozoan infections
- garlic – antibiotic for protozoan infections
- goldenseal – antibiotic for protozoan infections. *Caution:* Do not use if you are pregnant.
- turmeric – antibiotic for protozoan infections

Homeopathic Remedies
Seek the help of a homeopathic physician to determine the best homeopathic remedy for you. The following are several of the many possibilities.

- *Calcarea carbonica* – profuse, milky, itchy, burning discharge in young girls before puberty; in women before periods; burning with seminal emission; itching and burning in genitals.
- *Kreosotum* – profuse, watery, acrid, irritating and burning discharge causes soreness, smarting, and itching of the vulva; worse before a period; burning in male genitalia from contact with vaginal discharge during sex.
- *Mercurius* – acrid, burning, greenish-yellow discharge causing smarting and swelling of the vulva; worse at night; penis and testicles swollen.
- *Nitric acid* – chronic urethral discharge, may be bloody; non-specific urethritis; ulcers of genitals, ulcers or stricture in urethra with stitching pains; vaginitis, itching before or after menses; acrid vaginal discharge; worse with sex; sex drive excessive; itching, burning foreskin.
- *Sepia* – yellow-green, offensive discharge; worse before a period, with a bearing-down sensation in the pelvis; offensive perspiration on scrotum; genitals cold; sexual desire increased.

Other Therapeutic Measures
Use the following as a douche, for several days, or use a tampon saturated with the supplement, but it must be removed after four hours.

- zinc sulfate – 1 Tbsp. of a 2 percent solution in 1 pint of water (helps with wound healing; boosts immune system)
- *Lactobacillus acidophilus* – ½ tsp. in a cup of warm water as a douche, or use plain yogurt with live cultures (re-inoculates the vagina with beneficial bacteria)
- calendula, goldenseal, and echinacea combined as a douche (stimulates the immune system). *Caution:* Do not take goldenseal if you are pregnant.
- tea tree oil – soak a tampon with three drops of tea tree oil in 1 Tbsp. of yogurt (antiparasitic properties)

Add a few drops of lavender to douches, sitz baths, creams, lotions, and tampons (for trichomonas vaginitis).

Be treated by an environmental medicine physician with an extract for *Trichomonas vaginalis.*

Have NAET treatments for trichomonas (see Chiropractic section in chapter 9, Alternative Medical Disciplines).

Be sure that your sexual partner is also treated.

CHAPTER 23

Female Problems

Female problems are the special health problems that are directly related to female anatomy. The female genitalia consist of the vagina, vulva, uterus, and ovaries. During puberty the ovaries begin to secrete estrogen, which causes enlargement of the breasts, growth of pubic and underarm hair, and enlargement of the uterus. After the ovaries begin secreting hormones, the menstrual cycle begins.

THE MENSTRUAL CYCLE

The female cycle is a well-orchestrated sequence of rising and falling hormones. When the ovaries secrete estrogen, the endometrium (the lining of the uterus) thickens, preparing it to receive a fertilized egg. Estrogen levels peak before ovulation, together with leutinizing hormone (LH) and follicle stimulating hormone (FSH), which are secreted by the pituitary. At ovulation, which occurs about 14 days before the period begins, progesterone levels also begin to rise.

If no egg is fertilized, estrogen, FSH, and progesterone fall, and the sloughing of the inner lining of the uterus begins (menstruation). After menstruation, estrogen levels rise and the cycle begins again.

MENSTRUAL CRAMPS

Up to 60 percent of all women suffer from dysmenorrhea (menstrual cramps), which are described as sharp, viselike pains in the abdomen.

Cramps are not the same as PMS, although some women suffer from both. At least 10 percent of these women are so incapacitated by the severity of their pain that they have to stay home during their periods. Women who have cramps may also have backaches, and pinching and pain in the thighs.

Primary dysmenorrhea is not attributable to any condition other than the occurrence of a menstrual period. In secondary dysmenorrhea, however, the cramps are caused by endometriosis (a growth of cells from the inner lining of the uterus *outside* the uterus—in the abdominal cavity, on the ovaries, etc.) or some other pelvic disease.

Years ago it was felt that cramps were psychological, or "all in a woman's head." Since the 1970s, it has been known that women with cramps have high levels of a prostaglandin (a hormone-like fatty acid) in their menstrual blood, and it is the prostaglandin that causes the uterus to go into spasm.

MODERN MEDICAL TREATMENT

Diet
Women with cramps are told to eat a normal diet, and if they crave carbohydrates to eat them.

Exercise and Lifestyle
Women are encouraged to continue exercising during their menstrual period, as it may help to reduce or eliminate cramps.

Drug Therapy

The pain of menstrual cramps is treated with a non-steroidal anti-inflammatory drug (Aleve or ibuprofen or aspirin). Birth control pills are often prescribed, because women on the Pill generally do not have painful periods.

Non-steroidal anti-inflammatory medications help with pain, but they can cause heartburn, abdominal pain, nausea, stomach upset, diarrhea, mouth sores, ringing in the ears, and bruising.

Birth control pills can cause irregular vaginal bleeding or spotting, fluid retention with swelling of the fingers or ankles, high blood pressure, a spotty darkening of the skin, weight gain, depression, loss of scalp hair, vaginal infections, blood clots, heart attacks and strokes, gallbladder disease, liver tumors, and possible cancer of the reproductive organs.

SURGERY

If cramps are severe or chronic, women are offered laparoscopic surgery to check for endometriosis. In endometriosis, the lining of the uterus grows outside the uterus and causes severe cramps. Birth control pills frequently help control endometriosis. Surgical removal of the endometrium can also decrease cramps. Surgical removal of the uterus and ovaries may be performed in severe cases as a last resort.

ALTERNATIVE TREATMENT

Diet

For menstrual cramps, observe the following dietary guidelines. Stop eating dairy products, and avoid saturated fats, salt, alcohol, sugar, and caffeine. Eat a diet high in complex carbohydrates, low in fat, and low in protein (unless you have hyperinsulinemia). Eat seeds and nuts, which are high in essential fatty acids.

Exercise and Lifestyle

Do aerobic exercises three to four times a week consistently, not just during your period.

Try to minimize sources of stress in your life. If your time is overcommitted, look at which commitments you can drop.

Nutrient Therapy

Take nutritional supplements, as follows:

- multivitamin and mineral supplement – as directed on the label (decreases cramps)
- B-complex with 50 mg of each B vitamin – as directed on the label (diuretic; helps with congestion of pelvic area)
- vitamin B_6 – 100 mg a day (reduces water retention; increases oxygen to female organs; restores estrogen to normal levels)
- vitamin E – 400 IU a day (antioxidant; needed to balance extra essential fatty acids; helps PMS symptoms)
- calcium – 800 mg a day (antispasmodic; relaxes muscle of uterus)
- magnesium – 100 mg every two hours during your period, and three to four times a day during the rest of the cycle (antispasmodic; relaxes muscle of uterus)
- zinc picolinate – 15 mg a day (balances hormones)
- essential fatty acids (flaxseed oil, borage oil, and black currant seed oil) – 1 Tbsp. a day; or evening primrose oil, two capsules three times a day (antispasmodic; decreases prostaglandins that cause cramping)

Herbal Therapy

Take a botanical supplement:

- black cohosh – relieves cramps with back pain
- black haw – antispasmodic; relieves cramps
- chaste tree berry, red raspberry leaf, or hops – for cramps
- cramp bark – for cramps
- dandelion leaf – for water retention
- ginger capsule – for cramps
- skullcap – helps irritability and anxiety
- yarrow tincture – antispasmodic; diuretic; reduces inflammation

Homeopathic Remedies

Take a homeopathic remedy that best fits your symptoms, beginning one week before your period is due. If you do not obtain relief, seek the help of a trained homeopath. The following remedies are only a few of the possibilities.

- *Cactus grandiflorus* – pulsating pain in uterus and ovaries; menses early, dark and pitch-like; cease on lying down; menstrual disorders with heart symptoms; cry out with pain.
- *Chamomilla* – tearing pains, with a dark, clotted flow; with excessive irritability and impatience.
- *Cimicifuga* – pain shoots across the pelvis from side to side and down to the thighs, starting just before the period commences; sharp abdominal pains during a period make the patient double up; headache before the period starts.
- *Cocculus* – dysmenorrhea with profuse dark menses; painful pressing in uterine region followed by hemorrhoids; weak during period, barely able to stand; menses early, gushes out when standing on tiptoe.
- *Magnesia phosphorica* – cramp-like pains start several hours before the period begins and continue throughout; better warmth, better pressure, better from bending double.
- *Pulsatilla* – dark, delayed, and intermittent periods; the more the pain, the chillier the patient feels; the pain seems to move about, doubling the patient up so she becomes restless and tearful.
- *Sepia* – sharp clutching pain; gripping, burning, or sticking pain in uterus; menses either too late and scanty or early and profuse; irregular; bearing down sensation as if everything would escape through the vagina.

Many patients respond to complex homeopathic remedies. You may want to try Ovarian Drops, which provide specific tissue support for the ovaries, or Female Endocrine Axis, which helps normalize female function. Both are available from PHP (see Sources). Female+ by Vibrant Health is an adaptogen that assists in proper production and flow of female hormones (see Sources).

Other Therapeutic Measures

Try stress reduction measures, including meditation. Dr. Weil's breathing exercises can also be helpful (see p. 225).

It may help to change your view of your menstrual cycle, regarding it as a positive part of your life rather than a negative event.

To reduce cramps, use castor oil packs on your lower abdomen at least three times per week for several months. This will improve immune system function and decrease stress and adrenaline levels.

PREMENSTRUAL SYNDROME

Premenstrual syndrome results from an imbalance of the hormones estrogen and progesterone. The relative imbalance of the hormones is a dynamic, changing phenomenon that cannot be documented with currently available laboratory tests for hormone levels. High estrogen levels can cause a woman to feel anxious and irritable, while if progesterone levels are high, a women can become depressed. Progesterone affects those areas of the brain responsible for carbohydrate cravings. Dr. Christiane Northrup, past president of the American Holistic Medical Association and author of *Women's Bodies, Women's Wisdom,* observes that unresolved emotional problems may disrupt the hormone balance of the menstrual cycle.

There are more than a hundred known symptoms of PMS. The particular symptoms reported are not important for the diagnosis, but the cyclic fashion in which they occur *is* important. Symptoms of PMS include craving sweets and fats, mood swings from euphoria to depression without reason, abdominal bloating, being accident prone, food binging, headaches, insomnia, joint swelling and pain, migraine head-aches, nausea, coordination difficulties, breast swelling and pain, asthma, back pain, sinus problems, suicidal thoughts, urinary difficulties, and fluid retention. When the period begins, the symptoms are relieved. Not all women have the same symptoms, and not all women respond to the same treatment.

One-third to two-thirds of all North American women between the ages of 20 and 50 have PMS. Having delivered several children, living with someone, or being married seems to increase the risk of having PMS, and the tendency to have PMS seems to be inherited. Initially the symptoms last for a few days, but if nothing is done to change the pattern, these symptoms tend to become worse over time and to last longer.

PMS can be associated with menarche (when a woman begins to have periods) or it can begin one or two years before menopause. It may also begin after an interval without periods, for instance when a woman is coming off birth control pills, or after the birth of a child. PMS can also appear after pregnancies complicated by toxemia, tubal ligation, or stress such as a death in the family. Women who develop PMS tend to:

- consume a lot of dairy products and caffeine;
- consume excessive animal fat;
- eat excessive amounts of sugar;
- be overweight;
- have a relatively high level of estrogen and a low level of progesterone;
- have low levels of vitamins C and E, and selenium;
- have a deficiency of magnesium; and
- have a tendency toward seasonal affective disorder.

High estrogen levels are related to a decreased breakdown of estrogen in the liver and/or overproduction of the hormone. They are associated with B-complex deficiencies (es-pecially B_6 and B_{12}) which are needed by the liver to break down estrogen—as are vitamins C and E, magnesium, and selenium. Vegetarians excrete more estrogen in their feces than do non-vegetarians. Low progesterone levels also seem to be caused by a lack of production or by excess breakdown.

MODERN MEDICAL TREATMENT

Diet
Women are told to eat a well-balanced diet and to avoid alcohol, caffeine, sugar, and salt. They are also told to decrease fat intake.

Exercise and Lifestyle
A regular exercise program is encouraged.

Drug Therapy
Modern medicine uses medication to treat the symptoms of PMS, sometimes without considering the underlying physiology of the condition. Diuretics are prescribed for bloating (see p. 199 for side effects). Painkillers are prescribed for headaches and other pain (see pp. 115–16 for side effects), and Valium is used for anxiety (see p. 438 for side effects). Birth control pills are used to balance hormones. (Side effects of birth control pills are listed on p. 339.)

PSYCHOTHERAPY

Because PMS is considered by some physicians to be a psychological problem, patients may be advised to receive psychotherapy.

ALTERNATIVE TREATMENT

Diet
Observe the following dietary guidelines. Eliminate sugar and refined carbohydrates and decrease dairy. The lactose in dairy products can block absorption of magnesium, which helps regulate estrogen levels and increases its excretion. Cut back on animal fats, and eat a high–complex carbohydrate, low-fat diet (except in cases of hyperinsulinemia). Restrict salt intake,

eliminate caffeine from your diet, and avoid alcohol.

Eat high-fiber foods such as vegetables, beans, and whole grains. Have high-protein snacks. Drink 1 quart of pure, tolerated water a day for one week before and one week after your period.

Exercise and Lifestyle

Do 20 minutes of aerobic exercise three times a week. Exercise decreases many PMS symptoms and increases endorphins (naturally occurring narcotic-like substances that help decrease depression). Brisk walking is a good form of aerobic exercise.

Nutrient Therapy

Take nutritional supplements daily, as follows:

- multivitamin – as directed on the label of the product (all nutrients are needed for relief of symptoms)
- vitamin A – 10,000 IU a day. *Caution:* Do not take more than 8,000 IU a day if you are pregnant or might be pregnant (deficiency has been linked to PMS).
- beta carotene – 50,000 IU a day (antioxidant; precursor to vitamin A)
- B-complex, with 50 mg of most B vitamins – as directed on the label (combats depression; acts as a diuretic)
- vitamin B_6 – 50 to 200 mg a day (reduces water retention; increases oxygen flow to the female organs)
- vitamin C – 1,000 mg three times a day (relieves discomfort of breast swelling and pain)
- vitamin D – 400 IU a day (to aid absorption of calcium and magnesium)
- vitamin E – 400 to 800 IU a day (decreases symptoms, such as headache, fatigue, depression, insomnia)
- calcium – 1,000 mg a day (relieves backaches and nervousness)

- magnesium – 600 to 800 mg a day (antispasmodic; relaxes muscles; relieves cramping)
- zinc picolinate – 15 mg a day (balances hormones)
- essential fatty acids (borage oil, flaxseed oil, black currant seed oil, or evening primrose oil) – 500 mg three to four times a day (supply gamma-linolenic acid, important in relieving PMS symptoms and aiding glandular function)
- L-tyrosine – 500 mg a day (combats depression, anxiety, and headache)

Herbal Therapy

Take a botanical supplement three times a day.

- chasteberry – helps to balance hormones
- cramp bark – for cramps
- dandelion – for water retention
- skullcap – for irritability/anxiety

Homeopathic Remedies

Take the homeopathic remedy that best matches your symptoms. Start 10 days before your next period is due and take three times a day for 5 days. If you do not obtain relief, consult a homeopathic physician.

- *Lachesis* – headache, at its worst on waking; face appears and feels bloated; tight clothes cannot be tolerated, especially around the neck and waist; palpitations with a feeling of faintness; patient becomes jealous, vindictive, unreasonable, and talks excessively; much better as soon as the period starts.
- *Natrum muriaticum* – blinding headache, with a pale face, nausea, and vomiting; craving for salt; the abdomen becomes distended; with a "fluttery" heart and palpitations; worse from noise, mental exertion, and consolation; the worst about 10 to 11 A.M.; irritable, weary, selfish, withdrawn, and moody.
- *Pulsatilla* – lack of thirst with a partial loss of the sense of taste; shooting pain in the neck

and upper part of the back; very moody and changeable; cries a lot and requires much sympathy; much better out of doors.

- *Sepia* – severe headache; food tastes too salty; sensation of the pelvic contents about to drop out; cold, totally weary and tired; dislike of family, irritable, and very sad, but enlivened with exercise and movement.

Many patients respond to complex homeopathic remedies. You may want to try Female Liquescence by PHP, which contains potentized nutrients for balancing the female endocrine axis (see Sources).

Other Therapeutic Measures
Do not take diuretics, as they remove minerals from the body. Drink 1 quart of pure water a day, beginning a week before your period and ending a week after.

Do aerobic exercises for 20 minutes three times a week. Practice deep breathing, meditation, or deep relaxation. Decrease stress in your environment. Stick to a schedule to avoid being overwhelmed. Get more sleep when you anticipate having PMS.

Have a massage treatment. Take a mineral bath, using 1 cup of sea salt and 1 cup of baking soda in the tub. Soak for 20 minutes. Have sex with orgasm, or masturbate to orgasm. This helps move blood and other fluids away from the congested organs.

Expose yourself to full-spectrum light for two hours each evening or morning from natural or full-spectrum lights. Receive acupuncture treatments. Consult an Ayurvedic or Chinese medicine practitioner.

Have allergy testing, and be treated for sensitivity to hormones if the results warrant it. Use either allergy extracts for hormones from an environmental medicine physician or have NAET treatments for hormones.

If your PMS does not respond to lifestyle changes, take natural progesterone. Use progesterone cream, ¼ to ½ tsp. on the inner thighs, inner arms, face, neck, and abdomen. Rub in well one to two days before symptoms would ordinarily occur, and stop when the symptoms would normally end.

MENOPAUSE

Menopause occurs when the ovaries stop producing estrogen. It marks the end of a woman's menstrual bleeding and reproductive life. The output of hormones does not reduce gradually, but in stops and starts. Progesterone is no longer produced, and estrogen (still produced by fat cells, the tissue around the ovaries, and in the adrenal glands) predominates. The estrogen level reaches a plateau, and stays at the same level until about age 70. When no longer balanced by progesterone, estrogen can cause irritability, water retention, weight gain, mood swings, depression, memory loss, fibroids, fibrocystic breast disease, and, in some cases, breast cancer.

In North America menopause occurs (on average) between the ages of 48 and 52—although some women stop having periods in their late thirties or early forties, while others stop in their mid-fifties. The number of menopausal women will increase significantly by 2010, because of the aging population.

Perimenopause occurs about 5 to 10 years before menopause, and is a time of irregular cycles and (sometimes) heavy bleeding. PMS and fibroids (benign tumors of the uterus) are common during perimenopause. Once women go into menopause, these symptoms will subside, with the shrinking of fibroids, disappearance of PMS, and cessation of bleeding.

Artificial menopause occurs when the ovaries (and usually the uterus and fallopian tubes) are surgically removed because the ovaries are enlarged, or have large cysts. Menopause can occur with a hysterectomy even if the ovaries are not removed. It is speculated that disturbance of the blood supply to the ovaries is the cause in those cases. Tubal ligation may also bring on early menopause, and women who receive chemotherapy or radiation therapy to the pelvis usually undergo premature menopause. The symptoms of artificial menopause can be severe unless hormone levels are properly adjusted.

At least half of women who go through menopause have only mild symptoms or no symptoms at all. The severity of menopausal symptoms depends upon a woman's level of health, and her preconceived ideas about menopause. Forty percent of women in North America have symptoms severe enough to make them seek medical help. In other countries, such as Japan and Indonesia, women have fewer menopausal symptoms.

Hot flashes (also known as vasomotor flushes) are experienced by 80 to 90 percent of North American women during menopause; they can last for months or years. With hot flashes, women feel hot and may start to sweat, especially around the head and neck. At night, they may get so hot that they throw off their blankets and soak the bed with sweat, then they get cold and need more blankets. Hot flashes may be caused by norepinephrine metabolism in the brain, as a response to estrogen deprivation, or they may be caused by sudden drops in estrogen levels. Stress worsens hot flashes, and placebos help them. Hyperthyroidism, alcohol intake, out-of-control diabetes, and serotonin excess can all cause and exacerbate hot flashes.

Vaginal dryness and thinning are other common symptoms of menopause. The outer, tough cells of the vagina can be lost after menopause—perhaps caused by decreased estrogen levels, or perhaps because of higher pH levels. Bacterial vaginitis or yeast vaginitis is more likely to occur, as is atrophic vaginitis, which is related to the thinning of the vagina (see Vaginitis section, below). However, many women never have thinning of the vagina after menopause, even if they do not take estrogen. Some women may develop urinary frequency related to thinning of the tissue at the end of the urethra. This area is estrogen sensitive, and can be helped by using a small amount of estrogen cream.

Half of all menopausal women have no decline in sexual interest; estrogen is not associated with sex drive. Menopause also does not contribute to depression in most women. In those who do develop depression, it may be related to the socially defined loss of sexuality and youth, rather than to physiological changes. Some women are easily fatigued at menopause, and for some women, menopause is a time of emotional upheaval. Many women, however, experience increased energy, a greater focus on their life goals, and an increased interest in sex.

MODERN MEDICAL TREATMENT

Diet
Women are told to eat a well-balanced diet, as well as foods high in calcium, such as dairy products. They are also told to eat a low-fat, high-fiber diet.

Exercise and Lifestyle
Weight-bearing exercise (running or walking) is recommended for 20 minutes three to four times a week.

Hormone Therapy
Most gynecologists recommend that all women take estrogen replacement therapy (ERT—estrogen only) or hormone replacement therapy (HRT—estrogen and progesterone) after menopause to treat menopausal symptoms, and to prevent osteoporosis. Even though ERT has been approved by the FDA only for the prevention of osteoporosis, it may also improve elasticity of the skin, protect against senility, help prevent heart disease, help stop hot flashes, and prevent vaginal thinning and drying.

Contraindications for taking ERT include a history of heart disease, migraine headaches, significant liver disease, or a history of breast cancer. Women who have had blood clots in their legs or lungs, or who have had a heart attack or stroke while using birth control pills, should not take ERT.

Replacement estrogen causes weight gain, bloating, mood swings, and cravings. It has also been associated with a higher incidence of breast, uterine, and ovarian cancer. Other side effects of ERT include nausea and vomiting, breast tenderness or enlargement, a discharge from the breasts, benign tumors and enlargement of the liver, fibroid tumors, elevated blood pressure, a worsening of glucose tolerance, increased levels of calcium, excess fluid retention, a worsening of asthma, epilepsy, or kidney disease. Estrogen taken postmenopausally causes a decrease in dehydroepiandrosterone (DHEA— an adrenal hormone) and testosterone.

Premarin is the estrogen most commonly used for ERT. It is derived from the urine of pregnant horses, and only two types of estrogen in Premarin are similar to those that humans produce. If women who still have their uterus use ERT in the postmenopausal period for more than a year, their risk of endometrial cancer (cancer of the lining of the uterus) increases five- to ten-fold. The progesterone combined with estrogen in HRT helps to prevent endometrial cancer. Women who have bleeding after menopause should see their physician, as this can be a sign of endometrial cancer.

Estraderm (a transdermal patch) is another form in which estrogen can be taken for ERT. Estraderm produces high levels of estradiol, with lower circulating levels of estrone. It requires smaller total doses than oral estrogens. Estraderm has the same side effects as Premarin, although some physicians believe that because it bypasses the liver it does not influence blood clotting. Fifteen percent of women become sensitive to the adhesive used for the patch, and have to stop using it for that reason.

A recent study from the University of California at San Francisco, published in the *Archives of Internal Medicine*, December 1997, found that women taking only half the standard estrogen dose of 0.625 mg of esterified estrogen (Estratab) could preserve bone density and decrease LDL cholesterol (see p. 160). Women in the study did not have significant vaginal bleeding or breast tenderness.

There are no studies of women who have *not* gone on ERT. Women who opt not to go on ERT are sometimes made to feel that they have made the wrong decision. Dr. Robert Atkins notes that women who tend to gain weight (especially in the midsection), have high triglyceride levels, and display signs of insulin resistance do not do well on the supplemental estrogen. It aggravates these conditions and increases the risk of heart disease. In 1996, the Committee on Safety of Medicines in the United Kingdom issued a warning of a threefold risk of blood clots in women treated with conventional ERT.

Many studies now confirm that the use of ERT increases the risk of breast cancer. However, heart disease is the top killer of postmenopausal women, and women on ERT have been shown to have a decreased risk of dying from heart disease. In the large studies that have been carried out, though, women who were on ERT had a higher socioeconomic status (and likely a healthier lifestyle) than women who were not on ERT. Their generally better health may have been the factor that protected them rather than the ERT therapy itself.

A study in the *Journal of the American Medical Association* in 1996 showed that HDL to cholesterol ratios improved in women on ERT. However, estrogen therapy caused at least a 30 percent increase in triglycerides, and high triglycerides are a potent cardiovascular risk factor. Estrogen therapy also causes unstable blood sugar, high blood pressure, and Syndrome X (see Hyperinsulinemia, p. 232).

Provera is the most common progesterone agent used for hormone replacement therapy, and it is a synthetic progesterone (medroxyprogesterone). It can cause breast tenderness, production of breast milk, hives, itchy skin, swelling, rashes, bloating, acne, excess hair, hair loss, blood clots in the legs, blood clots in the lungs, spotting or periods, changes in weight, jaundice, depression, fever, insomnia, nausea, sleepiness, elevated blood pressure, and increased blood lipid levels.

Synthetic hormones are used by the drug companies because they are patentable. Natural estrogen and progesterone are not patentable, and are not used by the drug companies because they are not profitable. HRT with synthetic progesterone can cause cramps of the uterus, menstrual periods, sore breasts, bloating, and weight gain.

Women who still have a uterus are given progesterone (Provera) in combination with estrogen to prevent endometrial cancer. Women who do not have a uterus may be given either estrogen alone, or both estrogen and progesterone, depending on the philosophy of the physician.

If women have low libido after menopause, they may be given testosterone. Although females need only 10 percent of the testosterone men require, postmenopausal women who lack testosterone can find that their health suffers, since testosterone prevents bone loss and protects against breast cancer. Testosterone is often combined with estrogen in a combination known as Estratest. If women take testosterone, they should be observed for signs of virilization, (deepening of the voice, increased hair on the face, acne, and enlargement of the clitoris). Testosterone can also increase calcium levels and cause sodium and fluid retention. One form of testosterone, methyl testosterone, can cause liver toxicity.

Surgery

When there is excessive bleeding, women may have a surgical procedure (dilatation and curettage, commonly known as a D&C) to remove the inner lining of the uterus, which usually controls the bleeding. If the D&C fails to control bleeding, a hysterectomy is considered.

Other Therapeutic Measures

For a vaginal lubricant, women are given Replens (an over-the-counter lubricant that lowers the pH of the vagina), or other lubricating jellies.

Women with menopausal symptoms are also advised to stop smoking.

ALTERNATIVE TREATMENT

Diet

Observe the following dietary guidelines. Avoid sugar, caffeine, and alcohol, all of which can trigger hot flashes and make mood swings worse. Follow a diet high in complex carbohydrates (unless you have hyperinsulinemia) and low in fat, which helps prevent hot flashes. Avoid most dairy products, as dairy and meat can promote hot flashes and may contribute to loss of bone calcium. Add blackstrap molasses, broccoli, dandelion greens, kelp, salmon with bones, and sardines to your diet as sources of natural calcium. Also include seeds and nuts in your diet.

Phytoestrogens are less potent, estrogen-like compounds found in plant-based foods such as tofu, miso, cashews, peanuts, oats, corn, apples, and almonds. Soy-based diets also contain isoflavones, which are natural estrogens of plant origin. They exert weak estrogen effects, and may help prevent bone disease, promote a healthy heart, and maintain a healthy genito-urinary tract. They inhibit the growth of breast, prostate, and colon cancer, and lower blood cholesterol. Isoflavones can bind to estrogen receptors, and they can compete at these binding sites with synthetic estrogens. Animal studies demonstrate that soy isoflavones prevent bone loss over the short term, and there is a lower prevalence of osteoporosis-related fractures in postmenopausal women in Asia (where much soy is consumed) than there is in Western countries. Isoflavones also have an anti–blood clotting effect (in contrast to the blood-clotting potential of HRT).

Add one to two servings of soy and soybeans to your diet each day. A serving of soy is 1 cup of soy milk, ½ cup of tofu, ½ cup of tempeh, ½ cup of green soybeans, or a 3-ounce soyburger. Check the label on soyburgers to be sure they retain the isoflavones.

Exercise and Lifestyle
Do weight-bearing exercise for 20 minutes three to four times a week. Stop smoking and avoid the smoke of others.

Nutrient Therapy
Take nutritional supplements, as follows:

- vitamin A – 25,000 to 75,000 IU a day. *Caution:* Do not take more than 8,000 IU daily if you are or might be pregnant (for heavy periods; if you take the higher doses, have your levels monitored).
- B-complex with 50 mg of each B – as directed on the label (balances Bs)
- vitamin B_6 – 100 to 250 mg a day (decreases water retention; eases symptoms)
- vitamin C – 2,000 to 3,000 mg a day (for hot flashes)
- vitamin E – 400 IU two times a day (for hot flashes, libido, and to prevent blood clotting if you take estrogen)
- boron – 6 to 12 mg a day (for libido)
- copper – 1 to 2 mg a day (to balance zinc)
- zinc picolinate – 30 to 50 mg a day (helps protect against bone loss; reduces symptoms)
- arginine – 2,000 to 3,000 mg a day (for libido)
- cod liver oil – 1 Tbsp. a day (to reduce the risk of blood clotting if you take estrogen)
- DHEA – 5 to 25 mg a day (for libido—but have your levels monitored: too much DHEA can cause a slight increase in hair growth on the arms and legs)
- essential fatty acids (borage oil, black currant oil, flaxseed oil) – 1 Tbsp. a day (for hot flashes; important in production of estrogen)
- evening primrose oil – two capsules three times a day (supplies essential fatty acids; helps hot flashes; helps in production of estrogen)
- folic acid – 10 to 40 mg a day. This is a large dose of folic acid and is available only by prescription at compounding pharmacies (for libido).
- quercetin – 500 mg twice a day (for hot flashes)

Herbal Therapy
Take a botanical supplement.

- two parts licorice, two parts burdock root, two parts dong quai, one part wild yam, and one part motherwort as a mixture in a capsule – for vaginal dryness, hot flashes, palpitations, and increased energy
- alfalfa – helps with bloating and water retention
- black cohosh – an antispasmodic and estrogen enhancer
- calendula flowers – for vaginal dryness
- chamomile tea or lemon balm tea – before bedtime for insomnia or anxiety
- chasteberry – for hot flashes and anxiety and/or vaginal dryness and/or mood swings
- dong quai – for hot flashes and/or mood swings
- ginkgo – for mood swings
- gotu kola – for hot flashes
- marshmallow root – as a douche for vaginal dryness
- motherwort – for help with palpitations that accompany hot flashes
- oat straw – for libido or depression and vaginal lubrication

- Siberian ginseng *(Eleutherococcus senticosus)* – for hot flashes or depression
- skullcap – for anxiety, pain, and spasms
- St. John's wort – for mood swings
- valerian tincture – before bedtime for insomnia
- wild yam tincture – for vaginal dryness

Homeopathic Remedies
Twice a day, take the homeopathic remedy that best describes your menopausal symptoms. If your symptoms do not subside, seek the help of a homeopathic physician.

- *Bellis perennis* – excessive and permanent tiredness; backache.
- *Lachesis* – a general unwell feeling; with piles, vertigo, palpitations, and headaches; head may be flushed; the feet cold; worse after sleep; acts well in women who have had numerous pregnancies.
- *Pulsatilla* – mood is changeable, frequently weepy; feels better with an open window; hot flashes, desires consolation.
- *Sanguinaria* – hot flashes with right-sided headaches, the skin burns and itches all over the body; offensive, acrid vaginal discharge; periods may be profuse and offensive; breasts become sore.
- *Sepia* – in spite of frequent flushes, the patient feels cold and sweats from the slightest exertion; worse toward the evening; intercourse is painful.

Take a homeopathic remedy as needed for heavy periods sometimes associated with early menopause. Seek the help of a homeopathic practitioner if you do not obtain relief.

- *Belladonna* – bearing-down sensation, worse lying down; profuse, early, bright red periods; cramp-like back pain; cutting pelvic pain.
- *Calcarea carbonica* – profuse, irregular, long-lasting periods; feet feel cold and damp.

- *Cantharis* – black, early, profuse periods; bladder irritation.
- *Caulophyllum* – when periods are too frequent, with spasmodic pain.
- *Cimicifuga* – early, profuse periods with wandering backache and muscle ache; with gloom and dejection.
- *Magnesia carbonica* – dark, thick blood loss, chiefly at night.

Many patients respond to complex homeopathic remedies. You may want to try Fem Pro Drops from PHP, which aids in correcting severe female hormone imbalances, or Female+ by Vibrant Health, which is an adaptogen to assist in proper production and flow of female hormones (see Sources).

Other Therapeutic Measures
Expose the hands, face, and arms to the mid-morning or late afternoon sun for 15 to 20 minutes three days a week. This helps the body to manufacture vitamin D, which is needed to maintain strong bones and prevent osteoporosis. (A 30-minute sunbath will provide 300 to 350 IU of vitamin D.)

There are three types of estrogen: estrone, estradiol, and estriol. Estriol is the weakest of the estrogens, and studies have shown that the ratio of estriol to the other estrogens is low in women who have breast cancer. Vitamin E increases the ratio of estriol to estradiol and estrone. Estriol cream helps with vaginal symptoms, but it is not known if it has the same protective effects against heart disease as the other estrogens.

If hormones are necessary, use natural hormones of estrogen and progesterone. Dr. Jonathan Wright of the Tahoma Clinic in Kent, Washington uses a combination of 80 percent estriol, 10 percent estrone, and 10 percent estradiol, in a formula known as Triest (available at compounding pharmacies). If you take replacement estrogen, take 25 mg of vitamin B_6 a day.

The formula is taken on days 1 to 25 of the month, with natural progesterone taken on days 14 to 25 as well.

Natural progesterone has fewer side effects than synthetic progesterone: for example, it has fewer adverse effects on blood lipid levels than does Provera.

Women who have more body fat may produce enough of their own estrogen, and may just need to add natural progesterone.

Oral estrogens have to be metabolized by the liver, which increases the body's need for B-complex vitamins and some minerals. Dr. Christiane Northrup feels that women who have gone through surgical menopause should have hormone replacement until the average age of menopause.

If you cannot decide whether to take ERT (even natural ERT) and are having serious symptoms, try the natural hormones first and see how you feel. Remember that there are many different ERT regimens: a survey of 283 gynecologists in the Los Angeles area found 84 different patterns of estrogen use in their practices. You must find and use the regimen that works best for you.

Take DHEA and/or natural testosterone if you have symptoms and laboratory evidence of deficiencies.

Use natural progesterone cream to treat vaginal atrophy. Use ¼ to ½ tsp. on the face, neck, inner arms, abdomen, inner thigh, or soles of feet daily for 30 days, then for at least two weeks of each month after that. Alternate sites, and rub it in thoroughly.

If you need a vaginal lubricant, use one of the following: vitamin E oil, cold-pressed castor oil, or sesame or other high-quality oil.

Try a low-dose estrogen vaginal cream for vaginal dryness. It does not get absorbed systemically. (See Sources for compounding pharmacies that carry natural hormones.)

Try Ayurvedic medicine, or use traditional Chinese medicine.

Use stress reduction techniques such as meditation and progressive relaxation.

VAGINITIS

Vaginitis is an inflammation of the vagina that is marked by pain and a white viscid discharge. The most common symptoms of vaginitis are vaginal discharge, vaginal odor, itching, and painful urination (when it may be mistaken for a urinary tract infection). As many as 72 percent of young, sexually active females have had one or more forms of vaginitis. Vaginitis can be a symptom of a sexually transmitted disease, although many women can harbor diseases such as trichomoniasis for years with no symptoms. (See chapter 22, Socially Transmitted Diseases.)

CAUSES OF VAGINITIS

The most common cause of vaginitis is a disruption in the normal balance of bacteria in the vagina, or a change in the normal pH of the vagina. Vaginitis can be related to hormones, irritants, and infections, and postmenopausal women are prone to atrophic vaginitis, a condition caused by a decrease in hormones. The vagina is raw and sore. Physiological vaginitis is common in teenagers, and is a function of changes to the normal vaginal secretions that occur over the course of the menstrual cycle. Douching may alleviate symptoms temporarily, but may then cause an irritant vaginitis.

Irritant vaginitis can be caused by medication or hygiene products that directly irritate the vaginal tissue (for instance, perfumed toilet paper, scented sanitary tampons, and pads that contain deodorants). Chemicals in hot tubs and swimming pools can also irritate the vagina. Some women sweat excessively from the vulva when stressed, and this, combined with nonabsorbent, synthetic clothing can cause irritation. Allergic vaginitis can occur in some women in peak pollen season.

Repeated sexual intercourse over a short period of time can upset the pH balance of the vagina. Semen is very alkaline, with a pH of around 9, and it may take 24 hours for the normal pH of the vagina to recover. A vinegar douche can help speed the process.

MODERN MEDICAL TREATMENT

Drug Therapy
Modern medicine treats atrophic vaginitis with prescription estrogen ointments. This increases the body's need for vitamin B_6.

ALTERNATIVE TREATMENT

Diet
Avoid refined foods, sugar, simple carbohydrates, and food allergens. Keep fats to a minimum and consume fiber such as oat bran daily. Avoid citrus and acidic fruits such as oranges, grapefruits, lemons, limes, tomatoes, and pineapple when you have vaginal inflammation. Add them back into your diet slowly after the inflammation subsides. Include phytoestrogens in your diet (see Alternative Treatment for Menopause, above).

Exercise and Lifestyle
Do aerobic exercise for 20 minutes three times a week. Do not exercise wearing tight clothes or clothes that keep moisture in the crotch area. The increased moisture can increase the risk for vaginitis. Never sit around in a wet bathing suit for any length of time.

Wear white cotton underwear and avoid tight clothing and synthetic fabrics. Avoid bubble baths and douching with chemicals. Avoid intercourse to reduce trauma to inflamed tissue.

Nutrient Therapy
At the first sign of vaginal discomfort, take the following nutritional supplements:

- vitamin A – 50,000 IU a day. *Caution:* Do not take more than 8,000 IU a day if you are pregnant or might be pregnant (powerful antioxidant that aids in healing).
- beta carotene – 100,000 IU a day (converted to vitamin A)
- vitamin B-complex – 50 mg of most Bs a day (aids in reproduction of cells)
- vitamin C – 2,000 to 5,000 mg a day (necessary for tissue healing)
- vitamin E – 400 IU a day (powerful antioxidant that aids in tissue repair)
- vitamin E – topical cream (lubricates vagina)
- zinc picolinate – 15 mg a day (promotes proper utilization of vitamin A; promotes tissue repair)
- bioflavonoids – 1,000 mg a day (act synergistically with vitamin C)
- essential fatty acids – 500 mg four times a day (aids healing)

Herbal Therapy
Use the following botanical supplements as a douche or suppository. You may also use a tampon saturated with the substance, but it must be removed after four hours. Remember that it is not healthy to douche frequently as it disturbs the normal bacterial flora of the vagina. Recurrent douching has also been associated with ectopic pregnancy. Use douching for several days, but only for treating specific symptoms.

- calendula – soothes and heals irritated tissues
- comfrey – soothes irritation
- echinacea – anti-inflammatory properties
- goldenseal – anti-inflammatory and antibiotic properties; cleanses mucus membranes. *Caution:* Do not use if you are pregnant.
- marshmallow root – soothes and heals mucus membranes

Homeopathic Remedies
Take the homeopathic remedy that best describes your symptoms, twice a day. Unless you receive relief quickly, consult a homeopathic physician.

- *Arsenicum album* – acrid, corrosive, and yellow discharge; mainly in the elderly and people with chronic diseases.
- *Borax* – clear, copious, hot discharge, which is acrid and causes swelling of the labia and is at its worst mid-cycle.
- *Graphites* – profuse, thin, white mucus discharge which comes in gushes with back and lower abdominal pain; more profuse in the morning on rising; the patient is constantly cold.
- *Hydrastis* – tenacious, thick, ropy discharge; patient is weak and constipated.
- *Pulsatilla* – acrid, burning, creamy discharge with back pain.
- *Sepia* – yellow-green, offensive discharge; worse before a period, with a bearing-down sensation in the pelvis.

Other Therapeutic Measures

If at all possible, use natural therapies to clear your vaginitis. Take warm sitz baths with herbs, plain water, or Epsom salts.

Natural progesterone applied to the vagina is beneficial for atrophic vaginitis.

Use a retention douche of acidophilus powder or use an acidophilus capsule as a suppository to rebalance vaginal pH.

Use antibiotics only if the vaginitis or infection can cause pelvic inflammatory disease (see Chlamydia section in chapter 22, Socially Transmitted Diseases).

BREAST PROBLEMS

Breasts are complicated glandular organs composed of fat, connective tissue, milk glands, and ducts. They are sensitive to the hormones secreted by the ovaries. These hormones can affect glandular size, and an excess of estrogen can cause breast tenderness.

A discharge from the nipple can occur after nipple stimulation, and this is normal. After breast feeding, many women will have a milk discharge from their breasts for at least one year and often for two years. A rare type of tumor of the pituitary gland in the brain can cause a nipple discharge. If you have a discharge that is bloody, it should be checked to make sure it does not indicate the presence of a cancer.

BREAST EXAMS

It is very important that all women should have regular breast exams by their physician. In addition all women should examine their breasts regularly, beginning at age 20. Premenopausal women should examine their breasts five to seven days after they begin menstruation. Postmenopausal women should pick a specific time each month to examine their breasts.

The first goal of self-examination is to learn what normal breasts feel like. Breasts feel as if they contain tiny lumps or "BBs," and these are normal. Once you are comfortable with knowing what your breasts normally feel like, you should check for changes or new lumps each month.

According to Dr. K. M. Kash, in a 1992 article in the *Journal of the National Cancer Institute,* women at the highest risk for breast cancer are the ones least likely to examine their breasts, probably because they are anxious about breast cancer.

When you examine your breasts:

- Lie down with your right hand behind your head and a pillow supporting your right shoulder. This helps to flatten the breast against the chest wall.
- Feel the right breast with the flat part of the fingers of your left hand. Palpate superficially—then deeper. Examine the entire breast, including the area around the armpit. Divide the breast into four imaginary quadrants, and examine each quadrant, one at a time; or examine the breast in circular patterns, working from the nipple to the outside

or from the outside to the nipple. Breast tissue is densest in the upper, outer, quadrant.

- When you have finished examining your right breast, put your left hand behind your head, and examine your left breast with your right hand.
- Finally, examine the breasts while sitting or standing, watching for dimpling, changes in the shape of the breasts, and changes in the nipples.

If you feel a lump or note any dimpling of the skin, seek medical care. If you are pre-menopausal and the lump is tender, you may want to wait for one menstrual cycle to see if the lump goes away. Remember that most lumps in the breast are benign (non-cancerous). However, if a new lump persists in your breast, do not delay consulting a physician.

There are new devices on the market now that aid both self-breast examination and breast examinations by physicians. Sensor Pad is a silicone-filled device that looks like a deflated balloon (see Sources). It is placed over the breast to reduce friction and make it easier for women to feel shapes. Physicians can use a new product called BreastAlert, which is a differential temperature sensor. It is a cone-shaped device that fits inside the bra and records the temperature of the breasts. A difference of 2°F to 7°F between mirror-image areas of the breasts suggests underlying breast disease. In clinical studies done by the manufacturer (HumaScan—see Sources), temperature differentials of 2°F or more were found in a sample of women with biopsy-proven breast tumors less than 10 mm and as small as 5 mm. BreastAlert is appropriate for all patients, is non-invasive, and takes only 15 minutes to use.

FIBROCYSTIC BREAST DISEASE

Fibrocystic breast disease, also known as benign cystic mastitis, is the most common breast problem. The cysts are painful and tender, especially just before the menstrual period, and the breasts feel unusually lumpy on examination. Almost half of all women will have fibrocystic breast disease, usually between the ages of 30 and 50, and it can be one symptom of premenstrual syndrome (PMS).

The development of fibrocystic breast disease seems to be related to a predominance of estrogen over progesterone. Women who have a predominance of estrogen often have a sluggish liver detoxification system, and cannot break down estrogen normally.

About half of all women who go to physicians have some type of breast pain. Breast pain can be caused by too much estrogen, too much caffeine, an infection in a nursing mother, or too much stress. At least 70 percent of all American women have been told that they have fibrocystic breast disease, and at one time it was believed that this put them at higher risk of breast cancer. However, the U.S. National Cancer Association Consensus Committee noted in 1985 that about 80 percent of what is called fibrocystic breast disease is merely an expression of normal changes in breast anatomy. A biopsy done on fibrocystic breast tissue will show normal cells, and many physicians now believe that fibrocystic breast disease is not a true disease.

MODERN MEDICAL TREATMENT

Diet
There is strong evidence that the consumption of caffeine in tea, cola, chocolate, and caffeinated medications plays a role in fibrocystic breast disease. When these food substances (which contain methylxanthine) are limited or removed from the diet, fibrocystic breast disease usually improves.

Radiology
Modern medicine responds to breast lumps by sending patients for frequent mammograms and ultrasound studies. An ultrasound can help distinguish a solid lump from a cyst. If the lump is

not a cyst, the woman will have a mammogram and then see a surgeon. (See p. 206–7 for more information on mammograms.)

Surgery

A needle aspiration or needle biopsy will be performed if the mammogram or ultrasound is positive. The lump will be aspirated with a needle to see if it contains fluid. If the lump disappears when it is aspirated, it is a good sign that it is not a tumor. Many doctors then have the aspirated fluid sent to a lab to be checked for cancer cells.

If the lump is not fluid-filled, surgeons will often do a needle biopsy of the lump to determine if cancer is present.

If cancer is present, a lumpectomy may be performed, surgically removing the cancerous lump. Surgery may be followed by chemotherapy or radiation therapy. (For more information on breast cancer see chapter 17, Cancer.)

ALTERNATIVE TREATMENT

Diet

If you have breast lumps, stop ingesting food that contains caffeine: cola, root beer, chocolate, and caffeinated coffee. Also avoid dairy foods, alcohol, sugar, white flour products, heat- or chemical-processed cooking oils, fried foods, and foods high in salt.

Eat a high–complex carbohydrate, high-fiber, low-fat, vegetarian diet (unless you have hyperinsulinemia). Eat sea vegetables (for their iodine content), and also include in your diet foods that are high in organic germanium such as garlic, onions, and shiitake mushrooms (germanium improves oxygenation at the cellular level). Try to eat some foods raw, such as seeds, nuts, and grains.

Exercise and Lifestyle

Do aerobic exercise for 20 minutes three times a week. Exercise helps prevent breast cancer by strengthening the immune system.

Try to have a bowel movement daily. Women who have fewer than three stools a week have a higher incidence of fibrocystic disease than do women who have a stool at least once a day.

Nutrient Therapy

You should take the following nutritional supplements:

- vitamin A – 75,000 IU a day for three months (take this under supervision of a nutritional physician) then drop to 25,000 IU a day. *Caution:* Do not take more than 8,000 IU a day if you are pregnant or might be pregnant (supports mucus membranes of the breast's duct system; causes remission of breast cysts).
- beta carotene – 50,000 to 300,000 IU a day (this is a safer alternative to vitamin A and is converted to vitamin A)
- B-complex vitamins – 50 mg of most Bs a day (help regulate hormones)
- vitamin B_6 – 200 mg a day (helps fluid and hormone regulation)
- vitamin C – 2,000 to 3,000 mg a day (strengthens tissues; needed for hormone production)
- vitamin E – 400 to 600 IU a day (decreases cysts in breasts)
- magnesium chelate – 400 to 800 mg a day (decreases breast tenderness)
- SSKI (supersaturated potassium iodide) – 1 to 10 drops a day, or iodine – 0.25 mg a day (anti-inflammatory and anti-scarring effect; helps shrink cysts)
- selenium – 200 mcg a day (antioxidant; helps prevent cancer)
- evening primrose oil, borage oil, flaxseed oil, or black currant seed oil – 500 mg four times a day (reduces the size of cysts; normalizes hormonal levels)
- *Lactobacillus acidophilus* – ½ to 1 tsp. a day in divided doses (helps to metabolize estrogen)

Herbal Therapy

Take a botanical supplement. If your symptoms are not relieved, seek the help of a trained herbalist.

- chasteberry – for breast tenderness
- dandelion – for breast sores, tumors, and cysts
- echinacea – for mastitis
- goldenseal – for breast infections. *Caution:* Do not take if you are pregnant.
- mullein – relieves pain
- parsley – for swollen breasts
- red clover – estrogenic

Homeopathic Remedies

Take the homeopathic remedy that best fits your symptoms. Unless your symptoms resolve completely, consult a homeopathic practitioner.

- *Calcarea carbonica* – breasts swollen and painful, especially before menses; hot swelling breasts.
- *Carbo animalis* – fibrocystic breasts; abscess, tumors, or cysts, more often left-sided; hard painful nodes in breast.
- *Carsinosum* – swelling and tenderness of the breasts before menses; menses early; chronic mastitis; breast changes shape.
- *Lac caninum* – pain and swelling of breasts; worse before menses, jarring pressure; often alternating sides; feel full of very hard lumps.
- *Phytolacca* – fibrocystic breast disease; tenderness of breasts, worse before and during menses.

- *Silica* – fibrocystic disease; breast abscesses; breast nodules; hard lumps in breasts; sharp pains in breast; nipples sore, ulcerate easily.

Other Therapeutic Measures

Use natural progesterone on the skin from day 15 to 25 of the menstrual cycle. This will make cysts disappear.

Apply castor oil packs to help pull out toxins. Cold-pressed castor oil is poured onto a flannel or cotton cloth, and the cloth is applied to the area with heat, such as an electric heating pad or hot water bottle. Change or launder the cloth after every third use. Use the pack three times per week for one hour, for two to three months to help breast pain.

Investigate treatment for PMS (earlier in this chapter) and use the applicable portion of it.

Have thyroid function monitored. If needed, take a natural thyroid replacement. Thyroid supplements decrease pain and breast nodules, even in patients who have normal blood thyroid levels.

Avoid estrogen from drugs and contaminated foods. (Some meats contain added hormones.)

Use acupressure:

- Massage the area the width of two thumbs above the most prominent crease on the inner wrist, in line with the middle finger.
- Press on the top of the shoulder, midway between the tip of the shoulder and the neck.

Massage therapy can also be helpful.

Use stress reduction techniques (see Anxiety, p. 247).

CHAPTER 24

Male Problems

Male health problems are the unique health concerns that are directly related to male anatomy. The male genitalia consist of the penis, the scrotum with the testicles inside, the prostate gland, and other glands. The testicles produce sperm, which come out through the urethra in a milky fluid (semen) during ejaculation. The prostate gland secretes this fluid, which enhances the delivery and fertilizing ability of the sperm. The testicles secrete testosterone, the hormone that initiates the changes of puberty. The penis and testicles enlarge during puberty, and there is development of underarm and pubic hair and the beard.

PROSTATE PROBLEMS

Prostate problems are a significant health issue for males. The prostate gland is a chestnut-shaped gland located at the base of the bladder, which surrounds the beginning of the urethra.

The three most common prostate problems are infection, enlargement, and tumors. All of these conditions occur more commonly in older men.

The first sign of prostate disease is a need to urinate frequently during the night. In the next stage, there is slight or burning pain during urination, urgency, and a problem starting or stopping urine flow. The urine stream is reduced in force; it may appear in a split stream, and there may be a dribble after urinating. There can also be a feeling of having a full bladder together with dribbling, difficulty achieving or maintaining erections, painful sex, painful ejaculation, pus or blood in the urine, lower back pain, or a heavy, waterlogged feeling of the genitals. On physical exam the prostate is enlarged, but not tender. The symptoms are vague, and over 90 percent of prostatic growths are not detected until past the point at which they can be easily treated.

PROSTATITIS

Prostatitis is an inflammation of the prostate. It can be caused by several factors, including infection, dehydration, prolonged sitting, sexual activity levels (both too high and too low), irritation from vigorous exercise such as horseback riding or bicycling, or irritation from foods such as coffee and alcohol. Prostatitis may also be aggravated by estrogen.

The usual cause for prostatitis is infection. Infection often begins in another part of the body and spreads to the prostate. For example, recurrent bladder infections can spill over into the prostate and urinary tract. An infected prostate becomes swollen and blocks the passage of urine from the bladder through the urethra, and the infection can then spread to the kidneys.

Symptoms of a prostate infection are severe pain and tenderness in the region of the prostate, radiating into the genitals, pelvis, and back; fever; chills; and fatigue.

Prostate infection is most commonly seen in men between the ages of 20 and 50. It can be caused by several different organisms, including those that are sexually transmitted, such as chlamydia. Prostate infections can become chronic.

ENLARGED PROSTATE

Enlargement of the prostate is typically related to decreased production of the male hormone testosterone after the age of 40. At the same time, other hormones increase (prolactin, estradiol, luteinizing hormone, and follicle stimulating hormone), which raises the concentration of dihydrotestosterone (another male hormone) within the prostate. Cells in the prostate overgrow because of the high concentration of dihydrotestosterone. This condition is known as benign prostatic hyperplasia (BPH) or benign prostatic hypertrophy.

Dr. Denham Harman, professor emeritus of the University of Nebraska School of Medicine, notes that 90 percent of the population have insufficient zinc in their diet. Zinc helps to prevent or control BPH because it blocks the enzyme that facilitates the conversion of testosterone to dihydrotestosterone, and the prostate uses 10 times more zinc than any other part of the body. Zinc also increases the excretion of both testosterone and dihydrotestosterone. Zinc is depleted by caffeine, alcohol, and spicy foods.

Men with enlarged prostates are at risk for acute urinary retention, a condition in which the bladder outlet is blocked by the enlarged prostate so that it cannot be emptied. The signal to void becomes overwhelming and painful, but urine cannot be voided until a catheter is placed into the bladder to bypass the obstruction. This situation is a medical emergency.

Prostate enlargement is common in North America. Close to 60 percent of men between the ages of 40 and 59 have an enlarged prostate gland, and by the age of 65, nearly all men have enlarged prostates. An enlarged prostate can cause impotence and incontinence. It also can cause blockage of the bladder, infection, and spread of infection to the kidneys.

A 1995 study of 25,000 men, done by Harvard Medical School in Boston, found an increased risk of developing urinary problems with increased abdominal fat: a seven-inch increase in waist measurement was correlated with a 75 percent increase in urinary problems after age 50. Half of the men with a waist measurement over 43 inches either had severe urinary problems or had undergone prostate surgery. High-fat diets may be responsible for BPH. Dr. Camille Mallouh of the Metropolitan Hospital in New York examined 100 prostates of men of all ages at autopsy and found that the cholesterol content of BPH prostates was 80 percent higher than that of normal prostates.

MODERN MEDICAL TREATMENT

Drug Therapy

For a prostate infection, antibiotics are given. Proscar is used to shrink the prostate gland. Years ago natives of Santo Domingo, who lack an enzyme that is normally present in other populations, were found to have a low incidence of prostate enlargement due to the absence of that enzyme. Proscar acts by neutralizing this enzyme and thus preventing the buildup of dihydrotestosterone. Proscar is only marginally effective, and it sometimes takes six months for improvement to become apparent. It causes impotence in about 4 percent of men who take it. It can also cause decreased libido and decreased volume of ejaculate. It lowers prostate specific antigen (PSA) levels even in patients who have prostate cancer (for which a high level of PSA is a marker—see below). Proscar should not be handled by women who are pregnant, or who may become pregnant, as it can cause birth defects.

Phenoxybenzamine (Dibenzyline), terazosin (Hytrin), or prazosin (Minipress) are given at bedtime. They do not reduce the size of the prostate gland but do reduce the need to urinate frequently. Dibenzyline and Hytrin are alpha-receptor blocking agents that are used to control high blood pressure. Either can cause a drop of blood pressure when the patient stands up, or nasal congestion. Dibenzyline can also cause a rapid heart rate, inhibition of ejaculation, gastrointestinal irritation, drowsiness, fatigue, and small pupils. Hytrin can also cause fainting in the first few days of treatment, back pain, headache, swelling of the feet, dizziness, and impotence. Minipress is an antihypertensive. It can cause dizziness, headache, drowsiness, lack of energy, weakness, palpitations, and nausea.

Surgery

The usual approach to the treatment of non-infectious prostate problems is surgery. In fact, one-third of males in the U.S. have had their prostate gland surgically removed by the time they are 85 years old. Unfortunately, the major side effects of surgery are impotence and incontinence. Other possible side effects of surgery include perforation of the bladder, hemorrhage, and infection.

There are two surgical treatments for removal of an enlarged prostate. Transurethral resection of the prostate (TURP) is the most commonly used method. An instrument with a tiny light and a knife or a laser at its end is inserted into the penis, and the overgrown prostate tissue is removed. Recovery from this procedure can take up to eight weeks. The other method is called a suprapubic procedure. An incision is made in the lower abdominal wall and the obstructing prostate tissue is removed. It takes longer to recover from the suprapubic procedure than from a TURP. Parts of the gland are left behind in each of these procedures in an effort to minimize the chances of impotence.

Neither of these surgical procedures relieves the symptoms of an enlarged prostate in every case. Scar tissue may form in the urethra, and this can cause difficulty urinating even after the prostate is removed. The risk of post-surgical impotence is probably higher with the suprapubic procedure. After either form of surgery, the semen may travel backward into the bladder during ejaculation, instead of forward through the penis, but this does not affect the sensation of orgasm. Within five years, 20 percent of men who have had a TURP need another operation. The TURP does not prolong life, and in fact (for reasons which are not understood) may decrease life span by one year. As well, the part of the prostate gland left behind can become cancerous.

Other Therapeutic Measures

An experimental alternative to surgery is prostatic ballooning. A catheter with a cylindrical balloon at the end is inserted into the penis under local anesthesia. When it reaches the area of the enlarged prostate, it is inflated for 10 to 15 minutes, which compresses the prostate tissue. About 80 percent of men undergoing this procedure achieve 100 percent improvement in urine flow, and have to get up fewer times at night to urinate. This improvement usually lasts about three years.

ALTERNATIVE TREATMENT

Diet

Observe the following dietary guidelines. Avoid alcohol (especially beer), which increases the excretion of zinc. Also avoid eating fried foods, margarine, and partially hydrogenated vegetable oils, as well as spicy foods, chocolate, caffeine, and foods high in carbohydrates. Eat natural, organic whole foods. Add 1 to 4 ounces of raw pumpkin seeds to your diet every day. Pumpkin seeds are rich in zinc and will help almost any prostate problem.

Because prostatitis can be aggravated by estrogen, eating soy products that dampen the effects of estrogen can help prevent prostatitis. Drink 2 to 3 quarts of pure water a day to stimulate urine flow and help prevent cystitis.

Exercise and Lifestyle

Perform aerobic exercise for 20 minutes, three times a week.

Eliminate tobacco use. Avoid chlorinated and

fluoridated water and limit your exposures to toxins, pesticides, and environmental contaminants. Avoid exposure to very cold weather.

Nutrient Therapy
If you have an enlarged prostate, take the following nutritional supplements:

- vitamin A – 5,000 to 10,000 IU a day (has antioxidant and anti-cancer properties)
- B-complex – with 50 mg of each B vitamin, three times a day (balances the extra B_6)
- vitamin B_6 – 50 mg twice a day over and above the B-complex amount (reduces fluid retention and infection)
- vitamin C – 2,000 to 3,000 mg a day in divided doses (aids healing)
- vitamin E – 400 IU a day (antioxidant; balances the extra essential fatty acids)
- calcium – 1,000 mg a day (needed to improve prostate function)
- copper – 1 to 2 mg a day (to balance zinc)
- magnesium – 500 mg a day (needed to improve prostate function)
- zinc arginate, citrate, or picolinate – 60 to 80 mg a day (reduces the size of the prostate)
- glycine, alanine, and glutamic acid – 400 mg of each three times a day for two weeks, and 200 mg three times a day thereafter. For the best absorption, take with vitamin B_6 and vitamin C (reduce the size of the prostate)
- linseed oil, sunflower oil, evening primrose oil, or soy oil – 1 tsp. or 4,000 mg three times a day (reduce the size of the prostate)

Herbal Therapy
Take a botanical supplement. If you do not obtain relief from your symptoms, seek the help of a trained herbalist.

- echinacea – for prostatitis
- garlic in its natural form – to protect against infection
- ginseng *(Panax ginseng)* extract – for stimulating the prostate
- horsetail – for acute prostatic infection
- parsley, saw palmetto berries, cornsilk, buckeye leaves, cayenne, kelp, and pumpkin seeds (blend together in equal parts) – for enlarged prostate.
- pygeum – for BPH
- saw palmetto – to reduce inflammation. Avoid fluid extracts and tinctures because of alcohol content.

Homeopathic Remedies
Take the homeopathic remedy that best fits your symptoms. If you do not obtain relief, consult a homeopathic physician.

- *Baryta carbonica* – BPH, enlarged prostate in the elderly, with a frequent urge to urinate; the urethra burns on urination.
- *Chimaphila unbellata* – prostate enlargement and irritation; smarting from neck of bladder; loss of prostate fluid; acute prostatitis with retention and dysuria; feeling of a ball in perineum.
- *Conium maculatum* – BPH, enlargement of the prostate and difficulty in passing urine, which comes in stops and starts; testicles hard and enlarged; impotence; dribbling of prostatic fluid worse with stools.
- *Ferrum picricum* – prostate enlarged; frequent urination at night with full feeling and pressure in rectum; retention of urine; smarting at neck of bladder and penis.
- *Medorrhinum* – frequent urging with painful urination; urine flows slowly; worse during the night; prostatic hypertrophy; epididymitis.
- *Pulsatilla* – protatitis; prostatic hypertrophy; epididymitis, worse left side; high sexual energy; worse heat and sun; better open air.
- *Staphysagria* – prostate condition with fre-

quent urination and a burning sensation in the urethra when not urinating.

- *Thuja* – enlarged prostate; offensive smelling genitalia; semen offensive; bladder feels paralyzed; must wait for urination; sensation of trickling after urination; desire to urinate sudden and cannot be controlled.

Many patients respond to complex homeopathic remedies. You may want to try Male Endocrine Axis by PHP, for prostate support (see Sources).

Other Therapeutic Measures
Use one of the hydrotherapy procedures below:

- Sit in a tub with the hottest water tolerable for 15 to 30 minutes once or twice a day.
- Spray the lower abdomen and pelvic area with warm and cold water, alternating three minutes hot and one minute cold.
- Sit in hot water while placing the feet in cold water for three minutes. Then sit in cold water while immersing the feet in hot water for one minute.
- Take hot sitz baths (105° to 115°F) for three to ten minutes. Follow with cool sponging of the pelvic area.

Lower serum cholesterol levels (see chapter 15, Heart Disease), and if needed, lose weight. Reduce stress. Have acupuncture treatment.

Delay sexual activity until the prostate is better. Sex can retard recovery of an infected or irritated prostate.

TESTICULAR PROBLEMS

Men of all ages can develop testicular problems. Among these are testicular cancer (see chapter 17, Cancer) and epididymitis. The epididymis is a tube that attaches to the back of each testicle. If it becomes inflamed there may be pain and swelling at the back of the testicle, as well as heat and tenderness. The scrotum can swell, and there can be fever, chills, and pain in the groin area. Epididymitis (inflammation of the epididymis) can be caused by urinary tract infections, mumps, prostatitis, sexually transmitted diseases, tuberculosis, prostate surgery, or long-term use of a urinary catheter. In young men, a urinary tract infection is the most common cause of epididymitis.

Epididymitis mimics torsion of the testicle, a surgical emergency in which the testicle twists and cuts off its blood supply. The Doppler blood flow can differentiate between the two conditions by demonstrating blood flow using sound.

Epididymitis is usually accompanied by orchitis, an inflammation of the testicles. Orchitis is not common, but may accompany a variety of infectious diseases. Symptoms of acute orchitis are swelling of one or both testicles with pain and sensitivity to touch. With chronic orchitis there is no pain, but the testicles slowly swell and become hard.

All men of all ages should do regular testicular exams, as well as having regular physical examinations. These examinations can help identify problems with the epididymis, as well as locating testicular masses that could be testicular cancer.

For a testicular self-exam:

- Lie in bed when you are relaxed (perhaps after a warm shower).
- Examine each testicle by rolling it between your thumb, middle, and index fingers; check the entire area, including the ropelike epididymis.
- Watch for swelling, lumps, or changes in size, shape, or consistency.

MODERN MEDICAL TREATMENT
Drug Therapy
For cases of epididymitis, antibiotics are prescribed.

ALTERNATIVE TREATMENT

Diet

Observe the following dietary guidelines, which are helpful for most male problems.

Eliminate sugar, caffeine, and alcohol, and cut back on red meat and fat. Cut back on foods containing nitrites, such as luncheon meats.

Eat a diet high in soy, fiber, organic fruits, and organic vegetables that are red-orange in color and contain carotenes. Eat seafood, lean meats, and grain products to ensure an adequate intake of selenium (an anti-cancer mineral).

Drink bottled or filtered water daily (½ ounce per pound of body weight).

Exercise and Lifestyle

Exercise regularly.

Nutrient Therapy

The following nutritional supplements are helpful for most male problems.

- multivitamin – with 100 mg of each B (unless taking B-complex) (necessary for all cellular function)
- vitamin A – 10,000 IU a day (antioxidant)
- beta carotene – 15,000 IU a day (antioxidant)
- vitamin B-complex – 100 mg a day (for normal cell division and function)
- vitamin B_3 – a total of 100 mg a day, including that in B-complex (needed for circulation; synthesis of sex hormones)
- vitamin B_6 – 100 mg a day over and above B-complex (helps immune system; has anti-cancer properties)
- vitamin B_{12} – 2,000 mcg a day (for normal cell division)
- folic acid – 180 mcg a day (for normal cell division)
- vitamin C – 2,000 mg three times a day (antioxidant; aids healing)
- vitamin E – 400 IU twice a day (antioxidant; immune system enhancer)
- magnesium – 500 mg a day (necessary for prostate function)
- selenium – 200 mcg a day (antioxidant)
- zinc picolinate – 60 mg a day (aids healing)
- coenzyme Q_{10} – 100 mg a day (antioxidant; needed to produce energy)
- essential fatty acid such as flaxseed oil – 1 Tbsp. twice a day (aids in repair and production of new cells)
- copper – 1 to 2 mg a day (balances zinc)

Herbal Therapy

The following botanical supplements are helpful for male problems.

- barberry – strengthens immune system; protects against infection
- echinacea – strengthens immune system; protects against infection
- garlic – strengthens immune system; protects against infection

Homeopathic Remedies

Take the homeopathic remedy that best fits your symptoms. If you do not obtain immediate relief, consult a homeopathic physician.

- *Aurum metallicum* – problems of testes and epididymitis; pain especially in right testicle; undescended testicle; malignancy of testicle; high sex drive.
- *Belladonna* – epididymitis; cystitis; pyelonephritis; sex drive generally low to low-normal.
- *Medorrhinum* – epididymitis; orchitis; prostatitis; prostatic hypertrophy; sex drive extreme.
- *Pulsatilla* – epididymitis, worse left side; sexual energy generally high, excessive in some cases; bladder pain, worse at end of urination or if trying to retain urine.
- *Rhododendron* – epididymitis; pain in testicle, more often the right side, may be de-

scribed as if crushed; pain extends up into abdomen; swelling of testes and chronic
inflammation.

• *Spongia tosta* – swelling, inflammation, and
pain in testes or epididymis.

Other Therapeutic Measures
For epididymitis, rest in bed and use scrotal support. To reduce swelling use ice packs twice a
day for 10 minutes at a time, until the swelling is
gone.

Have acupuncture treatments.

IMPOTENCE

Impotence (the inability of a male to achieve or
maintain an erection of sufficient rigidity to successfully perform sexual intercourse) is a problem for more than 15 million North American
men. Impotence may occur in isolated incidents,
or it may be chronic or recurring. While most
men think of impotence as resulting from emotional problems, in fact 80 to 90 percent of impotence has a physical cause. Impotence is
associated with age. Approximately 2 percent of
40-year-olds experience the problem, and this
increases to 25 percent of 65-year-olds.

CAUSES OF IMPOTENCE

Vascular disease, which blocks blood flow, can
be a cause of impotence—arteriosclerosis is not
limited to just the vessels of the heart. Prostate
problems (such as BPH) can cause impotence,
and sexually transmitted disease can play a
role as well. The use of alcohol and cigarettes
can be a factor. Smokers have a 50 percent
higher risk of impotence than non-smokers and
past smokers. Hormonal disturbances (diminished levels of testosterone, or overproduction
or underproduction of thyroid hormone) may
cause impotence. Diabetes, in which atherosclerosis and impaired circulation are often a
problem, is probably the most common cause
of impotence.

In addition, there are over 200 drugs that can
cause impotence. Many of these are commonly
prescribed drugs, among them blood pressure
medication, diuretics, antidepressants, muscle
relaxants, tranquilizers, anti-anxiety drugs,
antispasmodics, antihistamines, cholesterol-
lowering drugs, female hormones, immunosup-
pressive drugs, anti-ulcer drugs, arthritis
medications, and medications to treat Parkinson's disease. Fortunately, the negative effects of
drugs on potency are nearly always reversible
when the drug is stopped. The dosage may need
to be adjusted, or the medication changed to
avoid the side effect of impotence. (*Caution:*
Medications should not be stopped or changed
without first checking with a physician.)

Any time impotence is persistent or becomes
worse, a man should consult his physician, particularly if he has diabetes or arteriosclerosis.
Because impotence can be caused by serious
physical problems, it is important to determine
the exact cause. Many times proper treatment
can eliminate the physical problems causing the
impotence. Even if the problem is wholly emotional, many times proper treatment can restore
function.

MODERN MEDICAL TREATMENT

Testing for Causes of Impotence
Patients are advised to have a Nocturnal Penile
Tumescence (NPT) test that measures frequency,
rigidity, and duration of nighttime erections.
This test is done at home. If nocturnal erections
are occurring, impotence is not as likely to be
physiological. If the cause of impotence proves
to be an emotional problem, patients are advised to seek counseling.

Drug Therapy
If the problem is physical, the possibility that a
side effect of a medication may be causing the
problem should be investigated.

Recently, the new drug sildenafil citrate (Viagra) has become a bestseller. It helps men who have physical causes of impotence to achieve an erection by maintaining increased blood flow to the penis. Side effects include abnormal vision, nasal congestion, headache, flushing, and gastric problems such as pain, burning, and belching. Viagra has caused death in some men who have heart disease.

Surgery

A patient can have a surgical implantation of a prosthesis that achieves an erection through mechanical means.

Other Therapeutic Measures

If there is no treatable physical cause, an external vacuum device that produces erections can be used. There is also an injection treatment that produces an instant erection that lasts from ten minutes to two hours.

ALTERNATIVE TREATMENT

Diet

Avoid animal fats, fried foods, sugar, or junk foods. Include pumpkin seeds in the diet, as they are high in zinc and many men are zinc deficient. Avoid alcohol, particularly when anticipating sexual encounters.

Exercise and Lifestyle

Do not use tobacco and avoid exposure to tobacco smoke. Do not use marijuana or cocaine.

Avoid exposure to extremely cold weather. Avoid hot tubs and saunas. Wear boxer shorts instead of briefs.

Exercise regularly, but avoid overtraining or vigorous, intense exercise. Aerobic exercise for 20 minutes three times a week is best. If you ride a bike and develop numbness in the groin or genital area, stop riding. These symptoms mean that there is pressure on a nerve.

Nutrient Therapy

Take the following nutrients.

- vitamin A – 15,000 IU a day (antioxidant; enhances immunity)
- vitamin B-complex – 50 mg three times a day (for healthy nervous system and cell function)
- vitamin B_6 – 50 mg a day over and above that in the B-complex (for cellular reproduction)
- vitamin E – 200 IU initially, increasing gradually to 400 to 1,000 IU a day (increases circulation)
- copper – 2 to 3 mg a day (to balance zinc)
- zinc – 80 mg a day (important in prostate function). *Caution:* Do not exceed this amount.
- coenzyme Q_{10} – 30 to 60 mg twice a day (increases cellular oxygenation)
- octacosanol – 1,000 to 2,000 mcg three times a week (for hormone production)

Herbal Therapy

Take an herbal remedy:

- damiana – improves blood flow to the genital area
- sarsaparilla – contains a testosterone-like substance
- saw palmetto – normalizes prostate function
- wild yam – contains natural steroids
- yohimbe – dilates blood vessels
- dong quai, gotu kola, hydrangea root, pygeum, and/or Siberian ginseng *(Eleutherococcus senticosus)* – all are helpful for impotence

Homeopathic Remedies

Consult a homeopathic practitioner to help you determine which of the following remedies is best for you.

- *Agnus castus* – cold and relaxed penis; lack of sexual desire; impotence with chronic urethral discharge.
- *Argentum nitricum* – erection fails when attempting intercourse; intercourse is painful; symptoms worse at night, warmth, and from sweets.

- *Baryta carbonicum* – impotence; atrophy or smallness of genitalia, testes; diminished sex drive or aversion to sex; prostate hypertrophy.
- *Caladium* – impotence; absolutely flaccid penis, often described as a "wet dish rag"; lascivious thoughts but unable to have slightest erection; nocturnal semen emissions with totally flaccid penis, sometimes without sexual desire.
- *Conium maculatum* – impotence; premature ejaculation, even during foreplay; high sex drive; prostate enlargement or cancer; weight or heaviness in the perineum; prostate discharge.
- *Lycopodium* – apprehension; cannot have an erection; erections lead to premature emission; impotency in old age.
- *Sabal serrulata* – impotency; genitals cold, testicles shrunk, penis shrunk and cold with urinary troubles.

Many patients respond to complex homeopathic remedies. You may want to try Male+ by Vibrant Health. It is an adaptogenic formula to assist in the proper production and flow of male hormones.

Other Therapeutic Measures
See your physician to rule out physical causes of impotence. Investigate medications as a cause of impotence.

Do an impotence self-test in which nocturnal erections are checked. Nocturnal erections still happen during sleep if the problem is emotional, while if impotence is physical in origin, there are usually no erections. You can test for nocturnal emissions by using a Snap Gauge kit from Urohealth Corporation. This kit detects and measures rigidity of erections during sleep (see Sources).

The most inexpensive way to test for nocturnal erections is using postage stamps. Before going to bed, glue a strip of stamps around the shaft of the penis. If the ring of stamps is broken the next morning, a nocturnal erection took place and the cause of impotence is likely psychological. If you repeat this test over several nights and the stamps remain unbroken, the impotence is likely physiological and you should visit your physician for further testing.

Investigate the possibility that you have hyperinsulinemia, and treat it if found.

Use Kegel exercises (see Stress Incontinence, p. 306) to strengthen the pelvic muscles. This technique can help mild cases of impotence.

Do daily thermal biofeedback (see p. 120 for more information). Obtain professional reflexology treatments.

If there is no physical cause of impotence, it may have an emotional cause. Practice relaxation and meditation techniques. Flower essences help emotional balance and can be helpful for impotence.

ANDROPAUSE

There is a type of menopause in men, which is called andropause. It is caused by declining levels of testosterone, the male hormone that gives a male his sex drive and male characteristics, such as a beard. Testosterone is essential to the function of the testicles and many health-related matters. Men who have had heart attacks tend to have low testosterone levels, and men who have higher testosterone levels also have higher levels of HDL cholesterol (the "good" cholesterol). Testosterone has an anticoagulant effect, and it has been proven to be protective against cancer. Studies done in Japan show a reduction in incidence and severity of stroke with testosterone therapy. Testosterone also helps to control blood sugar and can help in preventing diabetic retinopathy. It is a major regulator of sugar, fat, and protein metabolism. Andropause is not as dramatic as menopause in women, but can be devastating for a man affected by it.

Symptoms of andropause can include weakness, impotence, pain, stiffness, drooping muscles, depression, irritability, and excesssive sweating, with intolerance to heat. Most men and physicians accept these symptoms as the inevitable accompaniments of aging, and very little is done by most physicians to alleviate them.

MODERN MEDICAL TREATMENT

Drug Therapy
Men who have low levels of testosterone are given the hormone by injection. Testosterone (Andro 100, Delatestryl, Testein P.A.), methyltestosterone (Android, Viribon), and nandroline (Durabolin) are the pharmaceuticals typically used.

Side effects of these drugs include acne or oily skin, bloating, hair loss, and changes in mood. These drugs may magnify the effects of insulin or anti-clotting drugs. If taken in combination with steroids; anti-nausea, anti-thyroid, and anti-infective drugs; oral contraceptives; heart medications; gold; or large doses of acetaminophen, these drugs may cause liver damage. Improperly used, they can cause breast enlargement and increase the risk of prostate cancer, hypertension, and heart disease. The use of alcohol while taking testosterone is discouraged. The United States is the only country still using methyltestosterone, which has been shown to harm the liver.

Testosterone patches are also used by modern medicine. These include Testoderm and Androderm Transdermal Systems. Side effects are the same as for injectable testosterone.

ALTERNATIVE TREATMENT

Diet
Follow the dietary suggestions for Testicular Problems on Page 360.

Exercise and Lifestyle
Exercise to increase your general fitness level.

Examine your priorities, and make changes that will relieve stress and enrich your life.

Nutritional Therapy
Take a nutritional supplement.
- multivitamin and mineral – as directed on the label (all nutrients are necessary for hormone production)
- vitamin E – 400 to 1,000 IU a day (needed for hormone production)
- copper – 2 to 3 mg a day (to balance zinc)
- zinc – 50 to 80 mg a day (important for male reproductive organs)
- DHEA – 25 mg a day, have levels montiored (precursor for male hormones)
- essential fatty acids – 500 mg four times a day (essential for hormone production)
- octacosanol – 1,000 to 2,000 mcg three times a week (good for hormone production)
- raw orchic glandular – as directed on label (enhances testicular function)

Herbal Therapy
Take a botanical supplement.
- damiana – improves blood flow to genitals
- dong quai – increases effects of testicular hormones
- false unicorn – balances sex hormones
- sarsaparilla – contains testosterone-like substance

Homeopathic Remedies
Many patients respond to complex homeopathic remedies. You may want to try Male+ by Vibrant Health. It is an adaptogenic formula to assist in the proper production and flow of male hormones (see Sources).

Other Therapeutic Measures
When testosterone levels are too low, treatment with testosterone is extremely beneficial, if it is given in the proper form and doses. Use natural testosterone, obtained from compounding pharmacies. Be aware that you may have some erection difficulties during andropause (see Sources).

CHAPTER 25

Allergy

An allergy is an abnormal response to a substance that is well tolerated by most people. Allergy symptoms are caused by the immune system attacking harmless or even useful substances entering the body. Modern medicine considers allergy to be a reaction that is mediated by immunoglobulin E (IgE) only. Immunoglobulin E is the antibody that is responsible for immediate hypersensitivity (allergic reactions) and skin whealing (raised bump on the skin surface from injection of an antigen). It is the antibody that participates in the classic pollen reactions: sneezing and itchy, watery eyes. It is also the antibody responsible for food reactions (either asthma or hives) that occur immediately after eating. A host of adverse reactions are not IgE mediated, however. Most alternative practitioners believe that these are allergic reactions that are immunoglobulin G (IgG) mediated. Immunoglobulin G, also known as gammaglobulin, is the major antibody in the blood that protects against bacteria and virus. Reactions that may be mediated by IgG are frequently *delayed* reactions and include many of the adverse reactions that people have to foods and chemicals.

Varying estimates exist regarding the number of North Americans who suffer from allergies; most figures indicate that 13 percent of the population have allergies. However, these figures probably refer to pollen allergies only, and may not even include dander and mold allergies. In his newsletter, *Health and Healing,* Dr. Julian Whitaker states that 40 million Americans spend up to $2 billion annually on allergy treatments, and lose up to 3 million workdays each year because of sneezing, watery eyes, scratchy throats, and asthma. When food and chemical sensitivities are considered as well, the figures are much higher (though accurate statistics are not available). Some reports state that 20 percent of North Americans have allergies, but this estimate is probably quite low.

Some allergic people cough, sneeze, and wheeze only during pollen season; these are the people with pollen and inhalant allergies. Some allergic individuals have no seasonal symptoms, but have varying symptoms when they consume a food to which they are sensitive. People with chemical sensitivities will have problems when they are exposed to perfumes, gasoline, cleaning supplies, and many other chemicals. Still others suffer from symptoms that affect many body systems; these people have food and chemical sensitivities, in addition to pollen/inhalant allergies. The most sensitive people of all are those who are environmentally ill. They have such severe allergies and sensitivities overlaid with other health problems that they are considered to be "universal reactors."

TOTAL LOAD/OVERLOAD

There are many factors that work together to determine your level of health, and whether or not you are likely to develop allergies.

In our day-to-day living we are subjected to many stresses:

- physical stresses: infections, chronic disease, allergies, pregnancy, inadequate or excessive exercise, insufficient nutrition, hormonal imbalance, acid/alkaline imbalance, poor digestion, lowered immune system function, and insufficient rest and sleep.
- emotional stresses: job frustrations, marital problems, divorce, deaths of relatives or friends, criticism, rejection, sibling rivalry, abuse (past or present), insufficient acknowledgment and touching, and failure to succeed.
- environmental stresses: extremes of temperature or altitude; pollution of air, food, and water; radiation; toxic metals; pesticides; toxic cleaning products; tobacco and wood smoke; vehicular exhaust; cosmetics and toiletries; natural and propane gas; and new building materials.

Our bodies can adjust to a few of these stresses, but with the accumulation and repetition of stressors, our metabolism loses its adaptability. Normal control mechanisms of the immune, nervous, endocrine, respiratory, and digestive systems will be upset, and we will develop symptoms because our total body stress burden is too high. The collective effect of the stressors exceeds the threshold level that our body metabolism can tolerate.

When the immune system is stressed, we can develop allergies. Dr. William Rea (of the Environmental Health Center in Dallas, Texas, and author of a four-volume series on chemical sensitivity) compares our immune system to a rain barrel. Any combination of stressors can fill our rain barrels, and when they overflow, we exhibit the symptoms of an allergic reaction. If we can keep our rain barrel emptied by reducing our stresses, controlling our allergies, cleaning up our environment, improving nutrition, and exercising regularly, we can tolerate moderate stresses without having our rain barrel overflow. However, if our rain barrel is always full, the slightest additional stress factor will cause it to overflow, resulting in unpleasant symptoms.

This concept helps to explain why a particular allergen will sometimes cause symptoms, and other times it will not; it depends on how full our rain barrel was at the time of the stress. This concept is referred to as total load/overload. Heredity plays a role in the size of our rain barrels, and lifestyle determines how full they are. If we drain our rain barrels with proper treatment and lifestyle adjustments, our immune system will not be pushed to exceed its adaptive capacity and will begin to heal. Allergies *can* be controlled and in some cases eliminated.

ALLERGY TESTING

There are many methods of allergy testing; the accuracy of any method depends on the skill and competence of the technician, the testing laboratory, and the physician. Space permits only an overview of these techniques (for more detail, see *The Whole Way to Allergy Relief and Prevention* by Dr. Jacqueline Krohn, Frances Taylor, and Erla Mae Larson).

Fasting and deliberate food testing involves fasting for four to seven days, and then reintroducing pure foods one at a time to observe any resulting symptoms.

Deliberate chemical testing is performed inside a testing booth where the person is exposed to a specially prepared chemical allergen. Pulse, blood pressure, and symptoms are noted before and after exposure, to reveal sensitivity.

Pulse testing involves taking a resting pulse, exposing the patient to the suspected allergen, and then taking the pulse again at 10- and 30-minute intervals. A change in pulse or other symptoms indicates sensitivity to the test substance.

Several blood tests for detecting allergies and sensitivities are available:

- Cytotoxic testing exposes food allergies and some chemical sensitivities by showing adverse changes in the patient's white blood cells.
- The RAST (radioallergosorbent test) radioactively labels IgE and IgG antibodies. A Geiger counter–type of instrument that measures the amount of antibody in the blood in response to foods, pollen, mold, dust and dust mites, and danders.
- The ALCAT (antigen leukocyte cellular antibody test) uses a Coulter counter to count and size white blood cells and platelets before and after incubation with food or mold samples. Changes in size and numbers signify a reaction.

Other testing methods for allergies include:

- Scratch or prick test: A drop of concentrated antigen on the skin is pricked or scratched so that a minute amount of antigen is absorbed. A wheal surrounded by inflammation at the test site indicates a problem substance. This test is accurate only for pollen, mold, and dander allergy in people with high IgE levels.
- Patch test: A patch impregnated with a test antigen is applied to the skin. Lesions, rash, inflammation, or hardness of the skin under the patch 24 to 48 hours later indicates a problem substance.
- EAV (electroacupuncture according to Voll): Instrument testing that measures galvanic skin response changes on exposure to an antigen. A change in skin response indicates sensitivity. Foods, chemicals, inhalants, and other substances can be tested.
- Serial dilution endpoint titration: Similar to traditional skin testing by injection, but uses serially diluted antigens (1:5, 1:25, 1:125, etc.). A whealing pattern provides a precise treatment dose. This test is extremely accurate for IgE mediated inhalant allergies.

- Provocative neutralization testing: Changes in baseline symptoms are noted after intradermal or sublingual administration of an antigen. The skin wheal is measured, or pulse changes are noted, along with any change in symptoms, as progressively weaker dilutions are given. The dilution that produces no change from, or restores the baseline symptoms, is the neutralizing, or treatment, dose. This method tests foods, chemicals, and inhalants, and is accurate for both IgE and IgG mediated allergy.
- Kinesiology testing: In this form of muscle testing, relative weakness of the test muscle indicates sensitivity to the test substance. Variations of this technique include applied, clinical, and transformational kinesiology methods.
- NAET (Nambudripad's Allergy Elimination Technique): Kinesiology and acupuncture are combined to test and treat food, chemical, and inhalant allergy, as well as other problem substances. (See the Chiropractic section in chapter 9, Alternative Medical Disciplines.)
- NET (Neuro Emotional Technique): Kinesiology and acupressure are combined to remove emotional blocks. Advanced techniques can be used to test and treat for allergies. (See the Chiropractic section in chapter 9, Alternative Medical Disciplines.)

INHALANT ALLERGY

Inhalants are substances that are inhaled when we breathe. They include not only gases, but solid particles (we inhale more than two tablespoons of particulate matter a day). Common inhalants that cause allergies are pollens of grasses, weeds, and trees; mold; dust and dust mites; animal danders; fibers; feathers and down; tobacco; and other substances.

Common symptoms of inhalant allergy are sneezing, itchy and watery eyes, coughing, wheezing, scratchy throat, increased mucus production that causes a runny nose, sinus pressure, pain behind the eyeballs, headaches with head pressure, tenderness over the cheekbones, and aching teeth. There may also be itching of the palate, eyes, and ears, and edema (swelling) of the eyelids. Many people have "allergic shiners" (dark circles under the eyes), and some children may have a horizontal crease across their nose— a result of the "allergic salute" (wiping a runny nose upwards with the palm of the hand). These are the symptoms of allergic rhinitis, and are caused by IgE mediated allergic reactions. When people with these symptoms are skin tested, they will develop large, itchy skin wheals (lumps on the skin).

Allergic rhinitis (which affects one out of every ten Americans) is divided into two classes: people who have symptoms only during pollen season are said to have seasonal rhinitis; people who have symptoms year round suffer from perennial rhinitis and are more likely sensitive to dust; dust mites; cockroaches; molds; and a large variety of animal danders, feathers, and fibers. Equal numbers of men and women suffer from allergic rhinitis.

There are people who do not display the classic symptoms of rhinitis, but who do not feel well during pollen season. These people have low IgE levels in their blood, but nevertheless experience significant symptoms. They may have eczema, insomnia, fatigue, depression, cramps and diarrhea, cold and flu-like symptoms, headaches, hives, swollen lymph glands, skipped heart beats, panic attacks, and many other symptoms. Some women may experience uterine hemorrhaging, toxemia of pregnancy, and irregular periods during pollen season.

In these people, the allergic reactions are probably IgG mediated. They do not develop significant skin wheals when skin tested, and must be tested by a different method. They also require a different type of allergy extract for treatment.

POLLEN ALLERGY

Not all pollen is allergenic. Plants with beautiful, bright-colored, sweet-smelling flowers generally do not produce airborne, allergenic pollen; their pollen is usually heavy, and spread by birds and insects. It is typically the plants with tiny, plain flowers that have no odor of nectar that produce allergenic pollens. To be allergenic, a pollen must:

- be produced in large quantities and widely distributed;
- be light enough to be carried some distance by the wind; and
- contain specific antigens for hypersensitivity.

Trees, grasses, and weeds are the wind-pollinated plants that produce most allergenic pollens. There are about 15 different proteins in pollen, and people can be allergic to some or all of them (which means they can be allergic to some or all of the allergenic plants). Pollen grains are between 15 and 50 microns in diameter, and when inhaled, the grains enter the nose and pass into the small ducts of the bronchi.

People who are pollen sensitive will have symptoms:

- in the early spring when the trees pollinate
- in the late spring and early summer when grasses and early weeds pollinate
- in the autumn when the weeds peak

Symptoms that occur from spring to first frost, with a peak in the fall, are frequently caused by mold allergy. Symptoms that occur during the winter (when no pollen is being produced) may be caused by dust, dust mites, pets, and/or the gas furnace (due to combustion products and airborne allergens that are circulated by forced air).

Symptoms and indicators of pollen sensitivity are:

- itchy eyes and nose with thin, watery discharge from the nose
- condition worse when outdoors from 8 A.M. until noon
- condition is worse on clear, windy days; better on rainy days
- condition is better indoors, with the house closed and air-conditioning and filtration units on—and gets worse when going from an air-conditioned room to the open air during a period of high pollen count
- condition is worse at specific pollen peaks, and improves after the first frost

If the whole eye itches, pollen allergy is the likely culprit. If only the inner canthus (inside corner of the eye) itches, this suggests a food allergy even though it may occur during pollen season. The term "hay fever" is frequently used to describe the allergic rhinitis of pollen allergy (even though there usually is no fever involved) because people frequently have nasal symptoms during haying season.

MODERN MEDICAL TREATMENT

Drug Therapy

Modern medicine uses antihistamines as the main drug treatment for pollen allergies. The antihistamines of choice are prescription drugs that cause minimal or no sedation and include cetirizine (Zyrtec), fexofenadine (Allegra), loratidine (Claritin), and astemizole (Hismanal). Many other antihistamines are available, including non-prescription preparations, but more frequent dosing is required and sedation is a major side effect. Dry mouth, blurry vision, and trouble urinating are other possible side effects of antihistamines. Some prescription antihistamines can cause serious drug interactions if taken with erythromycin, ketoconazole, or itraconazole.

Decongestants, expectorants, nose drops, oral and nasal steroids, and anti-inflammatory medications are also used. Decongestants and expectorants are available both as prescription and non-prescription preparations. Dry mouth is the main side effect of decongestants, and nose drops may cause dryness and rebound swelling of the nasal passages. Oral steroid preparations can cause weight gain, elevated blood pressure, bone loss, cataracts, impaired immune response, shakiness, and heart palpitations. Nasal steroid preparations can cause irritation and burning of the nose, runny nose, bloody nose, and a yeast infection of the nose and throat. Side effects of anti-inflammatory medications can include dizziness, mental confusion, drowsiness, diarrhea, nausea, rashes and hives, dry eyes and mouth, and asthma.

Immunotherapy

Immunotherapy is the major modern medical treatment for pollen allergies. After scratch testing to determine the allergenic pollen, injections containing minute amounts of the allergens are given in increasing strengths to desensitize the person to the pollen. They block the body's immune reaction to the allergen. A reduction in sensitivity may not occur for as long as a year.

Exercise and Lifestyle

Patients are counseled to minimize contact with pollens. When pollen counts are high, they are told to stay indoors with the windows closed and air conditioners on. If traveling in the car, they are to keep the windows up and the air conditioner on.

They are advised to take a shower or bath at night or after coming in for the day, and to leave shoes at the door to avoid tracking in pollen and mold.

If possible, they should take a vacation during the worst part of pollen season.

Patients are advised to go outdoors only in late morning or afternoon, when there is less pollen in the air, and to avoid activities that involve contact with pollen, such as mowing the grass. Landscaping should be designed to eliminate the more allergenic plants, and weeds should be removed before they pollinate. A mask should be worn when doing yard work.

Diet

Avoid eating concomitant foods, which are foods that are a problem only when eaten while a given plant is pollinating. Common concomitant pollen/food combinations include juniper and cedar/beef; ragweed/milk and egg; grasses/grains and legumes; and sage/potato and tomato.

Drink pure, tolerated water—up to 3 quarts a day during pollen season.

Exercise and Lifestyle

Use the measures listed under modern medical treatment. As well, do not let pets in the house after they have been outside; they will bring in pollens and molds on their fur.

Consider moving. However, there may be only a short grace period before you develop allergies to the pollens in your new location.

Nutrient Therapy

Take the following nutrients.

- vitamin A – 100,000 IU a day for one month, then reduce to 25,000 IU a day. *Caution:* Do not take more than 8,000 IU a day if you are pregnant or might be pregnant (for proper immune function).
- beta carotene – 15,000 IU a day (free radical scavenger; stimulates immune response)
- vitamin B-complex – as directed on label of your product (balances other B vitamins; aids proper digestion and nerve function)
- vitamin B$_5$ – 100 mg three times a day over and above that in the B-complex (combats stress)
- vitamin B$_6$ – 50 mg twice a day over and

above that in the B-complex (aids in immune function)
- vitamin C – 3,000 to 10,000 mg three times a day (moderates inflammatory response; protects body from allergens)
- vitamin E – 400 to 800 IU a day (for proper immune function)
- calcium – 1,000 to 1,500 mg a day in divided doses (helps reduce stress)
- copper – 1 to 2 mg a day (to balance zinc)
- magnesium – 500 to 750 mg a day in divided doses (helps reduce stress)
- zinc – 50 to 80 mg a day (for proper immune function)
- coenzyme Q$_{10}$ – 30 mg twice a day (improves immune function and cellular oxygenation)
- proteolytic enzymes – take as directed on label with meals and between meals (destroy free radicals; reduce inflammation)
- quercetin – 400 mg twice a day between meals (start before and continue through allergy season) (decreases reactions to allergens; increases immunity)
- raw thymus glandular – 500 mg twice a day (stimulates proper immune function). *Caution:* Do not use for a child under 16 years of age.

Herbal Therapy

Take the following botanical substances.

- angelica – has significant effects for individuals sensitive to pollens, dust, and animal dander; treats hay fever, asthma, and eczema
- Chinese skullcap – has anti-inflammatory actions comparable to those of anti-inflammatory drugs
- ephedra – contains alkaloids effective in treating mild asthma and hay fever. Use with botanical or nutritional adrenal gland support such as vitamin B$_5$, as ephedra used over time can weaken the adrenal glands.

- licorice – has anti-inflammatory and anti-allergy activities
- stinging nettles – freeze-dried: one to two capsules every two to four hours (helps with hay fever)

Homeopathic Remedies

Take the homeopathic remedy that best fits your symptoms. The remedies listed below are but a few of the many possibilities. If you do not obtain relief, consult a homepathic practitioner.

- *Arsenicum album* – burning eyes and acrid tears; burning lid margins; hay fever; watery nasal discharge that drips forward; leaves the nose completely obstructed; general aggravation at midnight or from midnight to 1 or 2 A.M.
- *Arsenicum iodatum* – hay fever with frequent sneezing and copious acrid, watery nasal discharge that burns the lip; burning watery discharge from the eyes; swelling of the nasal tissues.
- *Euphrasia* – copious burning discharge from the eyes and bland discharge from the nose; allergy centered in the eyes; eyes burning and irritated; cough with great tearing; allergic asthma and hay fever; one of the most important hay fever remedies.
- *Natrum muriaticum* – hay fever; nasal discharge "egg white"; headaches; allergic shiners; tearing of eyes, worse open air or wind; sneezing early in the morning; little ulcers in the nose; loss of smell and taste; aggravation from the sun; allergy to ragweed pollen.
- *Sabadilla* – primary remedy for hay fever; sneezing primary complaint; violent sneezing, not knowing when it will end; worse cold, odors, and perfume; itching and tingling in the nose; generally thin and copious nasal discharge, often acrid; asthmatic form of hay fever.
- *Sinapis nigra* – mainly allergy and hay fever remedy; left-sided symptoms; intense sneezing, often worse at night; running nose alternating with obstruction; better sitting erect, lying down at night.

Many patients respond to complex homeopathic remedies. You may want to try BHI Allergy or Euphorbium Compositum nasal spray for relief of symptoms. Other effective complex remedies include PHP Grass and Weed Mix, Tree Mix I and II, which mitigate hypersensitivity to grasses, weeds, and trees, and P'llens Early, Mid, and Late from Vibrant Health, for allergies to seasonal pollens and dust (see Sources).

Other Therapeutic Measures

Have proper allergy testing done, and receive treatment for your type of pollen allergy from an environmental physician.

Take "rescues," which are substances that help turn off allergic reactions:

- buffered vitamin C – a vitamin C preparation containing calcium carbonate, magnesium carbonate, and potassium bicarbonate in addition to the ascorbic acid. As the name implies, the mixture is a buffer; it helps to restore body pH and stop the allergic reaction. The vitamin C (ascorbic acid) helps to stop the reaction through a different mechanism. Several companies make a buffered C product (see Sources).
- Tri-Salts – a buffer containing calcium carbonate, magnesium carbonate, and potassium bicarbonate.
- BiCarb Formula – a buffer containing equal amounts of sodium and potassium bicarbonate. *Caution:* Do not use if you have high blood pressure.
- "Magic Brew" – 1 tsp. of sea salt and 1 tsp. of baking soda in 1 quart of water. Chill and sip slowly. This mixture forms a buffer that

helps to stop reactions. *Caution:* Do not use if you have high blood pressure.

- Alka Seltzer Gold – a buffer that helps to stop reactions. Because it contains corn, some people are unable to use it.
- Bach Flower Rescue Remedy – several drops of this preparation will stop an allergic reaction.

Take bee pollen. Obtain local pollen (or use Aller-Bee-Gone, available from health food stores) and begin taking it four to six months before pollen season begins. Begin with one grain a day and work up to 1 tsp. a day. *Caution:* Be very careful. Many people do not tolerate bee pollen and have severe allergic reactions to it. Watch for any itching in your throat and stop the pollen immediately if this occurs.

Use a HEPA filter on the furnace, or an air cleaner containing a HEPA filter (see Sources).

Wash out your nose regularly with saline. Wash your face morning and evening in warm water to which a special solution that contains hydrogen peroxide, iodine, potassium, magnesium, zinc, and manganese (High Performance Hygiene System kit; see Sources). Dip your face into the water with your eyes, nose, and mouth submerged. Blink a few times and blow air out of your nose. This cleans out your tear ducts and stimulates the cilia in your nose and bronchi to eliminate allergens. Wash your hair frequently, particularly after having been outdoors.

Have acupuncture treatment, or press the following acupressure points:

- Hold the hand open, palm down, and press the point on the back of the hand in the center of the fleshy webbing between the thumb and index finger. *Caution:* Pregnant women should not use this pressure point.
- Press on top of the foot in the valley between the big toe and second toe.
- Hold the arm out, palm down. Press on top of the forearm two and a half fingers' width

above the wrist crease, between the two arm bones.

- Hold the arm out, palm down. Press the point on the outer elbow crease.
- Press the point on both sides of the spine, one finger's width below the base of the back of the skull on the muscles one finger's width from the spine.
- Press the point high on the chest in the hollow below the collarbone and next to the breastbone.
- Press the point two fingers' width directly below the navel.

Have enzyme potentiated desensitization (EPD) treatment. In this technique, small amounts of allergens and the enzyme beta glucuronidase are injected to desensitize people to the allergens. EPD can be used to desensitize to foods, inhalants, or chemicals. Strict dietary and environmental control must be exercised for two weeks before and two weeks after the injection.

Have NAET treatments (see Chiropractic section in chapter 9, Alternative Medical Disciplines).

To reduce allergies and help the immune system heal, take bowel tolerance vitamin C daily. Begin with 1,000 mg of ascorbic acid with each meal and at bedtime. Increase vitamin C intake by 1,000 mg a day, in divided doses spread throughout the day, until the dosage is high enough to cause diarrhea (bowel tolerance level). Then, back down by 1,000 mg and continue to take that amount daily in divided doses. Take ascorbic acid with meals and buffered vitamin C between meals. Bowel tolerance will increase during times of stress or illness and may have to be adjusted.

TERPENE ALLERGY

Terpenes are special hydrocarbons that are made by both animals and plants. They are more widely distributed in plants, occurring in all parts of a plant (including the pollen). However, the highest concentrations are found in stems, leaves, and flowers. Terpenes are responsible for the pine scent of all conifers, the smell of freshly cut grass, and the sweet smell of lilacs. The taste of meat broiled over charcoal comes from the wood terpenes of the charcoal, and the flavor of spices is caused by terpenes in the condiments.

Many sensitive people have adverse reactions to both terpenes and pollens. The terpene levels in plants rise about a month before the pollen appears, and many people develop what they think are their pollen symptoms at this time. People with terpene intolerance will also be chemically sensitive, particularly to perfumes and essential oils, and will have difficulty eating spicy foods and charcoal-grilled foods. They will be unable to tolerate live Christmas trees and sometimes cannot be in the same room with fresh-cut flower arrangements.

MODERN MEDICAL TREATMENT

Allergists trained only in modern medicine do not acknowledge or treat terpene allergy or sensitivity.

ALTERNATIVE TREATMENT

Diet
Avoid spicy foods, as spices contain terpenes. Also avoid smoked foods, which contain terpenes from the wood smoke.

Exercise and Lifestyle
Do not have a live Christmas tree or cut flowers in the house.

Do not wear perfumes or use scented products.

Nutrient Therapy
Take the nutrients recommended under Pollen Allergy, above.

Herbal Therapy
All herbs contain terpenes and may not be tolerated by terpene-sensitive people.

Homeopathic Remedies
Take a homeopathic remedy to relieve terpene symptoms. Those listed for Pollen Allergy may also help.

- *Allium cepa* – hay fever; worse from flowers; worse in warm rooms, on the left side, late afternoon or evening; better open air; profuse tearing of eyes which is usually bland; nasal discharge is acrid, excoriating, may excoriate the nose or upper lip; nasal discharge profuse, watery, "like a faucet"; patient stuffs tissue inside the nose to stop the flow (used for pollen allergy also).
- *Sanguinaria* – allergic asthma, hay asthma; asthma worse odors, flowers; hayfever, "rose colds," patient is very sensitive to odors, flowers, and airborne pollen; watery eyes and nose, right side affected; frequent sneezing; burning in nose, mouth, throat; cough, worse from lying down, worse irritation in throat (used for pollen allergy also).

Many people respond to complex homeopathic remedies. You may want to try PHP Flower Mix, which mitigates hypersensitivity to flowers (see Sources section at back of book).

Other Therapeutic Measures
Be tested for terpenes by an environmental medicine physician. If the test is positive, take terpene extracts for prevention and relief of symptoms.

Have NAET treatments for terpenes (see Chiropractic section in chapter 9, Alternative Medical Disciplines).

MOLD ALLERGY

Molds can grow in any place in any part of every continent; there is nowhere that molds can be totally avoided. They grow both indoors and outdoors, and are capable of growing on almost any substance at almost any temperature. They flourish in damp areas and send their spores into the air when it is humid, when it rains, and when snow thaws. These spores are easily carried by air currents and may outnumber pollens in the air. Peak spore production is usually from mid-summer through the fall.

Inhaled mold spores (and possibly mold fragments) cause nasal symptoms, but there is no itching of the eyes and nose. Dermatitis, hives, secretory otitis, gastrointestinal distress, cerebral (mental) symptoms, depression, and other complaints can be caused by mold sensitivity. Many people with sinus problems have mold colonizing their nasal passages, and organisms in the sinuses are frequently found in the lungs also. The possibility of mold colonizing in the lungs should always be investigated in people with bronchitis or asthma symptoms.

Mold can also cause cerebral symptoms, particularly depression. Anger, confusion, irritability, anxiety, hostility, and inability to concentrate are among the cerebral symptoms mold can trigger.

A mold-sensitive person will be:

- worse outdoors between 5 to 9 P.M., because as the air cools, more spores drop toward the ground where they can be more easily inhaled
- worse in damp places, both indoors and outdoors
- worse when mowing the grass, raking leaves, or playing on grass
- worse when exposed to hay
- distinctly worse from August until heavy frost
- symptomatic even after the ragweed season is over
- improved inside a closed house when the furnace or air conditioning is on
- improved when the temperature is below freezing and there is snow on the ground
- worse when eating foods made by fermentation such as beer, cheese, wine, sauerkraut, pickles, and vinegar
- worse after eating mushrooms, seaweed, and other fungi

- worse after eating malt, tea (black and herbal), dried fruit, peanuts and peanut butter, grapes, melons, and coffee
- worse after the weather has been damp for a number of days in succession

Molds cause other problems, in addition to allergic responses, in sensitive people. Some molds produce mycotoxins when they grow on particular food substances. These toxins can cause mild to severe symptoms, including destruction of blood vessel and liver tissues, overgrowth of fibrous tissue, convulsions, hematomas, vertigo, rashes, swelling of the heart, destruction of brain cells, hemorrhage, and even death.

MODERN MEDICAL TREATMENT
Drug Therapy
Oral and nasal steroids are prescribed for mold allergy. Side effects of oral steroids include weight gain, elevated blood pressure, bone loss, cataracts, impaired immune response, shakiness, and heart palpitations. Nasal steroids can cause irritation and burning of the nose, runny nose, bloody nose, and yeast infection of the nose and throat.

Immunotherapy
Immunotherapy based on scratch testing results is used to desensitize patients to molds. (See Modern Medical Treatment for Pollen Allergy, above.)

Exercise and Lifestyle
Non-medical measures are intended to minimize contact with molds. Consequently, patients are advised to stay indoors on wet, windy days, and avoid exposure to areas of high mold growth (compost piles, cut grass, wooded areas, fallen leaves, and barns).

Patients should not mow grass or rake leaves—or, if those tasks cannot be avoided, a mask should be worn while working on them.

People with mold allergies should not live in basement apartments or work in basement areas.

Crawl spaces should be sealed off, and a dehumidifier should be used to lower the humidity in the house. Exhaust fans should be used in the bathroom and kitchen to increase ventilation and keep humidity down. Leaks in roofs, walls, or plumbing should be repaired immediately, and mold and mildew removers should be used in the house to prevent mold growth. Household plants should be eliminated or kept to a minimum. And patients with severe mold allergies should not hike through the woods or camp out.

ALTERNATIVE TREATMENT

Diet
Do not eat foods that are moldy. Many people also do not tolerate foods that contain mold, such as blue cheese, or foods that have been prepared by fermentation, such as yogurt, wine, and yeast products.

Exercise and Lifestyle
Follow the measures under Modern Medical Treatment, above.

Use the following *indoor* mold control measures. Clean the basement regularly, and check it for mold. If you have a "swamp cooler" air conditioner, change the pads frequently. Dry towels and clothing before putting them into a dirty-clothes hamper. Do not leave wet clothes in the washer; keep the lid of the washer open when not in use to provide air circulation.

Clean the drip pan of a self-defrosting refrigerator regularly, and do not allow molded food to remain in the refrigerator. Wash dishes after each meal to prevent mold growth.

Discard moldy books, newspapers, magazines, old furniture, bedding, carpet, clothing, and pillows. Clean garbage cans regularly to prevent mold growth. Cover furniture and bedding made of latex rubber or urethane with barrier cloth.

For mold clean-up and control, use soap and water. Wash thoroughly and scrub with a brush if possible. Use bleach to kill mold, but if you are chemically sensitive avoid bleach or use a mask. Use Zephiran (17 percent aqueous solution) diluted one ounce per gallon of water. It will kill mold and is available at drugstores.

Avoid mold clean-up if you are extremely mold sensitive. If it is not possible to have someone who is not mold sensitive clean for you, wear a mask and gloves during the clean-up. Keep the area well ventilated, wash your clothing immediately, and take a shower and wash your hair when you are finished.

Treat houseplants by adding Impregnon (a fungal retardant) or Taheebo tea to plant water, to retard mold in the potting soil. Both are available at health food stores. Kill mold in the dirt under the house (pillar and post foundation) by spreading copper sulfate or borax crystals.

Sprinkle borax in moldy places to retard mold growth. Mix ½ tsp. borax with 1 cup water in a spray bottle, wash the walls of the shower or bathroom, and let it dry on the walls. Kill mold with heat. Use a hair dryer or a portable electric heater to kill mold. However, unless the heat is extremely high, it will not kill the spores.

Keep all areas of the house dry and well lit. Allow room for circulation behind furniture.

Run an air cleaner to remove mold spores from the air (see Sources). Air out houses or cabins that have been closed for the winter season.

Use the following *outdoor* mold control measures. Keep the exterior of the house free of leaves and debris; remove vines on the outside walls of your house, and shrubs resting against the walls. Clean leaves and debris from gutters. Avoid sweeping porches, basements, and garages (approximately one-third of cement dust is mold). Avoid stacking or playing on fireplace logs, and do not store them in the house. Avoid greenhouses.

Nutrient Therapy

Take the nutrients listed for Pollen Allergy, above, as they are also helpful for mold allergy.

Homeopathic Remedies

Take a homeopathic remedy to relieve mold symptoms.

- *Blatta orientalis* – general aggravation from moldy, damp environments; great allergy or sensitivity to molds, mildew, or rotting leaves; asthma with great wheezing, worse exertion; bronchitis; shortness of breath.

Many patients respond to complex homeopathic remedies. You may want to try BHI Allergy, which can help to relieve mold symptoms, or PHP Household Dust and Mold Mix, which mitigates hypersensitivity to household dust, molds, and dust mites. F'gus by Vibrant Health is for relief of symptoms caused by fungus, yeast, and molds (see Sources).

Other Therapeutic Measures

If a mold allergy is suspected, you should be tested by an environmental medicine physician and treated if an allergy is found.

Take "rescues" to turn off an acute allergic reaction (see Other Therapeutic Measures for Pollen Allergy, above).

Take bowel tolerance vitamin C (see Other Therapeutic Measures for Pollen Allergy, above).

Have NAET (see the Chiropractic section in chapter 9, Alternative Medical Disciplines) or EPD treatments for mold allergy (see Other Therapeutic Measures for Pollen Allergy, above).

Use an ozone generator to kill mold. These generators can be rented from some physicians, cleaning companies, or fire departments. They produce the gas ozone, which penetrates to all parts of the room and kills mold. People, animals, and plants must leave the room while the generator is producing ozone. They can return one hour after the generator turns off.

DUST AND DUST MITE ALLERGY

House dust contains so much organic matter that it is considered organic dirt. It is a very complex mixture containing plant fibers, food remnants, mold spores, pollen, animal hair and dander, insect parts, fabric fibers, fireplace soot, and many other substances.

No matter how clean we keep our houses, we are surrounded by dust and we breathe it continually. The average six-room house accumulates 40 pounds of dust in a year. This dust can produce allergic symptoms year round, but symptoms will be worse when the house is closed and the furnace is on.

People with a dust allergy (and possibly dust mite allergy) will be worse:

- indoors and better outdoors
- when the furnace is on
- while the house is being swept or dusted
- when the bed is being made
- when sitting on upholstered furniture
- in a library
- on arising in the morning, and better during the day
- when they have been in bed for 30 to 60 minutes

Dust mites are microscopic insects that live in dust and feed on animal dander (skin scales) in the dust. They occur around the world, but their numbers are lower in hot, dry climates, and at high altitudes. Dust mites colonize in mattresses, upholstered furniture, carpets, and stuffed toys. Mites are harmful only to people who are allergic to their feces and carcasses. These pellets of feces and carcasses float about and enter our lungs and noses when we breathe.

They trigger symptoms of rhinitis, sneezing, congestion, and itchy, watery eyes. The bronchial inflammation they cause can lead to asthma and other forms of breathing difficulty. People with a dust mite allergy will have persistently stuffy noses or ears, repeated sneezing on awakening, and worsening of symptoms when beds are made. They will improve outside the house.

Dust mites are not the only insects that contribute to allergies. Cockroaches, their body parts, and feces also cause allergic symptoms. The cockroach parts and feces are often a component of dust and play a large part in triggering asthma. This type of allergy is more common in damp climates, and in cities where there are large apartment buildings with poor insect control.

MODERN MEDICAL TREATMENT

Drug Therapy

The asthma triggered by dust, dust mites, cockroaches, cockroach body parts and feces is treated with oral and nasal steroids, as well as anti-inflammatory medications. Side effects of these medications are listed under Pollen Allergy, above. Antihistamines may be used for sneezing and watery eyes. For side effects of antihistamines see p. 369.

Immunotherapy

Modern medicine gives immunotherapy for dust mites only, based on scratch test results. (See Modern Medical Treatment for Pollen Allergy, above.)

Exercise and Lifestyle

Non-medical measures stress creating and maintaining a "dust-free" bedroom. This can be achieved by removing the carpet; keeping only one bed in the bedroom, and encasing the springs and mattress in a dust-proof or allergen-proof cover; keeping all animals with fur or feathers out of the bedroom; and using only washable materials on the bed. (Bedclothes must be washed frequently in water at least 130°F to kill dust mites.) Furniture and furnishings should be kept to a minimum and upholstered furniture and venetian blinds avoided. Curtains should be washable.

The room should be cleaned thoroughly once a week with a damp mop or damp cloth. An air filter should be used, either in the room or attached to the central heating and air conditioning unit. A dehumidifier should be used in areas of high humidity to lower the dust mite population.

Toys should be kept out of a child's bedroom, and stuffed toys should be avoided altogether. Use only washable toys made of wood, metal, rubber, or plastic, and store them in a closed toy chest or toy box.

Avoid using fuzzy wool blankets and feather- or wool-stuffed comforters. Store bedroom closet contents elsewhere. If this is not possible, put clothing in zippered plastic bags and shoes in boxes raised off the floor.

Dust control measures should also be used in other parts of the house.

ALTERNATIVE TREATMENT

Diet

Avoid eating concomitant foods, which are foods that are a problem only in combination with a specific allergy. Oysters, clams, and scallops are concomitant foods with dust.

Exercise and Lifestyle

Carry out the Exercise and Lifestyle suggestions for dealing with dust and dust mites outlined under Modern Medical Treatment, above.

Vacuum upholstered furniture and rugs daily for acute cases of dust allergy; one to two times per week for mild cases. Open the windows to blow away the dust raised when vacuuming. Discard vacuum cleaner bags as soon as you have finished vacuuming, to get rid of the dust mites and dust mite eggs inside.

Take carpets and rugs outdoors for four hours on a hot, sunny day to kill mites and their eggs. Use a prepared tannic acid solution for rugs and carpets that cannot be taken outside. This can reduce dust mites in carpets by 92 percent. It also inactivates the enzyme coating on dust mite feces so that it will not trigger an aller-gic reaction.

Do not sit on upholstered furniture if you have a dust or dust mite allergy. Avoid knick-knacks and do not use brooms or feather dusters. Spend most of your time in the cleanest, barest rooms in the house, usually the bedroom and the kitchen. Avoid attics, closets, base-ments, or storerooms. Replace furnace filters twice a year.

Do not use a live Christmas tree and exercise caution when bringing stored ornaments into the house. Keep stored ornaments covered so they do not get dusty, and throw away the dusty cover.

Nutrient Therapy
Take bowel tolerance vitamin C daily (see Other Therapeutic Measures for Pollen Allergy, above).

Herbal Therapy
Herbs that help pollen allergy will help sneezing caused by dust allergy (see Pollen Allergy, above).

Homeopathic Remedies
Take the homeopathic remedy that best de-scribes your symptoms.

- *Bromium* – left-sided headaches; allergy to dust; rawness and mucus throughout the air-ways; cough worse swallowing, worse dust or smoke, worse exertion; asthma; bronchitis; hoarseness or cough from being over-heated.
- *Silica* – sinusitis with thick postnasal dis-charge; chilly and aggravation from cold weather; aggravation from drafts and dust; weakness and fatigue; eyes tender to the touch; cough with expectoration in day; shortness of breath from manual labor; frothy nasal discharge; sneezing in the morn-ing; itching at tip of nose; nose obstructed and loss of smell.

- *Sulphuricum acidum* – asthma, worse from dust; general aggravation from dust; chilly and worse from cold; hurriedness; tendency to bruising; small painful ulcers on the tongue, inner cheeks, and gastrointestinal tract; flow of water from nose; nosebleeds in the evening.

Many patients respond to complex homeo-pathic remedies. You may want to try BHI Al-lergy for relief of symptoms, or PHP Household Dust and Mold Mix, which mitigates hypersen-sitivity to household dusts, molds, and dust mites (see Sources).

Other Therapeutic Measures
You should be tested for allergy to dust and dust mites by an environmental medicine physician, and treated for the allergy if the tests are posi-tive.

Use an air cleaner with a dust filter and change the filters or clean them as needed.

Take "rescues," which are substances that help turn off an allergic reaction (see Other Therapeutic Measures for Pollen Allergy, above).

Have NAET treatment for dust (see the Chi-ropractic section in chapter 9, Alternative Med-ical Disciplines), or have EPD treatment (see Other Therapeutic Measures for Pollen Allergy, above).

ANIMAL DANDER ALLERGY
All animals, including humans, shed dander or skin scales and scurf (all known as dandruff) into the air. Dander is light and airy, and can float about freely. It can remain in an area for days after the animal has been removed. (Cat dander can remain in a home for years.) People can be allergic to both human and animal dan-der, as well as animal saliva and serum. Fleas carried by pets can also cause allergic symp-toms. Symptoms to animal dander and saliva can include difficulty breathing, hives, head-

aches, loss of voice, itching or watering of the eyes, and sneezing.

Both cat and dog dander and saliva are allergenic to people, but cats generally produce a worse reaction, and cat saliva is more allergenic than the dander. Horse dander can also be a potent allergen, but it is not the problem that it was at the turn of the century when people had more contact with horses. Rabbit dander and fur may also cause allergic reactions, as can that of hamsters and gerbils. Sensitivities to cattle, pig, and goat hair and dander are also possible, as are sensitivities to sheep wool, dander, and lanolin.

You should suspect an animal dander sensitivity if you are worse when:

- you are exposed to animal hair in blended form in articles such as sweaters, gloves, rug padding, furniture stuffing, and other items;
- you are exposed to animals; or
- you are licked by an animal.

MODERN MEDICAL TREATMENT
Drug Therapy
Antihistamines and decongestants are used to treat animal dander allergy. For severe cases, oral and nasal steroids may be prescribed as well as anti-inflammatory medications. Side effects of these medications are described earlier in this chapter under Pollen Allergy.

Immunotherapy
Medical measures generally undertaken for modern treatment of animal sensitivities include desensitization shots based on scratch test results. Some traditional allergists use these injections, while others do not.

Exercise and Lifestyle
Other measures to deal with severe animal allergies often start with finding new homes for pets. Improvement may not be noticeable for as much as six months after the animal is gone.

Where allergies exist but are not as severe, pets should be kept out of the bedroom. People who have animal allergies should never sleep with an animal. All pets (including cats) should have regular baths—weekly, if possible. And people who are allergic to pets should avoid being licked by an animal.

ALTERNATIVE TREATMENT
Exercise and Lifestyle
Carry out the approaches to dealing with animal allergies outlined under Modern Medical Treatment, above.

Nutrient Therapy
Take bowel tolerance vitamin C daily (see Other Therapeutic Measures for Pollen Allergy, above).

Homeopathic Remedies
Take a homeopathic remedy to relieve your symptoms.

- *Dulcamara* – allergy to cats; general aggravation from damp or cold, damp weather, change of weather; worse drafts; cough, asthma, bronchitis; hay fever at the end of summer or in the fall.
- *Tuberculinum* – hay fever and allergicasthma; tremendous reaction to animal danders, especially cats, lids swollen, tearing of eyes.

Many patients respond to complex homeopathic remedies. You may want to try BHI Allergy for relief of symptoms; PHP Animals Mix, which mitigates hypersensitivity to animal feathers, hair, dander, and other residues; or P'ts by Vibrant Health for allergies to pets, furs, feathers, dust, and saliva (see Sources).

Other Therapeutic Measures
You should be tested for allergy to animal dander by an environmental medicine physician, and treated for the allergy if the test is positive.

Take "rescues," which are substances that help turn off an allergic reaction (see Other Therapeutic Measures for Pollen Allergy, above).

Have NAET treatment for dander (see the Chiropractic section in chapter 9, Alternative Medical Disciplines), or have EPD treatment (see Other Therapeutic Measures for Pollen Allergy, above).

FEATHER ALLERGY

Many people are allergic to feathers—all kinds of feathers, including those from chickens, geese, and ducks. Feather allergens are usually the decomposition products of the feathers, and most feather-sensitive people are able to eat the meat and eggs of the fowls without symptoms. They also usually do not have problems from egg-containing vaccines. In today's urban society, most exposure to feathers comes from comforters, pillows, quilts, jackets, sleeping bags, and beds, rather than from live animals.

Suspect a feather allergy if symptoms are worse when:

• you are exposed to feathers in the above items;
• you are exposed to chickens, geese, or ducks;
• you are exposed to someone who works with fowl.

MODERN MEDICAL TREATMENT

Exercise and Lifestyle
The approach to dealing with feather allergies includes avoiding down-filled articles such as feathers, comforters, and garments with feather trim.

ALTERNATIVE TREATMENT
Exercise and Lifestyle
Follow the guidelines for Modern Medical Treatment, above.

Nutrient Therapy
Take bowel tolerance vitamin C daily (see Other Therapeutic Measures for Pollen Allergy, above).

Homeopathic Remedies
Take the following homeopathic remedy.

• *Sulphur* – for hay fever or asthma from feathers or the use of feather pillows.

Many patients respond to complex homeopathic remedies. You may want to try BHI Allergy for relief of symptoms; PHP Animal Mix, which mitigates hypersensitivity to animal feathers, hair, dander, and other residues; or P'ts by Vibrant Health, for allergies to pets, furs, feathers, dust, and saliva.

Other Therapeutic Measures
You should be tested for allergy to feathers and fibers by an environmental medicine physician, and treated for the allergy if the test is positive.

Take "rescues," which are substances that help turn off an allergic reaction (see Other Therapeutic Measures for Pollen Allergy, above).

Have NAET treatment (see the Chiropractic section in chapter 9, Alternative Medical Disciplines), or have EPD treatment (see Other Therapeutic Measures for Pollen Allergy, above).

TOBACCO

Tobacco smoke is a major contributor to air pollution in North America. About one-third of the adult population smokes tobacco, and everyone around those people is exposed to tobacco to some degree. Mainstream smoke is the smoke that is drawn through the tobacco during inhalation (active smoking) and sidestream smoke is the smoke that arises from smoldering tobacco. Ninety-six percent of the gases and particulates (small solid particles) produced when tobacco burns are found in the sidestream smoke, and it is unpleasant to everyone, including the smoker. The smoke from one cigarette contains three mg of carbon monoxide and 70 mg of dry particulate matter. Cigar and pipe smoke is even more irritating to the nose and upper respiratory tract.

Burning cigarettes generate over 4,000 known compounds. The specific contents of tobacco smoke vary with the type of tobacco, the soil in which it was grown, the curing method, and the temperature reached by the tobacco product during smoking. Pesticide and fertilizer residues, smoke residues from the curing process, the contents of the cigarette paper used, and the sugar mixed with the tobacco also affect the ingredients of the smoke.

Over 350,000 people die prematurely each year from smoking-related diseases. Many studies have shown that "passive" smoking is even more dangerous than active smoking, and many spouses and co-workers of smokers have died from lung cancer that is a direct result of the smoke they inhaled from cigarettes others were smoking. Secondhand smoke causes more lung cancer than all other air pollutants in the environment, and medical researchers estimate that at least 120,000 people will die each year as a result of breathing in secondhand smoke. Even children are affected by cigarette smoke. Children of smokers have more upper respiratory problems and behavior problems than do children of nonsmokers.

It is now well known to the public at large that tobacco smoking (particularly cigarette smoking) is strongly implicated in cancers of the larynx, pharynx, lung, and respiratory tract, but it is not as well known that smoking also causes cancer of the bladder, esophagus, mouth, and pancreas, and increases the risk of breast cancer and diabetes. It also plays a large role in chronic obstructive lung disease (emphysema) and cardiovascular diseases, including aortic aneurysms, coronary heart disease, and atherosclerotic peripheral vascular disease (deposits in the arteries of the extremities).

MODERN MEDICAL TREATMENT

Drug Therapy

While modern medicine does not acknowledge tobacco allergy, physicians do advise people not to smoke and prescribe nicotine gum and nicotine patches to help them stop smoking.

Exercise and Lifestyle

Patients are told to avoid any exposure to tobacco by not allowing people around them to smoke. They are also advised not to use smokeless (or chewing) tobacco, as it can cause oral cancer.

ALTERNATIVE TREATMENT

Exercise and Lifestyle

Do not allow smoking in your house or your car. Do not use smokeless (or chewing) tobacco. Dine only in non-smoking restaurants or in restaurants with a large non-smoking section. Stay only in hotels or motels with non-smoking rooms and floors. Insist on good air quality in your workplace.

Nutrient Therapy

Take the following nutrients to help overcome a tobacco addiction and allergy:

- vitamin A – 25,000 IU a day. *Caution:* Do not exceed 8,000 IU a day if you are pregnant or might be pregnant (antioxidant that aids in healing mucus membranes).
- beta carotene – 15,000 IU a day (important for lung protection)
- vitamin B-complex – 100 mg a day (necessary for enzyme systems, often damaged from smoking)
- vitamin B_{12} – 1,000 mcg twice a day, over the amount in B-complex (needed for liver function)

- folic acid – 400 mcg a day, over the amount in B-complex (needed to form red blood cells)
- vitamin C – 5,000 to 20,000 mg a day, to bowel tolerance (important antioxidant; smoking depletes vitamin C)
- vitamin E – start with 200 IU a day and increase by 200 IU monthly until you are taking 800 IU a day (protects cells and organs from damage by tobacco smoke)
- copper – 2 mg a day (to balance zinc)
- zinc – 50 to 80 mg a day (aids immune function)
- coenzyme Q_{10} – 200 mg twice a day (aids in oxygen flow to the brain; antioxidant to protect the lungs)
- L-cysteine, L-methionine, and glutathione – as directed on label (to detoxify, and to protect tissues from cigarette smoke)
- pycnogenol or grape seed extract – as directed on the label of your product (antioxidants; free radical scavenger)

Herbal Therapy

Take the following botanical medicines.

- cayenne – desensitizes the respiratory tract cells to tobacco smoke irritants
- catnip, lobelia, skullcap, hops, and/or valerian root – reduce the nervousness and anxiety of tobacco withdrawal
- milk thistle and dandelion root – protect the liver against toxins from cigarette smoke
- slippery elm – helps lung congestion and cough
- ginger – causes perspiration, helping the body to get rid of poisons ingested through smoking
- oat straw – helps to stop smoking

Homeopathic Remedies

Take the following homeopathic remedy.

- *Natrum arsenicosum* – sensitivity to cigarette or tobacco smoke.

Many patients respond to complex homeopathic remedies. You may want to try PHP Anti-Smoking I and II, which can reduce addictive behavior from smoking; T'batox by Vibrant Health helps remove residues and buildup of smoke and cigarette substances (see Sources).

Other Therapeutic Measures

Be tested for a tobacco allergy by an environmental medicine physician, and be treated for tobacco allergies if the test is positive. Most people who smoke are allergic to tobacco, and the testing and treatment may help them stop smoking. Treatment for tobacco allergy also helps nonsmokers who are allergic to and bothered by tobacco smoke.

Take "rescues," which are substances that help turn off an acute allergic reaction (see Other Therapeutic Measures for Pollen Allergy, above).

Have an NAET treatment for tobacco allergy (see the Chiropractic section in chapter 9, Alternative Medical Disciplines).

FOOD ALLERGY

Problems that arise after ingesting food have been described for centuries, but it was only in the 1940s that the late Dr. Theron Randolph (one of the founding fathers of environmental medicine and author of several books, among them *An Alternative Approach To Allergies*) described physical and mental disorders that can be caused by an allergic response to food. Food allergy and undernutrition are the most common undiagnosed health problems in North America. Some experts estimate that 60 percent of all the people visiting physicians have symptoms caused by (or complicated by) food allergy. Most physicians are not trained to recognize food allergy unless it takes the form of an immediate reaction resulting in wheezing, hives, or anaphylaxis. The causes of the more subtle symptoms of food allergies are not obvious either to most physicians or to most patients.

Food allergy/addiction and "masking" are the main reasons these food allergies are not more obvious. In food allergy/addiction, people crave the food they are allergic to, and the lift they get from it. The person is addicted to the food, and can have withdrawal symptoms if the food is not available. When the food is eaten regularly, "masking" occurs. There are chronic, low-grade symptoms such as "spaciness," temporary sleepiness after a meal, or postnasal drip—and these may be the only evidence of a problem. Avoiding the suspect food for 4 to 10 days will unmask the allergy, and subsequent re-exposure to the food will produce acute symptoms that are more easily recognized as symptoms of food sensitivity.

The body copes with food allergy by producing an adaptation response, which minimizes the symptoms. However, this adaptation will not last indefinitely; when it eventually breaks down, there will be full-blown allergic symptoms.

SYMPTOMS OF FOOD ALLERGY

Symptoms of food allergy vary according to the target organ affected, and this can vary from person to person. If the brain is affected, the person will have cerebral (mental and emotional) symptoms. The person may be easily angered, quarrelsome, easily hurt, depressed, restless, tense, nervous, fearful, erratic, uncooperative, or jumpy.

If the gastrointestinal tract is the target organ, ulcers, diverticulitis, colitis, Crohn's disease, diarrhea, and constipation may be the chief symptoms. If the respiratory system is the target, the person may develop asthma, bronchitis, or recurrent upper respiratory infections. Food allergies can be expressed by still other symptoms, among them bedwetting, arthritis and joint pain, bad breath, eczema, hives, hyperactivity, headaches and migraines, obesity, acne, eye pain, conjunctivitis, restless legs, fatigue, excessive perspiration, abnormal body

odor, and learning disorders. In some people, many different foods will cause the same symptoms, while for other people, each food allergen will cause a different symptom.

CLASSIFICATION OF FOOD ALLERGIES

Food allergy can be classified in several different ways, and the American Academy of Allergy and Immunology Committee on Adverse Reactions to Food (a modern medicine organization) has proposed standard terminology for describing these reactions:

- food anaphylaxis – a classic allergy, showing an (immediate) hypersensitivity reaction to food or food additives involving IgE antibody and the release of chemical mediators;
- food hypersensitivity – an immunologic reaction (often delayed) to the ingestion of a food or food additive; may or may not involve IgE antibody; and
- food intolerance – an abnormal physiological response to an ingested food or food additive, including idiosyncratic, metabolic, pharmacologic, or toxic reactions.

While alternative practitioners basically accept these definitions, a slightly different perspective is more generally used for defining food reactions:

- immediate – these are the IgE mediated food reactions mentioned above. Symptoms are obvious within minutes of eating the food, and may include hives, wheezing, eczema, rhinitis, swelling of the lips and face, or anaphylactic shock. Anaphylactic shock (usually a reaction to foods such as shellfish or peanuts) is rare, but can be fatal.
- delayed – these are the food reactions that are probably IgG mediated, and in which the symptoms are delayed—sometimes not appearing until the next day or for several days. Most food allergies fall into this category, and symptoms include chronic headaches

(frequently migraine); chronic indigestion or heartburn; fatigue; depression; failure to thrive; joint or arthritis-type symptoms; recurrent abdominal pain; canker sores; wheezing or bronchitis; and bowel problems such as diarrhea, constipation, and colitis.

- synergistic – symptoms occur when two specific foods are eaten within the same meal—but not when they are eaten separately. Corn and banana, egg and apple, and beef and yeast are examples of foods proven to have synergistic allergic effects.
- concomitant – food reaction that occurs when another non-food allergen (a chemical or a particulate inhalant, for instance) is present. Milk, milk products, or mint consumed during ragweed season can cause an allergic reaction, but will not elicit a reaction when ragweed is not in season. Concomitant food reactions can occur up to six weeks after pollen season is over.

According to modern medicine allergists, 5 percent of children and 2 percent of adults have food allergies; but these figures include only the IgE mediated food reactions. Alternative practitioners consider food hypersensitivity reactions as probably being IgG mediated, and there are many more of these reactions than there are IgE mediated reactions. Alternative practitioners also consider any adverse response to food to be a problem, regardless of its mediation. Patients who experience problems with foods do not care how their reactions are mediated; they just want relief from their symptoms. In this book, we use the term "food allergy" to refer to any adverse reaction to a food.

The late Dr. Herbert Rinkel (former associate instructor of medicine at the University of Oklahoma School of Medicine, and one of the authors of a landmark book called *Food Allergy*) classified food allergies as being *cyclic* or *fixed*. A cyclic food allergy is an allergy that is dependent on the frequency with which the food is eaten. The more exposures and the closer together the exposures to the food, the worse the allergy becomes. Total avoidance reinstates tolerance, with the length of avoidance time depending on the individual and the severity of the allergy. Once the food can again be tolerated, re-sensitization can be prevented by avoiding overexposure.

However, if after a two-year period of total avoidance the food still elicits symptoms when it is reintroduced, the food allergy is considered to be a permanent or fixed allergy. Eating the food will always trigger an allergic reaction unless food extracts are taken to prevent or block the symptoms (see Other Therapeutic Measures, below). Fortunately, most food allergies are cyclic rather than fixed.

ALLERGENICITY OF FOODS

Any food can cause an allergic reaction, producing any symptom, depending on the target organ affected. In general, protein is more allergenic than fats or carbohydrates because it is more difficult to digest. If digestion of a food is not complete, the molecule eventually absorbed into the bloodstream is larger than most food molecules. The immune system recognizes it as a foreign substance rather than a food, and sets up a chain reaction to destroy the supposed invader. This produces the symptoms of an allergic reaction.

People with food allergy should have their digestive system evaluated for stomach acid levels, pancreatic enzyme production, small intestine bicarbonate levels, condition of the digestive tract, possible infections in the digestive tract, and nutritional imbalances. (See Sources for information on how to have these evaluations carried out.) Problems in any of these areas can result in disordered digestion and play a major role in food allergy.

Meats, grains, vegetables, and fruits—ranked here in descending order—tend to be permanent or fixed allergies. Allergenicity of a food is affected by cooking, which reduces it by half. Allergenicity is also affected by the purity of the food. Foods contaminated by additives, preservatives, dyes, flavorings, pesticides, antibiotics, bacteria, and hormones are more likely to cause problems than pure foods. Some prescription drugs can provoke reactions to foods that would normally be "safe" foods.

We refer to the most common food allergens as the "sinister seven," because they are in almost all processed food products, and most North Americans eat all of them every day. These foods include wheat, yeast, corn, soy, egg, cow's milk, and sugar.

The allergy-producing proteins of some foods are identical to those in certain pollens. This means that a person who is sensitive to a particular pollen could react to the food containing the same allergen the first time it is eaten. Such cross-reactivity occurs between ragweed and bananas, watermelon, zucchini, honeydew, cucumber, and other members of the gourd family; and birch and potatoes, carrots, celery, hazelnuts, and apples.

Because so many allergies are masked, and because of delayed food reactions, allergy testing is of benefit in confirming or eliminating food allergy as a health problem. There are many techniques available for this testing (see Allergy Testing earlier in this chapter).

MODERN MEDICAL TREATMENT

Food Testing
The scratch test or prick test is the form of testing generally used by modern medicine for food testing, and these tests will pick up only IgE mediated food reactions. Most food reactions are IgG mediated and are not found by these testing methods, nor are they recognized by most modern medicine physicians.

Diet
Because modern medicine allergists recognize only IgE food mediated reactions, both their testing and treatment for food allergies is limited.

Most physicians recommend avoidance of the offending food, either alone or in combination with other foods.

Drug Therapy
Adrenaline for anaphylactic reactions, and oral steroids to minimize hives and asthma are given for immediate hypersensitivity allergic reactions to foods. Benadryl is used orally and intravenously to stop allergic reactions.

ALTERNATIVE TREATMENT

Diet
Allergy diets are designed to identify and/or control food allergies. Often food allergies are difficult to identify, because reactions can take place many hours after the food is consumed, and because of combination (synergistic) reactions, in which foods eaten together cause a problem, although they cause no symptoms when eaten separately.

If you are sensitive to only a few foods, the best route to take is to simply avoid those foods. If you are allergic to a number of foods, follow a rotation diet.

The rotation diet was developed in the 1930s by the late Dr. Herbert Rinkel of Missouri, and serves both to identify foods that cause problems, and to control allergic reactions. Its efficacy is based on the fact that it takes four days for most people to clear a food from the body; on this diet, a food is eaten no more than once every four days. This prevents the development of cumulative effects from offending foods. Some extremely sensitive people require 7 to 10 days to clear a food from their bodies, and these people will have to use a 7- or 10-day rotation diet.

In the rotation diet, both animal and vegetable foods are grouped into "families" according to their biological and botanical characteristics. Each of these families is assigned to a specific rotation day—distributed over the four days so that some meats, fish, vegetables, and fruits are available each day. Each rotation day also offers spices, teas, and oils from which to choose. It is like a menu in a restaurant: each day you may select only from what is listed for that day; you may not eat anything listed for another day. After four days, the cycle begins again with Day One.

The rotation diet prevents the development of new food allergies because of overexposure to a given food. It helps identify hidden food allergies, protects the immune system, and allows it to repair by preventing allergic reactions. It also allows enzyme systems to repair.

Rotation days may be handled two different ways. In one, you can begin the rotation day with breakfast and go through to the evening meal; under that system, leftovers must be frozen and used on the next rotation cycle. Alternatively, you can begin the rotation day with the evening meal and go through lunch the next day; with this schedule, leftovers from the evening meal may be used for breakfast or lunch the next day.

In a strict rotation diet, grains may be eaten only on the day for which the grass family is listed. However, for people whose sensitivities will permit it, grains may be eaten every other day—or daily, if you alternate gluten and non-gluten grains. (Corn, rice, millet, and teff are non-gluten grains; amaranth and quinoa are gluten-free seeds that can be used as grain substitutes.)

Alcoholic beverages do not fit well into rotation diets, because they have many ingredients and many of them are grain-based. Butter is allowed only on beef/milk day, and because most margarines contain whey combined with a vegetable oil, they do not fit on any rotation day. An interesting substitute for margarine or butter is the oil of the day, in which spices of the day have been marinated. Cheese made from cow's or goat's milk is allowed only on the beef/milk day. Soy cheese may be used on legume day.

It is important to read labels carefully—not only those on food products, but also labels on anything you put in your mouth or on your skin. Even minor ingredients can cause severe problems. Most fast foods and prepared foods must be avoided because many of their ingredients will not fit in a rotation diet.

The rotation diet is a balanced nutritional diet, and is very helpful in restoring health and controlling food allergies. There are several good books that expand on the brief information that appears here, providing "how to" guidance as well as excellent recipes. Some are available at health food stores and bookstores; others can be obtained directly from the authors (see Suggested Reading).

An allergy elimination diet is a technique to help identify food allergens. In this diet, all suspect food is avoided completely for four to seven days. At the end of this period, one of the suspect foods is reintroduced. It must be free of chemical contaminants and prepared with no seasonings, as both seasonings and contaminants can confuse the results. Foods are reintroduced one at a time, one test food a day. Symptoms will appear when the offending food is eaten.

Pulse changes can be used as an additional indicator of a problem food. When all suspect foods have been eliminated, and before the test day, the pulse should be taken two to three times a day to obtain an average pulse rate. On the day of the test, the resting pulse is taken after the patient has been sitting quietly for 10 minutes; the suspect food is then eaten, and the pulse is taken again after 10 minutes and after 30 minutes. A pulse change (either up or down) indicates that the food is a problem. However, some people are not "pulse changers," and other symptoms will have to be used to identify problem foods.

Nutrient Therapy

Take the following nutritional supplements, making certain that the supplements are free of the common food allergens. This must be stated on the label. (If you tolerate multivitamin and multimineral supplements, you will not need all of these.)

- vitamin C – 1,000 to 15,000 mg a day (protects body from allergens; moderates inflammation)
- coenzyme Q_{10} – 100 mg a day (improves cellular oxygenation and immune function)
- quercetin – 500 mg twice a day between meals (increases immunity; decreases reactions to foods)
- vitamin B-complex – 100 mg a day (this preparation is not tolerated well by some sensitive individuals) (for proper digestion and nerve function)
- calcium – 1,000 mg a day (reduces stress)
- copper – 2 mg a day (to balance zinc)
- magnesium – 500 to 1,000 mg a day, depending on need (balances calcium)
- proteolytic enzymes – take with meals as directed on the label (aid digestion; destroy free radicals)
- betaine hydrochloride – take with meals as directed on label. *Caution:* Do not use if you have an ulcer (aids digestion, but use only if stomach acid is low).
- vitamin A – 10,000 IU a day. *Caution:* Do not exceed 8,000 IU a day if you are pregnant or might be pregnant (for proper immune function).
- vitamin E – 600 IU a day (for proper immune function)
- zinc – 50 mg a day (for proper immune function)
- chromium – 200 mcg a day, particularly if you are hyperinsulinemic or have blood sugar problems (helps stabilize blood sugar)
- amino acid supplement – as directed on your product's label. Use a preparation of free amino acids that is extremely pure and free of the common food allergens. (important if food intake, particularly protein, is severely restricted)

Homeopathic Remedies

Take the homeopathic remedy that best matches your symptoms. If you do not obtain results, consult a homeopathic practitioner.

- *Chamomilla* – coffee headache.
- *Ferrum metallicum* – allergy to eggs.
- *Lycopodium* – allergy to oysters.
- *Natrum muriaticum* – allergy to eggs, starches, milk, honey, ragweed pollen, onions, wheat, meat.
- *Nux vomica* – too much spicy food, alcohol, coffee, or fat.
- *Psorinum* – wheat allergy that causes eczema.
- *Pulsatilla* – allergy to cod-liver oil, fats, and orange juice; sensitive to fat containing protein.
- *Staphysagria* – allergic headache after eating beef.
- *Sulphur* – allergy to milk, eggs, sardines, cooked meat, chocolate.
- *Thuja* – allergy to onions.
- *Tuberculinum* – allergy to milk, eggs, sardines, cooked meat.
- *Urtica urens* – allergy to milk, which causes hives; allergy to shellfish.

Many patients respond to complex homeopathic remedies. Depending on your sensitivities, you may want to try PHP Dairy Mix, Meat and Poultry Mix, Nightshade Mix, Nut Mix, Sugar Mix, Grain and Seed Mix, Shellfish and Fish Mix, Fruit and Berry Mix, and Caffeine Mix; F'ds by Vibrant Health for food allergies, digestive intolerance, or Da'ry by Vibrant Health for dairy sensitivities, allergies, food intolerances, and digestive problems.

PHP Opsin I assists in reversing maladaptive responses to autotoxins and food allergens.

Other Therapeutic Measures

To diagnose food allergies, have allergy testing done by an environmental medicine physician or an alternative practitioner.

If you are allergic to many foods, take allergy extracts to control food reactions. Allergy extracts will block the food reaction, allowing you to safely eat the offending food. These extracts allow you to eat more normally and at the same time take the stress off the immune system, allowing it to heal.

Have NAET or NET treatments (see the Chiropractic section in chapter 9, Alternative Medical Disciplines). Have EPD testing and treatment (see Other Therapeutic Measures for Pollen Allergy, earlier in this chapter).

Have your digestion evaluated for the following conditions (see Sources).

- stomach acid levels and small intestine bicarbonate levels: pH as determined by a Heidelberg gastrogram
- pancreatic enzyme production: amylase levels
- condition of the digestive tract: Stool Analysis, Digestive Function, Intestinal Permeability
- possible infections in the digestive tract: bacterial and parasitic examinations
- nutritional imbalances: vitamin, fatty acid, amino acid, and mineral profiles

Take a plain water enema to clear your body of the offending food.

Detoxify the liver by taking one of the following: Liver Liquescence by PHP; Hepatatox by BioActive; Dandiplex by BioActive; or Hepatica from Marco Pharma (see Sources).

Take "rescues," which are substances that help turn off an allergic reaction (see Other Therapeutic Measures for Pollen Allergy, above).

CHEMICAL SENSITIVITIES

The chemical revolution that has taken place since World War II has resulted in the manufacture of *500 billion* chemicals each year; 500,000 of them have found their way into our homes, food, water, and air, and more than 400 chemicals have been identified in human tissue. Over 3,000 chemicals are added to foods, 700 are added to water supplies, and over 10,000 are used to process and extend the storage life of food. These figures represent only those chemicals that are deliberately added; they do not reflect chemicals that turn up in foods by accident. Both because of the sheer numbers of substances involved and because of their intimate roles in our everyday lives, these chemicals are now dramatically affecting our lives and health. Many people experience symptoms when exposed to common everyday articles, including cleaning supplies, insecticides, cosmetics and toiletries, building supplies, cigarette smoke, combustion products, and consumer products.

Because very few chemical sensitivities and reactions are IgE mediated (alternative practitioners believe most are IgG mediated) modern medicine does not acknowledge the existence of chemical sensitivities or allergies. It classifies most substances as "minor irritants," and in most cases does not recognize the many reactions and symptoms produced by exposure to chemicals. Unless they are dealing with a known toxic chemical in high concentrations, most physicians do not consider chemicals to be a health problem. Nevertheless, the number of individuals complaining of adverse symptoms triggered by chemical exposures is rising steadily.

A chemical sensitivity or allergy is manifested as an adverse reaction to chemicals in the air, food, or water. Reactions can occur to either inorganic or organic chemicals, indoors and outdoors.

Chemical sensitivity develops in several different ways. It may result from an overwhelming exposure to a chemical, such as pesticide exposure when a building is sprayed for insect control. In that case, a person with chemical sensitivities will initially have acute symptoms, and may later develop chronic symptoms. Subsequent exposures to small doses of the same (or other) chemicals will trigger additional and/or enhanced symptoms. This is known as the "spreading phenomenon," in which increased sensitivities to new substances and new target organs will occur over time unless treatment is obtained.

Other people become chemically sensitive after a series of cumulative, subacute toxic exposures over a long time period. Because the development of chemical sensitivity may be slow and insidious, many people are unaware that a problem is evolving until the point at which very small amounts of a chemical trigger their symptoms.

Chemical sensitivity may occur after exposure to small amounts of chemicals following a traumatic event such as a severe injury, childbirth, immunizations, or surgery.

Chemical sensitivity may also develop after an acute infection (bacterial, viral, fungal or parasitic). Dr. William Rea of the Environmental Health Center in Dallas, Texas reports that 1 percent of his chemically sensitive patients trace the origins of their sensitivity to such an infection.

The specific symptoms of chemical reactions (which are usually multiple) depend on:

- the tissues or organs involved
- the type of chemical causing the reaction
- the concentration of the chemical
- the length of the exposure
- the susceptibility of the exposed person
- the person's total load/overload at the time of the exposure (see p. 366)

Most chemicals are lipid (fat) soluble, and therefore many of the chemicals to which we are exposed are deposited in the fat cells and cell membranes of the body. The brain is the primary target organ in chemical sensitivity because of its high fat content. Cerebral symptoms such as confusion, depression, anger, inability to concentrate, apathy, emotional instability,

lethargy, and many other symptoms are common when the brain is affected.

However, any system or organ of the body can be affected by chemical reactions, and the symptoms vary according to the tissue affected. Other systems and organs affected, and the symptoms caused, include:

- gastrointestinal system: excessive thirst, eating or drinking binges, diarrhea, constipation, nausea and vomiting, gas, dry mouth, bad or metallic taste in the mouth, abdominal pain, difficulty swallowing, heartburn, and gallbladder symptoms
- cardiovascular system: heart pounding, racing palpitations, irregular beats, edema, chest pain, phlebitis (vein inflammation), purpura (hemorrhaging under the skin)
- musculoskeletal system: fatigue, muscle pain, weakness, joint pain, cramps, stiffness, lack of coordination, arthritis
- respiratory system: coughing, bronchitis, asthma, "air hunger"
- ear, nose, and throat: dizziness, cough, itching inside ears, ringing in ears, hypersensitivity to noise, rhinitis, nasal obstruction, stuffy nose
- eye: vision disturbances, watery eyes, light sensitivity, eye pain, swelling around eyes
- neurological: headaches, neck aches, nerve pain, muscle pain, arthritis, fainting, restless legs, and numbness
- urinary tract: urgency and frequency of urination
- skin: hives, acne, eczema, blisters, itching, burning

Chemically sensitive people can be "masked" to chemicals just as people with food allergies are masked to foods. For example, they may recognize symptoms from the smell of fresh paint, but will not be able to tell that the odor of their gas cookstove is a problem because they are exposed to it daily. Even though they may not detect the chemical or odor that is triggering a reaction, chemically sensitive people frequently have a very acute sense of smell, and are more aware of odors than people who are not affected. They often love the smell of the chemical that causes them problems, and may even crave the odor of the substance.

People with chemical sensitivities are probably the most misdiagnosed and misunderstood of all patients. Their symptoms may cause them to be labeled as lazy, troublemakers, or even "crazy." Most physicians recommend psychiatric help or counseling when they cannot find a physical cause for such a patient's symptoms. Employers seldom recognize chronic chemical exposure at the workplace as the cause of their employee's symptoms; they usually suspect psychological problems. Chemically sensitive people can have severe health problems unless they receive an accurate diagnosis and appropriate treatment. They can become incapable of working, and even finding a safe place to live can become very difficult.

Many people are beginning to recognize the causes of their symptoms, and are beginning to clean up their environments. They are also insisting that others not contribute to their problems. For example, people who are sensitive to perfumes and scented items are requesting that magazines not include scented advertising. Similarly, non-smoking areas (in airports, restaurants, and public gathering places of all kinds) are becoming larger, more comfortable, and more numerous.

MODERN MEDICAL TREATMENT

Because modern medicine does not acknowledge chemical sensitivities, it provides no treatment for this problem.

ALTERNATIVE TREATMENT

Diet
Eat organic foods, free of pesticides, chemical fertilizer residues, ripening agents, protective waxes, and dyes. Eat fiber (such as oat bran or apple pectin) to help remove toxic metals.

Do not eat processed foods, any foods containing artificial coloring, flavors, or sweeteners, or foods to which preservatives and other chemicals have been added.

Exercise and Lifestyle
Clean up your home environment to lower your chemical exposures. Run an air cleaner continuously and change the filters regularly. Activated charcoal filters must be used to remove chemicals.

Create a bedroom oasis free of chemical, inhalant, or food exposures.

Do not use a natural gas clothes dryer, water heater, or furnace. If you have no choice, move them to an outbuilding.

Use a water filter in the shower and kitchen. Better still, use a whole house water purification system.

Do not use a natural gas cookstove, and use appliances with the least amount of interior plastic. Avoid aluminum and Teflon coatings on all appliances and cookware.

Cook in glass, enamel, or stainless-steel cookware. Store food in glass or cellophane containers, or in aluminum foil with the shiny side next to the food. Do not use plastic wrapping.

Clean the house with safe cleaning products, such as lemon and baking soda.

Remove all chemicals from the house, including "unsafe" cleaning supplies, paints, detergents, fabric softeners, perfumes, and other scented products, solvents, glues, lighter fluids, shoe polish, mothballs, and rubber and soft plastic items. (Even if these items are stored in containers with lids, small amounts of the chemicals will escape.)

Do not use aerosol products (anything from paint to hairspray) and remove any aerosols you have in the house. Do not use any insecticides or pesticides in the house, and do not store these products in the house.

Do not smoke or allow anyone else to smoke

in your house. Do not use a fireplace, wood-burning or pellet stove, candles, or incense.

Do not idle vehicles in an attached garage or carport. Weatherstrip the door between the house and the garage.

Wear natural fibers as much as possible, and do not wear dry-cleaned clothes or leather garments.

Select personal care products carefully, avoiding those that are scented.

Stop using standard commercial mouthwash, deodorant, and toothpaste; use baking soda as both an underarm deodorant and a toothpaste.

Do not use bleach, scented laundry soap, and fabric softener. Use ½ to 1 cup of baking soda in the rinse water as fabric softener.

Clean up your work environment, following the guidelines for household cleanup. Do not allow people to smoke around you, and run an air cleaner in your work area. See Sources. Use nontoxic office supplies whenever possible. If your job involves chemicals that can get on your skin, wear protective clothing. Wear a mask containing activated charcoal if you are exposed to chemical fumes.

Avoid chemicals in the course of driving, shopping, and spending time in public places. Use an air cleaner in your car, and if you cannot find a full-service gas station, exercise care when putting gasoline in your car; wear a mask if you are very sensitive to chemicals, and wash your hands afterward. Stay away from the detergent aisle in the grocery store. If you are extremely sensitive, wear a mask or respirator containing activated charcoal when you think you might be exposed to chemicals. Be particularly careful to wear the mask in malls and stores where new merchandise is displayed, as these are full of potentially harmful chemicals (especially formaldehyde).

Do not use solvents, chemical pesticides, or chemical fertilizers. Use nontoxic building materials, paints, and floor coverings if remodeling or building a new house.

Nutrient Therapy

Take the following nutritional supplements to replace any depletion caused by chemical exposures:

- vitamin A – 50,000 IU a day for 30 days, then reduce to 25,000 IU a day. *Caution:* Do not take more than 8,000 IU a day if you are pregnant or might be pregnant (powerful antioxidant).
- vitamin B-complex – 100 to 200 mg a day (protects the liver and body functions)
- niacinamide – 500 mg three times a day, over and above the amounts in B-complex. *Caution:* Do not substitute niacin (large doses help control histamine release during an allergic reaction).
- vitamin B_6 – 100 mg three times a day, over and above the amounts in B-complex (aids in detoxification; natural antihistamine)
- vitamin C – 5,000 to 20,000 mg a day (or bowel tolerance—see p. 372) in divided doses. Use both ascorbic acid, and a buffered form between meals (protects the body from pollutants; aids in elimination of toxic substances).
- vitamin E – 400 to 800 IU a day (powerful antioxidant)
- copper – 2 to 3 mg a day (balances zinc)
- selenium – 200 mcg a day (helps detoxify; essential for immune function)
- zinc – 50 mg a day. *Caution:* Do not exceed a total of 100 mg a day (for proper immune function).
- bioflavonoids – 500 mg a day (protects the body from pollutants; aids in elimination of toxic substances)
- coenzyme Q_{10} – 60 mg a day (provides oxygen to the tissues; helps rebuild the immune system; counters the histamine released in allergic reactions)
- garlic (Kyolic) – two capsules three times a day (an immunostimulant)
- L-cysteine, L-methionine, and L-glutamic acid – 500 mg each, a day (remove toxins)

- proteolytic enzymes – as directed on the label of your product, three times a day between meals (for proper digestion; control of inflammation)
- pycnogenol or grape seed extract – as directed on the label of your product (powerful antioxidant)
- superoxide dismutase (SOD) – as directed on the label of your product (powerful destroyer of free radicals)
- taurine – 500 mg a day (most important antioxidant and immune regulator)
- raw thymus glandular – as directed on the label of your product (important for immune function)

Herbal Therapy
Use the following herbal products:

- Natureworks Marigold Ointment from Abkit – for skin rashes caused by metal allergy (see Sources)
- calendula, chamomile, elder flower, and tea tree oil – as a wash for skin rashes

Homeopathic Remedies
Take the homeopathic remedy that best fits your symptoms. If you do not obtain relief, consult a homeopathic practitioner.

- *Arsenicum album* – sensitivity to pesticides; anxiety, exhaustion, and restlessness; burning pains; sudden great weakness; shortness of breath.
- *Phosphorus* – great sensitivity to odors; chemical sensitivity; suggestible and anxious; mentally distractible and "spacey"; easily dehydrated; general aggravation at night; thirst for cold drinks.
- *Sulphuricum acidum* – cures chemical hypersensitivity; tremendous sensitivity to fumes and smoke; asthma made worse from smoke, fumes, and dust; general aggravation from car exhaust, smoke, dust, and aromatics; hur-

riedness; tendency to bruising; small ulcers on the tongue, inner cheeks, and gastrointestinal tract.

Many patients respond to complex homeopathic remedies. You may want to try BHI Body Pure, which assists in detoxifying environmental chemicals and lowering total load, or Chem'ls by Vibrant Health for toxicity caused by chemicals and drugs. Environmental by Vibrant Health helps eliminate toxins from the environment.

The following PHP products help with sensitivities to specific substances.

- Beautox – detoxification of materials used in cosmetology
- Envirotox – detoxification of hydrocarbons and miscellaneous air and water pollutants
- Industriox – detoxification of industrial toxins
- Metox – elimination of heavy metals
- Mertox – drainage and detoxification of mercury and related compounds
- Addex – aids in drainage, and helps relieve the effects of pesticide and insecticide exposure

Other Therapeutic Measures
Be tested and treated for chemical sensitivities by an environmental medicine physician.

Take detoxification baths or participate in a detox program at a detoxification center (see Sources).

Detoxify the liver and lower the chemical load of the body by taking one of the following: Liver Liquescence by PHP, Hepatatox by BioActive, Dandiplex by BioActive, Karzan by BioActive, and Hepatica from Marco Pharma.

Consider having your mercury amalgam fillings removed. Locate a biological dentist to advise you. Take H Metals and Dent'l by Vibrant Health—complex remedies for heavy metal toxicity and dental and chemical poisoning.

Take a coffee enema to clear a chemical reaction and to help the liver detoxify (see pp. 119).

Have NAET treatments (see Chiropractic section in chapter 9, Alternative Medical Disciplines), or EPD treatments (see Other Therapeutic Measures for Pollen Allergy, earlier in this chapter).

Take "rescues," which are substances that help turn off an allergic reaction (see Other Therapeutic Measures for Pollen Allergy).

ALLERGIES TO MICROORGANISMS

Bacteria, viruses, parasites, molds, and yeast are all microorganisms. They can cause infections, but they also affect us in many other ways. They can attack the immune system, exacerbating sensitivities. Some emit toxins that can poison us. We may also be allergic or sensitive to some toxins—as well as to the bodies of the organisms themselves, cell fragments of the organisms, and inactive organisms.

Many symptoms of an acute infection actually result from an allergic response to the infecting organism. When symptoms of an infection are unusually severe or prolonged, or when they occur in an allergic person, an allergic response to the organism should be suspected as a complication of the infection. Eggs released by egg-producing parasites frequently trigger allergic symptoms, and many symptoms that occur during a viral infection are caused by an allergic reaction to the protein of the viral body.

Even after an infection has subsided, a continued allergic response to the cellular debris of the organism, and to excess circulating antibodies, can cause low-grade symptoms. Organisms produce and release metabolic products as they grow in our bodies. When the organisms die as a result of treatment, all of their metabolic products are released as their cell walls rupture. These metabolic products are toxic to us, and we can be allergic to these also.

MODERN MEDICAL TREATMENT

Modern treatment for microorganisms deals only with eliminating the infection, usually by prescribing an antibiotic. Except in the case of the Jarisch-Herxheimer reaction seen with syphilis (chills, fever, headache, muscle pain, and rapid heartbeat that may develop after treatment is begun as a response to the antigens released when the syphilis spirochetes are killed), modern medicine seldom acknowledges the role of allergy in infection.

ALTERNATIVE TREATMENT

Nutrient Therapy
- vitamin C – bowel tolerance each day (protects against infection; enhances immunity)
- *Lactobacillus acidophilus* – as directed on your product (replaces helpful bowel bacteria; has natural antibiotic action)

Homeopathic Remedies
Many patients respond to complex homeopathic remedies. The following PHP products aid in eliminating infection, stimulating the defense systems, and dealing with allergic reactions to infecting organisms:

- Bacterial Immune Stimulator – balances the antibacterial systems of the body.
- Viral Immune Stimulator – assists in eradication of viral infection.
- Virox – assists in eradication of viral infections.
- Mycological Immune Stimulator – assists in the eradication of fungal infections.
- Mytox – assists in eradication of fungal infections.
- Mycotoxin Inhibitor – assists in eradication of mycotoxin (mold) infections.
- Vermex – assists in eradication of intestinal parasites.
- Amebex – assists in eradication of amebic infection.

The following products from Vibrant Health also help with specific conditions.

- B'terias – for bacterial contamination; chronic disposition for illness.
- Ep'tein – for Epstein-Barr Virus; an immune stimulant; aids in lymph drainage.
- F'gus – for fungus, yeast, and mold contamination.
- Herps – for Herpes II, retroviruses, vaccine, flu shots.
- V'rus – for flu and viral conditions; aids in immune support.

Other Therapeutic Measures
Be tested for sensitivity to microorganisms and their toxins by an environmental medicine physician. If the tests are positive, follow the recommendations for treatment including an allergy extract for the organism(s) involved.

Allergy extracts for microorganisms and their toxins can relieve both acute and chronic, low-grade allergic symptoms caused by the organisms and their metabolic products. They also help release the cellular debris from the organisms that may remain, and stimulate the immune system to fight the infecting organisms.

Have NAET treatment (see Chiropractic section in chapter 9, Alternative Medical Disciplines).

If you have an infection, take the appropriate antimicrobial treatment, below (see also Parasites, chapter 20, and Upper Respiratory Infections in Respiratory System Problems, chapter 13).

Take the following antibiotic substitutes:

- colloidal silver – follow the directions on the label for your product
- NK 9-1-1 – a colostrum/echinacea combination made by Biotics Code and distributed by Super Life (see Sources).

Take an antibiotic only if alternative treatments do not eliminate the infection.

CHAPTER 26

Attention-Deficit Hyperactivity Disorder

Our society is overstimulated, and places little value on quiet and solitude. Children spend hours in front of the television, receiving constant stimulation. We eat in fast-food restaurants. The use of drugs, legal and illegal, is increasing.

Many people, both children and adults, appear to be overstimulated and overactive. These people have been described as hyperactive or hyperkinetic, and may have attention-deficit hyperactivity disorder.

Attention-deficit hyperactivity disorder (ADHD) affects over 15 million North Americans. It is an inherited neurological syndrome characterized by easy distractibility, low tolerance for frustration or boredom, impulsivity, and a penchant for situations of high intensity. (In the past, this syndrome was usually called minimal brain dysfunction, or attention deficit disorder.) The syndrome reflects attention *inconsistency* rather than true attention *deficit,* since people with ADHD can focus intently at times. Hyperactivity may not always occur, and some people with ADHD—especially girls—can be quiet and retreat into daydreams. People with ADHD have high energy, and are intuitive, creative, and enthusiastic, but they have difficulty with appropriate behavioral inhibition.

Dr. Russell Barkley of the University of Massachusetts Medical Center states that the primary problem in ADHD is a deficit in the neurological motivation system, which makes it impossible to stay on task for any length of time unless there is constant feedback and reward. Other symptoms of ADHD in children can include lack of concentration, a tendency to disturb other children, self-destructive behavior, disorders of speech and hearing, absentmindedness, forgetfulness, difficulty solving problems or managing time, learning disabilities, low tolerance for stress, inability to sit still even at mealtime, sleep disturbances, and failure in school despite average or above average intelligence. No individual will have all of these symptoms, and the particular combination of symptoms will vary from person to person.

ADHD is typically associated with at least normal intelligence, and most people with the disorder are above average in intelligence. However, as many as 80 percent of people with ADHD have a specific learning disability. An evaluation by a physician is necessary to confirm the diagnosis of ADHD.

ADHD is typically first noted in childhood, and about 5 to 10 percent of school-aged children have ADHD. About 20 to 30 percent of those who have ADHD in childhood outgrow the condition, but in others ADHD remains a problem throughout adult life. About 40 percent of children with ADHD have at least one parent who has the trait, and 35 percent have a sibling with the trait. Some people who have had

ADHD all their lives recognize only as adults that they have the condition. In those cases, there is a childhood history which may include behavior problems in school, impulsivity, overexcitability, or temper outbursts, and an adult history with at least two of the following symptoms: changeable moods, hot temper, stress intolerance, disorganization, and impulsivity.

Adults with ADHD may not do well with routine desk jobs, and are often considered chronic underachievers. Half of all adults with ADHD do well in the workplace, but the other half have work problems, psychiatric problems, or difficulties with drug abuse. They may be clumsy or awkward, and they often engage in risky behavior (such as gambling or fast driving).

As adults, 25 to 30 percent will have substance-abuse problems with marijuana, alcohol, or other depressants. Initially these drugs calm them and help them to focus. However, secondary psychological problems frequently also develop.

Depression is biologically linked with ADHD, and half of all patients with ADHD become depressed at some time during their lives. Drs. James Hudson and Harrison Pope at the Harvard Medical School in Boston have demonstrated that ADHD, depression, bulimia, obsessive-compulsive disorder, cataplexy, migraine headaches, panic disorder, and irritable bowel syndrome are all physiologically linked.

Children with ADHD often have social problems because of their distractibility or impulsivity. They may be bored with school, or exhibit depression, frustration, fear of learning new things, impaired peer relations, or even violent behavior. Dr. Barkley notes that half to two-thirds of ADHD children between five and seven years old are hostile and defiant. By the time ADHD children reach the age of 10 to 12, many will have developed a conduct disorder.

Conduct disorder is estimated to affect 4 to 10 percent of all children. These children steal, are aggressive, set fires, run away, lie, do not go to school, are cruel to animals or people, use a weapon in fights, and initiate fights. They tend to be likeable and charming but as adults would be diagnosed as sociopaths (people who have an antisocial personality).

Children with ADHD often have "oppositional defiant disorder" in addition, but children may have only one of these conditions. They get into frequent fights, cannot obey rules, resist limits, disrupt the work and play of others, and may break the law. They deliberately do things that annoy other people and blame others for their own mistakes. They often swear and use obscene language.

DIAGNOSIS

There is no blood test, EEG, or CAT scan that can definitively make the diagnosis of ADHD. Instead, a diagnosis is based on a cluster of symptoms and on behavior, so the most reliable way to diagnosis ADHD is through a history taken from the child, the parents, and teachers. Because of the difficulty in making a diagnosis of ADHD, it is frequently either overdiagnosed or not recognized. When ADHD children are tested in a one-on-one situation, they often focus well and are intrigued by the novelty of the testing situation, and so perform well on the tests. A high IQ can delay the diagnosis of ADHD.

Hyperthyroidism can mimic ADHD, as can some learning disabilities, speech and language disorders, pervasive developmental disorders (autism), conduct disorder, depression, chronic fatigue, fetal alcohol syndrome, lead poisoning, obsessive-compulsive disorder, personality disorders, post-traumatic stress disorder, seizure disorder, substance abuse, mental retardation, or situational disturbances such as family dysfunction. Dr. Stanley Greenspan, professor of Clinical Psychiatry and Behavioral Science in Pediatrics at George Washington University Medical School in Washington, D.C., notes that attention problems can be caused by visual, auditory, motor, and spatial processing difficulties.

The diagnosis of ADHD in children is based on the American Psychiatric Association's *Diagnostic and Statistical Manual of Mental Disorders*. Health care professionals consider the criteria are met only if the behavior is considerably more frequent than that of most people of the same mental age. The children must have six or more of the following symptoms of inattention for a period of at least six months to meet the criteria.

- carelessness in schoolwork
- difficulty sustaining attention to task or play
- not listening when spoken to directly
- not following through on instructions
- failing to finish schoolwork or chores
- problems organizing tasks
- avoiding tasks that require sustained mental effort
- losing things needed for tasks
- distraction by extraneous stimuli
- often being forgetful in daily activities

Children may instead fulfill criteria for the hyperactivity/impulsivity type (a variant of ADHD) if six or more of the following symptoms persist for at least six months.

- fidgeting with hands or feet or squirming in their seat in the classroom
- leaving their seat in the classroom when being seated is expected
- running or climbing excessively in inappropriate situations
- difficulty playing quietly
- often being on the go or acting as if driven by a motor
- often talking excessively
- blurting out the answer before a question has been completed
- having difficulty awaiting a turn, or interrupting or intruding on others

Symptoms of inattention or hyperactivity must have been present before the age of seven years, and they must be present in two or more settings. As well, there must be evidence of impairment in social, academic, or occupational functions. The symptoms should not occur exclusively during the course of a pervasive developmental disorder, schizophrenia, or a mood or personality disorder.

NUTRITIONAL FACTORS IN ADHD

There is much controversy about whether and how diet affects children's activity levels. Within a few hours of eating sugar, children release large amounts of epinephrine (adrenaline). This causes shakiness, anxiety, excitement, and problems with concentration. EEG testing has confirmed the problems with concentration.

Barbara Reed, a probation officer from Ohio and author of *Food, Teens and Behavior,* found that most of her young adult clients had diets extremely high in sweets; many would begin the day with doughnuts and soft drinks. She found that these patients had fluctuating blood sugar levels, which contributed to their violent behavior. When they changed their diets, their rate of recidivism plummeted.

Dr. Doris Rapp (a pediatric allergist, former Clinical Assistant Professor of Pediatrics at the State University of New York at Buffalo, and author of *The Impossible Child*) has co-authored several studies which demonstrate that food sensitivities can cause hyperactivity and violent behavior. She has videotaped allergy testing on some of these children, showing that a certain dose of food extract can provoke abnormal behavior, and that a neutralizing dose of food extract can stop the abnormal behavior—almost like flipping a switch.

Dr. Marvin Boris and others at the North Shore University Hospital in New York demonstrated in a double-blind placebo study that foods and food additives are common causes of ADHD in children.

The Feingold diet (developed by the late Dr. Ben F. Feingold, who was attending physician at

Los Angeles Children's Hospital and author of numerous papers) treats hyperactivity by eliminating all foods containing additives, including coloring, flavoring, and preservatives, from the diet. The diet also eliminates foods containing salicylates. Fifty percent of the hyperactive children in his practice improved on Dr. Feingold's diet, and in many cases allowed the ADHD child to stop medication.

Dr. William Walsh of the Carl Pfeiffer Treatment Center in Napierville, Illinois has done many hair analysis studies, and has found that certain mineralization patterns fit certain behaviors. For instance, his group has found very abnormal hair analyses in such criminals as Jeffrey Dahmer and Charles Manson. Some minerals were abnormally high; others very low. Based on these findings, he prescribes various minerals to balance the body chemistry, including calcium, copper, magnesium, and zinc. He has been very successful in treating patients who exhibit violent behavior.

MODERN MEDICAL TREATMENT

Drug Therapy
Stimulant Medication
According to the International Narcotics Control Board of the United Nations, at least two million children in the United States—more than one in every 30 children between the ages of 5 and 18—are taking stimulant medications, and the number of children taking stimulants has been doubling every two years. Production of the stimulant Ritalin has increased almost 500 percent in the last five years, and Dr. James Swanson, director of the Child Development Center at the University of California at Irvine, notes that the sudden increase in Ritalin use is cause for alarm. He estimates that one-third of the children now on Ritalin should not be taking it.

Stimulants are the medication used for ADHD treatment. These medications include dextroamphetamine (Dexedrine), cylert (Pemoline) and methylphenidate (Ritalin). Stimulants are effective in controlling ADHD 60 to 80 percent of the time. They act on neurotransmitters to activate or stimulate the central nervous system, and this helps the patient to focus. Stimulants also even out moods without making the person taking them feel drugged, and they are not addictive in the doses prescribed for ADHD. Despite this, many high school seniors admit to abusing Ritalin, using it to study more effectively and to get high. Several deaths have been caused by Ritalin abuse.

Stimulants improve attention span, handwriting, compliance, and motor coordination, and they diminish impulsivity and aggressiveness. They do not stifle creativity. There is no significant improvement in reading skills, athletic or game skills, or positive social skills. Long-term academic achievement, antisocial behavior, and arrest rates have not been shown to be affected by use of the medication.

The most common side effects of stimulant medication are loss of appetite and sleep problems. Blood pressure and heart rate can be increased, but these effects can be decreased or avoided by lowering the dose. Nausea, stomach aches, headaches, drowsiness, irritability, depressed mood, and moodiness can occur.

When the medication wears off, there can be a letdown or mood change. In children who are very active, rebound hyperactivity can occur as the medication wears off. Tolerance occurs almost universally, which means that children require increases in dosage over time and as they grow. Too high a dose can put the patient in a "zombie-like" state, which makes the child easier to control in the classroom.

Ritalin, Dexedrine, and Pemoline can cause nervousness or jitteriness; frequent involuntary muscle twitching can occur while a patient is on stimulant medication. These medications also cause growth suppression in children, but rapid growth when medication is discontinued compensates for this. The blood count can be affected, as can other blood chemistries, although they return to normal when the medication is discontinued. High doses of Ritalin can cause liver cancer in mice. Stimulants in high doses can cause strokes, hyperthermia, hypertension, and seizures. Pemoline has caused liver damage, which is usually reversible when the medication is stopped.

Short-acting Ritalin and Dexedrine last about four hours; the dose must be repeated when the person needs to be focused again. Sustained-released Ritalin or Dexedrine is available, but the sustained-released Ritalin does not work as well as the short-acting Ritalin. Brand name Ritalin seems to work better than generic methylphenidate.

It often takes weeks or months to find the right dose and the right dosage schedule for a given child. Sometimes adding another medication will enhance the action of the first medication. The person taking the medication may not be able to tell that the drug is working, but teachers, parents, friends, and others may notice improvements. Stimulants should be discontinued for about a week every four to six months to see if the medication is still needed.

A study by Dr. Alan Zametkin and colleagues at the National Institute of Mental Health demonstrated that adults with ADHD who had not been treated with stimulant medication had abnormal brain scans, showing abnormalities in the areas of the brain that are involved in the control of attention, impulses, and motor activity. Studies demonstrate that the outcomes for people treated with stimulant medication are no better than for those not treated with it. Children who take stimulant medication tend to rely upon it as a crutch. About 15 percent of adults do not respond to stimulant medication, and some people stop taking the drug because they experience side effects that they cannot tolerate.

Antidepressants

Antidepressants are the second most commonly used medications for ADHD. Desimipramine (Norpramin), a tricyclic antidepressant, is the drug most frequently used to treat ADHD. Nor-

pramin can be taken in one dose a day. It has a smoother action than the stimulant medications, and since it is not a controlled substance, prescriptions are easier to fill.

Norpramin can be used either in high or low dosages, but high doses need to be monitored with blood tests. Side effects may include dry mouth, mild urinary retention, and transient lowering of the blood pressure with standing up. Norpramin can also cause irregular heart rhythms, and it has caused sudden death in a few children. Other side effects include palpitations, confusional states, insomnia, nightmares, blurred vision, constipation, loss of appetite, breast enlargement in males and females, and elevation or depression of blood sugar.

Other antidepressants—nortriptyline (Pamelor), imipramine (Tofranil), bupropion (Wellbutrin), maprotiline (Ludiomil), and fluoxetine (Prozac)—have also been successfully used to treat ADHD. Prozac does not have an effect on attention, but does treat depression by acting on the serotonin system (see p. 406).

Antihypertensive Medication

Alpha-agonist hypertensive medications have been used for very impulsive children with attention-deficit hyperactivity disorder. These agents reduce sympathetic output from the brain (affecting the "fight or flight" response) and decrease peripheral resistance (pressure and tone in blood vessels), heart rate, and blood pressure. Clonidine (Catapres) and guanfacine (Tenex) are some of the drugs used in children.

Side effects of these preparations include headaches, depression, dry mouth, heart problems, itching or hives, drowsiness, low blood pressure, and weight gain. Children may develop tolerance to the antihypertensive effects of alpha-agonist agents.

Beta Blockers

Beta blockers have been used to treat the nervousness or anxiety that some people experience when they take stimulant medication. Beta blockers such as nadolol (Corgard) and propranolol (Inderal) also help to reduce explosive rage. Beta blockers can cause depression, slow heartbeat, difficulty exercising, fatigue, dizziness, insomnia, triggering of asthma (in people with asthma), shortness of breath, and constipation (see p. 190 for more information on beta blockers).

EDUCATION

People with ADHD need structure. They need concrete tools such as lists, reminders, simple filing systems, appointment books, goals, and daily planning. It helps to make a master calendar, and fill in times daily so that they become regular appointments. People with ADHD are helped by structured group therapy or a coach to keep them on task. This also helps them develop insight into their disorder.

Drs. Edward Hallowell and John Ratey (of Boston and authors of *Driven to Distraction*) suggest the following tips for adults who want to achieve non-medicated management of ADHD:

1. Try to join or start a support group.
2. Try to get rid of the negativity that you have heard all your life. Realize that you are a capable person.
3. Make lists, files, reminders, etc. to structure your life.
4. Handle papers only once; take care of papers as soon as you receive them.
5. Make deadlines.
6. Do what you are good at, and do not spend time at what you do badly.
7. Develop ways to manage mood changes.
8. Expect to become depressed after success.
9. Be an advocate for yourself, and speak up about what you can do well.
10. Joke with yourself and others about various symptoms.

They have a similar list for non-medicated management of children with ADHD:

1. Write down the problem and what the problem areas are.
2. Decide upon specific remedies for problems.
3. Use lists, schedules, reminders, etc.
4. Use incentive plans, and give the child a reward for accomplishments.
5. Give the child responsibility wherever possible.
6. Use praise and positive feedback.
7. Arrange for a coach or tutor to help with schoolwork.
8. Provide the child with any tools that can help (using a word processor works for some children).
9. Negotiate with the child; do not struggle.

Three of the best approaches to use for children with ADHD are one-on-one tutoring, high motivation, and novelty.

SUPPORT GROUPS

Support groups exist for parents of children with ADHD, and for adults with ADHD. The best known such group is called Children and Adults with Attention Deficit Disorder (C.A.A.D.D.), based in Plantation, Florida. This group is underwritten by a drug company, and does not support alternative treatment.

Other Therapeutic Measures

Physicians also recommend behavior modification, cognitive therapy, family therapy, and social skills training.

ALTERNATIVE TREATMENT

There are several alternative treatments that are effective for ADHD; they can be used either alone or in combination with each other.

Diet

Observe the following dietary guidelines for children as well as adults with ADHD. Avoid MSG and other additives such as artificial colors, flavorings, and preservatives. Avoid carbonated beverages, which contain high amounts of phosphates. Excessive phosphates combined with low calcium and magnesium creates potential for hyperactivity and seizures. Avoid caffeine and eliminate sugar, chocolate, and candy from the diet.

Avoid eating fruits and vegetables containing salicylates, such as apples, apricots, almonds, all berries, cherries, grapes, peaches, plums, prunes, tomatoes, cucumbers, and oranges. Do not eat cloves, mint, or wine vinegars. Breads should contain only rice and oats. Do not eat any processed, manufactured, or prepared foods such as ketchup, hot dogs, luncheon meats, salami, soy sauce, and similar foods.

Have food allergy testing performed and be treated for any allergies or sensitivities that are found. Either avoid the foods, be desensitized to them, and/or follow a rotation diet. If food testing is not available from a physician, use an elimination allergy diet (see chapter 25, Allergy). Have NAET (see p. 80) or EPD treatments for food allergy (see p. 372).

Regardless of the diet followed, the whole family should participate to eliminate temptation for the person being treated.

Exercise and Lifestyle
Do patterning exercises such as cross crawl, marching, and figure 8s to reprogram the brain. When they were infants, some children with ADHD did not crawl well, or for long enough, and these exercises seem to help both adults and children to correct deficits that have occurred because of this.

Help the child to be as active as possible and participate in sports such as track, football, volleyball, skiing, and rugby to burn up the excess energy. Classes such as dance, martial arts, fencing, gymnastics, and wrestling are also good.

Be aware that common toiletries may contain substances that can contribute to hyperactivity.

Do not use antacid tablets, cough drops, perfume, throat lozenges, or commercial toothpaste.

Alcohol and drugs must be avoided.

Nutrient Therapy
The following supplements are helpful.

- B-complex – with 25 mg of each B once a day (acts on nervous system; promotes relaxation)
- vitamin B_6 – 15 mg per kg of body weight a day, up to 300 mg maximim (helps with attention and focus; increases serotonin levels)
- vitamin C – at least 1,000 mg a day in divided doses. If allergies are present, 2,000 mg a day (antihistamine; affects neurotransmitters, especially acetylcholine).
- calcium – 750 mg a day (has a calming effect; works with magnesium)
- magnesium – 400 mg a day (combats mood swings, irritability, anxiety, hyperactivity)
- zinc – 15 mg a day (needed to produce norepinephrine and dopamine; for proper B_{12} functioning in brain)
- essential fatty acids – 1 to 2 tsp. three times a day (building blocks of cell membranes and nerve endings)
- GABA – 750 mg a day (calms the brain)
- glutamine – 500 mg in the morning and at noon for children. For teenagers, 200 mg a day in divided doses (essential for cerebral function; increases GABA levels).
- pycnogenol or grape pips – one capsule two times a day (helps with attention and focus)
- taurine – 1,000 to 1,500 mg a day (protective effect on the brain; helps reduce hyperactivity)
- tyrosine – 500 mg a day (acts as a mood elevator; precursor to norepinephrine and dopamine)

Use Balanced Neurotransmitter Complex formulated by Dr. Billie J. Sahley of the Pain and Stress Center in San Antonio, Texas (see Sources).

This formulation helps to restore neurotransmitter balance and function. It contains L-phenylalanine, L-leucine, L-valine, L-histidine, L-arginine, L-lysine, L-isoleucine, L-alanine, L-glutamine, L-methionine, L-threonine, GABA, alpha-ketoglutaric acid, pyridoxal 5-phosphate, and chromium picolinate.

Caution: If the child is taking MAO inhibitors or tricyclic antidepressants, do not use tyrosine or Balanced Neurotransmitter Complex.

Herbal Therapy

The following herbs have been found to be helpful in some cases of ADHD.

- catnip – calms and relieves stress
- chamomile – nerve tonic; helpful for stress, anxiety and insomnia. Do not use on an ongoing basis, or if allergic to ragweed.
- hops – good for restlessness; helps hyperactivity
- passionflower – gentle sedative, helps hyperactivity
- skullcap – aids sleep, fatigue, hyperactivity, and nervous disorders
- valerian – acts as a sedative; good for anxiety
- wood betony – good for hyperactivity; relaxes muscles

Homeopathic Remedies

Homeopathy has been used very successfully in children with ADHD and other behavioral and learning problems. Drs. Judyth Reichenberg-Ullman and Robert Ullman of Edmonds, Washington (co-authors of *Ritalin Free Kids*) have had about a 70 percent success rate among patients who have continued homeopathic treatment for at least one year. Prescribing homeopathic remedies for ADHD is complex, and we strongly suggest that you consult a qualified and experienced homeopathic practitioner for this condition. (*Caution:* The remedies listed below should not be tried without consultation. They are cited only to illustrate how precise the association can be between symptoms and the various homeopathic remedies.)

- *Cina* – among the most irritable of children, do not seem to know what they want and reject what they are given; want to be rocked but do not like to be touched, looked at, or carried (except over the shoulder); pinch, kick, and hit out of irritability and contradiction; worms are a causative factor in some cases, especially pinworms; children pick or bore into their nose or ears, scratch their bottoms, grind their teeth at night; fussy, obstinate, throw tantrums, and do not want to be touched when angry; child may be precocious and hard; will not tolerate parental authority; may have convulsions from being scolded or disciplined; tendency for yawning.
- *Stramonium* – a mixture of extreme fear and violence; afraid of the dark, especially when alone, and can become extremely clingy; may become violent if provoked; fear animals, water, and violent death; often have nightmares or terrors with shrieking; they stammer, curse, develop rage and jealousy; very intense children; violent abuse or birth trauma may push a child into a Stramonium state; has the capacity to commit murder; night terrors; craving for sweets; rage is uncontrolled and impulsive, rage comes in an outburst.
- *Tarentula hispanic* – these children love music and rhythmic activities such as dancing, tapping, or drumming; tell lies, are cunning and mischievous; love to hide; hurried and impatient; can be destructive and will break anything they can get their hands on; impulsive and distractible; muscles twitch and jerk; attracted to bright colors; manipulate conversations and situations to bring about their wants by cunning or even lying rather than by persuasion.
- *Tuberculinum* – like to travel, desire constant change; often allergic to cats and other ani-

mal dander; strong fear of cats and animals and can be cruel to them; irritable and mean to other children; can break their parents' favorite things just to get back at them; very restless; can be sensitive, artistic, and bright; throw tantrums; coldly and deliberately destructive and malicious; completely indifferent to punishment or reprimand; useful in cases of mental retardation and even autism; compulsive and ritualistic behavior; grinding teeth; sleep in knee-chest position; long, fine eyelashes especially in children.

- *Veratrum album* – patient overly intellectual and not connected to those around him; often harshly critical; child curious and almost adult level in conceptual ability; great restlessness; inner frustration which leads to disobedient and behavior problems; child has tremendous restless feeling, which is expressed by senseless, repetitive behavior such as stacking things or cutting paper into ever smaller bits; may be so restless he cannot sit down to eat; shows no emotion when reprimanded or punished; seems to know it all and can be bossy, self-righteous, and debative; often touch, hug, and kiss inappropriately; often chilly and may have very cold hands and feet that turn white or blue.

Some people with ADHD respond well to complex homeopathic remedies. PHP Learning Disability Drops, a complex homeopathic remedy, helps increase mental clarity. Neuro, by Vibrant Health, addresses sleep and behavior challenges, and Neuro 3 assists in proper production and flow of neurotransmitters (see Sources).

Other Therapeutic Measures

Be tested and treated for neurotransmitter imbalance and sensitivity by an environmental medicine physician. In addition, use nutritional supplements to compensate for low neurotransmitter levels. Have an NAET treatment for neurotransmitters.

Have a hair analysis to rule out toxic heavy metal levels.

See an osteopath for craniosacral therapy, in which imbalances in cranial (head) bones are corrected. This allows the physiology of the nervous system to function more efficiently and can help to correct or minimize ADHD.

Investigate biofeedback training.

CHAPTER 27

Mood Disorders

Just as people can suffer from physical disorders, they can have mood disorders. Mood disorders affect over 16 million North Americans and range from mild conditions to serious disorders that may require institutionalization. All mood disorders involve mental and emotional states, and many are whole-body illnesses, involving the body, nervous system, moods, thoughts, and behavior. They can affect every aspect of people's lives, including the way they think, eat, sleep, react to themselves and others, and conduct their lives.

While there are many mood disorders, we are presenting only the most common disorders of depression, anxiety, and panic attacks.

DEPRESSION

Depression is a total body illness, affecting physical well-being, the nervous system, behavior, thoughts, and moods. Signs of depression include loss of pleasure in life, early morning awakening and problems sleeping, physical inactivity, feelings of guilt and worthlessness, lack of desire to socialize, irritability, memory problems, crying spells, loss of self-esteem, thoughts of suicide, and difficulty concentrating. According to the National Institute of Health in Rockville, Maryland, at least two-thirds of depressed patients are not properly diagnosed by their family physician.

Unipolar depressive disorder is the name given to episodes of depression that occur several times during a person's lifetime; it is the most common type of depression. A major depression is a combination of symptoms that interfere with working, sleeping, eating, and enjoying pleasant activities. Less severe depression, dysthymia, is characterized by long-term symptoms that do not disable, but prevent the person from feeling well and performing at maximum ability. Some people have bipolar disorder, also known as manic depression, which begins with episodes of depression but progresses to cycles of depression alternating with mania. When people with this disorder are in the manic phase of the cycle, they are self-confident, make grandiose plans, and exhibit extravagant behavior. They have great energy (including sexual energy) but their mood can change in a matter of minutes from happy and expansive to irritable or frustrated.

Depression is becoming more and more common in our society. More than 20 million Americans (twice as many women as men) will suffer an episode of depression at some point in life. In Canada, three million people suffer from depression, but fewer than one-third seek help. Depression is the number one mental health problem in the United States, and of all behavioral diagnoses, it accounts for the highest medical plan costs. The length of disability and the relapse rate for depression is greater than that for other medical problems.

Depression tends to run in families, probably because of similarities in metabolism and neurotransmitter problems. Around 50 percent of people who suffer from recurrent depression have parents who have also dealt with depression.

Elderly people with depression may experience insomnia, low energy, loss of memory, and weight loss. Depressed teenagers may just be less communicative than usual, more withdrawn, and more irritable. Children with depression may have symptoms of abdominal pain, headaches, loss of appetite, and bedwetting. Dr. Martin Seligman, professor of psychology at the University of Pennsylvania and author of *Learned Optimism,* notes that depression is more prevalent in children nowadays, and that prevention is critical because "...we can't give Prozac to a whole generation."

DIAGNOSIS

There is no blood test or neuro-imaging test that can diagnose depression. Depression is typically identified when a certain cluster of symptoms has been present for at least one month. If a person has five of the eight symptoms listed below over that time period, he or she meets the criteria for depression, while four symptoms over the same time period indicate probable depression. The following criteria are taken from the *American Psychiatric Association Diagnostic and Statistical Manual of Mental Disorder (DSM-IV):*

- poor appetite with weight loss, or increased appetite with weight gain
- insomnia or hypersomnia (sleeping too much)
- loss of interest or pleasure in usual activities, or decrease in sexual drive
- loss of energy and feelings of fatigue
- feelings of worthlessness, self-reproach, or inappropriate guilt

- diminished ability to think or concentrate
- recurrent thoughts of death or suicide
- physical hyperactivity or inactivity

Dr. James Gordon, a psychiatrist in Washington, D.C., feels that depression is a signal that your life needs to be re-evaluated. He feels that you need to investigate *why* you are depressed, rather than just treating the symptom. Depression can indicate a problem in a belief system, physical health, lifestyle habits, or relationships with others. Dr. Gordon feels that if people take antidepressants, they will not learn what made them depressed, and other problems will develop from the same root cause.

CAUSES

There are many causes for depression and much controversy in both modern and alternative medicine about its causes. Even within these branches of medicine, there is disagreement about the roles that various factors play in depression. We have attempted to present the major causes of depression, and because there are overlaps, have roughly classified them within the belief systems of modern and alternative medicine.

Situational

Depression can be situational. It can be triggered by a death in the family, a divorce, serious financial problems, or loss of a job. Doctors and psychologists feel that if depression is not situational, it is related to a biochemical imbalance in neurotransmitters, which are also known as biogenic amines. These include serotonin, melatonin, dopamine, adrenaline (epinephrine), and noradrenaline (norepinephrine).

Drugs

Depression can be associated with taking certain drugs: oral contraceptives, corticosteroids, beta blockers and other blood pressure medications, cholesterol-lowering medications, H2 blocker medications, and antibiotics such as Cipro and Floxin. When used for a long period of time, antidepressants themselves can cause depression.

Some drugs cause nutrient deficiencies which then can cause depression. Oral contraceptives are a well-known cause of nutrient deficiencies (especially folic acid, vitamin B_{12}, riboflavin (B_2), pyridoxine (B_6), ascorbic acid, and zinc). Excess estrogen disrupts vitamin B_6, blood sugar metabolism, and tryptophan metabolism. Antidepressants can also cause depletion of certain nutrients.

Alcohol and cigarette smoking can cause depression. Alcohol is a known depressant, and in addition, it can cause nutrient deficiencies. Cigarette smoke contains nicotine, which stimulates increased secretion of adrenaline and cortisol. It also lowers levels of ascorbic acid (vitamin C).

Neurotransmitters

Neurotransmitters are chemicals that facilitate how the brain communicates internally and to other parts of the body. Neurotransmitters are manufactured in the body and are very closely linked to mood—in particular, the neurotransmitters serotonin, norepinephrine, and dopamine control mood. When the brain produces serotonin, tension eases, while norepinephrine and dopamine allow us to be more alert, and to act and think more quickly.

Serotonin is frequently found in reduced quantities in depressed patients. The amino acid tryptophan is the precursor for serotonin, and raising tryptophan levels raises the level of serotonin. The body makes serotonin from dietary tryptophan and requires vitamin B_6, magnesium, and other nutrients to do so. In 1989, tryptophan manufactured by one company for use as a nutritional supplement became contaminated in the manufacturing process, and caused the eosinophilic myalgia syndrome, in which a type of white blood cell (eosinophils) count is high and

muscle pain is experienced. Since then, the Food and Drug Administration (FDA) has banned over-the-counter tryptophan sales, and it is now sold only by prescription from compounding pharmacies, which formulate nonstandard medications. The pharmaceutical Prozac is widely used as a medication to raise serotonin levels. Prozac works by preventing the re-uptake of serotonin by nerve cells, thereby increasing the amount of the neurotransmitter that remains available.

Norepinephrine is very important to mood, because low levels of norepinephrine lead to generalized slowing and impairment of function, expressed as symptoms of depression. The amino acid L-phenylalanine is the precursor (a building block) for norepinephrine. Some people have greater mood improvement when they take L-phenylalanine together with vitamin B_6.

Dopamine, a precursor for norepinephrine, occurs primarily in the brain. The concentration of dopamine is directly related to the availability of dietary tyrosine. Dopamine and norepinephrine are part of the brain "reward system" that provides motivation. Lowered levels of these neurotransmitters are directly related to the lack of motivation that is common in depression.

Tyrosine is an amino acid that also functions as a neurotransmitter, and it improves mood, self-esteem, sleep patterns, and energy levels, and reduces anxiety. It increases the rate at which the brain produces dopamine and norepinephrine. Tyrosine is the precursor to dopamine, which is in turn a precursor to norepinephrine (noradrenaline) and epinephrine (adrenaline). However, it can push patients who are manic depressive into the manic state. Tyrosine is also the precursor to thyroid hormones.

Glutamine is an amino acid that improves mood and lightens depression. Glutamine is metabolized into two neurotransmitters: glutamic acid and GABA (gama-aminobutyric acid). GABA has a calming effect on the brain; levels of GABA are lower in depressed men as compared to controls. Supplementation with GABA improves memory and depression after strokes.

Modern medicine uses pharmaceuticals that act as antidepressants by crossing readily over the blood-brain barrier, affecting neurotransmitter levels. They prevent reuptake of the neurotransmitters produced by the brain, thus increasing their levels and helping the patient to feel less depressed. Most physicians believe that precursors to neurotransmitters, many of which are amino acids, cross over into the brain poorly and are not worthwhile supplementing. They also do not acknowledge that neurotransmitters or their building blocks can be depleted, and need to be replenished.

The alternative approach to treating depression is by increasing neurotransmitter manufacture by the body. Alternative practitioners use supplementation of amino acids, vitamins, and minerals to supply the building blocks that will allow the body to restore depleted precursors and to manufacture sufficient neurotransmitters. When neurotransmitter levels are sufficient and balanced, mood is elevated and depression lifts.

Hormonal

Many different hormones in the body can cause depression when there is an excess or deficiency of these hormones.

Hypothyroidism can cause depression, but in most people additional symptoms (cold intolerance, fatigue) ensure that the hypothyroidism is diagnosed and treated. Elderly people, however, often do not have other symptoms, and if they are depressed, they should be screened for hypothyroidism. Hyperthyroidism can also cause depression, but is a less common cause than hypothyroidism.

Sex hormones play a role in depression. Along with hot flashes, menopause can cause a depression (see p. 343 for more information on menopause). A deficiency of estrogen, proges-

terone, and testosterone can cause depression in women, and many women experience depression with hormonal changes related to their menstrual cycle (see p. 340–41 for information on PMS). Although it is less well known, both men and women can also suffer from depression if their testosterone level is low.

Some patients who are depressed have disorders of their adrenal system, with abnormal patterns of cortisol release. Steroids, even those made by the body, interfere with the metabolism of serotonin from tryptophan.

Nutrients

Although it is not commonly recognized by modern medicine, depression is one of the most common symptoms of any vitamin or nutrient deficiency. The Food and Drug Administration stated in 1986 that the average American diet contains less than 80 percent of the recommended daily allowance of one or more of the following nutrients: calcium, magnesium, iron, zinc, copper, and manganese. A study by Roubenoff reported in 1987 in the *Archives of Internal Medicine* found that 23 to 50 percent of patients admitted to hospitals had undiscovered nutrient deficiencies, and numerous other studies have verified nutrient deficiencies in the North American population.

Amino acids are nutrients, but also function as neurotransmitters that control mood. If one amino acid is deficient, it is likely that others are deficient as well. While amino acid deficiencies are not the leading cause of depression (food allergies and vitamin and mineral deficiencies are typically the more common causes of depression), they are usually accompanied by deficiencies of minerals and vitamins. When the mineral and vitamin deficiencies are corrected, the amino acid deficiency may correct itself. The most common mineral and vitamin deficiencies that affect amino acid metabolism are magnesium and vitamin B_6.

Folic acid deficiency, the most common nutrient deficiency in the world, is frequently seen in psychiatric patients, and is present even more often in elderly psychiatric patients. In one study, reported in the *British Journal of Psychiatry* in 1970, 25 percent of 100 consecutive patients admitted to hospital with depression had low serum folic acid levels.

Vitamin B_{12} or folic acid deficiency can occur without causing anemia and without causing an enlargement of the red blood cells. Vitamin B_{12} deficiency is often caused by a lack of a stomach enzyme known as intrinsic factor. It can also be caused by long-term use of H_2 acid blockers such as Tagamet and Zantac (see Peptic Ulcer Disease, p. 258).

A deficiency of vitamin B_1 can cause depression, a skin rash, and diarrhea. Vitamin B_6 is necessary to convert tryptophan into serotonin. It is also needed to convert the amino acid phenylalanine into tyrosine and then into norepinephrine.

Vitamin E is a potent antioxidant that protects the cell membrane and helps it to function properly. It decreases the turnover of serotonin and the loss of brain chemicals (such as ATP and glucose) that occur with stress and increase depression.

If vitamin C is deficient, the brain does not receive the signal to turn on the neurotransmitters that affect happiness. There are many people who eat little fresh fruit and vegetables and who are vitamin C deficient—but at a level without obvious symptoms such as scurvy.

Magnesium deficiency, which occurs in at least 80 percent of the North American population, can cause irritability, anxiety, agitation, and panic attacks. Stress causes a loss of magnesium, which in turn signals the brain to make more stress hormones.

Zinc deficiency is common worldwide, and zinc levels are lower in depressed patients than they are in study group controls. Zinc is a coenzyme (a substance needed for an enzyme to par-

ticipate in biochemical reactions) for the enzyme that is necessary for the production of norepinephrine from dopamine. People who are zinc deficient often have white spots on their fingernails.

Depression typically has more than one cause. If you find one cause and correct it, but still have some problems with low mood, examine other treatment options. If you take nutrients and feel better for weeks to months, then later do not feel well again, it is likely that you have uncovered a hidden nutrient deficiency.

Diet

Hypoglycemia can be a cause of depression, but this is not recognized by most physicians as valid. Some people do not have the acute symptoms of hypoglycemia, but nevertheless can develop dizziness, headache, confusion, emotional instability, depression, violent behavior, and poor concentration. Most people who have hypoglycemia have food allergies or hyperinsulinemia, and correcting the diet will help prevent these problems (see Food Allergy, pp. 385–86 and Hyperinsulinemia, pp. 235–36)

Food allergies or sensitivities can cause depression; wheat, milk, sugar, dyes and additives, MSG, and aspartame are common triggers for depression. Foods that contain mold antigens (fermented foods such as pickles and vinegar) can trigger depression, as can environmental molds and mold that occurs naturally in refrigerated foods that are several days old.

Caffeine causes a decrease of blood flow to the brain and can cause generalized anxiety, panic, depression, nervousness, heart palpitations, irritability, recurrent headaches, and twitching. In addition, it can cause hypoglycemia, and makes people more aware of their hypoglycemia symptoms.

The quality of your diet can affect depression, since neurotransmitters are controlled by what we eat. The typical North American habit of snacking on junk food, as well as the poor nutritional quality of much of the food we consume, are major contributors to depression.

Chemical Exposures

The effect of chemical exposures is controversial. Alternative physicians think that exposure to organic solvents or pesticides can trigger depression, as well as contributing to poor memory, anxiety, irritability, and loss of problem-solving capabilities in some people. Solvent exposure is most commonly experienced when new carpets are installed, new buildings are inhabited, or houses are remodelled.

Pesticide poisoning is usually chronic, and not always recognized as a trigger of mental changes. Dursban (chlorpyrifos), the most commonly used indoor and outdoor pesticide, inhibits conversion of tryptophan to serotonin. Dieldrin, another pesticide, depletes the neurotransmitters norepinephrine and dopamine. Toxic metals, such as lead, can also cause depression.

Seasonal Affective Disorder

Seasonal affective disorder (SAD) is a controversial disorder, related to the lack of sunshine during winter months. People with this disorder have normal moods during the summer months, but as the days become shorter in the fall they become more and more depressed. Food allergies, carbohydrate craving, and nutritional deficiencies are commonly associated with SAD. (See Light Therapy in chapter 10, Alternative Therapies.)

Diseases

Arteriosclerosis that affects the arteries in the brain (or those that go to the brain) can cause depression, and elevated homocysteine is one cause of arteriosclerosis (see Heart Disease, p. 182).

Depression also accompanies other diseases, including ankylosing spondylitis, cancer, fibromyalgia, lupus, and others. Most people assume that the disease is the cause of the depression, but for some people the depression preceded the illness.

MODERN MEDICAL TREATMENT

Modern medical care deals with depression by checking for a medically recognized cause for the condition. If such a specific cause is found, patients are told to take appropriate action: for example, they may be told to stop taking medications that are known to cause depression. In general, however, people are told to take an antidepressant.

Drug Therapy

The major treatment for depression offered by modern medicine is the prescription of antidepressants. The first antidepressants were the monoamine oxidase (MAO) inhibitors, which are enzymes that help break down some of the neurotransmitters. This raises the levels of gamma-aminobutyric acid (GABA), an inhibitory neurotransmitter that has a calming effect on the brain (see Insomnia, p. 438). MAO inhibitors include medications such as phenelzine (Nardil) and tranylcypromine (Parnate) and they can have serious side effects. The most dangerous is a hypertensive crisis (extremely high blood pressure), which can cause bleeding in the brain and may be life-threatening. Symptoms of hypertensive crises are a headache in the back of the head that may radiate to the front, palpitations, neck stiffness or soreness, nausea, vomiting, sweating (sometimes with fever and sometimes with cold, clammy skin), dilated pupils, constricting chest pain, and sensitivity to light.

People taking MAO inhibitors have to avoid pickled herring, liver, dry sausage, fava bean pods, sauerkraut, cheese, yogurt, beer and wine, yeast extract, excessive amounts of chocolate and caffeine, and cold and cough preparations. They must also avoid nasal decongestants, hay fever medications, asthma inhalers, weight-reducing preparations, and tryptophan, because these substances can trigger high blood pressure. Certain prescriptions and other drugs also have to be avoided. These include narcotics, alcohol, adrenaline, amphetamines, cocaine, and methylphenidate (Ritalin), which can also cause high blood pressure. MAO inhibitors combined with fluoxetine (Prozac) have caused high body temperature, rigidity, and uncontrolled muscle movement.

The next group of antidepressants to be developed were the tricyclic antidepressants, including imipramine (Tofranil), amitriptyline (Elavil), amoxapine (Asendin), doxepin (Sinequan), and trazodone (Desyrel). Tricyclic antidepressants are potent antihistamines, as much as 100 to 200 times more potent than most marketed antihistamines. Tricyclic antidepressants inhibit the mechanisms responsible for the uptake of norepinephrine and serotonin in their respective nerve cells, resulting in increased levels of these neurotransmitters. They also raise dopamine levels. They cannot be given with MAO inhibitors, as the combination can precipitate a hypertensive crisis or an attack of glaucoma. In high doses, tricyclic antidepressant drugs can produce heart rhythm disturbances, fast heart rates, heart attacks, and stroke. Several children taking tricyclic antidepressants have died suddenly, apparently from heart rhythm disturbances.

Tricyclic antidepressants can also cause seizures, hallucinations, tremors, high fever, urinary retention (especially in men with enlarged prostates), disturbed concentration, problems with memory, numbness, sensitization of the skin to the sun, nausea, abdominal pain, mouth sores, diarrhea, enlarged breasts in the male, impotence, elevated blood sugar levels, and weight gain (or loss). Overdoses (which may be taken by suicidal patients) can cause heart rhythm disturbances, convulsions, low blood pressure, muscle rigidity, vomiting, high fever, coma, and death.

Bupropion (Wellbutrin) is an antidepressant related to phenylethylamine, a chemical related to the active ingredient in chocolate. Wellbutrin raises norepinephrine and dopamine levels. Its side effects can include seizures, agitation, dry mouth, insomnia, headache, nausea, tremor, changes in mental status, and electrocardiogram abnormalities.

The most recent class of antidepressants to be developed is the selective serotonin-reuptake inhibitors (SSRI), such as fluoxetine (Prozac), sertraline (Zoloft), and paroxetine hydrochloride (Paxil). This new class of antidepressants, developed in the 1980s, is related to the tricyclic antidepressants, and their action blocks the reuptake of serotonin. Side effects can include nervousness, insomnia, fatigue, diarrhea, headache, sweating, chest pain, painful menstruation, tremor, stuffy nose, dizziness, increased appetite, hypothyroidism, blackouts, impaired judgment, abnormal dreams, agitation, impotence, loss of appetite, activation of mania, seizures, and suicide. These drugs can also cause rapidly cycling bipolar disorder, and can have serious side effects if used in conjunction with MAO inhibitors.

In its first year on the market, the amount spent on Prozac was more than the total sum spent annually by Americans on all other antidepressants combined. However, in a double-blind placebo-controlled study, Prozac performed no better than the other antidepressants, and the benefits of Prozac were shown to decrease over time. Prozac and other SSRIs are used more frequently than the tricyclic antidepressants simply because they do not have the annoying side effects of the other classes of antidepressants (such as dry mouth and urinary retention) and they often work faster. There have been more than 28,000 reports of adverse reactions to Prozac in North America. More than 1,885 patients on Prozac have attempted suicide. As well, 1,734 people on the drug had died as of September 1995. (The cause of these deaths is not known.)

Effexor belongs to a new class of drugs. It raises both serotonin and norepinephrine levels by blocking their reuptake. It also blocks the reuptake of dopamine, but more weakly, and it does not have MAO inhibitor activity. Psychiatrists refer to it as "side effexor" because of all the side effects that it causes. These can include headaches, chills, chest pain, sweating, nausea, constipation, dry mouth, sleepiness, sexual dysfunction, frequent accidental injury, migraine headaches, difficulty swallowing, swallowing of air, burping, swelling of the hands and feet, weight gain, emotional lability, dizziness, clenching of the jaw, bronchitis, shortness of breath, abnormal vision, ear pain, blood in the urine, pain with urination, and vaginitis.

If you are taking antidepressants and want to switch to an alternative treatment, do not suddenly stop taking the drugs. Instead, gradually wean yourself from them with the help of a qualified health professional as you begin the alternative treatment. *Caution: If you have suicidal thoughts, seek help immediately from a qualified medical practitioner.*

Electroconvulsant Therapy
In rare cases, people are given electroconvulsant therapy for severe depression that does not respond to the typical antidepressants. Although used more extensively in the past, this therapy is now not common, and is used less than 10 percent of the time.

Cognitive Therapy
Pessimists are people who believe that there will always be trouble and that the fault is often theirs. This can lead to feelings of helplessness and depression, and cognitive therapy is useful in dealing with this type of depression. Cognitive therapy teaches coping skills that allow people to turn pessimism into optimism.

Dr. Martin Seligman formulated the theory of "learned helplessness," which says that the experience of failure causes people to feel that they cannot accomplish their goals, and therefore that they should avoid new or challenging situations. He and other psychiatrists practice cognitive therapy based on the following ABCDE model to combat this type of depression: Adversity (a negative event); Belief (the person's interpretation of the event); Consequences (how you feel and behave following an event); Disputation (arguments you make to yourself to counter the negative event); and Energization (the emotional and behavioral consequences of the Disputation). Using this model, people learn how to alter their responses to negative events.

ALTERNATIVE TREATMENT
Alternative medicine takes a multi-faceted approach to depression, based largely on supporting the body in manufacturing the neurotransmitters that induce a sense of well-being. However, some people entering therapy are so depressed that they cannot follow a healing program until their depression lessens. For those people, an antidepressant is prescribed on a temporary basis.

Diet
Because pesticides can affect the brain, include as much organic food in your diet as possible. Avoid sugar, refined flour, alcohol, tea, coffee, soda, chocolate, and processed foods, all of which are capable of causing depression. Avoid wheat also, because gluten has been linked to depressive disorders.

Eat complex carbohydrates to increase serotonin levels. Protein meals containing essential fatty acids will increase alterness. Eat foods high in tryptophan and protein, such as nuts, salmon, and turkey. To avoid the mild depression seen in people with low folic acid levels, eat spinach, dark green leafy vegetables, okra, kale, and beans, all of which are high in folic acid.

Drink only filtered or bottled water because city water that is chlorinated and fluoridated can be harmful.

Exercise and Lifestyle

Exercise, if done often and vigorously, will counteract depression. If possible, exercise outside for 30 minutes (or long enough to increase the heart rate by 50 percent) five times a week.

Keeping your knees bent, stand up and pump your arms up and down as you breathe in and out. Breathe through your nose as deeply as possible and focus completely on the act of breathing. Do this every morning for 5 to 10 minutes to increase energy levels.

Because balancing the body's energy is helpful in combating depression, try practicing Tai Chi or Qigong, or go through a daily yoga routine.

Stop smoking and avoid nicotine in all forms.

You can boost your own natural serotonin in a variety of ways: exercise; play a board game; talk to people who give you unconditional support; sit near water, especially running water; have sex or masturbate.

Nutrient Therapy

If possible, have vitamin and mineral assays performed at the appropriate labs that specialize in this type of testing. Supplement any nutrients that are at low levels. If an assay is too costly or not easily available, undertake a trial of any of the following nutrients that are appropriate.

Start with:

- magnesium – 400 mg a day (needed to convert tryptophan to serotonin)
- vitamin B_6 – 50 to 500 mg a day (needed to convert tryptophan to serotonin)

- B-complex – as directed on your product (for stress; to balance other B vitamins)

If you do not feel better, then add the following:

- vitamin A – 5,000 to 10,000 IU a day. *Caution:* Do not take more than 8,000 IU a day if you are or might be pregnant (helps to balance blood sugar and is an antioxidant).
- vitamin C – 1,000 to 8,000 mg a day (turns on neurotransmitters that affect happiness)
- vitamin E – 400 to 500 IU a day (decreases turnover of serotonin and loss of brain chemicals from stress)

If you do not continue to improve, add any of the following nutrients that will help your symptoms:

- vitamin B_{12} nasal spray – 250 to 1,000 mcg a day (reverses depression with memory loss and violent tendencies)
- folic acid – 400 mcg three times a day (reverses depression, particularly in people with heart disease)
- N-acetyl or L-carnitine – 250 to 500 mg twice a day (improves depression; boosts mood and disposition; vitalizes energy; improves memory, emotion, and alertness)
- PhosChol – 1 tsp. a day (precursor for acetyl-choline, a neurotransmitter that affects moods (American Lecithin Company—see Sources)
- L-glutamine – 500 mg twice a day between meals (precursor to glutamic acid and GABA, which are neurotransmitters; improves mood and lightens depression)
- coenzyme Q_{10} – 30 to 60 mg three times a day (provides energy to brain)
- glutathione – 10 to 50 mg a day in three divided doses (antioxidant; detoxifies chemicals)
- cold-pressed flaxseed oil – start with 1 tsp. a day and build up to 1 Tbsp. a day (needed

for proper functioning of cell membrane receptors)
- pycnogenol or grape pips – 200 to 300 mg two to three times a day (detoxifies chemicals)
- Norival—BH4 (tetrahydrobiopterin) – one to two capsules a day (functions as a coenzyme in the synthesis of several neurotransmitters) (Cardiovascular Research—see Sources). Or take tyrosine – 500 mg a day (improves mood, self-esteem, energy levels, and reduces anxiety; works best with lethargy and listlessness).
- tryptophan – start with 500 mg twice a day and build up to 6,000 mg a day as needed (precursor for serotonin, which helps nervousness and agitation)
- methionine – 500 mg twice a day (precursor to taurine, deficiency of which can cause depression; toxifies chemicals). Or take SAM (S-adenosylmethionine) – 400 mg orally twice a day (acts as an antidepressant).
- phenylalanine – 500 mg twice a day (precursor to norepinephrine; improves mood; works best with lethargy and listlessness)
- evening primrose oil – two capsules three times a day (for mental depression)
- DNZ-2 (dimethyl aminoethanol or deanol) – use 100 to 250 mg capsules to build up to the tolerated dose (increases action of acetylcholine; improves memory and fatigue) (Bio-Tech—see Sources)

The following combinations of nutrients are also helpful for depression:

- DLPA – 500 to 1,500 mg in the morning on awakening (together with 500 mg of vitamin C, 100 mg of vitamin B$_6$, and a small piece of fruit or fruit juice. Wait at least 45 minutes before eating breakfast. This can be taken even if you are on an SSRI medication.) (precursor to synthesis of neurotransmitters that increase wakefulness and energy)
- Emotional Aid Formula – contains St. John's wort, acetyl-L-tyrosine, B$_{12}$, methionine, and folic acid (Atkins Nutritionals, Inc.—see Sources)

If your depression is related to hypoglycemia or hyperglycemia, be sure to take the following nutrients, all of which stabilize blood sugar:

- chromium – 200 mcg one to two times a day (helps to control blood sugar)
- zinc – 30 mg a day (deficiency has been associated with problems with sugar metabolism; needed as a coenzyme to convert dopamine to norepinephrine)
- manganese – 10 to 15 mg a day (needed for repair of the pancreas; cofactor in enzymes for glucose metabolism)

Herbal Therapy
If the following botanical supplements do not relieve your depression, seek the help of a trained herbalist.

- cayenne – (should be used in gradually increasing doses, as your stomach tolerates, in capsules or as a food spice) triggers endorphin release by the brain; causes mild euphoria
- ginkgo – inhibits MAO
- kava kava – induces calm and relieves depression. Reduce dose if drowsiness occurs.
- Ma-Huang – for lethargic depression. *Caution:* Do not use this herb if you have anxiety disorder, glaucoma, heart disease, or insomnia, or if you are taking an MAO inhibitor.
- sage – for depression, nervous conditions, or trembling
- St. John's wort – inhibits monoamine oxidase (MAO). It may take a month to six weeks to start working.
- valerian root – for insomnia

Homeopathic Remedies
For serious depression, consult a homeopathic physician to determine the best remedy for you.

For mild, transient depression, try the remedy that best fits your symptoms. If you do not obtain relief, seek professional help from a trained homeopath.

- *Aurum metallicum* – disgusted with life and talks of committing suicide; oversensitive to noise; peevish at the least contradiction; feels no connection to life, existing in a dark and isolated void; people are very intense, idealistic, want to be the best, and set high goals; can be devastated by grief and disappointed love relations; deep religious convictions; desire for meditation and deep spiritual longings; suicidal impulses as jumping from a height or driving at break-neck speeds in a car, with an impulse to turn into oncoming traffic; outbursts of anger; everything seems sad and dark, as if there were a black cloud over everything; deep lover of music; anorexia.
- *Ignatia* – melancholic; full of contradictions, tearful, sighs a lot; element of spasticity and hysteria in the grief state; primarily a remedy for women; romantic and idealistic in dealing with the world; bitterness and hardness result from disappointments; oversensitive with easily hurt feelings; often difficult or even impossible to release the emotions that remain cramped inside, leading to defensiveness and causing the patient to act in a rude, suspicious, or challenging manner; lump in the throat; desire to avoid crying giving way to sobbing; aversion to consolation; stormy relationships filled with recrimination; grief occurs with shock after a loss, especially of a child, parent, friend, or pet.
- *Lycopodium* – extreme sadness in the morning on waking; loss of self-confidence; afraid to be alone; extreme apprehension; problems of self-esteem and low confidence; bullying, domineering, arrogant behavior to family and those with less authority; intellectual and withdrawn; depression and anxiety about health, conflicts, and career; weeps from sentimental events or upon being thanked; main fear is of people; sometimes patient becomes bombastic, egotistical, bragging, acting extroverted and assertive.
- *Natrum muriaticum* – depression because of a chronic illness; consolation makes the patient worse; closed, responsible, dignified, and much affected by grief; too serious and overly proper and responsible; easily offended or wounded; sad, yet unable to weep or involuntary and hysterical weeping; dwells on past griefs and humiliations; perfectionistic; sensitive to noise and music; uses alcohol to loosen inhibition; a new loss awakens the unexpressed sadness that originated from other losses that have not been dealt with.
- *Phosphoric acid* – remedy for grief, especially when the patient becomes overwhelmed by loss and is unable to respond – almost dead inside; becomes weak, apathetic, slow to answer, fatigued, and drained; patient is flat, indifferent or even lifeless; mental weakness after grief; wants to lie and watch TV.
- *Pulsatilla* – sad and cries easily; changeable, contradictory moods; much better out of doors; frequently weeps when talking about problems; strong desire for tenderness and reassurance; emotional, yet the moods are changeable; can become irritable; sadness, worse in warm room, worse before the period; feels forsaken, desires and ameliorated by consolation; feels much better after a good cry; depression can be caused by a loss, jealousy, or betrayal.

If you are unable to identify a homeopathic remedy that seems to match your symptoms, try a complex homeopathic remedy. PHP Anti-Depression Drops assist in recovery from and prevention of recurrent depression (see Sources).

Other Therapeutic Measures
Be tested by an alternative practitioner to identify any physical conditions that may be con-

tributing to depression. Assess toxic metal burden with hair mineral analysis, which is the most accurate test for this problem (see Sources). Undertake a detoxification program if a problem is found.

Find an environmental medicine physician to test you for food, mold, and chemical sensitivities. If you do have sensitivities, avoid the substances that can be avoided, be treated for those that cannot, and make any necessary environmental changes. Also have this physician test you to determine whether you have a neurotransmitter problem, and undergo treatment if needed. Have NAET treatments for your allergies.

Consider consulting an Ayurvedic practitioner.

Have a regular reflexology session, working either on yourself, or with the help of a practitioner. Have acupuncture, massage, or get a chiropractic treatment. Have NET treatments (see Chiropractic section in chapter 9, Alternative Medical Disciplines).

Use acupressure at the following points:

- two thumbs' width up from the palm wrist crease, toward the elbow, directly in the center between the two tendons
- three thumbs' width below the joint under the kneecap, lying on the outer side of the knee
- in between the tendons of the big toe and the second toe, two thumbs' width toward the top of the foot from the web.

If you have SAD, use special intense lights that duplicate bright daylight to treat it, and/or take melatonin at night (1 to 2 mg). Get out in the sun for half an hour each day, with no sunglasses and without sunscreen. (See Light Therapy in chapter 10, Alternative Therapies.)

Get counseling, but also use self-help tools to release any anger, hate, and fear. There are many of these tools available in self-help books and audiotapes, and actively using them can make counseling more effective. Practice reframing situations to discover the positive side of things. Be sure to laugh each day, and give and receive hugs daily. Meditate or pray regularly. Try sound therapy, using the type of music that lifts your spirits.

Take a flower remedy: fill a one-ounce brown bottle (to protect the mixture from light) with spring water and add several drops of up to four essences from the following list. Take several drops four times a day.

- gentian for hopelessness and despair, for worry or sorrow over small difficulties, or for depression following a long-term problem (for instance, unemployment)
- hornbeam if you are feeling blue and gloomy, or experience mental weariness
- mustard for deep depression with no apparent cause, and for dark but passing moods
- gorse if there are feelings of despair or despondency, or a sense of the inevitability of trouble or pain
- sweet chestnut for mental anguish and a feeling that the limits of endurance have been reached
- elm if you are feeling overwhelmed.

PANIC DISORDER

Each year, more people experience a panic disorder attack than have strokes, seizures, or AIDS. More than three million North American adults will have at least one panic attack at some point in life. Because symptoms of panic disorder mimic those of many other medical conditions, the disorder often goes undiagnosed. This is especially unfortunate because panic attacks can be prevented in most patients by the use of medication, nutrients, homeopathic remedies, or flower essences.

Panic attacks are episodes of sudden, extreme anxiety that erupt for no apparent reason. Symptoms of panic disorder include: difficulty breathing; dizziness or lightheadedness; racing or pounding heartbeat; trembling or shaking; sweating; choking; nausea or abdominal distress; numbness or tingling sensation in the hands; chills or hot flashes; weakness; chest pains; terror; feelings of unreality or being detached from oneself, dreamlike sensations or perceptual distortions; fear of dying; fear of losing control or fear of doing something embarrassing; fear of becoming insane; or a sense of impending doom. If you have at least four of these symptoms, you may be having a panic attack. On the other hand, you may be experiencing a major medical illness such as hyperthyroidism, stroke, or heart attack. Go to a physician or an emergency room at once for a diagnosis and treatment.

During a panic attack, people may feel the urge to flee, or the need to escape. People feel that something terrible might happen, that they may be dying or having a heart attack, suffocating, or losing control. People worry about these episodes and fear having another one—which often causes them to avoid places or situations that they think might have triggered an attack.

Patients with panic disorder often develop a fear of crowds (agoraphobia) and are unable to leave their homes. Panic disorder predisposes people to depression, substance abuse, obsessive-compulsive disorder, bipolar mood disorder, post-traumatic stress disorder, migraine headaches, asthma, and irritable bowel syndrome. They have a low tolerance for the body's normal physiological and psychological response to stress.

Some people have a great fear of being embarrassed or humiliated in a social situation. This is termed social phobia and can cause panic attacks. Nervous anticipation is normal the first time you do something new, and some degree of fear can provide positive energy to do your best. However, people with social phobia have intense anxiety and experience enormous dread before the feared event. They will be uncomfort-

able throughout the event and may have unpleasant feelings that linger afterward. One of the most common social phobias is the fear of speaking or performing in public; stage fright is a type of panic attack that can affect public performers, politicians, and public speakers.

Panic attacks often occur with no apparent trigger; they can even occur during sleep. Patients with panic disorder may go to the emergency department repeatedly, since the attacks can mimic heart attacks, heart rhythm abnormalities, mitral valve prolapse, hyperthyroidism, seizure disorder, respiratory problems, neurological disease, or gastrointestinal disease. Panic attacks sometimes occur for the first time within six months of stressful life events (the death of a loved one, divorce, moving, childbirth, or surgery), which appear to act as triggers. Large doses of caffeine, some cold medicines, cocaine, and marijuana can also trigger panic attacks.

Panic disorder tends to get worse if not treated. Anxiety and prolonged stress deplete the body of the nutrients it needs to make its own tranquilizers. Food allergies can also trigger panic attacks (see Food Allergy, pp. 385–86) as can sleep apnea (see Insomnia, pp. 435–36).

Dr. Robert Atkins, of the Atkins Center for Complementary Medicine in New York, states that 60 percent of patients who have panic attacks can be cured by correcting low blood sugar. Dr. Alan Gaby, of Bastyr University in Seattle, Washington, also notes that hypoglycemia is a common trigger for anxiety (see Hypoglycemia, pp. 241–42). As blood sugar levels drop suddenly, the body releases hormones that cause the heart and breathing rate to increase, and the patient experiences heart palpitations, sweating, hunger, irritability, tendency to fatigue easily, tense muscles, nausea, and shakiness. Dr. Atkins recommends first getting a glucose-insulin tolerance test. If this shows no abnormalities, then have a thyroid test (see Thyroid section in chapter 18, Metabolic Disorders).

ANXIETY

Many people do not have full-blown panic attacks, but do have anxiety disorders. Generalized anxiety disorder (GAD) is a chronic and exaggerated tendency to tension and worry with little or no provocation. It can be associated with mild depression. Anxiety disorder is the most common of all mental health problems: more than 65 million North Americans experience anxiety symptoms in any given year.

Anxiety can present as shortness of breath, rapid shallow breathing, fatigue, headaches, forgetfulness, nausea, twitching or trembling, palpitations, dizziness, and sweating. Other symptoms include blackouts, hot flashes, rectal bleeding, a racing pulse that will not slow, sweaty palms, chronic back and neck pain, chronic or severe headaches, hives, overwhelming anxiety, and insomnia. These symptoms may occur episodically, or they may be chronic.

Generalized, persistent anxiety is defined by the *American Psychiatric Association's Diagnostic and Statistical Manual III* as anxiety of continuous duration lasting for at least one month, with symptoms from at least three of the following four categories:

- Motor tensions: shakiness, jitteriness, jumpiness, trembling, tension, muscle aches, easily fatigued, inability to relax, strained face, restlessness, easily startled, fidgeting, eyelid twitching, furrowed brow.
- Autonomic hyperactivity: sweating, heart pounding or racing, cold clammy hands, dry mouth, dizziness, lightheadedness, tingling in the hands or feet, upset stomach, hot or cold spells, frequent urination, diarrhea, discomfort in the pit of the stomach, lump in the throat, flushing, pallor, high resting pulse rate, and high respiration rate.
- Apprehensive expectation: anxiety, worry, fear, rumination, and anticipation of misfortune to self or others.

- Vigilance and scanning: hyperattentiveness resulting in distractibility, difficulty in concentrating, insomnia, feeling "on edge," irritability, impatience.

STRESS

The most common trigger of anxiety is stress: a reaction to a stimulus that upsets normal functioning and disturbs mental or physical health. Between 70 and 80 percent of visits to physicians are for stress-related disorders, while almost 60 percent of women say stress is their number one problem. The most important point to remember is that stress itself is not the problem; the real issue is how a person *reacts* to stress. Some anxiety is normal, and helps to protect us in dangerous situations, but for some people too much stress can cause the disabling symptoms noted above. Anxiety can cause those effects when a person responds to situations that do not pose real threats with the biochemical changes of the "fight or flight response," releasing epinephrine (adrenaline) and other hormones that increase the heart rate and speed up breathing.

Stressors can include job pressures, deadlines, financial pressures, a new marriage, a job promotion, divorce, exposure to heat or cold, environmental toxins, physical trauma, nutritional deficiencies, substance abuse, toxins produced by microorganisms, and strong emotional reactions.

Stress triggers biological changes known as the general adaptation syndrome. As elucidated by the late Dr. Hans Selye (a physiologist who was Director of the Institute of Experimental Medicine and Surgery at the University of Montreal), there are three phases of the general adaptation syndrome: alarm, resistance, and exhaustion. The first response to stress is the alarm or "fight or flight reaction," which is stimulated by the release of epinephrine. The resistance phase allows the body to continue to counteract a stressor after the flight or fight response has worn off. The hormones secreted in this phase include corticosteroids, which stimulate the conversion of protein to energy, and mineralocorticoids, which help the body retain sodium to maintain appropriate blood pressure. In the alarm and resistance stages, the adrenal glands will be overactive. This will cause high blood pressure, anxiety, depression, elevated blood sugar, and elevated cholesterol levels.

Eventually chronic stress depletes the body's resources and its ability to adapt, and the last stage of the general adaptation syndrome is therefore exhaustion. Specific organs may collapse or the body functions may totally collapse. Hormones like cortisone, a glucocorticoid, become depleted. Potassium ions are lost, and this causes poor functioning and eventual death of the cells. Cancer or heart disease often develop.

EFFECTS OF ANXIETY

Chronic anxiety can worsen other health problems. Anxious people are five times more likely to develop colds. Anxiety can lead to high blood pressure, heart attacks, alcoholism, workaholism, other addictions, eating disorders, low self-esteem, emotional dependence, overconcern for others, premenstrual syndrome, and headaches. It may lead to broken relationships, violence, and emotional withdrawal.

MODERN MEDICAL TREATMENT
Drug Therapy
Allopathic medical doctors treat patients with anxiety by prescribing an antidepressant (a selective serotonin-reuptake inhibitor, MAO inhibitor, or tricyclic antidepressant), or anti-anxiety agent (for example, Valium or Buspar). If anxiety is provoked by an impending public event (such as a stage performance), they may prescribe a beta blocker (such as propranolol).

Anti-anxiety agents (benzodiazepines such as Xanax and Valium) are often used in combination with some forms of antidepressants because they have a rapid onset of action, while many antidepressants take three to six weeks to achieve a therapeutic effect.

Benzodiazepines have a rapid onset of action, and can treat anticipatory anxiety or panic. However, they can have a sedative effect and cause psychomotor impairment, and they interact with alcohol. Some of these side effects go away after four to six weeks of treatment, but 15 percent of patients stop taking benzodiazepines because of their side effects. Physical dependence is very common, and withdrawal symptoms or recurrence of panic symptoms occur as dosages are reduced. Withdrawal from Xanax is particularly difficult because it wears off rapidly, so that people become anxious again and take more. Benzodiazepines should be used cautiously in patients who have a history of drug dependence (see Insomnia, pp. 438, regarding other side effects of benzodizepines.)

When tricyclic antidepressants are prescribed, the dosage needs to be increased gradually. These antidepressants have a low risk of dependence. Side effects include low blood pressure, overstimulation, and weight gain. Up to 35 percent of patients stop treatment due to side effects before they receive therapeutic benefits (see Depression for other side effects of antidepressants).

The MAO inhibitors have a low risk of dependence, but can cause sexual difficulties, especially problems achieving orgasm. They also lower blood pressure and induce weight gain. Patients taking MAO inhibitors must be very careful about their diet (see pp. 409–10).

Buspirone (Buspar) is an anti-anxiety agent that is not chemically related to the benzodiazepines or barbiturates. It can cause dizziness, drowsiness, nausea, dry mouth, headaches, non-specific chest pain, dream disturbances, ringing in the ears, sore throat, nasal congestion, impotence, or nervousness.

COGNITIVE BEHAVIORAL THERAPY

Cognitive behavioral therapy is often recommended for anxiety. This form of therapy teaches patients to identify, anticipate, and prepare for situations and bodily sensations that may trigger panic attacks. Patients are taught to become less sensitive to inappropriate bodily sensations and feelings of terror, and learn breathing exercises that prevent hyperventilation. Patients must be motivated to learn this, because it takes a lot of practice. Cognitive behavioral therapy to deal with panic attacks typically requires 8 to 12 weeks to complete.

ALTERNATIVE TREATMENT

Diet
Alternative approaches to dealing with anxiety focus first on diet control. Eat a low-carbohydrate diet if you have hypoglycemia. Eat foods high in potassium (vegetables and fruits) to help support the adrenal gland—make sure you eat 3,000 to 5,000 mg of potassium a day.

Avoid using caffeine and sugar. Caffeine is often a factor in anxiety; for some people, even a small amount of caffeine may cause problems.

If you have other symptoms as well as anxiety (migraine headaches, joint pains, or nasal congestion), arrange to be tested and treated for food allergies.

Exercise and Lifestyle
Exercise regularly to help keep stress levels low. Stretch and massage tight muscles. Try a yoga class, or practice Tai Chi or Qigong.

Avoid the use of tobacco, alcohol, and drugs, all of which can increase anxiety.

Be sure you do activities you enjoy. Take a walk, or do a craft. Restructure your lifestyle to include calming activities.

Nutrient Therapy
Use the following nutrients to help control anxiety and panic attacks.

- multiple vitamin and mineral supplement – as directed on the label of your product (provides all needed nutrients in balance)
- B-complex – 50 mg of each B a day (promotes relaxation; controls jittery nerves)
- niacinamide – 1,000 mg three times a day (promotes relaxation; regulates adrenal hormones). *Caution:* With this dose have liver tests periodically, as excessive amounts of niacinamide can cause liver problems.
- vitamin B_6 – 250 mg a day (exerts a calming effect; important in the production of certain brain chemicals)
- vitamin B_{12} – 1,000 mcg a day (combats fatigue, insomnia, jittery nerves)
- vitamin C – 1,000 mg a day (for proper function of adrenal glands and brain chemistry)
- pantothenic acid – 250 mg three times a day (for proper functioning of nervous system and adrenal glands)
- calcium citrate or lactate – 800 to 1,000 mg a day (balances magnesium; calming effect)
- chromium – 200 mcg twice a day (increases energy and endurance; prevents overeating)
- magnesium aspartate, citrate, or glycinate – 400 to 800 mg a day (also helps support the adrenal gland; combats muscle tension and lifts mood; deficiencies linked to irritability and depression)
- zinc picolinate – 30 mg a day (for proper immune and digestive function; depleted by stress)
- gamma-aminobutyric acid (GABA) – 500 to 4,000 mg a day (tranquilizing effect)
- glutamine – 500 mg one to three times a day (improves mood and depression; precursor for GABA)
- glycine – 500 mg one to three times a day (improves central nervous system function)
- inositol – 1,000 to 3,000 mg a day (tranquilizing effect)

Take Anxiety Control – two to four capsules twice a day. This product is specifically formulated to control anxiety and contains GABA, glycine, glutamine, vitamin B$_6$, and magnesium in optimal proportions. It is available from the Pain and Stress Therapy Center in San Antonio (see Sources).

Herbal Therapy

Use one of the following botanical supplements to help control mild anxiety. If you do not obtain relief quickly, or if you have severe anxiety problems, seek the help of a qualified herbalist.

- elm – reduces feeling of being overwhelmed
- kava kava – mild muscle relaxant; helps anxiety and insomnia
- Korean or Chinese ginseng *(Panax ginseng)* – reduces feelings of anxiety and fatigue
- passion flower – calming, relaxing, tranquilizing, but not sedating
- Siberian ginseng *(Eleutherococcus senticosus)* – protects against effects of physical and mental stress
- spicy floral and apple – lower blood pressure and heart rate
- valerian root – treats anxiety, sleepiness, muscle tension
- ylang ylang – relaxing; balances extreme emotions, including anger and fear

Homeopathic Remedies

Consult a homeopathic physician to help you find the best remedy for your anxiety.

- *Aconite* – acute anxiety with agonizing terrors and fear of death; frequent palpitations, patient is inconsolable and restless.
- *Argentum nitricum* – anticipatory anxiety, with diarrhea; hurried, irritable, nervous, and lacking in self-confidence; for pre-exam nerves.

- *Arsenicum album* – intense anxiety with great restlessness; fear something terrible will happen, worse after midnight; fastidious, exacting and fault-finding.
- *Calcarea carbonica* – the patient thinks he has done something wrong; uneasy and anxious with palpitations; fears loss of reason.
- *Natrum muriaticum* – anxious about everything and has anxious dreams; patient is certain something terrible will happen; dwells on past griefs and humiliations, perfectionistic; averse to consolation; uses alcohol to loosen inhibition, bites fingernails.
- *Pulsatilla* – anxiety after bad news or an emotional upset; patient is weepy, touchy, and needs company; feels better in open air or in breezes; soft, timid, easily influenced and dependent; changeable moods; desires consolation.

Other Therapeutic Measures

Be tested and treated for allergies by an environmental medicine physician, as allergic reactions to many different substances can manifest as panic attacks or generalized anxiety. Have NAET treatments for allergy.

There are many self-help tools that can help to relieve anxiety and panic attacks. You can practice meditation, biofeedback, or progressive relaxation.

Progressive relaxation is an easy technique to learn: a muscle is contracted forcefully for one to two seconds, and then relaxed. (You can start by contracting the muscles of the face and neck, or the toes.) Contract as many of the muscle groups in the body as possible, one at a time; repeat two or three times.

Have bodywork done, as emotions are often stored in muscles. Old or repressed emotions associated with physical or emotional trauma can be released through massage. Have NET treatments.

Take a hot bath, using essential oils.
Use acupressure to relieve anxiety:

- Press on the temples (or press in the indentation of your breastbone at the level of your heart) and hold for two minutes while you take long, slow, deep breaths.
- Press on the crease of the inner wrist (in line with the smallest finger) for anxiety and stage fright, but avoid deep stimulation.
- Press on an imaginary line drawn between the crown of the inner ankle and the tip of the heel, the width of two thumbs from the tip of the heel.

Use breathing techniques to release stress. Dr. Robert Ivker, author of *Thriving* and president of the American Holistic Medical Association, states that forming healthy breathing habits is likely to produce the greatest relief of anxiety. Most people take shallow breaths when they are stressed, only filling the top part of their lungs with oxygen. Dr. Ivker suggests the following one-minute exercise be carried out daily for three weeks to increase the amount of oxygen you receive.

1. Sit in a chair, with your feet flat on the floor. Hold your back straight, and place your palms on your thighs.
2. Inhale through your nose, breathing deeply and expanding your abdomen.
3. In a continuous breath, imagine filling your chest and lungs. Feel your chest expand fully and your shoulders rise slightly.
4. Exhale slowly through your nose, taking longer than you did to inhale. Exhale completely, pulling in your stomach.
5. Repeat steps 1 through 4 for one minute or longer.

Dr. Andrew Weil has also developed a useful breathing exercise (see p. 225).

Learn about your physical symptoms, and try to let go of your worry about them, knowing that the sensations will pass. Think, "I can handle this. This is anxiety, and it won't hurt me." Reduce panic attacks by doing the following:

- Look for a pattern in your panic attacks.
- If you have recognizable warning signs of a panic attack, stop them before they begin: eat, count, sing, breathe deeply.
- Pause and relax before responding to something. This helps you feel in control.
- Avoid hurry and worry.
- Identify your fears.

Schedule worry time for half an hour a day. During that time, you may write down solutions to your problems if they occur to you, but otherwise *spend your time worrying*. If something new develops during the day, write it down, and then distract yourself by refocusing on what you are doing. *Worry about it only during your worry time.*

Learn to desensitize yourself. In order to do this, you first need to be practiced in a relaxation technique and in countering negative thoughts with constructive ones. Once you know how to do that:

- First imagine the worst and best scenarios for something that's worrying you—and picture yourself coping with both.
- Then close your eyes and relax yourself completely.
- See the situation in great detail, and let yourself feel the anxiety it arouses.
- Counter the anxiety by breathing deeply, and counter negative thoughts with constructive ones. Do not run away from the image.
- If you feel overwhelmed, temporarily visualize a calming, peaceful scene.

Repeat this exercise daily for about 15 minutes, and then move to a more frightening situation, finally progressing to the one that most frightens you. Then go out and face the frightening situations for real.

Counseling can be an important part of treating anxiety and panic attacks. A trained counselor can help you learn to control worry, to work on communication skills, and to examine your relationships. People tend to be less anxious when they have positive and fulfilling relationships.

Start to take control of the stress in your life. When you realize you are under stress, deliberately think about something else, or recite an anti-stress litany, like this one suggested by Dr. Emmett Miller, medical director of the Cancer Support and Education Center in Menlo Park, California, and a nationally known expert on stress:

> There's no place I have to go at this
>   moment in time.
> There's no problem I have to solve at this
>   moment in time.
> There's nothing that I have to do at this
>   moment in time.
> The most important thing that I can
>   experience at this moment in time is
>   relaxation.

Use affirmations when you feel stressed. Try saying: "I can handle this." "It will turn out okay." "I'm a good, capable person." "I've done

things like this before." Turn negative thoughts into more productive ones. Keep your thoughts in the present, focused on what you can do now.

Make sure to distinguish what you *can* control from what you *cannot*. Identify the situations or triggers that cause stress, and then manage them. Look away from the problem that is causing stress—or get up and leave it. Learn how to say "No."

Stage fright is a special form of anxiety or panic attack. To help with stage fright, think positively before a presentation. Try relabeling the fear sensations as those of "excitement" or "anticipation." Join a group such as Toastmasters, which gives members training and support for public speaking. Practice talking while making eye contact in a mirror.

For additional help in controlling anxiety, use prayer and guided imagery (see Preparing for Surgery in chapter 5, Surgery). Use visualization to take a mini-vacation in your mind, imagining a place where you'd like to be. Picture the scene in detail, and allow yourself to feel the relaxing emotions and sensations. Listen to a relaxation tape or music.

CHAPTER 28

Fatigue

Everyone gets tired occasionally, but with adequate rest, most people recover quickly. If fatigue comes on suddenly with no cause, does not improve with adequate rest, or starts to interfere with normal activities, then it should be investigated.

Fatigue lasting more than two weeks affects more than 25 percent of all North Americans. Because it is so common, it is often dismissed as normal, especially since at least 60 percent of these people report that their physician can find no medical cause for their fatigue. Fatigue can be a sign of a minor illness, stress, or a serious illness. It is one of the most frequent reasons for a visit to a doctor, and women are seen for fatigue one and a half times more often than men.

CAUSES OF FATIGUE

There are many causes of fatigue, some implicated in more serious fatigue problems. The following causes are discussed in these chapters:

- Allergies—Allergy
- Cancer—Cancer
- Candida overgrowth—Gastrointestinal Problems
- Diabetes—Metabolic Disorders
- Depression—Mood Disorders
- Headaches—Headaches
- Hepatitis B or C—Socially Transmitted Diseases
- Hypothyroidism or hyperthyroidism—Metabolic Disorders
- Menstrual Problems—Female Problems
- Obesity—Metabolic Disorders
- Parasitic infections—Parasites
- Sleep habits—Insomnia
- Stress—Mood Disorders
- Viral infections—Socially Transmitted Diseases, Respiratory System Problems

A long list of drugs and vaccines can also cause fatigue. Other major causes of fatigue are as follows.

ANEMIA

Anemia occurs when there is a low red blood cell count (see Common Laboratory Tests in chapter 3, The Laboratory). The most common cause of anemia is iron deficiency, especially in women who are menstruating. More than three million women in the United States have iron-deficiency anemia. Pregnancy also causes a loss of iron stores.

A hematocrit of less than 36 percent (although the exact figure varies with altitude) indicates anemia. Iron supplements should not be taken without confirmation that the cause of the anemia is iron deficiency. Iron-deficiency anemia is sometimes seen in infants and toddlers, and can cause loss of cognitive abilities.

AUTOIMMUNE DISEASES

Autoimmune diseases can cause fatigue. In autoimmune diseases (rheumatoid arthritis, multiple sclerosis, and lupus erythematosus) the immune system starts to attack the body, not recognizing it as "self."

Symptoms include joint swelling, pain, and redness; skin rashes; anemia; fevers; double vision; and weakness on one side of the body. Autoimmune diseases are more common in women than men.

BACTERIAL INFECTIONS

Lyme disease is one of the bacterial infections that can cause fatigue. It is transmitted by the bite of an infected deer tick, and is reported mainly in the northeastern U.S., upper Midwest, and northern California. The most common early symptom of Lyme disease is a circular red rash, like a bulls-eye, around the bite. People then develop fatigue, fever, and eventually arthritis, heart problems, and neurological problems.

A blood test for Lyme antibodies helps to diagnose the disease, but a negative test does not rule it out. Antibiotics must be used to treat the disease.

HEMOCHROMATOSIS

Hemochromatosis is a disease of iron overload, and is the most common genetic disease in North America. One out of every two hundred people inherits the two genes that cause hemochromatosis, and 10 percent of people who do not have the disease are carriers for it.

In hemochromatosis the gastrointestinal tract absorbs too much iron from the diet, and over the years the excess iron builds up in body organs (the heart and liver). The iron buildup ultimately can cause liver failure, liver cancer, or heart failure. The effects of the disease do not usually show up in menstruating women because they have monthly blood loss (and therefore iron loss). However, men of all ages and postmenopausal women can show the results of the disease. It causes chronic fatigue, arthritis, diabetes, anemia, and then enlargement of the liver. Treatment for the disease is periodic removal of blood.

Hemochromatosis can be diagnosed with a blood test that measures iron levels, iron binding capacity, and transferrin saturation. If the transferrin saturation is 60 percent or greater, have the test repeated. If the level still tests high, a liver biopsy is recommended. The College of American Pathologists recommends that doctors screen for hemochromatosis at age 20 (or younger if there is a family history of the disease).

Patients with hemochromatosis typically have a mild anemia, probably because the excess of iron causes a decrease in the production of red blood cells. Many doctors recommend an iron supplement for this anemia, thereby worsening the problem. If you are a young man and show a mild anemia on a blood count, have a transferrin saturation test done.

INACTIVITY

Fatigue can be induced from inactivity that results in boredom. A sedentary lifestyle perpetuates fatigue and the negative feelings that accompany it. Inactivity or low activity reduces energy and aggravates aches and pains that cause people to consult their physician.

Exercise is the key for increasing energy and reducing fatigue. Aerobic exercise (exercising so that the heart rate is increased, increasing oxygen use), resistance (pushing or pulling against resistance), and flexibility (stretching) exercises can all help to combat fatigue.

METAL TOXICITY

The presence of heavy metals in the body can be the cause of fatigue, from both acute and chronic toxicity. Common problems include mercury from dental fillings, fungicides, and the diet, especially fish contaminated from industrial discharge; aluminum from cookware, soft drink cans, antacids, paints, salt, deodorants, baking powder, and many other sources; cadmium from cigarette smoke, plastics, auto exhaust, fertilizers, coffee, and soft or acidic water; and lead from solder in plumbing pipes and from the soil, air, and water as a result of industry and manufacturing.

Detoxification procedures are the main treatment for this type of toxicity and include chelation procedures, nutrient and herbal therapy, and homeopathic treatment.

NUTRIENT AND NUTRITIONAL DEFICIENCY

Diet can be a source of fatigue, because of what the person is eating as well as what is not being eaten. Poor dietary habits that include a high consumption of refined carbohydrates and high fats can rob a person of energy.

Insufficient protein, whole grain, and vegetable intake can set up nutrient deficiencies that cause fatigue. For example, low levels of the B vitamins, particularly vitamin B_{12}, can result from not eating enough protein. A deficiency of any of the B vitamins can result in fatigue. Folic acid or folate deficiency results from not eating enough vegetables, particularly green vegetables. Vitamins B_1 and B_5, found in whole grains, legumes, and eggs, are essential for conversion of fats, carbohydrates, and protein to energy. Vitamin C, found in fresh fruits and vegetables, increases energy levels.

Mineral deficiencies can also contribute to fatigue. For example, low potassium levels cause a lack of energy.

Correcting dietary habits and nutrient supplementation can combat fatigue resulting from low vitamin and mineral levels.

STIMULANT OVERUSE

Stimulant overuse can cause fatigue because of the adrenal insufficiency triggered by the excessive use of such stimulants as tea, coffee, chocolate, cola, alcohol, tobacco, and drugs. When consumed, these substances increase energy by causing release of adrenalin from the adrenal glands. This pushes blood sugar out of the liver and muscles and into the bloodstream. The quick rise in blood sugar gives a quick boost. However, the increase in blood sugar causes the pancreas to release insulin, and the blood sugar to plummet, resulting in fatigue. Years of consuming these substances wears out the adrenal glands and pancreas, and they become unable to cope with these substances, increasing the frequency and intensity of the fatigue.

Drugs with a stimulant effect, such as amphetamine, cause a similar phenomenon. As soon as the drug wears off, acute fatigue occurs. Reducing and controlling consumption of these substances helps to combat this type of fatigue.

FIBROMYALGIA

More space is given here to fibromyalgia than to other causes of fatigue because it seems to be related to chronic fatigue syndrome, the most serious type of fatigue. In fact, some researchers and physicians believe they may be the same illness. However, in fibromyalgia, pain predominates over fatigue, whereas in chronic fatigue, fatigue is worse than pain. The cause or causes of fibromyalgia are not known. There are several theories about its cause, including immunologic abnormalities, a disturbance in brain chemistry, possible infections such as Epstein-Barr virus or *Candida albicans*, mercury poisoning from dental amalgams, anemia, parasites, hypoglycemia, and hypothyroidism. It may well have multiple causes.

Three to six million people in North America have fibromyalgia, the majority of them women of childbearing age. Symptoms are cyclic, but the major ones are aches and pains all over the body, with insomnia and non-restorative sleep. Other symptoms include irritability, nervousness, depression, headaches, dizziness, anxiety, nasal congestion, abnormal taste, ringing in the ears, numbness and tingling of the hands and feet, irritable bowel syndrome (see Gastrointestinal Problems, chapter 19), restless legs, and leg cramps.

Fibromyalgia is diagnosed based on history and physical exam. When the disease is present, at least 11 of 18 tender points (hard areas of swelling in muscles and tendons of the back, neck shoulders, buttocks, and chest) are found on physical exam. Non-steroidal medication or Tylenol do not relieve pain with fibromyalgia.

Dr. Ray Strand (a private practitioner from Rapid City, South Dakota) recently noted in *The CFIDS Chronicle* that athletes with overtraining syndrome had the same symptoms as patients with Chronic Fatigue Syndrome or fibromyalgia. Excessive free radicals or oxidative stress seem to be at the root of the problem for the three conditions. Dr. Strand has had success treating patients with antioxidants, though results are better if a patient is seen early in the course of the illness.

Dr. R. Paul St. Amand (Assistant Clinical Professor of Medicine/Endocrinology at the University of California in Los Angeles) has found a strong familial pattern in fibromyalgia. He feels that fibromyalgia is caused by an inherited abnormality in the excretion of phosphate, which causes an accumulation of phosphate and calcium within the mitochondria (the powerhouse of the cell) of each cell in the body. This leads to a deficit in adenosine triphosphate, the primary energy molecule of the body.

MODERN MEDICAL TREATMENT

Exercise and Lifestyle

Patients with fibromyalgia are told to exercise regularly.

Drug Therapy

Low-dose tricyclic antidepressants taken at bedtime are prescribed for fibromyalgia. (See Depression section in chapter 27, Mood Disorders for a discussion of these drugs.) They help with sleep and, in low doses, help with pain. Other drugs that may or may not help are often prescribed. These include muscle relaxants, local anesthetic sprays, injections for relief of pain, and the anti-anxiety drug lorazepam (Ativan). (See p. 438 for a discussion of this drug.)

ALTERNATIVE TREATMENT

Diet

Avoid white flour, sugar, caffeine, and foods high in fat. Also avoid red meats, gluten grains, dairy products, and processed foods. Eat high-protein foods, complex carbohydrate foods, vegetables, fruits, whole grains, raw nuts and seeds, skinless turkey or chicken, and deep-water fish. Eliminate food allergens.

Eat a series of small meals throughout the day to give the body a steady supply of protein. If the body does not have fuel for energy it will rob nutrients from the muscles, causing pain.

Drink 8 to 10 glasses of pure water a day.

Exercise and Lifestyle

Exercise regularly (many patients with fibromyalgia are not physically fit). Do aerobic exercise and gradually build up your exercise time to 20 minutes a day. Low-impact exercise is best, but 10 minutes of weight-bearing exercise can be added after you can easily do the initial 20 minutes of aerobic exercise.

Do not smoke and avoid all forms of tobacco, including secondhand smoke.

Nutrient Therapy

Take the following nutritional supplements:

- beta carotene – 100,000 IU a day (antioxidant; enhances immune system)
- B-complex – with 50 mg of each B (helps increase energy levels)
- vitamin C – 3,000 to 5,000 mg three times a day (antioxidant; enhances immune system)
- vitamin E – 400 to 800 IU a day (antioxidant; enhances immune system)
- magnesium malate – 300 to 600 mg of mag-

nesium and 1,200 to 1,400 mg of malic acid each day (helps with muscle pain)

- manganese – 15 mg a day (influences metabolic rate)
- selenium – 200 mcg a day (antioxidant)
- zinc picolinate – 15 mg a day (needed for proper function of the immune system)
- alpha-lipoic acid – 20 to 50 mg a day (antioxidant; helps to control blood sugar)
- cysteine – 500 mg twice a day (antioxidant)
- quercetin – 500 mg twice a day (works with vitamin C)
- coenzyme Q_{10} – 100 mg a day (enhances effectiveness of immune system; produces energy for immune system; improves oxygenation of tissues)
- Immunocal (a source of glutathione) – one packet a day (antioxidant) (see Sources)

Herbal Therapy
Take a botanical supplement.

- black cohosh – anti-inflammatory
- burdock tea – balances hormones; cleanses musculoskeletal system
- ginkgo – aids circulation
- rosemary – increases circulation
- turmeric – anti-inflammatory

Homeopathic Remedies
Take the homeopathic remedy that best describes your symptoms. If you do not obtain relief, seek the help of a homeopathic physician. Below are a few of the possible remedies.

- *Bryonia* – pain worse from the slightest motion, worse from a jar or being bumped, aggravation from any motion; amelioration from pressure; averse to being disturbed; must be left alone and quiet; preoccupied with business matters.
- *Cimicifuga* – rheumatism affecting the muscles; stitching pains, darting about; worse in cold, damp weather; fibrositis, muscle

twitches; neck spasms, spasms of the paraspinal muscles.

- *Nux vomica* – back pain, worse in bed at night; cramps and contractures of muscles; tremor and muscle spasms anywhere in the body; fibrositis, worse with cold, better with warmth.
- *Rhus toxicodendron* – stiffness and pains in the neck and back; worse cold damp, better heat; stiffness may go to the occiput and cause headache; joking, restless, cheerful patients; amelioration from motion; cannot sit still.
- *Ruta graveolens* – bruised or sore pains with stiffness; weakness and stiffness prevent rising from a chair; stiff through the body; easily fatigued, worse from exertion.

Other Therapeutic Measures
Use relaxation techniques, including meditation, guided imagery, yoga, biofeedback training, and progressive muscle relaxation.

Get regular massage or bodywork. Apply heat to painful areas.

Dr. St. Amand found that medications to lower uric acid in the blood (uricosuric medications) would help patients with fibromyalgia. His practice uses Guaifenesin (an ingredient in cough medications intended to loosen mucus) to help the body excrete uric acid. Salicylates block the benefit of Guaifenesin, and must be avoided—even the small amounts present in cosmetics, aloe creams, herbs, mouthwashes, lip and muscle balms, sunscreens, acne medications, shampoos, wart removal products, and Pepto Bismol.

Reversal of fibromyalgia with this treatment is a cyclical process. As the removal of abnormal chemicals occurs, the previous symptoms of severe muscle pain are periodically reproduced. However, good days gradually increase and cluster. About two months of treatment at the proper dosage reverses at least one year of accumulated disease effects.

Take 300 mg of guaifenesin, twice a day for two weeks. Depending upon the clinical response, increase the dose to 600 mg, twice a day; 30 percent of patients will need the higher dose. Guaifenesin is an over-the-counter drug, but the dosages used will probably have to be made up by a compounding pharmacy.

CHRONIC FATIGUE

Chronic Fatigue (immune deficiency) Syndrome (CFIDS or CFS; also known as myalgic encephalomyelitis in England) affects at least 3 million North Americans and 90 million people worldwide. Approximately one in one hundred adult patients seeking care have CFIDS. It affects mostly middle-class white people, and is most common in women 25 to 50 years old, but does affect all ethnic, racial, and socioeconomic groups. While it has been around for centuries, the incidence seems to be increasing. It seems to have a genetic link, because multiple family members can be affected.

CFIDS is a frustrating illness for both the patient and the doctor: the cause is not known, there is no definitive diagnostic test available, and many physicians still feel that CFIDS is not a "real" disease, but just an expression of depression.

Diagnosis of Chronic Fatigue

As there is no definitive lab test to diagnose this disease, it is diagnosed by the process of elimination. The Centers for Disease Control and Prevention, in Atlanta, Georgia, set forth a case definition in 1988, with a new definition in 1994, as follows:

1. Clinically evaluated, unexplained, persistent or relapsing chronic fatigue that is of new or definite onset (has not been lifelong); is not the result of ongoing exertion; is not substantially alleviated by rest; and results in substantial reduction in previous levels of occupation, educational, social, or personal activities; and

2. The concurrent occurrence of four or more of the following symptoms, all of which must have persisted or recurred during six or more consecutive months of illness and must not have predated the fatigue: self-reported impairment in short-term memory or concentration severe enough to cause substantial reduction in previous levels of occupational, educational, social, or personal activities; sore throat; tender cervical or axillary lymph nodes; muscle pain; multi-joint pain without joint swelling or redness; headaches of a new type, pattern, or severity; unrefreshing sleep; and postexertional malaise lasting more than 24 hours.

The case definition of CFIDS probably does not define a homogeneous group of patients. CFIDS seems to have different triggering factors, which share a pathway leading to the symptoms. CFIDS patients also report loss of appetite, nausea, drenching night sweats, dizziness, and intolerance to alcohol and medications that affect the central nervous system. Some CFIDS patients have light sensitivity and numbness of parts of the body.

Many patients with CFIDS have depression and anxiety, but their depression and anxiety develop after the onset of CFIDS—unlike the situation in many other physical conditions, in which depression and anxiety frequently predate the illness. Many patients who develop CFIDS are high-driving people who push themselves to their limit. Structured psychiatric interviews find no evidence of major depression in 25 to 60 percent of patients with CFIDS, before or after the onset of the disease.

Dr. Paul Cheney (of the Cheney Clinic in Charlotte, North Carolina and a leader in CFIDS research) finds that patients with CFIDS have three main complaints: fatigue, thought-processing and short-term memory problems, and pain. (Fibromyalgia symptoms overlap with CFIDS, but patients with fibromyalgia do not complain of thought-processing problems.)

Dr. Cheney has found subtle symptoms on physical exam of CFIDS patients. He notes puffiness of the left supraclavicular fossa (depressed area above the clavicle), because the thoracic duct (a major lymph carrier) is obstructed. Patients have discoid cervical nodes (disk-shaped neck lymph nodes), which are tender more than 90 percent of the time. Patients will have an oral temperature of 99.4°F or higher in the morning. Eighty percent of CFIDS patients have a dark red to dark pink coloration around the back of the soft palate and uvula. Most patients have evidence of neurotoxicity, as demonstrated by swaying on the Romberg test (feet together while standing, eyes closed) and tandem Romberg (one foot in front of the other while standing, eyes closed). Eighty percent of patients with CFIDS have hyperreflexia (exaggeration of reflexes) at the knees. Sophisticated neuropsychological testing demonstrates problems with memory and concentration. Signs of chronic immune activation, determined on more sophisticated tests, are also present.

Dr. Cheney and his group have also found typical lab test results that include a low sedimentation rate (a measure of inflammation in the body), low or low normal uric acid, increased cholesterol, a slight rise in liver tests, increased phosphate, elevated mean corpuscular volume (size of the cells), low white count (2,500 to 3,000), and an alkaline pH of the urine (8).

Dr. Cheney feels that the clinical symptoms, together with the laboratory test results, are consistent with an injury at the level of the hypothalamus, the master gland in the brain.

Screening tests (CBC, sedimentation rate, liver tests, albumin, globulin, alkaline phosphatase, calcium, phosphate, glucose, BUN, electrolytes, creatinine, TSH, and urinalysis) should be performed. These and additional tests may be performed, as needed, to make sure there is no liver disease, anemia, malnutrition, hypo- or hyperglycemia, kidney disease, autoimmune disease, or thyroid disorder.

Causes of Chronic Fatigue

Most cases of CFIDS develop suddenly after a viral infection; other cases occur after chemical exposure. Some cases develop gradually, especially after a series of stressful events, such as the death of a parent or spouse, a birth, marriage, or divorce. Over 60 percent of patients with CFIDS also have multiple chemical sensitivities.

Many medical researchers have tried to find a single cause for CFIDS. Dr. Murray Susser (Medical Director of the Omnidox Medical Group of Santa Monica, California) believes that it results from a combination of nutritional deficiency; toxicity from the environment, food, and drugs; poor stress-coping ability; parasites; and candida overgrowth—all causing a cycle of lowered immune function, allergy, and more infection.

Some researchers believe that CFIDS may be caused by a chronic malfunctioning of the hormonal system for dealing with stress, known as the hypothalamic-pituitary-adrenal (HPA) axis. In response to real or imagined stress, the HPA triggers the release of cortisol and other hormones (see Anxiety section in chapter oo, Mood Disorders).

Dr. Jesse Stoff (of the Soltice Clinical Associates in Tucson, Arizona, and coauthor of *Chronic Fatigue Syndrome*) notes that CFIDS is a multidimensional disorder involving many organs and systems, not just the immune system. There is an interrelationship between the nervous system and the immune system, because neurotransmitters such as serotonin, dopamine, and epinephrine are necessary to make the brain and the immune system work properly.

In patients with CFIDS, the autonomic nervous system, the system that controls heart rate, digestion, and automatic functions of the body, is abnormal. If these patients are placed on a tilt-table, and then stood upright for a controlled period of time, many patients will have a fall in blood pressure and almost black out. This is known as neurally mediated hypertension, and some physicians have postulated that this is one of the causes of CFIDS.

Dr. Jeffrey Bland, of HealthComm in Gig Harbor, Washington, believes that detoxification abnormalities are a common cause of CFIDS. He also feels that there are abnormalities of the mitochondria, the powerhouse of the cell.

Dr. Jay Goldstein, director of the Chronic Fatigue Syndrome Institute in Anaheim, California, postulates that CFIDS is a neurosomatic disease, because evidence shows abnormalities in a part of the brain of CFIDS patients. He believes CFIDS is a disorder of the management of sensory input to the brain, in which it misperceives sensory information. Information processing in the brain occurs appropriately, but the control of data input and output from processing centers is dysfunctional.

The cause of CFIDS remains unknown, but it clearly is *not* caused by a chronic infection with Epstein-Barr virus. The presence of the Epstein-Barr virus is just an indicator of a high level of chronic stress on the immune system, and elevated Epstein-Barr antibodies can be caused by an occult malignancy, AIDS, ankylosing spondylitis (a type of arthritis), multiple sclerosis, rheumatoid arthritis, and lupus.

MODERN MEDICAL TREATMENT

Exercise and Lifestyle

Patients are told to perform graded, modest, regular physical activity, working up to 20 to 30 minutes of aerobic exercise at least five days a week.

They are also to avoid unusual physical or emotional stress, to pace themselves, and to follow a regular daily routine.

Drug Therapy

There is no one treatment that helps all patients with CFIDS. Drugs commonly used for CFIDS are either ineffective or have side effects (or both).

Some patients are helped by Kutapressin, a liver derivative for complex infections that reduces inflammation and edema in a number of conditions. Side effects include a very occasional mild, allergic response.

Dr. Anthony Komaroff, professor of medicine at Harvard Medical School, states that in his (unpublished) studies, 12 percent of patients have returned to normal health at some time during a follow-up period that averaged eight and a half years. Half of these patients later relapsed after a period of at least six months of normal health. The typical progression is one of gradual improvement, but the illness can wax and wane. Some people who get better immediately go back to their previous lifestyle—and become ill again. From 40 to 60 percent of patients remain ill for 10 years or longer.

Tricyclic antidepressants are given to CFIDS patients at bedtime. If the response is not adequate, another antidepressant is given. (See Depression section in chapter 27, Mood Disorders, for a discussion of these medications.) Anti-inflammatory medication is given for muscle and joint pain (see Arthritis section in chapter 14, Musculoskeletal Problems). Klonopin and other similar medications are given for difficulties sleeping. Klonopin is a benzodiazepine drug that can cause drowsiness, loss of balance, behavior problems, abnormal eye movements, confusion, depression, chest congestion, palpitations, hair loss, loss of appetite, muscle weakness, pains, anemia, and transient elevations of liver enzymes. (See also chapter 29, Insomnia.)

Stimulant medication is given to improve energy (see chapter 26, Attention Deficit Hyperactivity Disorder). Non-sedating antihistamines are also prescribed (see chapter 25, Allergy). Acyclovir is given as an antiviral agent, 1,000 to

4,000 mg a day (see Vaginitis section in chapter 22, Socially Transmitted Diseases).

For neurally mediated hypotension, Florinef is prescribed. It is a cortisone derivative of the adrenal glands that helps the body retain salt and water. Florinef can raise blood pressure, and has to be increased gradually, with blood pressure being monitored. Some patients with CFIDS do not tolerate it. Patients are told to use salt liberally on food and to drink 10 to 12 glasses of fluid a day. One-third of patients make an almost complete recovery and one-third show moderate improvement. It is not a cure for CFIDS though, because if patients stop their drug and diet regimen, symptoms will return.

Other Therapeutic Measures

Cognitive behavior therapy, which teaches patients strategies for dealing with fearful thoughts, guilt, self-criticism, and performance expectations, is helpful for patients with CFIDS. (See Depression section in chapter 27, Mood Disorders.)

Support groups for chronic fatigue can be helpful if they are run by a skilled therapist. Without good management, chronic fatigue support groups may sometimes deteriorate into gripe sessions and people vying for the title of "the most sick." If you attend a support group for chronic fatigue, make sure the members have a positive attitude and a commitment to improve.

ALTERNATIVE TREATMENT

Diet

Avoid foods high in sugar and fat. Avoid gluten grains, dairy products, caffeine, alcohol, food additives, and refined carbohydrates. These foods negatively affect the immune system.

Eat high-protein, complex-carbohydrate foods. Eliminate food allergens. Drink 8 to 10 glasses of pure water a day.

Exercise and Lifestyle

Perform anaerobic exercise, such as light weight lifting and isometric exercise.

Engage in graded, modest, regular physical activity. Try to work up to 20 to 30 minutes of aerobic exercise at least five days a week.

Practice Tai Chi or Qigong.

Do not smoke, and avoid all forms of tobacco, including secondhand smoke.

Nutrient Therapy

Take the following nutritional supplements.

- beta carotene – 100,000 IU a day (protects the cells; enhances immune function to fight viruses)
- vitamin B_1 – 50 to 100 mg a day (increases energy)
- vitamin B_5 (pantothenic acid) – 150 mg a day, but not at bedtime (supports adrenal gland during stress)
- vitamin B_{12} – 1,000 to 5,000 mcg intramuscularly or subcutaneously, three times a week to once a month (helps with fatigue)
- B-complex with 50 mg of each B vitamin, two capsules twice a day (essential for increased energy levels)
- vitamin C – 3,000 to 5,000 mg three times a day (powerful antiviral effect; increases energy level)
- vitamin E – 400 to 800 IU a day (antioxidant)
- a multivitamin/mineral supplement as directed on the label of your product (helps immune system; increases energy level)
- calcium – 1,000 mg a day (balances magnesium)
- magnesium malate – 300 to 600 mg of magnesium and 1,200 to 1,400 mg of malic acid each day (helps with muscle pain, fatigue)
- manganese – 15 mg a day (influences metabolic rate)
- potassium/magnesium aspartate – four capsules of 500 mg of each, twice a day (increases energy level)
- selenium – 200 mcg a day (powerful antioxidant)
- zinc picolinate – 15 mg a day (essential for immune system function)

- adrenal extract – one to two tablets three times a day (supports adrenal gland)
- thymus gland extract – one to two tablets three times a day (immune system support)
- spleen extract – as directed on your product (immune system support)
- coenzyme Q_{10} – 100 to 200 mg a day for at least two months (enhances effectiveness of immune system)
- L-carnitine – 500 to 1,000 mg a day (increases energy level)
- cysteine – 500 mg twice a day (powerful antioxidant)
- quercetin – 500 mg three times a day (works with vitamin C)
- dimethylglycine – 50 to 100 mg a day (enhances oxygen utilization; destroys free radicals)
- alpha-lipoic acid – 20 to 50 mg a day (antioxidant)
- Immunocal – one packet a day (see Sources) (source of glutathione; antioxidant)
- Mitochondrial Resuscitate by HealthComm – as directed (helps mitochondria, which produce energy for the cells) (see Sources)
- Ultraclear or Nutriclear – as instructed (balanced nutrients with detoxification vitamins) (see Sources)
- amino acid supplements – based on blood testing of amino acids

Herbal Therapy
Take a botanical supplement.

- astragalus – enhances immune system
- echinacea – enhances immune system
- garlic – antiviral, enhances immune system
- ginseng *(Panax)* – improves energy
- goldenseal – enhances immune system. *Caution:* Do not use if you are pregnant.
- licorice root – strengthens adrenals
- maitake mushroom – strengthens immune system

- olive leaf extract – strengthens immune system
- shitake mushroom – improves immune system
- Siberian ginseng *(Eleutherococcus senticosus)* – improves energy; increases stamina
- wild indigo root – strengthens immune system

Homeopathic Remedies
Consult a homeopathic physician to prescribe the homeopathic remedy that best fits your symptoms. The following remedies are but a few of the possibilities.

- *Baptisia* – confusion; dullness of mind; falls asleep mid-sentence; bruised pains; uncomfortable in any position; sore all over the body, especially the part which is lain upon; dusky red inflammation of the throat, which is remarkably pain free.
- *Gelsemium* – trembling from exertion, especially the legs; chills begin in the hands or feet; heavy head, feels as if he can hardly lift it; eyelids heavy and drooping; timid, quiet, reserved; chills running up and down the back.
- *Mercurius corrosivus* – acute or chronic pharyngitis; tremor, especially of the hands; patient oversensitive to heat and cold, and to many other changes in the environment; introverted, closed, emotionally intense and suspicious; aggravation at night; night sweats; offensive breath.

Many patients respond to complex homeopathic remedies. You may want to try Aletris Heel by BHI for all types of fatigue, weakness, and exhaustion.

Other Therapeutic Measures
If candida overgrowth is present, treat it (see Gastrointestinal Problems, p. 273), and rule out

the presence of parasites. Eliminate any hidden bacterial infections (Lyme disease, abscesses in the teeth or cavitations in the jaw, chronic prostatitis, chronic sinusitis, and chronic gastritis).

Make positive changes in relationships or at work to alleviate stress.

Receive IV nutrients or rectal nutrients, such as BottomsUp by Nutricology (see Sources).

Receive IV gamma globulin. If you cannot afford IV, receive IM gamma globulin, 2 to 3 ml twice weekly for four to six months.

Have acupuncture treatment, or consult an Ayurvedic physician.

Receive artificial hyperthermia under medical direction to enhance the immune system. Dr. Bruce Milliman (Associate Professor of Medicine at Bastyr College, Seattle, Washington) has patients soak in a tub of water as hot as can be tolerated for five minutes, while drinking a 12-ounce glass of tepid water mixed with 2,000 mg of vitamin C. Then the patient gets into a bed with flannel sheets and wool blankets, putting a hot water bottle under the breast in women or over the liver in men, and staying under the blankets for 20 minutes. *Caution:* This procedure should not be used if patients have diabetes or certain endocrine problems.

Receive chelation therapy after testing for metal toxicity.

Receive bodywork, such as manual lymph drainage or massage.

Receive hydrotherapy with hot and cold applications to painful areas.

Perform a day deep breathing and relaxation exercises, or structured meditation techniques.

Practice Dr. Weil's breathing exercises (see p. 225).

Try home oxygen. Inhale it for 15 to 20 minutes, once or twice a day.

CHAPTER 29

Insomnia

More than 50 million North American adults have sleep problems at one time or another. Insomnia ranks high among the disorders for which patients seek help from physicians, and each year four to six million prescriptions are written for sedative hypnotics (sleeping pills).

Insomnia is closely related to the degree of emotional stress and lifestyle changes that occur from age 20 to about age 65. After that, insomnia is commonly caused by sleep disorders, such as sleep apnea and periodic movements in sleep. There is no evidence that sleep loss leads to long-term medical problems, but it does cause psychological suffering, and insomniacs are more likely to report poor health. It is estimated that 1,500 people die and 76,000 people are injured each year in car accidents caused by driver fatigue largely due to lack of sleep.

There is no "normal" amount of sleep for adults. The *average* amount of sleep required by adults is seven to eight hours, but some people need only five hours of sleep each night, and others need up to ten. If you cannot fall asleep easily or stay asleep throughout the night for a period of a month or more, it is probably time to consult your physician.

CAUSES OF INSOMNIA

Insomnia is a symptom, not a disease. Some of the underlying reasons for insomnia are anxiety, fear, depression, a poor sleep environment that may be too noisy or too hot, poor sleep habits and bedtime habits, and physical conditions.

Over 300 drugs can interfere with sleep, including amphetamines, corticosteroids, blood pressure medication, oral contraceptives, certain asthma inhalers, decongestants such as phenylpropanolamine and pseudoephedrine, appetite suppressants, alpha methyldopa (Aldomet, used to control hypertension), phenytoin (Dilantin, an anticonvulsant), and propanolol (Inderal, a beta blocker used for hypertension and heart disease). Taking too much thyroid supplement can also disrupt your sleep. Diuretics can affect sleep because they may make you need to urinate during the night.

Shift work is a common cause of insomnia. Over 60 percent of shiftworkers complain of sleep disturbances, including difficulty in falling asleep or staying asleep, habitually waking up too early, difficulty in waking up, and poor-quality sleep. About 15 percent of newly hired shiftworkers develop gastrointestinal complaints, most commonly gastric and peptic ulcers. Many shiftworkers rotate through different shifts. A steady shift, even at night, has been shown to be better than a continually changing shift. If the shift is rotating, it should rotate forward at each shift change (day to evening to night to day), rather than backward.

TYPES OF INSOMNIA

There are five major categories of chronic insomnia: psychiatric insomnia, stress-conditioned insomnia, physiologic insomnia, insomnia caused by poor sleep habits, and pseudo-insomnia.

PSYCHIATRIC INSOMNIA

Psychiatric insomnia is associated with depression and anxiety, and is the most common category of insomnia.

In depressed people, REM (rapid eye movement) sleep is unusually brief and light and begins abnormally early in the sleep cycle. During REM sleep, a group of brain cells block signals to voluntary and skeletal muscles to prevent the body from reacting to images during dreams. Only tiny twitches of the face and fingers and the constant darting of eyeballs beneath the lids are discernible. Eye movements are more intense in depressed people. REM sleep is essential for sound physical and mental health, and people deprived of sufficient REM sleep for more than a few nights become anxious and irritable.

STRESS-CONDITIONED INSOMNIA

In stress-conditioned insomnia, patients have no underlying psychiatric disorder. Their symptoms fluctuate as reactions to stressful events. Once their sleep patterns are disturbed, people worry about whether they will sleep well and perform well the next day. They try hard to fall asleep, but anxiety about insomnia and its effects arouses them further.

PHYSIOLOGICAL INSOMNIA

Physiological insomnia includes sleep problems caused by periodic leg movements, sleep apnea, and medical disorders. About 30 percent of people with chronic insomnia have a physiological cause for their sleep disorder.

Periodic Leg Movements

Some people have periodic involuntary leg movements during sleep (nocturnal myoclonus). Their legs jerk frequently throughout the night, often resulting in brief arousals or full-blown awakenings. Other people, in addition to having periodic leg movements when asleep, have "restless leg syndrome" (the sensation of ants crawling in the calf, or electricity in the legs) that delays sleep onset.

Sleep Apnea

Sleep apnea is a major cause of daytime sleepiness. People with sleep apnea may have enlarged tonsils; may be overweight; may have an enlarged tongue, excessive fat tissue in the throat, or other anatomical abnormalities of the face, chest, back, or neck that create a narrow airway when they are asleep.

These people tend to snore loudly. As people with sleep apnea fall into a deeper sleep, there is a significant decrease in breathing, with sounds of grunting, snorting, and gasping. There are pauses in breathing that can last 30 seconds to a full minute. The heart may slow down or skip a few beats, and the amount of oxygen in the person's bloodstream drops to a low level. The brain then awakens the sleeper for 5 to 10 seconds, the sleeper takes a deep breath, and goes back to sleep. The apnea can repeat 400 to 500 times a night. People affected by sleep apnea do not remember the brief arousals, but they are very sleepy in the daytime, and will fall asleep during conversations or even at stop signs when they are driving.

Severe sleep apnea affects 1 percent of the population. Studies of healthy senior citizens have found that over a third of them have sleep apnea. About 40 percent of sleeping pill prescriptions are written for people over 60, although people in that age group make up only 15 percent of the population. Sleeping pills change a sleeper's arousal threshold, and may prevent the brain from awakening the sleeper during an apnea episode. As a result, apneas may happen more frequently and each episode may last longer. Elderly people who use sleeping pills have a higher death rate than those in the same age group who do not use sleeping pills.

A report published in the *Southern Medical Journal* in 1988 (and other studies) suggests that for many people, subacute hypothyroidism may be the cause of sleep apnea. If thyroid hormone levels are too low, the soft tissues of the throat are abnormally relaxed. If symptoms of hypothyroidism are present together with sleep apnea, thyroid function should be investigated.

Medical Disorders

Many medical disorders can cause sleep problems. People with arthritis, chronic pain, fibromyalgia, and biological rhythm disorders may have insomnia. Low blood sugar levels at night can cause insomnia in the middle of the night, because a drop in blood sugar causes release of such stimulating hormones as adrenaline and cortisol. The hormonal problems of menopause can also contribute to insomnia.

Many people suffer from delayed-phase sleep syndrome. They tend to have a 25-hour clock, as opposed to the normal 24-hour rhythm. These people tend to go to bed later on Friday, Saturday, and Sunday night. They sleep later on Saturday and Sunday morning. On Sunday evening they are not tired at their normal weekday bedtime, and so stay up later; then they have a difficult time getting up on Monday morning.

When children become teenagers, their biological clock often changes so that they do not get sleepy until late in the evening, then have a hard time getting up in the morning. In response to this common problem, a school system in Minnesota is experimenting with having high school start later in the morning than elementary school.

POOR SLEEP HABITS

Poor sleep habits are related to alcoholism, addiction to sleeping pills or other drugs, marijuana use, excessive caffeine use, and irregular sleep schedules. The bedroom can become associated with sleeplessness, and that can trigger a phobic response.

For some people, sexual intercourse can be stimulating, and may be better moved away from bedtime. For others, sex may help enhance sleep. Insomniacs often sleep better alone than with a partner. Sleeping in a room warmer than 75°F may disturb some sleepers.

PSEUDO-INSOMNIA

Pseudo-insomnia now accounts for about 10 percent of chronic insomniacs. These people sleep seven to eight hours with normal brain tracings at night, but then say that they had no sleep at all—or a few hours of sleep at best. They may have underlying psychological problems, or there may be physiological arousals or perhaps brain activity that cannot be picked up by measuring devices.

MODERN MEDICAL AND ALTERNATIVE PREVENTION

Sleep hygiene is essential for good sleep. The following procedures help most people within three to five weeks.

Avoid naps longer than an hour or after 4 P.M., and keep a sleep diary.

Go to bed when you are sleepy. If you cannot fall asleep in about 15 minutes and are anxious, use relaxation techniques or breathing exercises in bed. If you are still anxious, get up and do something monotonous; read a boring article, watch television, or balance the checkbook. When you get sleepy, get back into bed. Regardless of what time you return to bed, get up at your usual time.

Take some quiet time before bed. About an hour before bedtime, sit down for at least 10 minutes to review your stresses and schedule. Focus on peaceful thoughts before bedtime. Play soft, soothing music or nature sounds. Learn and practice relaxation and breathing techniques.

People with insomnia often concentrate too much on their sleep. Learn how to turn off unpleasant thoughts as they pop into your mind, and how to remember enjoyable experiences. Counting sheep works for some people, or counting backwards from 1,000 or backwards from 100 by threes.

Make sure that your mattress is comfortable and that the temperature of the bedroom is appropriate. Redecorate the bedroom with your favorite, soothing colors. If necessary, soundproof the room and hang dark curtains to keep out light. If clocks distract you at night, remove them from view. Use earplugs to block out unwanted noise, and eyeshades to screen out unwanted light. Wear loose-fitting clothes. If you are cold, use an electric blanket or hot water bottle to warm the bed. (Turn off the blanket before going to bed.) Do not watch television, read, eat, or perform other activities in bed. Use the bedroom only for sleep and sex.

If you have persistent active thoughts near bedtime, set aside a 20-minute period after dinner when you try to worry as much as you can. Write the worries down, along with possible solutions.

Do not exercise within two hours of bedtime. Instead, exercise in the afternoon or early evening, not too strenuously. That will raise body temperature, and when the temperature later begins to fall, you will feel drowsy. A warm bath about four or five hours before bedtime will do the same thing.

Do not drink a lot of fluid before bedtime, as you may have to wake in the middle of the night to urinate. Do not consume caffeine-containing drinks or food (coffee, tea, colas, and chocolate) after 4 P.M. Avoid alcohol at dinner or in the evening, as alcohol disrupts sleep: it makes people sleepy at first, but then wakes them in the middle of the night. Do not smoke before bedtime, because nicotine can keep you awake. Also avoid spicy meals near bedtime.

MODERN MEDICAL TREATMENT
Drug Therapy

When patients have tried all possibilities for relaxation and still cannot fall asleep, they are advised to take an over-the-counter sleeping pill. After two consecutive nights of poor sleep, patients are told to take one sleeping pill on the third night 30 minutes before bedtime. Short-acting medications are the best choice, except for patients who have significant anxiety during the day.

Over-the-counter sleeping pills contain the antihistamines diphenhydramine or doxylamine, which produce a level of sedation that will allow the average person to get about four hours of sleep a night. Try Sominex, Nytol, Sleepinal, Compose, or Benadryl, but be aware that antihistamines can cause a rash, dry mouth, urinary problems (in men with enlarged prostates), and confusion.

The next step would be to take an antidepressant such as amitriptyline (Elavil) at a dosage of 25 to 100 mg at bedtime. Taking an antidepressant helps if the insomnia is caused by depression.

Most sleeping pills were not specifically developed to promote sleep, and it is not known how they work. They are derived from medications that were incidentally found to have sedative effects and to decrease arousal from sleep. In general, sleeping pills initially reduce sleep latency (the time from lights out to the initiation of sleep) and decrease night-time awakenings, causing an overall increase in total sleep time. They lose their effectiveness after two to four weeks of use. Often, the patient's response is to increase the dose.

Sleeping pills are most effective for short-term, transient insomnia, or as an adjunct to a sleep hygiene program. Drug-induced sleep is not normal, and it decreases dream activity. If people rely on a sleeping pill to get to sleep for a long time, when they stop taking medication it takes about a month for the body to adjust and develop good sleep habits. All sleeping pills should be avoided in the first three months of pregnancy and while nursing.

Abrupt withdrawal from sleeping pills causes rebound insomnia and may even cause a night of total insomnia. Patients then assume that they cannot sleep without medication, so they continue to use it. It is necessary to withdraw gradually and substitute sleep hygiene techniques for medication.

Some physicians recommend benzodiazepines, which act to induce sleep by enhancing the action of the neurotransmitter gamma-aminobutyric acid (GABA). This blocks the arousal of brain centers. Benzodiazepines also suppress REM (rapid eye movement) sleep, during which we dream and our body undertakes repair and rejuvenative processes. Benzodiazepines include diazepam (Valium), flurazepam (Dalmane), triazolam (Halcion), clonazepam (Klonopin), lorazepam (Ativan), oxazepam (Serax), clorazepate (Tranxene), alprazolam (Xanax), or temazepam (Restoril).

Dalmane may cause a hangover. Halcion can cause amnesia for events that occur after it is taken. It may also cause "traveler's amnesia," when the person awakens before the effect of the drug has worn off. The benzodiazepines that are eliminated rapidly, such as Halcion, tend to cause less drowsiness the next day, but may cause withdrawal problems the day after use.

Flurazepam is active for at least 80 hours, so that it promotes daytime sleepiness, which is undesirable except for an extremely anxious patient. Its hypnotic effect is equally potent at midnight and at 10 A.M. the next day. After a good night's sleep, patients who have taken flurazepam are sleepier the following day than they would have been after a night of insomnia. Patients taking this drug will often deny that they feel sleepy during the day, however, since they are happy to have slept all night without awakening.

Benzodiazepines may produce psychological and physical dependence. People who have been dependent on alcohol or other drugs may be at particular risk of becoming dependent on drugs in this class, but all people appear to be at some risk, especially when the drug is used regularly for more than a few weeks, or at high doses. Withdrawal symptoms such as convulsions, tremor, abdominal and muscle cramps, vomiting, sweating, mood changes, and insomnia have occurred following abrupt discontinuance of benzodiazepines.

Abnormal thinking and behavior changes have been reported with the use of benzodiazepine sleeping pills. Confusion, bizarre behavior, agitation, hallucinations, depersonalization, and worsening of depression (including suicidal thinking) have been associated with benzodiazepines. In combination with alcohol and other central nervous system depressants these drugs can exacerbate depression, and the combination with alcohol can cause brain damage.

Benzodiazepines can cause allergic reactions, headaches, blurred vision, nausea, indigestion, diarrhea or constipation, and lethargy. When administered during the early months of pregnancy, certain benzodiazepines have been linked to birth defects, while the use of benzodiazepines during the last weeks of pregnancy has been associated with sedation of the fetus. After ingesting a benzodiazepine, patients should not operate machinery or drive a motor vehicle. The development of oversedation, dizziness, confusion, and/or loss of balance is more common in elderly patients who take these drugs.

Barbiturates—phenobarbital, pentobarbital (Nembutal), and secobarbital (Seconal)—may be recommended instead of benzodiazepines, and they, too, are very addicting. Tolerance, psychological dependence, and physical dependence can occur with continued use. Barbiturates lose most of their effectiveness for inducing and maintaining sleep at a fixed dose by the end of two weeks of continued use. Barbiturates reduce REM sleep, and if they are stopped suddenly, the patient has increased dreaming, nightmares, and/or insomnia. The patient may also have withdrawal symptoms, including delirium, convulsions, and even death. It is recommended that withdrawal take place over a five- to six-day period.

In some people, barbiturates produce excitement rather than depression. Elderly people may react to barbiturates with marked excitement, depression, and confusion.

Barbiturates may impair mental and/or physical abilities required for the performance of potentially hazardous tasks such as driving and operating machinery. Like benzodiazepines, barbiturates can worsen depression when combined with alcohol and other central nervous system depressants. Barbiturates can cause fetal damage when given to pregnant women.

Other Therapeutic Measures

Modern medicine treatment of psychiatric insomnia involves treating the depression and anxiety with medication. The patient also obtains counseling, and is taught to focus on the underlying causes of the insomnia rather than on the sleep problems.

Stress-conditioned insomnia is treated with behavioral change techniques.

Sleep apnea is best treated by recommending weight loss, encouraging changes in sleeping positions, prescribing tongue-restraining devices, performing surgery, or prescribing a nasal pressure mask to keep the airway open. Supporting thyroid function will often help resolve sleep apnea.

For delayed-phase sleep syndrome, people are to sit in the sun or get some bright light as soon as they wake up. In the evening, they are to keep lighting dimmed or even wear dark glasses so that the body knows it is time to begin to wind down. They should try to get up at the same time, even on weekends.

People with poor sleep habits who get out of bed when they cannot sleep should not perform goal-oriented tasks (such as laundry or housework) while they are up. When they start to feel drowsy again, they should go back to bed, and always wake up at the same time in the morning. A program directed by a doctor, nurse, or counselor is helpful for people with this problem.

ALTERNATIVE TREATMENT

Diet

Eat foods that help trigger sleep, such as bananas, figs, dates, yogurt, milk, tuna, soybeans, turkey, eggs, whole grain crackers, and nut butters. They are rich in natural L-tryptophan, an amino acid that acts on the brain to cause drowsiness. These foods work well, particularly when combined with a simple carbohydrate such as orange juice.

Avoid snacks high in refined sugar and heavy meals before bedtime. Avoid high-tyramine foods such as bacon, cheese, chocolate, eggplant, ham, potatoes, sauerkraut, sugar, sausage, spinach, tomatoes, and wine close to bedtime. Tyramine increases the release of norepinephrine, an excitatory neurotransmitter. If you drink coffee or other caffeinated beverages, drink them only in the morning. Also avoid alcohol at bedtime; it may help induce sleep, but will disrupt deeper sleep cycles later.

Exercise and Lifestyle

Perform aerobic exercise for 20 minutes a day, at a heart rate between 60 and 75 percent of your maximum (but not within five hours of bedtime).

Avoid tobacco in all forms. Even though smoking may seem calming, nicotine is a long-acting neurostimulant and can adversely affect sleep.

Nutrient Therapy

Take the following nutrients to help with insomnia.

- tryptophan – 1,000 to 5,000 mg at bedtime (helps to shorten the time it takes to get to sleep and increases total sleep time). Take magnesium (250 to 400 mg a day) and vitamin B$_6$ (25 mg) as cofactors. Take tryptophan with a carbohydrate source, not with protein. (Tryptophan is available in the U.S. by prescription through compounding pharmacies.)
- 5-hydroxytryptophan – 50 to 100 mg a day at bedtime (has same action as tryptophan; substitute if tryptophan not available)
- folic acid – 35 to 60 mg a day. This is a very large dose of folic acid and is available only by prescription at compounding pharmacies (helps with periodic leg movements).
- vitamin B$_{12}$ – 500 mcg a day (taken with folic acid helps with periodic leg movements)
- vitamin E – 400 to 800 IU a day (for periodic leg movements)
- niacin – 100 mg a day; decrease the dose if this causes flushing (for nightmares)
- calcium lactate or calcium chelate – 1,000 to 1,500 mg a day in divided doses with 400 to 800 mg of magnesium a day (has a calming effect)
- inositol – 100 mg a day at bedtime (enhances REM sleep)
- melatonin – 1.5 to 5 mg two hours before bedtime—use synthetic form only (helps regulate sleep cycles by correcting imbalances in the body's circadian rhythm). It may take two months to notice improvement in sleep patterns. Do not take melatonin if you have night terrors, as it may make them worse.
- DLPA – 500 mg at bedtime (for pain if pain prevents sleep)
- GABA – 500 mg at bedtime, taken with 500 mg glycine (helps if hypoglycemic)

Herbal Therapy

Take a botanical supplement 20 to 30 minutes before bedtime.

- California poppy – has sedative, sleep promoting, and anti-anxiety properties
- chamomile – has a calming effect on smooth muscle tissue
- hops – has a calming effect on the body
- kava kava – has sedative properties
- passion flower – has sedative properties that promote sleep and relaxation
- peppermint – relaxes muscles and has a calming effect on the body
- St. John's wort – can relieve chronic insomnia caused by a brain chemistry imbalance
- skullcap – reduces aches and pains that can keep you awake
- valerian – improves sleep quality and relieves insomnia
- wild lettuce – calms restlessness and relieves insomnia

Homeopathic Remedies

Try the homeopathic remedy that best fits your symptoms. The following are but a few of the many possibilities. If you do not obtain relief, consult a homepathic practitioner.

- *Arsenicum album* – sleeplessness from fears; panic attacks, especially after midnight, or from 12 to 2 A.M.; restless, goes from bed to chair to sofa.
- *Calcarea carbonicum* – sleepless from rush of ideas; aroused from sleep by disagreeable ideas; nightmares in children who scream after midnight and cannot be pacified; fantastic, frightening dreams; horrible vision on closing eyes.
- *China officinalis* – sleep disturbed by slight noises; sleeplessness from excited thoughts and heroic fantasies.
- *Coffea* – wide-awake condition; cannot close

the eyes; physical excitement through mental exaltation, after happy news, after overwork that brings joy, and after pleasant surprise, but not from discomfort or pain; insomnia from good or bad news.

- *Kali carbonica* – wakes during the night, especially 2 to 4 A.M.; wakes four hours after falling asleep; sleeplessness without cause – just cannot let go; jerks or twitches on falling asleep or in sleep; talks in sleep; starts up in sleep.

- *Lachesis* – sleep impossible on left side, must sleep on right side; starts up in sleep as if suffocating; sleep apnea; nightmares; sleeplessness from cerebral irritation; frightful dreams of snakes; children toss, moaning in sleep; insomnia before midnight; sleepy but unable to fall asleep.

- *Nux vomica* – sleeplessness caused by abuse of coffee or tea or drugs; wakes especially at 3 or 4 A.M. and cannot sleep because of thoughts about work or how to accomplish tasks; sleepiness during day; worse eating, when sitting, watching TV; sleeplessness from mental strain, excessive study.

- *Pulsatilla* – sleep disturbed by a fixed idea or a particular song or phrase of a song running through the head; weeps from inability to go to sleep; worse warm room, large or rich meal.

Many patients respond to complex homeopathic remedies. You may want to try PHP Insomnia Drops, which help to stimulate natural sleep mechanisms.

Other Therapeutic Measures

If you cannot sleep because of physical discomfort, try a new mattress or consider having an adjustment from a chiropractor or an osteopath.

Avoid taking aspirin at night. It interferes with melatonin secretion, which in turn affects sleep.

Also avoid nasal decongestants and other cold medications late in the day. Although they cause drowsiness in some people, they have the opposite effect on others, acting as a stimulant.

If you have hyperinsulinemia, have it properly treated (see pp. 235–36).

If you snore, elevate your head, lose some weight, and do not sleep on your back. Even if your snoring does not cause you insomnia, it may be contributing to your mate's sleep problems.

Instead of using earplugs at night, run a white-noise generator; this new technology actually cancels out sound waves.

Obtain counseling to determine if emotional problems are contributing to your insomnia, and to learn how to deal with stress.

Try "virtual dreaming," in which you think about whatever you would most like to dream about. Visualize a pleasurable activity at length, and savor each detail.

Use stress reduction techniques such as biofeedback, progressive relaxation, yoga, hypnotherapy, and massage therapy.

Deep breathing and other breathing techniques can all help people fall asleep, as well. Take three deep breaths very slowly, exhaling fully each time. After the third exhalation, stop breathing for as long you can. This has a tranquilizing effect because it causes carbon dioxide to accumulate in the blood.

Take Bach Flower remedies (see chapter 10, Alternative Therapies).

Once a normal sleep pattern has been established, wean yourself from the botanicals, homeopathic remedies, or nutritional supplements. However, patients with restless legs and periodic leg movements may not be able to stop their supplements. If you are unable to stop completely, reduce the amounts you are taking or use the supplements only periodically.

CHAPTER 30

Conclusion

We hope that after reading this book, you have come to several conclusions. The first conclusion we hope you have reached is that neither modern medicine nor alternative medicine has all of the answers. Each type of medicine has many strengths, and each has weaknesses. We have attempted to add to your knowledge of the strengths and weaknesses of both modern medicine and alternative medicine. We have endeavored to spark your interest, so that you will investigate all the medical facilities available to you (both traditional and alternative). In order to protect and improve your health, it is imperative that you become an informed medical consumer, and learn to use the best of both worlds. For any given medical problem, traditional care, alternative care, or a combination of both will prove to be the right treatment.

We hope that you now realize some things about modern medicine you may not have been aware of before, among them that vaccinations may not be the preventative they are presented as being, and surgery may not always be necessary and may not be the only or best treatment. You may not have considered the active role you must play to help assure successful and safe hospital stays for you or your family.

There is no "magic pill" that is going to cure you. We hope you have come to realize that if you do indeed take pills (which are sometimes necessary, and which may provide some benefit)

you will have to be aware of their side effects. You should now better understand the attitudes of modern medicine practitioners, as well as the basic philosophy of modern medicine.

In our discussion of alternative medicine, we have endeavored to make you aware that there are many nontoxic and natural methods of treating diseases and health problems. Before reading this book, some of you may not have known that there are alternative total health care systems, and that modern medicine is not the only system available to you. There are also many alternative treatment techniques that can be helpful (even curative) that are not part of a total health care system. We hope that you will go on to a deeper investigation of the alternative treatments and health care systems than we have been able to present in this book.

There is no magic cure that requires no effort on your part; good health does not "just happen." You must take an active role in maintaining and promoting your health and that of your family. You must find health care that addresses your personal needs, goals, and expectations. Finding and using the best treatment will help you to recover and maintain your health. This can decrease the need for expensive and invasive treatments, which will in turn decrease the frequency and severity of complications, improving the overall effectiveness of your medical care.

The second conclusion we hope you have reached is that prevention of illness is of paramount importance. Modern medicine, as it is practiced today, is strictly rescue medicine—and sometimes rescue is difficult (if not impossible) when health has deteriorated beyond a certain level. Prevention is not just a matter of regular laboratory tests (although laboratory tests can be helpful). Prevention is living a healthy lifestyle to preserve and improve health, making rescue medicine largely unnecessary except in cases of accident or other trauma. There is no substitute for a healthy lifestyle in the quest to obtain and maintain good health.

As we have noted throughout the book, most of the degenerative diseases of today are lifestyle diseases. A sad example of this can be found among the Pima Indians of Arizona. The Pima today are more obese than almost any other group in the world. Fifty percent of the Pimas over 35 have diabetes (eight times the national average). Young men and women are disabled by diabetes; they have lost limbs, become blind, or are confined to a wheelchair.

All this is in stark contrast to the Pima Indians of Mexico—people of the same tribe. Although these Pima eat slightly more calories than the Arizona Pima, they are slender. Their diet consists almost entirely of beans, potatoes, and corn tortillas, with chicken perhaps once a month, while the diet of the Arizona Pima is the standard American diet: high in sugar and carbohydrates, and close to 40 percent fat. The Mexican Pima also put in 23 hours of moderate to hard physical labor each week, whereas the Arizona Pima put in two hours. Clearly lifestyle differences have played a role in the current health of each group.

There are uncontrollable risk factors that affect your health, such as family history, gender, and age. However, there are also many controllable risk factors such as diet, smoking, sedentary living, obesity, psychological stress, environmental exposures, and other variables.

Even our personality and character affect our health, as the way we handle our feelings and emotions directly relates to health. With the proper care and changes in lifestyle, controllable risk factors can be directed toward optimum health. Even the uncontrollable risk factors can be minimized.

Dr. Stephen Sinatra asks in his book, *Optimum Health,* "If you wear out this body, where are you going to live?" We urge you to take care of your body by taking charge of your health. Consider carefully each point listed below.

- Eat a diet appropriate to your health needs. In addition, eat quality food and avoid refined sugar, excess fats, excess salt, alcohol, and junk food. Keep your body hydrated by drinking ample pure water.
- Take nutrients, including vitamins, minerals, amino acids, fatty acids, antioxidants, and enzymes. Positive health benefits have been demonstrated from the use of nutrients, but they are not a substitute for proper diet. They can help to make up for deficits in our diet and to compensate for metabolism defects and problems.
- Detoxify your body. Our bodies labor under a toxic load caused by a polluted environment and unhealthy lifestyle, and until the toxins are removed from our bodies we cannot enjoy good health.
- Strengthen your immune system. A strong immune system makes you less vulnerable to disease, and being disease free is necessary for health. An intact and healthy immune system forms a strong base for optimum health.
- Exercise regularly. Exercise has physical and mental benefits, including relieving stress. The physical benefits are multiple, including increased energy and retardation of the aging process. Mental benefits can include improved self-concept and lower levels of anxiety and depression.
- Clean up your environment. Clean air, food,

and water, as well as a clean home and a safe work environment are essential to optimum health.

- Attend to your spirituality. Spirituality is belief in the life force and energy both inside you and beyond yourself. Have faith in those powers and turn to them for strength and courage. In addition to being a physical condition, health is also a mental, emotional, and spiritual condition.
- Find the right treatment. After intelligent investigation on your part, have your health problems treated by the best possible method with the help of an appropriate practitioner—whether it be a modern medicine practitioner, an alternative practitioner, or one who combines both worlds.

Prevent and correct health problems by changing your lifestyle to one that promotes good health. Strive for and maintain the best health possible, in order to enjoy the happiest and most fulfilling life possible.

RECOMMENDED SOURCES
AND ORGANIZATIONS

The following sources and organizations are those listed in the text of this book. They represent only the products and companies with which we are familiar. Certainly there are other sources and other products that would be of benefit to use in restoring and maintaining health.

AIR CLEANERS

AllerMed
31 Steel Road
Wylie, TX   75098
(972) 442-4898

Foust Air Purifiers
E. L. Foust Company, Inc.
P.O. Box 105
Elmhurst, IL   60126
(800) 225-9549

COMPOUNDING PHARMACIES

Abrams Royal Pharmacy
8220 Abrams Road
Dallas, TX   75231
(214) 349-8000
(800) 458-0804
Fax: (214) 341-7966

Apothe' Cure
13720 Midway Road
Suite 109
Dallas, TX   75244
(972) 960-6601
(800) 969-6601
Fax: (972) 960-6921
From Canada:
(800) 203-2158
Fax: (972) 490-7438

College Pharmacy
3505 Austin Bluff Pkwy #101
Colorado Springs, CO   80918-5072
(719) 262-0022
(800) 888-9358
Fax: (800) 556-5893

Kripps Pharmacy
994 Granville Street
Vancouver, BC   V6Z 1L2
Canada
(604) 687-2564
Fax: (604) 685-9721

Wellness, Health, and Pharmaceuticals
P.O. Box 59402
Birmingham, AL   35259
(800) 227-2627
Fax: (800) 369-0302

Women's International Pharmacy
13925 W. Meeker Blvd., Ste. #13
Sun City West, AZ   85375
(800) 699-8143
Fax: (800) 330-0268

CHIROPRACTIC TECHNIQUES

NAET
Nambudripad's Allergy Elimination
    Technique
Dr. Devi Nambudripad
6714 Beach Blvd.
Buena Park, CA   90621
(714) 523-8900
Fax: (714) 523-3068

NET
NeuroEmotional Technique
Dr. Scott Walker
524 Second Street
Encinitas, CA   92024
(619) 944-1030
(800) 888-4638
Fax: (619) 753-7191

DETOXIFICATION CENTERS

Center for Occupational and
    Environmental Medicine
Dr. Allan Lieberman
7510 Northforest Drive
North Charleston, SC   29420
(803) 572-1600
Fax: (803) 572-1995

Environmental Health Center
Dr. William Rea
8345 Walnut Hill Lane, Suite 205
Dallas, TX   75235
(214) 368-4132
Fax: (214) 691-8432

The Northwest Healing Arts Center
Dr. Walter Crinnion
1200 112th Ave. N.E., Suite A100
Bellevue, WA   98005
(206) 747-9200

Preventive Medical Center of Marin
Dr. Elson Haas
25 Mitchell, #8
San Rafael, CA   94903
(415) 472-2343
Fax: (415) 472-7636

Robbins Environmental Medicine Clinic
Dr. Albert Robbins
400 S. Dixie Highway, Building 2,
    Suite 210
Boca Raton, FL   33432
(561) 395-3282
Fax (561) 395-3304

HERBAL SUPPLIES

Abkit Inc.
207 East 94th Street, 2nd Floor
New York, NY   10128
(800) 226-6227
(212) 860-8358
(Natureworks Marigold Ointment)

BioActive Nutritional Inc.
1803 N. Wickham Rd., Suite 6
Melbourne, FL   32935
(800) 288-9525
Fax: (407) 254-6505
(Hepatatox, Dandiplex, Karzan)

Botanical Laboratories
P.O. Box 1596
Ferndale, WA   98248
(800) 232-4005
(360) 384-5656
Fax: (360) 384-1140
(Natra-Bio Bladder Irritation)

Eclectic Institute
14385 S.E. Lusted Rd.
Sandy, OR   97055
(503) 668-4120
(800) 332-4372
Fax: (503) 668-3227
(Herbal Products)

Gaia Herbs
108 Island Ford Rd.
Bervard, NC   28712
(828) 884-4242
(800) 831-7780
Fax: (828) 883-5960
(Herbal Products)

Herbs Etc. of Santa Fe
1345 Cerrillos Rd.
Santa Fe, NM   87505
(505) 982-1265
(Stomach Tonic)

Marco Pharma
15810 West 6th Avenue
Golden, CO   80401
(303) 277-9553
(800) 999-3001
Fax: (303) 277-9623
(Hepatica)

Nutricology, Inc./Allergy Research Group
P.O. Box 489
San Leandro, CA   94577
Information: (800) 545-9960
Orders: (800) 782-4274
Fax: (800) 688-7426
International Orders: (570) 639-4572
International Fax: (570) 635-6730
(ParaMicrocidin, ParQing)

UniKey Health Systems
P.O. Box 7168
Bozeman, MT   59771
(800) 888-4353
Customer Service: (406) 586-9424
(Herbal Parasite Treatment)

HOMEOPATHIC SUPPLIES

BHI Homeopathic Products
11600 Cochiti, S.E.
Albuquerque, NM   87123
(505) 293-3843
(800) 621-7644
Fax: (505) 275-1642
(Complex Homeopathic Remedies)

Boiron
East Coast:
Campus Boulevard Building A
Newtown Square, PA   19073
West Coast:
98C W. Cochran St.
Simi Valley, CA   93065
(800) BLU-TUBE
(Classical Homeopathic Remedies)

CompliMed
1441 West Smith Road
Ferndale, WA   98248
(800) 232-4005
Fax: (360) 384-1140
(Complex Homeopathic Remedies)

Dolisos America, Inc.
3014 Rigel Ave.
Las Vegas, NV   89102
(702) 871-7153
(800) 365-4767
Fax: (702) 871-9670
(Classical Homeopathic Remedies)

Homeopathic Educational Services
2124 Kittredge Street
Berkeley, CA   94704
(510) 649-0294
Orders: (800) 359-9051
Fax: (510) 649-1955
(Homeopathic Books and Literature)

Natural Health Supply
P.O. Box 6033
Santa Fe, NM   87502
(505) 474-9175
Fax: (505) 473-0336
(Homeopathic Supplies)

PHP Professional Health Products Ltd.
211 Overlook Drive
Suite 5
Sewickley, PA   15143
(800) 929-4133
(Complex Homeopathic Remedies)

Vibrant Health
150 des Grands Couteau
St. Mathieu de Beloeil, PQ   J36 2C9
Canada
(450) 536-1295
Fax: (450) 536-1294
(Complex Homeopathic Remedies)

LABORATORIES

Doctor's Data, Inc.
P.O. Box 111
West Chicago, IL   60185
(800) 323-2784
Fax: (630) 231-9190
(Nutritional Testing, Hair Analysis)

Great Smokies Diagnostic Laboratory
63 Zillicoa Street
Ashville, NC   28801
(704) 253-6621
(800) 522-4762
Fax: (704) 253-1127
(Nutritional Testing, Parasite Testing,
    Intestinal Permeability)

Meridian Valley Clinical Laboratory
515 W. Harrison St.
Suite 9
Kent, WA   98042
(253) 859-8700
Fax: (253) 859-1135
(Nutritional Testing, Parasite Testing)

Meta Matrix Medical Laboratory
5000 Peachtree Industrial Blvd.
Suite 110
Norcross, GA   30071
(770) 446-5483
Fax: (770) 441-2237
(Nutritional Testing)

Oncolab, Inc.
36 The Fenway
Boxton, MA   02215
(800) 922-8378 (answering service)
(AMAS Test)

Dr. O.M. Amin
Institute of Parasitic Disease
Diagnostic and Educational Laboratory
3530 E. Indian School Road
Phoenix, AZ   85018
(602) 955-4211
(Parasite Testing)

SpectraCell Laboratories
515 Post Oak Boulevard
Suite 830
Houston, TX   77027
(713) 621-3101
(800) 227-5227
Fax: (713) 621-3234
(Nutritional Testing)

Urokeep, Inc.
P.O. Box 2094
Chandler, AZ   85244
(602) 545-9236
(Distributor of parasite test kits—works
   with Dr. Amin)

MISCELLANEOUS

Aerobic Life Industries
2916 N. 35th Ave., Ste. 8
Phoenix, AZ   87017
(602) 455-6380
(800) 798-0707
(Aerobic 07)

Advanced Health Products
24000 Mercantile Rd., Ste. 7
Beachwood, OH   44122
(888) 262-5700
Fax: (216) 514-9904
(High Performance Hygiene Systems)

Heidelberg International, Inc.
933 Beasley Street
Blairsville Industrial Park
Blairsville, GA   30514
(706) 745-9698
(800) 241-7517
(Heidelberg gastrogram pH system)

Himalayan International Institute
RR1 Box 405
Honesdale, PA   18431
570-253-5551
Fax 570-253-9078
E-mail: himalayaninstitute.org
(Neti Pot)

HumaScan
125 Moen Ave.
Cranford, NJ   07016
(908) 709-3434
(888) HUMASCAN
Fax: (908) 709-4646
(Breast Alert)

Hydro Med, Inc.
4419 Van Nuys Blvd.
Suite 310
Sherman Oaks, CA   991403
Phone (800) 560-9007
Fax (818) 377-3426
(Grossan Nasal Irrigator Tip)

Inventive Products
1450 E. North St.
Decatur, IL   60521
(800) 356-6911
Fax: (217) 423-7282
(Sensor Pad)

N.E.E.D.S.
(National Ecological and Environmental
   Delivery System)
527 Charles Ave., 12-A
Syracuse, NY   13209
(800) 634-1380
Fax: (315) 488-6336 or (800) 295-NEED
(Environmental and Health Supplies,
   Somes #7)

NeoLife
GNLD Distributor Services
3500 Gateway Blvd.
Fremont, CA   94538
(510) 651-0405
(800) 432-5848
(NeoLife Green)

Urohealth Corporation
3050 Redhill Avenue
Costa Mesa, CA   92626
(714) 708-7748
(800) 328-1103
(Snap Gauge Kit)

Wilson's Syndrome Foundation
P.O. Box 539
Summerfield, FL   34492
(800) 621-7006 (voice mail)
www.wilsonssyndrome.com
(Thyroid Protocol)

NUTRIENTS

American Lecithin Company
115 Hurley Rd. Unit 2B
Oxford, CT   06478
(800) 364-4416
Fax: (203) 262-7101
(Phos-chol Concentrate)

AMNI
Advanced Medical Nutrition, Inc.
2247 National Ave.
Hayward, CA   94545
(800) 437-8888
Fax: (510) 783-8196
(Oral Chelation Pack, Organic
   Germanium)

Atkins Nutritionals, Inc.
125 Wilbur Place
Bohemia, NY   11710
(800) 628-5467
Fax: (888) 728-5467
(516) 563-9280
Fax: (516) 563-8943
(Emotional Aid Formula)

BioTech
P.O. Box 1992
Fayetteville, AR   79702
(800) 345-1199
Fax: (501) 443-5643
(DNZ-2)

Biotics Research Corporation
4850 Wright Rd., Ste. 150
Stafford, TX   77477
(281) 240-8010
(800) 231-5777
Fax: (281) 240-2304
(NutriClear)

Ecological Formulas
(Cardiovascular Research/Arteria)
1061 B Shary Circle
Concord, CA   94518
(800) 351-9429
(Hypoallergenic Nutrients, Tri-Salts,
   Norival, Monolaurin)

HealthComm International, Inc.
5800 Soundview Dr.
Gig Harbor, WA   98335
(800) 843-9660
(253) 851-3943
Fax: (253) 851-9749
(UltraClear, Mitochondrial Resuscitate)

Immunotec Research Ltd.
292 Adrien Patenaude
Vaudreuil—Dorion, PQ   J7V 5V5
Canada
(514) 424-9992
Fax: (514) 424-9993
(Immunocal)

Klaire Laboratories (Vital Life Products)
1573 W. Seminole
San Marcos, CA   92069
(760) 477-9680
(800) 533-7255
(Hypoallergenic Nutrients, BiCarb
   Formula)

Longevity Plus
814 N. Beeline, Suite I
P.O. Box 3660
Payson, AZ   85541
(800) 580-PLUS
(520) 474-3684
Fax: (520) 474-3819
(Beyond Chelation)

Marco Pharma
15810 West 6th Avenue
Golden, CO   80401
(303) 277-9553
(800) 999-3001
Fax: (303) 277-9623
(Protozymes)

Nutricology, Inc./Allergy Research Group
P.O. Box 489
San Leandro, CA   94577
Information: (800) 545-9960
Orders: (800) 782-4274
Fax: (800) 688-7426
International Orders: (570) 639-4572
International Fax: (570) 635-6730
(Hypoallergenic Nutrients, Organic
   Germanium, Oxynutrients,
   BottomsUp, Buffered C)

Rexall Showcase International
853 Broken Sound Parkway NW
Boca Raton, FL   33487-3694
(561) 994-2090
(BiosLife 2)

Pain and Stress Therapy Center
Dr. Billie Sahley
5282 Medical Drive #160
San Antonio, TX   78229-6023
Orders: (800) 669-2256
Consultations: (210) 614-7246
Fax: (210) 614-4336
(Specialty Nutrients, Balanced
   Neurotransmitter Complex, Anxiety
   Control)

Scientific Botanicals
P.O. Box 31131
Seattle, WA   98113
(206) 527-5521
Fax: (206) 526-7948
(Hydroxyfolate)

Super Life Inc.
P.O. Box 261280
San Diego, CA   92196-1280
Credit card orders only:
   (888) 4-MINERAL
Customer Service: (800) 359-3245
Fax: (619) 693-1330
(Biotic Code NK 9-1-1)

Thorne Research
P.O. Box 25
Dover, ID   83825
(208) 263-1337
(Hypoallergenic Nutrients, Formula
   SF722)

Twin Labs
150 Motor Parkway
Hauppauge, NY   11788
(516) 467-3140
Outside NY: (800) 645-5626
Fax: (516) 630-3488
(Hypoallergenic Nutrients, Allergy C)

William Wallace Marketing
P.O. Box 836
Cave Junction, OR   97523
(888) 840-4460
(541) 592-3495
Fax: (541) 592-6773
(Cetyl myristoleate)

PROFESSIONAL ORGANIZATIONS

American Academy of Biological
   Dentistry
P.O. Box 856
Carmel Valley, CA   93924
(408) 659-5385
Fax: (408) 569-2417

American Academy of Environmental
   Medicine
c/o American Finance Center
7701 East Kellog, Suite 625
Wichita, KS   67207
(316) 684-5500
Fax: 316-684-5709
E-mail: aaem@swbell.net

American Association of Acupuncture
   and Oriental Medicine
4101 Lake Boone Trial, Ste. 201
Raleigh, NC   27607
(919) 787-5181

American Association of Naturopathic
   Physicians
201 Valley St., Ste. 105
Seattle, WA   98109

(206) 298-0126
Fax: (206) 298-0129

American Botanical Council
P.O. Box 201660
Austin, TX   78720
(512) 331-8868

American Chiropractic Association
1701 Clarendon Blvd.
Arlington, VA   22209
(703) 276-8800
Fax: (703) 243-2593

American College for Advancement in
   Medicine
P.O. Box 3427
Laguna Hills, CA   92654
(714) 583-7666
(800) 532-3688

American Massage Therapy Association
820 Davis Street, Ste. 100
Evanston, IL   60201
(847) 864-0123
Fax: (847) 864-1178

American Osteopathic Association
142 East Ontario Street
Chicago, IL   60611
(312) 202-8000

American School of Ayurvedic Sciences
2115 112th Ave. NE
Bellvue, WA   98004
(425) 453-8022
Fax: (425) 451-2670

Canadian Chiropractic Association
1396 Eglinton Ave. W.
Toronto, ON   M6C 2E4
Canada
(416) 781-5656
Fax: (416) 784-7344

Canadian College of Naturopathic
   Medicine
2300 Yonge Street, 18th Floor
P.O. Box 2431
Toronto, ON   M4P 1E4
Canada
(416) 484-6821
Fax: (416) 486-8584
Email: Info@www.ccnm.edu

International Society for Orthomolecular
   Medicine
16 Florence Ave.
Toronto, ON   M2N 1E9
Canada
(416) 733-2117
Fax: (416) 733-2352
www.orthmed.org
E-mail: centre@orthmed.org

National Center for Homeopathy
801 North Fairfax, Suite 306
Alexandria, VA   22314
(703) 458-7790
Fax: (703) 548-7792

Ontario Massage Therapist Association
365 Bloor Street E., Suite 1807
Toronto, ON   M4W 3L4
Canada
(416) 968-6487

Shiatsu School of Canada
547 College Street
Toronto, ON   M6G 1A9
Canada
(416) 323-1703
(800) 263-1703
Fax: (416) 323-1681

RECOMMENDED READING

BOOKS

You may want to read some of these books to increase your knowledge regarding your health problems, and to help you find the right treatment.

Alternative Medicine—The Definitive Guide, Burton Goldberg Group. Future Medicine Publishing, Inc., Puyallup, WA, 1993.

A comprehensive, educational tool to acquaint the reader with alternative methods for the maintenance of good health and the treatment of illness. It presents an explanation of disease processes, the philosophy of alternative medicine, and many alternative treatments.

An Alternative Medicine Definitive Guide to Cancer, W. John Diamond and W. Lee Crowden with Burton Goldberg. Future Medicine Publishing, Tiburon, CA, 1997.

Tells how cancer can be reversed using clinically proven complementary and alternative therapies. The successful treatments used by 37 doctors for reversing cancer are presented, as well as information for locating both treatment centers and physicians.

The Best Treatment, Isodore Rosenfield. Simon and Schuster, New York, NY, 1991.

Dr. Rosenfield describes the standard medical treatment for over 100 diseases. The book is well written and easily read by the non-medical person.

The Carbohydrate Addict's Diet, Rachael Heller and Richard Heller. Signet, NY, 1993. This book discusses the physical addiction to carbohydrates and its effects on health, including obesity, hypertension, and cardiovascular disease. A diagnostic test is included as well as a diet plan, menus, and recipes.

Depression Cured at Last, Sherry A. Rogers. SK Publishing, Sarasota, FL, 1997.

Delves into the biochemistry of depression, illustrating with numerous scientific references why depression needs to be treated by correcting biochemical imbalances in the body. "Depression is not a Prozac deficiency."

Encyclopedia of Natural Medicine, Michael Murray and Joseph Pizzorno. Prima Publishing, Rochelin, CA, 1991.

This book explains disease processes in a very detailed and understandable way. It then discusses herbal and supplement treatment for the diseases.

Healthy for Life, Richard Heller and Rachael Heller. Plume/Penguin, NY, 1995.

Written more scientifically than their first book, the Hellers tell how to reduce obesity and the risk of serious illness and early death by controlling hyperinsulinemia. A diet plan, menus, and recipes are included.

Living Pain Free, Devi Nambudripad. Delta Publishing Co., Buena Park, CA, 1997. A handbook of acupressure points for treating pain arising in various parts of the body. It is helpful for the non-medical person who would like to use self-treatment of minor problems at home.

Prescription for Nutritional Health, James F. Balch and Phyllis A. Balch. Avery Publishing Group, Garden City Park, NY, 1997.

This encyclopedic book discusses nutrients, herbs, remedies and therapies, and their uses for over 100 medical conditions. Easy for the non-medical person to understand and use.

Rotation Isn't Just for Tires, Frances Taylor, Deborah Brandt, and Jacqueline Krohn. Los Alamos, NM, 1995.

A how-to rotation diet cookbook that takes the reader step-by-step through using a rotation diet. Several variations of rotation diets are included, complete with suggested menus and accompanying recipes for appetizers, main dishes, salads, dips, sauces, snacks, desserts, and vegetable/vegetarian dishes.

The Staying Healthy Shopper's Guide: Feed Your Family Safely, Elson Haas. Celestial Arts, Berkeley, CA, 1999.

Dr. Elson Haas guides you through the modern American grocery store, helping you avoid all the common nutritional pitfalls from additives and dyes to pesticides and preservatives. Explores how and why our foods are processed, and how pollutants and other toxic substances enter the food chain, ending up on your table.

The Whole Way to Allergy Relief and Prevention, Jacqueline Krohn, Frances Taylor, and Erla Mae Larson. Hartley and Marks Publishers, Inc., Point Roberts, WA, 1996.

A comprehensive book about allergies. This book discusses chemical, food, and inhalant allergies, and treatment and prevention of allergies.

The Whole Way to Natural Detoxification, Jacqueline Krohn, Frances Taylor, and Jinger Prosser. Hartley and Marks Publishers, Inc., Point Roberts, WA, 1996.

An encyclopedic coverage of detoxification and cleansing, balancing, and preventive methods. Nutritional, homeopathic, and herbal methods of detoxification are discussed.

NEWSLETTERS

All of the following newsletters are an excellent source of information regarding health problems and alternative treatment for them.

Health and Healing, Julian Whitaker, editor. Phillips Publishing, Inc., Potomac, MD.

Dr. Whitaker discusses common diseases and scientifically based treatment with herbs, nutrients, and diet. He includes sources for obtaining the products he discusses.

Nutrition and Healing, Jonathan A. Wright, editor. Nutrition and Healing, Inc., Phoenix, AZ.

Dr. Wright is one of the leading experts on nutrient supplementation in North America. In this newsletter, he features a disease and its nutritional treatment, a vitamin, and an herb each month. Scientific references and studies are also included.

Dr. Andrew Weil's Self Healing, Andrew Weil. Thorne Communications, Inc., Watertown, MA.

A leader in integrative medicine, Dr. Weil knows what conventional medicine can and cannot do, and he also knows alternative medicine. His newsletter gives advice on how to get well and stay healthy by relying on your body's innate healing powers.

Dr. Robert Atkins' Health Revelations, Robert C. Atkins. Agora Health Publishing, Baltimore, MD.

In this newsletter Dr. Atkins discusses his treatment of many different diseases and health problems, and the scientific basis for his use of complementary medicine. He gives many case histories to illustrate his points.

Second Opinion, Dr. William Campbell Douglass. Second Opinion Publishing, Inc., Atlanta, GA.

Written by a pioneer alternative physician,

this newsletter discusses health problems, medical treatments, laboratory tests, and nutritional treatments. He cites studies as well as drawing from his own medical practice and experience.

Prescriptions for Healthy Living, Dr. James Balch. Weiss Research, Palm Beach Gardens, FL.

The emphasis of this newsletter is alternative choices for health and longevity. Dr. Balch devotes each issue of this informative newsletter to a particular health problem, describing it completely and offering suggestions for alternative and nutritional treatment.

BIBLIOGRAPHY

BOOKS

Ackerknecht, Erwin H. *A Short History of Medicine.* New York: The Ronald Press Company, 1968.

Ader, R., ed. *Psychoneuroimmunology.* New York: Academic Press, 1981.

Altman, N. "Cancer." *Oxygen Healing Therapies.* Rochester, VT: Healing Arts Press, 1995.

Altman, N. "Hydrogen Peroxide." *Oxygen Healing Therapies.* Rochester, VT: Healing Arts Press, 1995.

Arky, Ronald, Medical Consultant. *Physicians' Desk Reference.* Montvale, NJ: Medical Economics Company, Inc., 1998.

Atkins, Robert C. *Dr. Atkins' Health Revolution.* New York: Bantam Books, 1989.

Atkins, Robert C. *Dr. Atkins' New Diet Revolution.* New York: Avon Books, 1997.

Atkins, Robert C. *Dr. Atkins' Vita-Nutrient Solution.* New York: Simon & Schuster, 1998.

Balch, James F., and Phyllis A. Balch. *Prescription for Nutritional Healing.* Garden City Park, NY: Avery Publishing Group, 1997.

Barnes, Broda. *Hypothyroidism: Unsuspected Illness.* New York: Harper Collins Publishers, Inc., 1976.

Batmanghelidj, F. *How to Deal Simply with Back Pain and Rheumatoid Joint Pain.* Falls Church, VA: Global Health Solutions, 1991.

Batmanghelidj, F. *Your Body's Many Cries for Water.* Falls Church, VA: Global Health Solutions, 1995.

Beaver, Paul Chester; Rodney Clifton Jung; and Eddie Wayne Cupp. *Clinical Parasitology.* Philadelphia, PA: Lea & Febiger, 1984.

Blake, Michael. *The Natural Healer's Acupressure Handbook, Vol. I; Basic G–Jo.* Fort Lauderdale, FL: Falkynor Books, 1983.

Blau, Sheldon P., and Elaine Fantle Shimberg. *How to Get Out of the Hospital Alive.* New York: Macmillan, 1997.

Bosker, Gideon. *Pills That Work—Pills That Don't.* New York: Harmon Books, 1997.

Bradford, T.L. *The Logic of Figures of Comparative Results of Homeopathic and Other Treatments.* Philadelphia, PA: Boericke and Tafel, 1990.

Braverman, Eric R., with Carl Pfeiffer. *The Healing Nutrients Within.* New Canaan, CT: Keats Publishing, 1987.

Brostoff, Jonathon, and Stephen J. Challacombe, eds. *Food Allergy and Intolerance.* London, England: Bailliere Tindall, 1987.

Brown, Harold W., and Franklin A. Neva. *Basic Clinical Parasitology.* Norwalk, CT: Appleton-Century-Crofts, 1983.

Budavari, Susan, ed. *The Merck Index.* Rahway, NJ: Merck & Co., Inc., 1989.

Burger, Alfred. *Drugs and People.* Charlottesville, VA: University Press of Virginia, 1988.

Burton Goldberg Group. *Alternative Medicine—The Definitive Guide.* Puyallup, WA: Future Medicine Publishing, Inc. 1993.

Castleman, Michael. *Nature's Cures.* Emmaus, PA: Rodale Press, 1996.

Castleman, Michael. *The Healing Herbs.* Emmaus, PA: Rodale Press, 1991.

Chabner, Bruce A., and Jerry M. Collins. *Cancer Chemotherapy.* Philadelphia, PA: J.B. Lippincott Co., 1990.

Cheraskin, Emanuel; Marshal W. Ringsdorf, Jr.; and

Emily L. Sisley. *The Vitamin C Connection*. New York: Harper and Row, 1983.

Chopra, Deepak. *Perfect Health—The Complete Mind/Body Guide*. New York: Harmony Books, 1991.

Christopher, John R. *Herbal Home Health Care* (Formerly *Childhood Diseases*). Springville, UT: Christopher Publication, 1976.

Clendening, Logan. *Source Book of Medical History*. New York: Dover Publications, 1942.

Coleman, Richard M. *Wide Awake at 3 A.M. by Choice or by Chance*. New York: W.H. Freeman and Company, 1986.

Cooper, Kenneth H. *Controlling Cholesterol*. New York: Bantam Books, 1988.

Coulter, Harris L., and Barbara Loe Fisher. *A Shot in the Dark*. Garden City, NY: Avery Publishing Group, Inc., 1991.

Cranton, Elmer. *Bypassing Bypass*. New York: Stein and Day, 1984.

Cukier, Daniel, and Virginia E. McCullough. *Coping with Radiation Therapy*. Los Angeles, CA: Lowell House, 1993.

D'Adamo, Peter J., and Catherine Whitney. *Eat Right 4 Your Type*. New York: C.P. Putnam's Sons, 1996.

Das, Rai Bahadur Bishamber. *Select Your Remedy*. New Delhi, India: Vishwamber Free Homoeo Dispensary, 1991.

DeBakey, Michael E; Antonio M. Golto, Jr.; Lynne W. Scott; and John P. Foreyt. *The Living Heart Diet*. New York: Raven Press, 1984.

Diamond, W. John, and W. Lee Cowden, with Burton Goldberg. *An Alternative Medicine Definitive Guide to Cancer*. Tiburon, CA: Future Medicine Publishing, Inc., 1997.

Dossey, Larry. *Healing Words*. San Francisco, CA: Harper, 1993.

Dossey, Larry. *Prayer is Good Medicine*. New York: Harper and Collins, 1996.

Douglass, William Campbell. *Hormone Replacement Therapies: Astonishing Results for Men and Women*. Altanta, GA: Second Opinion Publishing, Inc., 1996.

Duke, James A. *The Green Pharmacy*. Emmaus, PA: Rodale Press, 1997.

Eades, Michael R., and Mary Dan Eades. *Protein Power*. New York: Bantam Books, 1996.

Editors. *The Big Book of Health Tips*. Peachtree City, GA: FC & A Publishing, 1996.

Editors. *5-Minute Cures*. Emmaus, PA: Rodale Press, 1998.

Editors. *1,001 Home Health Remedies*. Peachtree City, GA: FC & A Publishing, 1993.

Editors. *Natural Medicines and Cures Your Doctors Never Tells You About*. Peachtree City, GA: FC&A Publishing, 1995.

Editors. *Prevention's New Encyclopedia of Common Diseases*. Emmaus, PA: Rodale Press, 1984.

Editors. *The Prevention How-To Dictionary of Healing Remedies and Techniques*. Emmaus, PA: Rodale Press, 1992.

Editors. *30 Foods that Fight Disease*. San Francisco, CA: Health by Time Publishing Ventures, Inc., 1997.

Editors *801 Prescription Drugs*. Peachtree City, GA: FC&A Publishing, 1996.

Editors of *Prevention Magazine*. *The Doctor's Book of Home Remedies for Children*. New York: Bantam Books, 1994.

Editors of *Prevention Magazine Health Books*. *High-Speed Healing*. Emmaus, PA: Rodale Press, Inc., 1991.

Editors of *Prevention Magazine Health Books*. *Prevention's Healing with Vitamins*. Emmaus, PA: Rodale Press, Inc., 1996.

Editors of *Prevention Magazine Health Books*. *The Complete Book of Natural and Medicinal Cures*. Emmaus, PA: Rodale Press, Inc., 1994.

Editors of *Prevention Magazine*. *The Doctor's Book of Home Remedies*. Emmaus, PA: Rodale Press, 1990.

Editors of *What Doctors Don't Tell You*. *Medicine: What Works and What Doesn't*. Baltimore, MD: Wallace Press, 1995.

Faelton, Sharon, and the Editors of *Prevention Magazine*. *The Complete Book of Minerals for Health*. Emmaus, PA: Rodale Press, 1981.

Feltman, John, ed. *Prevention How-To Dictionary of Healing Remedies and Techniques*. Emmaus, PA: Rodale Press, 1992.

Fischbach, Frances. *A Manual of Laboratory Diagnostic Tests*. Philadelphia, PA: J.B. Lippincott Company, 1984.

Freese, Arthur. *Managing Your Doctor: How to Get the Best Medical Care*. Briarcliff Manor, NY: Stein and Day, 1974.

Fuch-Berman, Adriane. *Alternative Medicine: What Works*. Tucson, AZ: Odonian Press, 1996.

Fulder, Stephen. *How to Survive Medical*

Treatment. New York: Barnes and Noble Books, 1994.

Galland, Leo. *The Four Pillars of Healing.* New York: Random House, 1997.

Gerras, Charles; Joseph Golant; and E. John Hanna, eds. *The Complete Book of Vitamins.* Emmaus, PA: Rodale Press, 1977.

Gittleman, Ann Louise. *Guess What Came to Dinner?* New York: Avery Publishing Group, Inc., 1993.

Gottlieb, Bill, ed. *New Choices in Natural Healing.* Emmaus, PA: Rodale Press, 1995.

Haggard, Howard W. *Mystery, Magic, and Medicine.* Garden City, NY: Doubleday, Doran, & Co., Inc., 1933.

Hallowell, Edward M., and John J. Ratey. *Driven to Distraction.* New York: Touchtstone, 1995.

Harvey, A. McGehee, and Richard Johns, et al. *The Principles and Practice of Medicine.* New York: Appleton-Century-Crofts, 1972.

Haas, Elton. *Staying Healthy with Nutrition: The Complete Guide to Diet and Nutritional Medicine.* Berkeley, CA: Celestial Arts, 1992.

Haas, Elton. *The Detox Diet: The How-To and When-To Guide for Cleansing the Body. A key to healing and preventing chronic disease for 21st Century Medicine!* Berkeley, CA: Celestial Arts, 1997.

Heller, Rachael F., and Richard F. Heller. *Healthy for Life.* New York: Plume, 1995.

Heller, Rachael F., and Richard F. Heller. *The Carbohydrate Addict's Diet.* New York: Signet, 1993.

Hobbs, Christopher. *Super Immunity—Herbs and Other Natural Remedies for a Healthy Immune System.* Capitola, CA: Botanica Press, 1985.

Hoffer, Abram. *Orthomolecular Medicine for Physicians.* New Canaan, CT: Keats Publishing, 1989.

Hoffer, Abram, and Morton Walker. *Orthomolecular Nutrition, New Lifestyle for Super Good Health.* New Canaan, CT: Keats Publishing, Inc., 1978.

Hoffman, David. *The Herbal Handbook: A User's Guide to Medical Herbalism.* Rochester, VT: Healing Arts Press, 1987.

Hoffman, Matthew; William LeGro; and the editors of *Prevention Magazine Health Books. Disease Free.* Emmaus, PA: Rodale Press, 1993.

Hoffman, Ronald L. *7 Weeks to a Settled Stomach.* New York: Pocket Books, 1990.

Imrie, David, and Lee Barbuto. *The Back Power Program.* New York, NY: General Publishing Company, Limited, 1983.

Inlander, Charles B., and Ed Weiner. *Take This Book to the Hospital with You.* Emmaus, PA: Rodale Press, 1985.

Ivker, Robert. *Thriving.* New York: Crown Publishing Group, 1998.

James, Walene. *Immunization: The Reality Behind the Myth.* South Hadley, MA: Bergin and Garvey Publishers, Inc., 1988.

Joklik, Wolfgang K., et al. *Zinsser Microbiology.* Norwalk, CT: Appleton and Lange, 1988.

Kastner, Mark, and Hugh Burroughs. *Alternative Healing.* La Mesa, CA: Halcyon Publishing, 1996.

Kelley, William Donald. *One Answer to Cancer: An Ecological Approach to the Successful Treatment of Malignancy.* Grapevine, TX: Wedgestone Press, 1969.

Kenyon, Julian. *Simply a Safer Way.* Altrincham, Cheshire, UK: Dove Marketing, Ltd., 1997.

Krohn, Jacqueline, et. al. *A Guide to the Identification and Treatment of Biocatalyst and Biochemical Intolerances.* Los Alamos, NM: J. Krohn, 1994.

Krohn, Jacqueline; Frances Taylor; and Erla Mae Larson. *The Whole Way To Allergy Relief and Prevention.* Point Roberts, WA: Hartley & Marks, 1996.

Krohn, Jacqueline; Frances Taylor; and Jinger Prosser. *The Whole Way to Natural Detoxification.* Point Roberts, WA: Hartley & Marks, 1996.

Kushi, Michio. *The Macrobiotic Way: The Complete Macrobiotic Diet and Exercise Book.* Wayne, NJ: Avery Publishing Group, 1985.

Lonsdale, Derrick, M.D. *Why I Left Orthodox Medicine.* Norfolk, VA: Hampton Roads Publishing Co., 1994.

Lust, John. *The Herb Book.* New York: Bantam Books, 1974.

Lust, John, and Michael Tierra. *The Natural Remedy Bible.* New York: Pocket Books, 1990.

Martin, Eric W. *Hazards Of Medication.* Philadelphia, PA: J.B. Lippincott Co., 1978.

Marrougelle, Jeffrey L., and Gregory S. Ellis. *The Stress-less Eating Plan.* Schuyllkill Haven, PA: Schuyllkill Bio-Nutritional, 1995.

McGilvery, Robert W., and Gerald W. Goldstein. *Biochemistry—A Functional Approach.* Philadelphia, PA: W.B. Saunders Company, 1983.

McGrew, Roderick Erle. *Encyclopedia of Medical History*. New York: McGraw Hill, 1985.

McTaggart, Lynne. *Medical Madness*. Baltimore, MD: What Doctors Don't Tell You, LLC, 1995.

Mein, Carolyn. *Different Bodies, Different Diets*. Women's and Men's Editions. San Diego, CA: Vision Ware Press, 1997.

Mendelsohn, Robert S. *How to Raise a Healthy Child in Spite of Your Doctor*. New York: Ballantine Books, 1984.

Mendelsohn, Robert S. *Confessions of a Medical Heretic*. Chicago: Contemporary Books, Inc., 1979.

Miller, Benjamin F., and Claire Brackman Keane. *Encyclopedia and Dictionary of Medicine, Nursing, and Allied Health*. Philadelphia, PA: W.B. Saunders Company, 1978.

Miller, Neil Z. *Vaccines: Are They Really Safe and Effective?* Santa Fe, NM: New Atlantean Press, 1992.

Milne, Robert, and Blake More, with Burton Goldberg. *An Alternative Medicine Definitive Guide to Headaches*. Tiburon, CA: Future Medicine Publishing, Inc., 1997.

Mindell, Earl. *Earl Mindell's Herb Bible*. New York: Simon & Schuster, 1992.

Mindell, Earl. *Earl Mindell's Secret Remedies*. New York: Fireside, 1997.

Mindell, Earl. *Earl Mindell's Vitamin Bible*. New York: Warner Books, 1991.

Morgan, Brian L.G. *Nutrition Prescription*. New York: Crown Publishers, Inc., 1987.

Morrison, Roger. *Desktop Companion to Physical Pathology*. Nevada City, CA: Hahnemann Clinic Publishing, 1998.

Morrison, Roger. *Desktop Guide to Keynotes and Confirmatory Symptoms*. Albany, CA: Hahnemann Clinic Publishing, 1993.

McBean, Eleanor. *The Poisoned Needle*. Mokelumne Hill, CA: Health Research, 1974.

McBean, Eleanor. *Vaccinations Do Not Protect*. Manachaea, TX: Health Excellence Systems, 1991.

McDonagh, E.W., and Charles Rudolph, ed. *A Collection of Published Papers Showing the Efficacy of EDTA Chelation Therapy*. Gladstone, MO: McDonagh Medical Center, Inc. ND.

Moss, Ralph. *"Essiac." Cancer Therapy: The Independent Consumer's Guide*. New York: Equinox Press, 1992.

Moss, Ralph. *The Cancer Industry*. New York: Paragon House, 1991.

Mowrey, Daniel B. *The Scientific Validation of Herbal Medicine*. New Canaan, CT: Keats Publishing, 1986.

Murphy, Robin. *Homeopathic Medical Repertory*. Pagosa Springs, CO: Hahnemann Academy of North America, 1993.

Murphy, Robin. *Lotus Materia Medica*. Pagosa Springs, CO: Lotus Star Academy, 1995.

Murray, Michael, and Joseph Pizzorno. *Encyclopedia of Natural Medicine*. Rocklin, CA: Prima Publishing, 1991.

Nambudripad, Devi S. *Living Pain Free*. Buena Park, CA: Delta Publishing Co., 1997.

Neustaedter, Randall. *The Vaccine Guide*. Berkeley, CA: North Atlantic Books, 1996.

Northrup, Christiane. *Women's Bodies, Women's Wisdom*. New York: Bantam Books, 1994.

Page, Linda Rector. *Healthy Living*. Carmel Valley, CA: Healthy Healing Publications, 1997.

Papolos, D., and J. Papolos. *Overcoming Depression*. New York: Harper Perennial, 1997.

Philpott, William H., and Dwight K. Kalita. *Victory Over Diabetes*. New Canaan, CT: Keats Publishing, Inc., 1982.

Podell, Richard N., and William Proctor. *When Your Doctor Doesn't Know Best*. New York: Simon & Schuster, 1995.

Rapp, Doris. *Is This Your Child?* New York: William Morrow and Company, 1991.

Rapp, Doris, and Dorothy Bamberg. *The Impossible Child*. Buffalo, NY: Practical Allergy Research Foundation, 1986.

Rea, William J. *Chemical Sensitivity*, vol. 1–4. Boca Raton, FL: Lewis Publishers, 1992–96.

Reed, Barbara. *Food, Teens, and Behavior*. Manitowoc, WI: Natural Press, 1983.

Reichenberg, Judyth, and Robert Ullman. *Ritalin Free Kids*. Rocklin, CA: Pima Publishers, Inc., 1996.

Rogers, Sherry A. *Depression Cured At Last*. Sarasota, FL: SK Publishing, 1997.

Rogers, Sherry A. *Wellness Against All Odds*. Syracuse, NY: Prestige Publishing, 1994.

Rose, Barry. *The Family Health Guide to Homeopathy*. Berkeley, CA: Celestial Arts, 1992.

Rosenfield, Isadore. *The Best Treatment*. New York: Simon & Schuster, 1991.

Scheibner, Viera. *Vaccination: The Medical Assault*

on the Immune System. Santa Fe, NM: New Atlantean Press, 1983.

Schmidt, Michael A. *Healing Childhood Ear Infections*. Berkeley, CA: North Atlantic Books, 1996.

Sears, Barry. *The Zone*. New York: Harper Collins, 1995.

Sears, Barry. *Mastering the Zone*. New York: Regan Books, 1997.

Seligman, Martin E.L. *Learned Optimism*. New York: Simon & Schuster, 1990.

Sigerist, Henry E. *A History of Medicine*, vol. I and II. New York: Oxford University Press, 1951.

Sinatra, Stephen. *Optimum Health, A Cardiologist's Prescription*. Gatlinburg, TN: Lincoln Bradley, 1996.

Sobel, David S., and Robert Ornstein. *The Healthy Mind, Healthy Body Handbook*. Los Altos, CA: DRX, 1996.

Spence, Alexander, and Elliott B. Mason. *Human Anatomy and Physiology*. Menlo Park, CA: The Benjamin/Cummings Publishing Company, Inc., 1987.

Stoff, Jesse A., and Charles Pellegrino. *Chronic Fatigue Syndrome*. New York: Random House, 1988.

Tyberg, Theodore, and Kenneth Rothaus. *Hospital Smarts*. Paramus, NJ: Prentice Hall, 1995.

Ullman, Dana. *Discovering Homeopathy*. Berkeley, CA: North Atlantic Books, 1991.

Vander, Arthur J.; James H. Sherman; and Dorothy S. Luciano. *Human Physiology*. New York: McGraw-Hill Book Co., 1985.

Walker, Morton. *The Chelation Way*. Garden City Park, NY: Avery Publishing Group, 1990.

Wallach, Jacques. *Interpretation of Diagnostic Tests*. Boston, MA: Little, Brown, and Company, 1992.

Weil, Andrew. *Health and Healing—Understanding Conventional and Alternative Medicine*. New York: Dorling Kindersley, 1995.

Weil, Andrew. *Natural Health, Natural Medicine—A Comprehensive Manual for Wellness and Self-Care*. New York: Dorling Kindersley, 1995.

Werbach, Melvyn R. *Healing Through Nutrition*. New York: Harper Collins Publishers, 1993.

Werbach, Melvyn R. *Third Line Medicine*. New York: Arkana, 1986.

Wild, Gaynor, and Edward C. Benzel. *Essentials of Neurochemistry*. Boston, MA: Joues and Bartlett Publishers, 1994.

JOURNALS

Allen, Allen B. "Is RA27/3 a cause of chronic fatigue?" *Medical Hypothesis* 27: 217–20 (1988).

Altura, B.M., and Altura, B.T. "New perspectives on the role of magnesium in the pathophysiology of the cardiovascular system." *Magnesium* 41: 226–44 (1985).

Apffel, C.A. "Nonimmunological Host Defense: A Review." *Cancer Research* 36(5): 1526–37 (1976).

Austin, et al. "Long-term Follow-up of Cancer Patients Using Contreras, Hoxsey, and Gerson Therapies." *Journal of Naturopathic Medicine* 5(1): 74–76 (1994).

Baraff, L.J.; W.J. Ablon; and R.C. Weiss. "Possible Temporal Association Between Diphtheria-Tetanus Toxoid-Pertussis Vaccination and Sudden Infant Death Syndrome." *Pediatric Infectious Diseases* 2: 7–11 (1983).

Bendich, Adrianne; Rajiv Mallick; and Shelah Leader. "Potential Health Economic Benefits of Vitamin Supplementation." *West J Med.* 166: 306–11 (1997).

Bierman, C.W.; W.E. Pierson; and J.A. Donaldson, "The Evaluation of Middle Ear Function in Children." *Am J. Dis Child* 120: 233–36 (1970).

Blennow, M., and M. Granstrom. "Adverse reactions and serological response to a booster dose of acellular pertussis vaccine in children immunized with acellular or whole-cell vaccine as infants." *Pediatrics* 84: 62–67 (1989).

Bodner, E.E.; G.G. Browning; F.T. Chalmers; and T.C. Chalmers. "Can Meta-Analysis Help Uncertainty in Surgery for Otitis Media in Children." *J. Laryngol Otol.* 105: 812–19 (1991).

Boris, M., and F.S. Mandel. "Food and additives are common causes of attention deficit hyperactivity disorder in children." *Ann Allergy* 72: 462–68 (1994).

Brooks, D.N. "Otitis Media with Effusion and Academic Attainment." *Intl J. Ped Otorhinolaryngol* 12: 39–47 (1986).

Brown, Burnell R., Jr. "Clinical Significance of the Biotransformation of Inhalation Anesthetics." *Resident and Staff Physicians* 72–77 (August 1978).

Brown, M.J.; S.H. Richards; and A.G. Ambegaoken. "Grommets and Glue Ear; A Five-Year Follow-Up of a Controlled Trial." *J Roy Soc Med.* 71: 353–56 (1978).

Brunell, P.A. "Chickenpox—Examining Our Options." *New England Journal of Medicine* 325: 1577–79 (1991).

Burzynski, S.R., et al. "Antineoplaston A in Cancer Therapy (I)." *Physiological Chemistry and Physics* 6: 485–500 (1977).

Caracciolo, E.A., et al. "Comparison of surgical and medical group survival in patients with left main equivalent coronary artery disease. Long term CASS experience." *Circulation.* 9: 2335–44 (1995).

Carter, J.P., and G.P. Saxe, et al. "Dietary management may improve survival from nutritionally linked cancers based on analysis of representative cases." *J Amer Coll Nutr.* 12: 209–26 (1993).

Cashin, W.L., et al. "Accelerated progression of atherosclerosis in coronary vessels with minimal lesions that are bypassed." *NEJM.* 304: 824–28 (1981).

CASS Principal Investigators and Their Associates. "The Coronary Artery Surgery Study (CASS): A Randomized Trail of Coronary Artery Bypass Surgery." *Journal of American College of Cardiology* 3: 114–28 (1984).

Cass, Hyla. "Talking Back to Prozac." *Journal of Longevity Research* 22–46 (1996).

Cathcart, Robert F. "Vitamin C: The Nontoxic, Nonrole Limited, Antioxidant Free Radical Scavenger." *Medical Hypothesis* 18: 61–77 (1985).

Chapat de Saintonge, D.M., and D.F. Levine, et al. "Trial of Three-Day and Ten-Day Courses of Amoxycillin in Otitis Media." *Br Med J.* 284 (April 10, 1982).

Cherry, J.D. "The 'new' epidemiology of measles and rubella." *Hospital Practice.* 49–57 (1980).

Cherry, J.D.; P.A. Brunell; G.S. Golden; and D.T. Karzon. "Report of the Task Force on Pertussis and Pertussis Immunization—1988." *Pediatrics* 81 (supp): 939–84 (1988).

Chiebowski, R.T., et al. "Hydrazine Sulfate's Influence on Nutritional Status and Survival in Non-small-cell Lung Cancer." *Journal of Clinical Oncology* 8(1): 721–26 (1990).

Clement, R.J., et al. "Peritoneal Mesothelioma." *Quantum Medicine* 1: 68–73 (1988).

Cody, C.L.; L.J. Baraff, and J.D. Cherry, et al. "Nature and rates of adverse reactions associated with DTP and TD immunizations in infants and children." *Pediatrics.* 68: 650–60 (1981).

Cohen, S.; D.A.J. Tyrell; and A.P. Smith. "Psychological stress and susceptibility to the common cold." *New Engl J Med* 325: 606–12, 1991.

Cordova, C., A. Musea, and F. Viola, et al. "Influence of ascorbic acid on platelet aggregation in vitro and in vivo." *Atherosclerosis* 41: 15–19 (1982).

Corti, M.C., et al. "Serum albumin level and physical disability as predictors of mortality in older persons." *JAMA* 272: 1036–42 (1994).

Coulter, Kevin P. "How to Short-Circuit Family-Spread URIs." *Pediatric Management* 41–45 (November 1991).

Curtis, R.E., et al. "Risk of Leukemia Associated with the First Course of Cancer Treatment: An Analysis of the Surveillance, Epidemiology and End Results Program Experience." *Journal of the National Cancer Institute* 72: 531–54 (1984).

DePalma, Louis, and Naomi L.C. Luban. "Transfusion-transmitted Diseases: CMV to Syphilis." *Contemporary Pediatrics.* May 1991: 87–97.

Diamant, M., and B. Diamant. "Abuse and Timing of Use of Antibiotics In Acute Otitis Media." *Arch Otolaryngol.* 100: 226–32 (1974).

Diamond, J.; J. Wadsworth; and E. Ross. "Pertussis Immunization and Serious Acute Neurological Illnesses in Children." *British Medical Journal.* 307: 1171–76 (1993).

Dohlman, Ann; Mary Pat Hemstreet; Gregory Odrezin; and Alfred Bartolucci. "Subacute sinusitis: Are antimicrobials necessary?" *J Allergy Clin Immunol.* 91: 1015–23 (1993).

Edwin, E., et al. "Vitamin B_{12} hypovitaminosis in mental diseases." *Acta Med Scand.* 177: 689–99 (1965).

Eisenberg, L. "Preventive Pediatrics: The Promise and the Peril." *Pediatrics* 80 (3): 415–16 (1987).

Ernster, D.L., et al. "Cancer Incidence by Martial Status: U.S. Third National Cancer Survey." *Journal of the National Cancer Institute* 63: 567–85 (1979).

Ettinger, Bruce. "Maintaining Skeletal Health Among Postmenopausal Women." *America Journal of Managed Care* 4: 387–96 (1998).

Filov, V.A., et al. "Results of clinical evaluation of hydrazine sulfate." *Vaprosy Onkologii.* 36 (6): 721–26 (1990).

Fitzpatrick, A.L. et al. "Use of calcium channel blockers and breast carcinoma risk in postmenopausal women." *Cancer* 80: 1438–47 (1997).

Follingstad, Alvin H. "Estriol, the Forgotten Estrogen?" *JAMA* 239: 29–30 (1978).

Fukuda, K.; S. Straus; and Ian Hickie, et al. "The Chronic Fatigue Syndrome: A Comprehensive Approach to Its Definitive and Study." *Annals of Internal Medicine* 121: 953–59 (1994).

Gagnon, Daniel. "Healing Herbs for the Lungs." *NFM's Nutrition Science News* March 1996: 20–21.

Gerber, Michael. "Strep Pharyngitis: Update on Management." *Contemporary Pediatrics* 14: 156–65 (1997).

Graboys, T.M., et al. "Results of a second opinion program for coronary artery bypass graft surgery." *JAMA* 258: 1611–14 (1987).

Graham, I.M., et al. "Plasma homocysteine as a risk factor for vascular disease." *JAMA* 277: 1775–86 (1997)

Grant, Kathryn L. "Loratidine-Related Heptatoxicity." *P&T*, August 1997: 406.

Greer, S., and T. Morris. "Psychological Attributes of Women who Develop Breast Cancer: A Controlled Study." *Journal of Psychosomatic Research* 19: 147–53 (1975).

Griffin, M.R.; W.A. Ray; and E.A. Mortimer, et al. "Risk of Seizures and Encephalopathy After Immunization With the Diphtheria-Tetanus-Pertussis Vaccine." *JAMA* 263: 1641–45 (1990).

Haynes, S.G. "Type A behavior, employment status, and coronary heart disease in women." *Behavioral Medicine Update* 6: 11–15 (1984).

Helfand, S.L., et al. "Oxygen Intermediates Are Required for Interferon Activation of NK Cells." *Journal of Interferon Research* 3(2): 143–51 (1983).

Hoffman, H.J.; J.C. Hunter; and K. Damus, et al. "Diphtheria-tetanus-pertussis immunization and sudden infant death: result of the National Institute of Child Health and Human Development Cooperative Epidemiological Study of Sudden Infant Death Syndrome Risk Factors." *Pediatrics* 79: 598–611 (1987).

Holt, Stephen, "Phytoestrogens for a Healthier Menopause." *Alternative and Complementary Therapies* 187–193 (June 1997).

Horrobin, D.F. "Abnormal membrane concentration of 20 to 22—carbon essential fatty acids: a common link between risk factors and coronary and peripheral vascular disease?" *Prostagl Leukotr Ess Fatty Acids* 53: 385–96 (1995).

Jarvis, Kelly B; Reed B. Phillips; and Elliott K. Morris. "Cost per Case Comparison of Back Injury Claims of Chiropractic versus Medical Management for Conditions with Identical Diagnostic Codes." J Occup Med. 33: August 1991, 847–52.

Jenson, Clyde B. "Common Paths in Medical Education." *Alternative and Complementary Therapies* 276–280 (August 1997).

Kash, K.M., et al. "Psychological distress and surveillance behaviors of women with a family history of breast cancer." *Journal of National Cancer Institute* 84: 24–30 (1992).

Katz, S.L. "Polio vaccine policy—time for a change." *Pediatrics* 98: 116–17 (1996).

Kemper, Kathi J. "A Practical Approach to Chronic Asthma Management." *Contemporary Pediatrics* 14: 86–107 (1997).

Kiene, H. "Clinical Studies on Mistletoe Therapy for Cancerous Diseases: A Review." *Therapeutikon* 3(6): 347–533 (1989).

Kirkwood, C.R., and M.E. Kirkwood. "Otitis Media and Learning Disabilities: The Case for a Causal Relationship." *J. Fam Prac.* 17: 219–27 (1983).

Kitchell, J.R., et al. "The Treatment of Coronary Artery Disease with Disodium EDTA. A Reappraisal." *American Journal of Cardiology* 11: 501–6 (1963).

Klein, S., and R.L. Loretz. "Nutritional Support in Patients with Cancer: What Do the Data Really Show?" *Nutrition in Clinical Practice* 9(3): 91–100 (1994).

Kleinman, L.C.; J. Kosecoff; R.W. Dubois; and R.H. Brook. "The Medical Appropriateness of Tympanostomy Tubes Proposed for Children Younger than 16 Years in the United States." *JAMA* 271 (16): 1250–55 (1994).

Komaroff, Anthony, "A 56-Year-Old Woman With Chronic Fatigue Syndrome." *JAMA* 278: 1179–85 (1997)

Krumholz, Harlan M., and Teresa Seeman, et al. "Lack of association between cholesterol and coronary heart disease mortality and morbidity and all-cause mortality in persons older than 70 years." *JAMA* 272: 1335–40 (1994).

Landrigan, P., and J. Witte. "Neurologic disorders following measles virus vaccination." *JAMA* 223: 1459 (1973).

Leroi, R. "Fundamentals of Mistletoe Therapy." *Krebsgeschehn* 5: 145–46 (1979).

Levine, P.H., et al. "Clinical Epidemiologic Envirologic Studies in Four Clusters of the Chronic Fatigue Syndrome." Arch Int Med. 152: 1611–16 (1992).

Lieberman, A.D. "The role of the rubella virus in the chronic fatigue syndrome." *Clinical Ecology* 7: 51–54 (1991).

MacDonald W., et al. "Effect of Frequent Prenatal Ultrasound on Birthweight: Followup at One Year of Age." *Lancet* 348: 482 (1996).

Mandel, E.M., et al. "Efficacy of Myringotomy with and without Tympanostomy Tubes for Chronic Otitis Media with Effusion." *Pediatric Infect Dis J* 11: 270–77 (1992).

Manna, V., and N. Martucci. "Effects of short-term administration of cytidine, uridine, and L-glutamine, alone or in combination on the cerebral electrical activity of patients with chronic cerebral vascular disease." *Int J Clin Pharm Res* 8: 199–210 (1988).

McWhirter, J.P., and C.R. Pennington. "Incidence and recognition of malnutrition in hospital." *Br Med J* 308:945–48 (1994).

Mechcahe, Elizabeth. "Treating Neurally Mediated Hypotension in CFS." *Pediatric News* January 1977: 8–9.

Merz, Beverly. "Malignant hyperthermia: Nightmare for anesthesiologists—and patients." *JAMA* 255: 709–14 (1986).

Miller, D.L.; Ross, E.M.; Alderslade, R.; Bellman, M.H.; and Rawason, N.S.B. Pertussis immunisation and serious neurological illness in children. *Br Med J.* 282: 1595–99 (1981).

Morazzoni, P., and Malandrino. "Anthocyanins and Their Aglycons as Scavengers of Free Radicals and Antilipoperoxidant Agents." *Pharmacology Rees Commission* 20(2): 254 Suppl. (1988).

Muhlestein, Joseph. "The link between *Chlamydia pneumoniae* and atherosclerosis." *Infect. Med.* 14: 380–82 (1997).

Multiple Risk Factor Intervention Trial Research Group: Baseline rest electrocardiograph abnormalities, antihypertensive treatment and mortality in the Multiple Risk Factor Intervention Trial. *Am J Cardiol* 55: 1–15 (1985).

Myginal, N.; K.I. Meistrap-Larsen; and J. Thomsen, et al. "Penicillin in acute otitis media: a double-blind placebo-controlled trial." *Clin Otol.* 6: 5–13 (1981).

Nakamura, M. "Effect of vitamin E deficiency on the level of SOD, glutathione peroxidase, catalase, and lipid peroxide." *Int J. Vit Nutr Res.* 46: 187–91 (1976).

Newman, T.B., et al. "Carcinogenicity of Lipid-lowering Drugs." *JAMA* 275: 55–60 (1996).

Nienhaus, J. "Tumor Inhibition and Thymus Stimulation with Mistletoe Preparation." *Elemente Naturowissenschaft* 13: 45–54 (1970).

Nsouli, T.M., et al. "Role of Food Allergy in Serous Otitis Media." *Ann Allergy* 73: 215–19 (1994).

Oakley, Deborah. "Quality of Condom Use as Reported by Female Clients of Family Planning Clinic." *American Journal of Public Health* 85: 1526–30 (1995).

Okuma, N.; H. Takayma; and H. Uchino. "Generation of prostacyclin-like substance and lipid peroxidation in vitamin E deficient rats." *Prostaglandis* 19: 527–53 (1980).

Olszewer, E., et al. "A pilot double-blind study of sodium-magnesium EDTA in peripheral vascular disease." *J Natl Med Assoc.* 82: 173–177 (1990).

Olszewer, E., et al. "EDTA Chelation Therapy in Chronic Degenerative Disease." *Med Hypothesis.* 27: 41–49 (1988).

Osterholm, M.T., and J.H. Rambeck, et al. "Lack of efficacy of *Haemophilus B* polysaccharide vaccine in Minnesota." *JAMA* 260: 1423–28 (1988).

Paradise, J.L. "Management of Secretory Otitis Media: State of the Art." *Adv. Oto-Rhino-Laryng.* 40: 99–109 (1988).

Parfentjev, I.A., and Goodhing M.A. Good. "Histamine Shock in Mice Sensitized with *Haemophilus Pertussis* Vaccine." *J Pharm Exp Therap.* 92: 411–13 (1948).

Pashki, L.L. "Cancer Chemoprevention with Adrenocortical Steroid Dehydroepiandrosterone and Structural Analogs." *Journal of Cell Biochemistry.* Suppl. 17G: 73–79 (1993).

Pennington, J.A., and B.E. Young. "The selected minerals in foods surveyed from 1982–1984." *J Am Dietetic Assoc.* 86: 867–76 (1986).

Petty, F., et al. "Low plasma gamma-aminobutyric acid levels in male patients with depression." *Biol Psychiatry.* 32: 354–63 (1992).

Philpot, Edward. "The Costs of Allergic Rhinitis." *Allergy and Asthma* 10–11 (Fall 1997).

Prudden, J. "The Treatment of Human Cancer with

Agents Prepared from Bovine Cartilage." *Journal of Biological Response Modifiers* 4(6): 590–95 (1985).

Prenner, Bruce M. "Allergies for All Seasons." *Allergy and Asthma* 8–9 (Fall 1997).

Psaty, D.M., *et al.* "The Risk of Incident Myocardial Infarction Associated with Antihypertensive Drug Therapies (abstract)." *Circulation* 91: 925 (1994).

Reynolds, E.H., *et al.* "Folate deficiency in depressive illness." *Br J Psych* 117: 287–92 (1970).

Richards, Cassandra. "Pediatric Drug Trials Raise Several Questions." *Infectious Diseases in Children.* 63 (April 1998).

Ringsdorf, Wm., Jr., and E. Cheraskin. "Nutritional aspects of urolithiasis." *South Med J.* 74: 41–44 (1981).

Roberts, J.E.; M.A. Sanyai; and M.R. Burchinal, *et al.* "Otitis Media in Early Childhood and in Relationship to Later Verbal and Academic Performance." *Pediatrics* 78 (September 1986).

Robbin, Anthony R., and Sandra M. Gawchilk. "Allergic Rhinitis—it's that time again!" *Contemporary Pediatrics* 11: 19–41 (1994).

Roubenoff, R., *et al.* "Malnutrition among hospitalized patients: problems of physician awareness." *Arch Intern Med* 147: 1462–65 (1987).

Ruokenen, J.; Paganus, A.; and Lehti, H. "Elimination Diets in the Treatment of Secretary Otitis Media." *Intl J Ped Otorhinolaryngol* 4: 39–46 (1982).

Schick, Robert M. "Scrotal Imaging." *Hospital Practice* 142–49 (September 15, 1985).

Seelig, M.S. "Nutritional Status and Requirements of Magnesium." *Mag Bull* 8: 170–85 (1986).

Shampault, G., *et al.* "A double-blind trial of an extract of the plant Serenoa repens in benign prostatic hyperplasia." *Brit J Clin Parm.* 18: 461–62 (1984).

Skolnick, Andrew A. "Transfusion Medicine Faces Time of Major Challenges and Changes." *JAMA* 268(6): 697–700 (1992).

Spiegel, D., *et al.* "Effect of Psychosocial treatment on Survival of Patients with Metastatic Breast Cancer." *Lancet* 2 (8668): 881–91 (1989).

Steele, Russell W., and Walter R. Wilson. "Challenges in the Management of Upper Respiratory Tract Infection." *Infections in Medicine Supplement* 26–32 (N.D.).

Thompson, N.P., and S.M. Montgomery, *et al.* "Is measles vaccination a risk factor for inflammatory bowel disease?" *Lancet* 345: 1071–73 (1995).

Thompson, N.P., and S.M. Montgomery, *et al.* "Measles vaccination as a risk factor for inflammatory bowel disease (letter)." *Lancet* 345: 1364 (1995).

Topol, E.J., *et al.* "A comparison of directional atherectomy with coronary angioplasty in patients with coronary artery disease." *NEJM* 329: 221–27 (1993).

Torch, W. "Diphtheria-Pertussis-Tetanus (DTP) Immunization: A Potential Cause of the Sudden Infant Death Syndrome (SIDS)." *Neurology* 32: A169 (1982).

Totsi, A.; L. Guerra,; and F. Bardazzi. "Hyposensitizing therapy with standard antigenic extracts: An important source of thimerosal sensitization." *Contact Dermatitis* 20: 173–76 (1989).

Towbin, Richard. "What's New in Interventional Radiology." *Contemporary Pediatrics* September 1995: 87, 89, 94, 98, 102, 104.

Vag, Rosalind; Deborah L. Best; Stephen W. Davies; and Michael Kaiser. "Evaluation of a testicular cancer curriculum for adolescents." *Journal of Pediatrics.* 114: 150–53 (1989).

Van Buchem, F.L. "Therapy of Acute Otitis Media: Myringotomy, Antibiotics, or Neither? A Double-Blind Study in Children." *Lancet* 883: (October 24, 1981).

Van Buchem, F.L.; M.F. Peeters; and M.A. Van't Hof. "Acute otitis media: a treatment strategy." *Br M J* 290: 1033–37 (1985).

Varro, J., edited by J. LaRaus. "Ozone Applications in Cancer Cases." *Medical Applications of Oxone.* Norwalk, CT: International Ozone Association Pan American Committee, 97–98 (1983).

Wakefield, A.J., and A Ellbon, *et al.* "Crohn's disease: pathogenesis and persistent measles virus infection." *Gastroenterology* 108: 911–16 (1995).

Wald, Ellen R.; Nancy Guerra; and Corol Byers. "Upper Respiratory Tract Infections in Young Children: Duration and Frequency of Complications." *Pediatrics* 87: 129–33 (February 1991).

Walker, A.M.; H. Jick; and D.R. Pervera, *et al.* "Diphtheria-tetanus-pertussis immunization and sudden infant death syndrome." *Am Journal of Public Health* 77: 945–51 (1987).

Wasserman, M., *et al.* "Organochlorine Compounds in Neoplastic and Adjacent Apparently Normal Breast Tissue." *Bulletin of Environmental Contaminants and Toxicology* 15: 478–84 (1976).

Weiner, L.P., and R.M. Herndon, *et al.* "Isolation of virus related to SV40 from patients with progressive multifocal leukoencephalopathy." *NEJM* 286: 385–89 (1972).

Weinstein, A.L., *et al.* "Breast Cancer Risk and Oral Contraceptive Use: Results from a Large Case-Control Study." *Epidemiology.* 2: 353–58 (September 1991).

Weiss, R. "Measles battle loses potent weapon." *Science* 258: 546–47 (1992).

Wentz, K.R., and E.K. Mareuse. "Diphtheria-Tetanus-Pertussis Vaccine and Serious Neurologic Illness: An Updated Review of the Epidemiologic Evidence." *Pediatrics* 87: 287–97 (1991).

Westin, J., and E. Richter. "Israeli Breast Cancer Anomaly." *Annals of New York Academy Science* 609: 269–79 (1990).

Winslow, C.M., *et al.* "The appropriateness of performing coronary artery bypass surgery." *JAMA* 260: 505 (1988).

Wiseman, A., *et al.* "Long-term prognosis after myocardial infraction in patients with previous coronary artery surgery." *J Am Coll Cardiol.* 12: 873–80 (1988).

Wright, D.J., and C.B. Mueller. "Screening Mammography and Public Health Policy: The Need for Perspective." Lancet 346 29–32 (July 1995).

Yiamouyiannis, J., and D. Burk. "Fluoridation and Cancer; Age-Dependence of Cancer Mortality Related to Artificial Fluoridation." *Fluoride* 10 (3): 102–23 (1977).

Young, Linda R; Douglas Wurtzbacher; and Crystal S. Blankenship. "Adverse Drug Reactions: A Review of Healthcare Practitioners." *The American Journal of Managed Care* 1884–1905 (December 1997).

OTHER

Abramson, R. "EPA Officially Links Passive Smoke, Cancer." *Los Angeles Times.* A27 (January 12, 1993).

Alderslade, R.; M.H. Bellman; N.S. Rawson; *et. al.* "The National Childhood Encephalopathy Study in Whooping Cough: Reports from the Committee on Safety of Medicines and the Joint Committee on Vaccinations and Immunization."

London, Department of Health and Social Security, Her Majesty's Stationary Office, 1981, 79–154.

Ali, Majid. "Why Are the Obese Obese?" Excerpts from *The Butterfly and Life Span Nutrition. Lifespanner.* ND: 15–17.

Alschuler, Lise. "Heal Hot Flashes Naturally." *Let's Live.* Nov. 1997: 40–127.

American Institute of Homeopathy: Special Reports of Homeopathic Yellow Fever Commission Ordered by AIH for Presentation to Congress. Philadelphia and New York: Boericke and Tafel: 1880.

American Lung Association. "What's Ailing You?" *Albuquerque Journal.* January 5, 1998: C1–2.

Anonymous. *Effective Hypertension Control Requires a Lifetime Commitment.* Pfizer, Inc., 1997.

Atkins, Robert. *Dr. Atkins' Health Revelations.* Baltimore, MD: Agora Health Publishing, 1995–1998.

Balch, James. *Prescriptions for Healthy Living.* Palm Beach Gardens, FL: Weiss Research, 1998–1999.

Barnard, Neal D. "Real Men Eat Tofu." *Vegetarian Times.* May 1997: 67–70.

Barr, Stephen. "How Safe Is Our Blood Supply?" *Good Housekeeping.* January 1997: 113–114.

Bechtel, Stefan. "The 'Space Age' of Diagnosis Has Arrived." *Prevention.* May 1983: 124–133.

Benson, Donna. "Vaccine Aftermath." *Health Freedom News.* July/Aug. 29, 1984 from *Science,* March 26, 1977.

Bland, Jeffrey. *Glandular-based Food Supplements: Helping to Separate Fact from Fiction.* Tacoma, WA: Bellevue-Redmond Medical Laboratory, Department of Chemistry, University of Puget Sound, 1980.

Borneman, John A. "Homeopathy and Naturopathy—Gentle Partners for Healing." *Let's Live.* April 1993: 16–25.

Burzynski, S., M.D. "Antineoplastons." From a lecture presented at the Oct. 7, 1990 World Research Foundation Congress. Los Angeles, CA.

Bushkin, Gary, and Estitta Bushkin. "Nutrition Questions and Answers." *Health & Nutrition Breakthroughs.* January 1998: 42.

Butterworth, Charles E. "The Skeleton in the Hospital Closet." *Nutrition Today.* 4–8 (March/April 1974).

Cairns, J., M.D. "The Treatment of Diseases and the

War Against Cancer." *Scientific American*. Nov. 1985.

Cantekin, E. "The Case Against Aggressive, Expensive, and Ineffective Treatment of a Benign Disease: Comments on the Clinical Practice Guidelines on Otitis Media." Report submitted to the U.S. Congress and the Department of Health and Human Services. 51 (1994).

Casura, Lily Giambarba. "Interview with Jesse Stoff, M.D." *Townsend Letter for Doctors & Patients*. 64–65 (July 1996).

Cichoke, Anthony J. "Estrogen Replacement Therapy: A Woman's Dilemma." *Let's Live*. November 1994: 41–44.

Cohn, Victor. "How to Survive the Hospital." *American Health*. 98–108 (March 1987).

Colt, George Howe. "The Magic of Touch." Unknown. 54–57, 60, 62 (n.d.).

Committee on Diet, Nutrition and Cancer, Assembly of Life Sciences, Nutritional Research Council. *Diet, Nutrition and Cancer*. Washington, D.C. National Academy Press, 1982.

Congress of the United States, Office of Technology Assessment. *Assessing the Efficacy and Safety of Medical Technologies*. #052-003-00593-0, Government Printing Office, Washington, D.C. 1978.

Connolly, Maureen. "Alcohol rubs reduce fever…and other myths you should ignore." *Child*. 93. (February 1998).

Couldwell, Clive, and Lynne McTaggart. "Radiotherapy." *What Doctors Don't Tell You*. Vol. 7(4): 2–4 (1996).

Coulter, H.L. "Review of Marie R. Griffin DTP Study." Unpublished, 1990.

Cowley, Geoffrey. "Cardiac Contagion." *Newsweek*. April 28, 1997, 69–70.

Croce, P. "Think Before You Sweeten." *Eating Clean: Overcoming Food Hazards*. Washington, D.C. Center for the Study of Responsive Law: 52 (1990).

Dean, Carolyn. "Mind Over Back Pain." *Let's Live*. March 1997: 34–37.

Dickey, Marilyn. "Anxiety Disorder." NIH Publication No. 95–3879. 1994 and 1995.

Division of STD Prevention. *The Challenge of STD Prevention in the United States*. in the United States. htm.

Donoghue, Elizabeth. "BCA reader survey results are in." *Breast Cancer Action Newsletter*. 38: 5 (Oct/Nov 1996).

Douglass, William Campbell. *Dr. William Campbell Douglass' Second Opinion*. Atlanta, GA: Second Opinion Publishing, 1996–1998.

Editors. "Guided Imagery Speeds Surgical Recovery." *Mind/Body Health Newsletter*. V1(3): 7 (1997).

Editors. "Hospital Food: As Bad As It Tastes." *Vegetarian Times*. (June 1997), 20.

Editors. "Pain Relievers: Go Easy or Else." *Health*. January/February, 1998: 15.

Editors. "Rethinking the Physician Visit." *Mind/Body Health Newsletter*. Vol. V(3): 7(1996).

Editors. "Rhinovirus receptor found; colds carry on." *Science News*. 135: 165 (March 18, 1989.)

Editors. "Vaccine Against the Common Cold Now Thought Possible." *Doctor's Infection Newsletter*. Vol. 1(2): 9–10 (May 1990).

Editors. "Washing Away the Common Cold." *Being Well. Qualmed's Magazine of Healthy Living*. 4 (N.D.)

Editors. "What's Wrong with Banking Your Blood." *Health*. January/February 1997: 24, 26.

Farley, Dixie. "FDA's Tips for Taking Medicines." Publication No. (FDA) 96–3221. U.S. Government Printing Office, 1996.

Fisher, Barbara Loe. Letter to Donald A. Henderson, Chairman of the National Vaccine Advisory Committee, p. 2, 1990.

Fitzgerald, Frances E. "Alternative Therapy." *Health Counselor*. Vol. 5(3): 33–36 (n.d.).

Fox, Arnold, and Barry Fox. "Doctors' Dialogue— Alternative Approaches to Treating an Enlarged Prostate." *Let's Live*. August 1995, 96.

Frishman, Ronny G. "Am I Sick Or Am I Tired?" *Ladies' Home Journal*. May 1998: 54–198.

Gale, J.L; P.B. Thapa; and J.R. Bobo, *et al*. "Acute Neurological Illness and DTP: Report of a Case-Control Study in Washington and Oregon." In Manclark., C.R., ed. Sixth International Symposium on Pertussis. Abstracts, Bethesda, Maryland: Department of Health and Human Services, 1990: 228–29 (DHSS Publication No. (FDA) 90–1162).

Gardner-Gordon, Joy. "Learning to Use the Sound That Heals." *Natural Health*. 46–48 (May/June 1994).

Gordon, James S. "Alternative Medicine, Major Medical Schools, National Institute of Health… and You." *Bottom Line*. June 15,1993: 11–13.

Hall, Stephen S. "Vaccinating Against Cancer." *Atlantic Monthly.* 66–84. April, 1997.

Hawk-Cromin, Kyle. "Alternatives to Treating Asthma." *Let's Live.* Sept. 1997: 30–34.

Hendrix, Mary Lynn. "Panic Disorder." NIH Publication No. 95-3508. 1993 and 1995.

Hershoff, Asa. "Breathe Easy With Homeopathy." *Let's Live.* April, 1997: 73–76.

Hobbs, Christopher. "Herbal Nightcaps for Sweet Dreams." *Let's Live.* April 1997: 78–83.

Hobbs, Christopher. "Herbs Make the Heart Grow Stronger." *Let's Live.* May 1997: 76–81.

Huemer, Richard. "Fibromyalgia: The Pain That Never Stops." *Let's Live.* Nov. 1996: 34–36.

Ivker, Rob. "Man to Man." *Natural Health.* March–April 1998: 34–38.

Janson, Michael, "Hypertension." *Health & Nutrition Breakthroughs.* January 1998: 24.

Johnson, Kent T. "Generic Drugs Are Good Medicine." PSC Health System 7: 1997.

Kamen, Betty. "Winter Wellness; The 'Cold' Wars." *Let's Live.* January 1991: 59–61.

Keating, Peter. "Why You May Be Getting the Wrong Medicine." *Money.* 142–152 (June 1997).

Keville, Kathi. "Herbs to Erase Stress." *Let's Live.* Sept. 1997, 83–86.

Khalsa, Karta Purkh Sigh. "Menopause Made Easy." *Let's Live.* April 1997: 57–62.

Kelley, Barbara Bailey. "Running on Empty." *Health.* May/June 1997: 64–68.

Lane, I.W. *Shark Cartilage Update Newsletter.* 1(3): 1 (1994).

Levin, Warren M. "Lowering Lipoprotein A—Letter to the Editor of *JAMA.*" *Townsend Letter for Doctors and Patients.* (August/September 1997) 122.

Malesky, Gale. "Music That Strikes Healing Chord." *Prevention.* 57–63. (October, 1983).

Maugh, T.H. "Invasive heart attack treatment questioned." *Los Angeles Times.* March 20, 1997.

Maugh, T.H. II. "Experts Downplay Cancer Risk of Chlorinated Water." *Los Angeles Times.* July 2, 1992.

McDonald, Claire and Susan McDonald. "A Woman's Guide to Self-Care." *Natural Health.* Jan.–Feb., 1997: 121–42.

McDowell, Baynon. "Andrew Weil M.D. Championing Integrative Medicine." *Alternative & Complementary Therapies.* Oct., 1994: 8–13.

Maradine, Cristin. "ERT Overdose?" *Vegetarian Times.* April 1998: 112–13.

McIssac, Warren J. Presentation at Interscience Conference on Antimicrobial Agents and Chemotherapy. 1998.

Morgan, Peggy. "Unmasking Thyroid Trouble." *Prevention.* March 1997: 87–165.

Moss, Jeffrey. "Hyperinsulinemia and Insulin Resistance—A Missing Link in Obesity and Cardiovascular Disease." *Townsend Letter for Doctors & Patients.* May 1997: 125–29.

Murphy, Robin. "H.A.N.A. Certificate Class Home Study Tapes 1–21." Santa Fe, NM: Hahnemann Academy of North America, 1991–92.

Murphy, Robin. "H.A.N.A. Certificate Homeopathy Classes Tapes 1–18." Santa Fe, NM: Hahnemann Academy of North America, 1991–92.

Murray, Patricia. "Vegetarian Diets in Children." *Small Talk.* 9(4): 10–11 (n.d.).

Naessens, G. "714X: A Highly Promising Non-Toxic Treatment of Cancer and Other Immune Deficiencies." In *Patron of Writers* Enterprise and Research Institutional Review Board. 10th ed. Jan. 1993.

Nash, J. Madeline. "Every Woman's Dilemma." *Time.* June 30, 1997: 60.

Newmark, Gretchen Rose. "Eat With Awareness." *Let's Live.* Dec. 1994: 24–27.

O'Conner, Amy. "High Touch, High Tech in the OR." *Vegetarian Times.* (October 1996) 18.

Radetsky, Peter. "Taming the Wily Rhinovirus." *Discover.* 38–43 (April 1989).

Randal, Judith. "Zinc Gluconate Nothing to Sneeze At." *Albuquerque Journal.* C1 and C5 (N.D.).

Robbins, John. "Recess for Ritalin." *Natural Health.* March–April 1997: 60–63.

Rock, Andrea. "Vaccine Business." *Money.* Dec. 1996: 149–163.

Sargent, Marilyn. "Plain Talk About Depression." National Institute of Mental Health. NIH Publication No. 94-3561. 1994.

Scheibner, Viera. "Evidence of the association between non-specific stress syndrome, DPT injections, and cot death." Proceedings of the 2nd National Immunisation Conference, Canberra. May 90–91 (1991).

Schwieger, Alice Burdick. "The 5 Most Common Drug Mistakes." *Woman's Day.* 10/7/97: 66, 68, 70.

Shambaugh, G.E., Jr. "Serous Otitis: Are Tubes the

Answer?" Paper presented at the Society for Clinical Ecology, New York, October 24, 1982.

Shannon, Salley. "The New Diet Pills." *Woman's Day*. June 24, 1997: 18–24.

Siegel, Paula M. "How to Finally Get Rid of That Cold." *Redbook*. 53–56 (November 1995).

Sobel, David S., and Robert Ornstein. "Rx: Preparing for Surgery." *Mind/Body Health Newsletter*. Vol 5(2): 3–6 (1996).

Spence, Annette. "How to Prevent Another Ear Infection." *Child*. Oct. 1997: 97–100.

Stabile, Toni. "Help for a Crippling Disease." *Reader's Digest*. April 1998: 93–97.

St. Amand, R. Paul. "Fibromyalgia." Patient Literature. Marina del Rey, CA: 1–4, 1996.

St. Amand, R. Paul. "The Use of Uricosuric Agents in Fibromyalgia." Patient Literature. Marina del Rey, CA: 1–5, 1996.

Stoller, Kenneth. "The Real Heart of Heart Disease." *Let's Live*. Aug. 1997: 88.

Stout, David. "Direct Link Found Between Smoking and Lung Cancer." *New York Times*. Oct 18, 1996.

Strand, Ray. "A Physician's Story." *CFIDS Chronicle*. March/April 1998: 16–18.

Strauss, Ronald G. "The Diminishing Risks of Blood Transfusion in the United States." Presented at Current Concepts and Controversies in Perinatal Care. Albuquerque, NM, 1992.

Streit, Rachel. "The Flipside of Depression: Anxiety." *Natural Health*. July–Aug. 1997: 103.

Sullivan, Charles. "Multiple Drug Prescribing Unscientific." *Townsend Letter for Doctors & Patients*. August/September, 1997: 121.

Thomsen, Bill. "Change of Heart." *Natural Health*. Sept.–Oct. 1997: 96–159.

Thomsen, Bill. "The Right Doctor." *Natural Health*. Jan.–Feb. 1997: 81–83, 140–49.

Trichopoulos, Dimitrios; P.L Frederick; and David I. Hunter. "What Causes Cancer?" *Scientific American*. Sept. 1996. 80–87.

Ullman, Dana. "Breathe Easier with Homeopathy." *Let's Live*. Sept. 1997: 30–34.

Weil, Andrew. *Dr. Andrew Weil's Self Healing*. Watertown, MA: Thorne Communications, 1996–1998.

Werbach, Melvyn R. "Nutritional Influences on Illness." *Townsend Letter for Doctors and Patients*. 56 (June 1997).

Whitaker, Julian. "EDTA Chelation Therapy: Your Safe Alternative to Surgery." *Health and Healing*. 2(4): 1–4 (April 1992).

Whitaker, Julian. *Health and Healing*. Potomac, MD: Phillips Publishing, 1995–1998.

White, Linda B. "Honk If You've Got Sinusitis." *Vegetarian Times*. Aug. 1996: 76–81.

Wolf, Robert V. "A Cut Above: Kinder Surgery." *Vegetarian Times*. September 1997: 36–41.

Wood, Stephanie. "Is Stress Making You Sick?" *Woman's Day*. Nov. 18, 1997: 50–59.

Wright, Jonathan. *Dr. Jonathan V. Wright's Nutrition and Healing with Alan R. Gaby, M.D.* Phoenix, AZ: Publishers Mgt. Corp., 1994–1998.

Zuger, Abigail. "Pharmaceutical Advertising Aimed Straight at Consumers May Educate Them—or Dangerously Misinform Them." *Los Alamos Monitor*. August 8, 1997: 7.

INDEX